EQUINE PEDIATRIC MEDICINE

EQUINE PEDIATRIC MEDICINE

Second Edition

Edited by

William V. Bernard
DVM, DipACVIM
Equine Internal Medicine
Lexington, Kentucky, USA

Bonnie S. Barr
VMD, DipACVIM
Rood and Riddle Equine Hospital
Lexington, Kentucky, USA

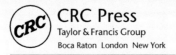

CRC Press
Taylor & Francis Group
Boca Raton London New York

CRC Press is an imprint of the
Taylor & Francis Group, an **informa** business

CRC Press
Taylor & Francis Group
6000 Broken Sound Parkway NW, Suite 300
Boca Raton, FL 33487-2742

First issued in paperback 2020

© 2018 by Taylor & Francis Group, LLC
CRC Press is an imprint of Taylor & Francis Group, an Informa business

No claim to original U.S. Government works

ISBN-13: 978-0-367-57140-5 (pbk)
ISBN-13: 978-1-4987-7600-4 (hbk)

Visit the Taylor & Francis Web site at
http://www.taylorandfrancis.com

and the CRC Press Web site at
http://www.crcpress.com

CONTENTS

PREFACE

This is the second edition of *Equine Pediatric Medicine.* As with the first edition, our hope is to provide useful information to the equine practitioner and to students regarding problems in the equine pediatric patient. In addition to written text, this book includes tables, figures, and numerous photographs to illustrate details of specific diseases. The aim of this book is to provide the practitioner with the information needed to make a presumptive diagnosis from physical and clinical examination findings, to consider the relevant pathophysiology of the conditions detailed, to compile a list of differential diagnoses, to confirm the diagnosis with laboratory testing and advanced diagnostics, and to plan the therapeutic course to be taken.

All of the chapters that appeared in the first edition have been updated and two new chapters—"Pediatric Nutrition" and "Case Studies"—have been added. The organization of the book is system based. Chapter 1 details the physical examination of the foal and the Chapter 2 reviews important aspects of identifying and managing shock in the critical pediatric patient. The rest of the chapters detail each organ system, highlighting diseases encountered in the pediatric equine patient and outlining diagnoses and management.

Chapter 18, "Pediatric Nutrition," begins with key points regarding the normal feeding behavior of the pediatric patient but primarily focuses on the nutritional needs of the sick foal. There is discussion regarding the two routes in which nutrition can be provided and reasons for choosing one over the other. Chapter 19, "Case Studies," includes 10 common problems encountered in the pediatric patient, ranging from the weak neonatal foal to the suckling foal with respiratory problems. The aim of this chapter is to provide the clinician with an example of physical examination findings and diagnostics, along with initial triage and management of certain problems in the pediatric patient.

Remember a wealth of information can be gained from a thorough physical examination so make this the first thing you do when presented with a patient. Base your treatment on the entire picture, including historical information, physical examination findings, and diagnostics results. Celebrate your successes, learn from your failures, and, above all, do no harm.

William V. Bernard
Bonnie S. Barr

CONTRIBUTORS

BONNIE S. BARR
Rood and Riddle Equine Hospital
Lexington, Kentucky

WILLIAM V. BERNARD
Equine Internal Medicine
Lexington, Kentucky

KEVIN T.T. CORLEY
Veterinary Advances, Ltd.
County Kildare, Ireland

MARY LASSALINE
Department of Surgical and Radiological Sciences
School of Veterinary Medicine, University of California, Davis
Davis, California

CLAIRE LATIMER
Rood and Riddle Equine Hospital
Lexington, Kentucky

LAURIE METCALFE
Rood and Riddle Equine Hospital
Lexington, Kentucky

JOHANNA M. REIMER
Reimer Ultrasound
Georgetown, Kentucky

TROY N. TRUMBLE
College of Veterinary Medicine
Department Veterinary Population Medicine
University of Minnesota
St. Paul, Minnesota

Physical Examination

William V. Bernard and Johanna M. Reimer

INTRODUCTION

Physical examination of the foal does not differ tremendously from that of the adult horse; however, laboratory values, vital signs, and disease processes can vary widely between horses and foals. If these differences are kept in mind, then the thought processes used for diagnosis in the adult can be applied to the foal. The basic physical examination provides the majority of information needed to make a presumptive diagnosis, provide a direction for ancillary tests, and formulate a plan for emergency therapy. If the patient is a neonate, the examination should include a detailed evaluation of the mare and placenta and a history of the events leading up to and including parturition. If the patient is an older foal, a complete medical history, including that of other foals on the farm, can be invaluable. The examination technique varies with individual preference; however, a routine should be established so that the evaluation is complete and individual areas are not omitted. In an emergency, the cardiovascular and respiratory systems should be the initial focus. In a nonemergency, it is good practice not to focus attention on the presenting complaint in order to reduce the risk of overlooking additional problems. As veterinary medicine has advanced and diagnostic aids have improved, the veterinarian's ability to diagnose and treat diseases has progressed. At the same time, these advances do not replace the physical examination as the primary and most valuable diagnostic aid available to the practitioner.

When presented with a neonatal foal, a physical examination and a complete history of the mare and periparturient events provide useful information. The mean gestational length in the mare is 335–342 days; however, the range of normal is considered to be 305–365 days. Knowledge of a mare's prior foaling history helps estimate the date of parturition, as mares that foal early or late may do so again in subsequent years. Mares bred later in the year generally have shorter gestations than mares bred in February or March (in the northern hemisphere). Maternal conditions that can influence fetal health and development of the foal include past reproductive problems such as dystocia, premature placental separation, uterine inertia, advanced maternal age, concurrent medical problems during gestation, musculoskeletal problems, and poor nutritional status. Premature lactation has been associated with placental and fetal abnormalities.

Examination of the reproductive tract should be performed if there is a history of dystocia, vaginal discharge, or retained placenta. The examination should include evaluation of the mammary gland. An enlarged, firm mammary gland may indicate mastitis or that the foal is not nursing adequately. A flaccid gland suggests inadequate milk production. Milk production can be evaluated by muzzling the foal for 1–2 hours while measuring the amount of milk produced.

Adequate colostrum and subsequent passive transfer of immunoglobulin (Ig) is very important to the health of the newborn foal. Colostrum is usually creamy yellow, with a thick and sticky consistency. However, visual inspection is not an adequate evaluation. Poor-quality colostrum, assessed directly by determining Ig content or measuring colostral specific gravity (SG), suggests the need for colostrum supplementation or plasma transfusion. The Ig content of colostrum should be >30 g/L (3,000 mg/dL). The SG of colostrum is directly related to Ig concentration and is considered adequate if greater than 1.060. The colostrometer, used to measure colostral SG, provides an immediate stall-side evaluation of colostral quality.

The fetal membranes consist of the allantochorion, amnion, and umbilical cord. In healthy Thoroughbred mares the weight of the placental membranes is approximately 11% that of the foal. Fetal membranes weighing >6.4 kg (14 lb) suggest the presence of uterine disease. If available, the allantoic fluid and amniotic fluids should be evaluated for character and color. Cloudy or discolored fetal fluid suggests infection. Culture of fetal fluids may identify the source of uterine infection and provide guidelines for treating a potentially infected foal. Often, the umbilical cord is twisted spirally, and severe twisting into a tight spiral can produce fetal compromise.

Examination of the placenta should include a systemic evaluation of the both the allantoic (inner-fetal side) and chorionic (outer-maternal side) surfaces. The placenta should be inverted and the chorionic surface examined carefully for evidence of bacterial placentitis, which may lead to weak, underdeveloped, or infected foals. A heavy, thickened, edematous, and discolored placenta is suggestive of bacterial placentitis, which is usually the result of ascending infection that frequently involves the cervical star area. Culture of the placenta may identify the cause of bacterial disease in the neonate. Submission of placental membranes for histopathology can confirm bacterial placentitis or identify other causes of placental/uterine disease. When fresh samples cannot be submitted, refrigerated or formalin-fixed sections should be saved.

NORMAL PARAMETERS

Vital parameters in the newborn foal vary significantly from those of the older foal or adult horse. These parameters change rapidly over the first hours of life and reflect the neonate's ability to adapt

Table 1. Evaluation of neonatal foal distress (performed 1 and 5 minutes after delivery)

Parameter	0	1	2
Heart rate	Absent	<60 bpm	≥60 bpm
Respiration	Absent	Slow, irregular	≥60 bpm
Muscle tone	Limp extremities	Some flexion of limbs	Sternal
Nasal stimulation	No reflexes	Grimace, slight rejection	Cough or sneeze

A total score or 7 or 8 indicates a normal foal, 4 to 6 indicates depression, and 0 to 3 indicates marked depression. From Martens RJ (1982) Neonatal respiratory distress: a review with emphasis on the horse. *Compendium on Continuing Education for the Practicing Veterinarian* 4:S23, with permission.

to its new environment. The average foal can maintain sternal recumbency within 1–2 minutes and stand within 1 hour of birth. A suckle reflex should be present within the first 30 minutes, and the average foal should be nursing the mare within 2 hours. A foal that takes longer than 3–4 hours to nurse and longer than 2 hours to stand is considered abnormal. The rectal temperature of the foal ranges between 37.2°C (99°F) and 38.6°C (101.5°F). A scoring system (*Table 1*) can help evaluate the severity of neonatal depression and asphyxia. These scoring systems can be helpful, but they should not replace the clinician's own interpretation of the physical examination findings. The heart rate and respiratory rate are the two most useful indicators of neonatal well-being immediately after birth and these are discussed in detail later in this chapter (pp. 4, 6). If the rates are within normal limits, then the foal should be monitored until it stands and nurses. Persistent increases or decreases in heart and/or respiratory rates should alert the clinician to existing or impending problems.

HEMATOLOGIC AND CHEMISTRY VALUES

Packed cell volume (PCV) and hemoglobin (Hb) concentrations increase during fetal development and reach adult values at approximately 300 days of gestation. PCV and Hb increase shortly after birth and gradually decrease over the first few weeks of life (*Table 2*). As with neonates of other species, foals may have lower red blood cell (RBC) indices than young adults. This is considered a physiologic anemia and should not be considered pathologic unless values continue to decrease or do not increase with age. At birth, the total white blood cell (WBC) count of the foal is similar to that of the adult horse (*Table 2*), although considerable individual variations occur in total leukocyte, lymphocyte, and neutrophil numbers. In the fetus there are more lymphocytes than neutrophils. Lymphocyte numbers decrease shortly after birth to a mean of 1,400 cells/µL. Adult levels are attained during the first 3 months of life. Low lymphocyte counts during the first few days

of life should not be used as an indicator of combined immune deficiency. However, persistent lymphopenia (i.e., <500 cells/µL) creates an index of suspicion in breeds at risk for combined immune deficiency.

At birth, there is a wide variation in plasma protein concentration (52–80 g/L [5.2–8.0 g/dL]). After nursing and Ig absorption, total plasma protein concentrations increase, but a wide range of values persists; therefore, plasma protein concentrations are not a reliable indicator of colostral absorption.

Although neonatal icterus may indicate disease, newborn foals frequently have elevated levels of bilirubin and mild icterus (*Table 3*). This physiologic icterus is a result of increased total and unconjugated bilirubin; the cause is not well documented in veterinary medicine, but it is likely the result of several factors including increased bilirubin load and immature hepatic metabolism or bilirubin. If icterus is severe or conjugated bilirubin is a large percentage of the total increase, then other causes of bilirubinemia, including neonatal isoerythrolysis (NI), septicemia, and hepatitis, must be considered.

Serum enzymes may be elevated in the first few days to weeks of life (*Table 4*). Occasionally, creatine kinase (CK), an indicator of muscle damage, is elevated in the newborn foal; this is likely the result of trauma during parturition. Alkaline phosphatase (ALP) is increased throughout the first few weeks to months of life. This is thought to be due to high metabolic bone activity during rapid growth and development, intestinal pinocytosis, and/or hepatic maturation. Gamma glutamyltransferase (GGT), sorbitol dehydrogenase (SDH), and aspartate aminotransferase (AST) may be increased transiently in the first few weeks after birth. This increase is thought to be related to hepatocellular maturation. Therefore, increased serum enzyme concentrations should be interpreted carefully in conjunction with clinical signs. Serial laboratory results are useful as an indicator of trends; increasing serum enzymes or marked elevations are indicative of a disease process. Occasionally, serum creatinine is elevated in the first 24–48 hours of life; this is discussed in Chapter 9 (Urinary and Umbilical Disorders, p. 175).

Table 2. Normal ranges for erythrocyte parameters and leukocyte counts in foals

Age	PCV l/L (%)	Hb g/L (g/dL)	RBCs ×10¹²/L (×10⁶/µL)	Total leukocytes ×10⁹/L (×10³/µL)	Neutrophils ×10⁹/L (×10³/µL)	Lymphocytes ×10⁹/L (×10³/µL)	Monocytes ×10⁹/L (×10³/µL)	Eosinophils ×10⁹/L (×10³/µL)	Basophils ×10⁹/L (×10³/µL)
1 day	0.32–0.46 (32–46)	120–166 (12.0–16.6)	8.2–11.0	4.9–11.7	3.36–9.57	0.67–2.12	0.07–0.39	0–0.02	0–0.03
3 days	0.30–0.46 (30–46)	115–167 (11.5–16.7)	7.8–11.4	5.1–10.1	3.21–8.58	0.73–2.17	0.08–0.58	0–0.22	0–0.12
1 week	0.28–0.43 (28–43)	107–158 (10.7–15.8)	7.4–10.6	6.3–13.6	4.35–10.55	1.43–2.22	0.03–0.54	0–0.09	0–0.18
2 weeks	0.28–0.41 (28–41)	101–153 (10.1–15.3)	7.2–10.8	5.2–11.9	3.99–9.08	1.32–3.12	0.07–0.58	0–0.10	0–0.10
3 weeks	0.29–0.40 (29–40)	105–148 (10.5–14.8)	7.8–10.6	5.4–12.4	3.16–8.94	1.47–3.26	0.06–0.69	0–0.16	0–0.09
1 month	0.29–0.41 (29–41)	109–153 (10.9–15.3)	7.9–11.1	5.3–12.2	2.76–9.27	1.73–4.85	0.05–0.63	0–0.12	0–0.08
2 months	0.31–0.44 (31–44)	116–160 (11.6–16.0)	9.1–13.2	5.4–13.5	2.70–9.46	2.37–4.72	0.05–0.61	0–0.28	0–0.10
3 months	0.32–0.42 32–42	117–153 11.7–15.3	9.2–12.0	6.7–16.8	3.92–10.35	2.88–7.15	0.12–0.76	0–0.55	0–0.07

Source: Harvey, J.W., Normal hematologic values. In: *Equine Clinical Neonatology*, A.M. Koterba, W.H. Drummond, P.C. Kosch (Eds.), Lea & Febiger, Philadelphia, PA, p. 563, 1990.

Table 3. Foal serum chemistry concentrations

Age (days)	Glucose mmol/L (mg/dL)	Blood urea nitrogen mmol/L (mg/dL)	Creatinine µmol/L (mg/dL)	Total bilirubin µmol/L (mg/dL)	Conjugated bilirubin µmol/L (mg/dL)	Unconjugated bilirubin µmol/L (mg/dL)	Cholesterol mmol/L (mg/dL)	Triglycerides µmol/L (mg/dL)
1	6.7–13.0 (121–233)	3.2–14.3 (9–40)	106–380 (1.2–4.3)	22–76 (1.3–4.5)	5–12 (0.3–0.7)	17–64 (1.0–3.8)	2.8–14.5 (110–562)	034–2.18 (30–193)
3	5.6–12.6 (101–226)	0.7–10.4 (2–29)	35–185 (0.4–2.1)	8–66 (0.5–3.9)	3–14 (0.2–0.8)	3–56 (0.2–3.3)	3.7–9.0 (142–350)	0.7–3.86 (63–342)
5	–	–	–	20–61 (1.2–3.6)	2–12 (0.1–0.7)	14–47 (0.8–2.8)	3.3–9.3 (127–361)	0.58–3.8 (52–340)
7	6.7–10.7 (121–192)	1.4–7.1 (4–20)	88–150 (1.0–1.7)	14–51 (0.8–3.0)	5–12 (0.3–0.7)	8–39 (0.5–2.3)	3.6–11.5 (139–445)	0.34–2.7 (30–239)
14	7.6–11.4 (137–205)	2.1–4.6 (6–13)	80–159 (0.9–1.8)	12–37 (0.7–2.2)	5–10 (0.3–0.6)	8–27 (0.5–1.6)	4.2–7.4 (164–287)	0.44–2.26 (39–200)
21	7.2–13.3 (130–240)	2.1–5.0 (6–14)	53–177 (0.6–2.0)	8–27 (0.5–1.6)	3–8 (0.2–0.5)	3–19 (0.2–1.1)	1.9–7.1 (74–276)	0.38–1.40 (34–124)
28	7.2–12.0 (130–216)	2.1–7.5 (6–21)	97–159 (1.1–1.8)	8–29 (0.5–1.7)	2–10 (0.1–0.6)	7–20 (0.4–1.2)	2.1–6.0 (83–233)	0.51–1.75 (45–155)
60	6.6–11.3 (119–204)	2.1–3.9 (6–11)	97–185 (1.1–2.1)	8–34 (0.5–2.0)	3–8 (0.2–0.5)	5–25 (0.3–1.5)	2.5–6.2 (98–242)	0.11–1.67 (10–148)
90	4.9–10.0 (88–179)	2.5–7.1 (7–20)	62–195 (0.7–2.2)	7–34 (0.4–2.0)	2–12 (0.1–0.7)	7–24 (0.4–1.4)	2.8–5.8 (110–226)	0.32–1.71 (28–151)

Source: Bauer, J.E., Normal blood chemistries, In: *Equine Clinical Neonatology*, A.M. Koterba, W.H. Drummond, P.C. Kosch (Eds.), Lea & Febiger, Philadelphia, PA, p. 608, 1990.

EXAMINATION OF THE FOAL BY BODY SYSTEM

CARDIOVASCULAR SYSTEM

Rate and rhythm

The heart rate of the foal is normally 40–80 beats per minute (bpm) in the immediate postpartum period; it increases to 120–150 bpm during the next few hours and then stabilizes at approximately 80–100 bpm within the first week of life. Sinus arrhythmias were noted relatively frequently during an electrocardiographic study of foals in the immediate postpartum period. Various other arrhythmias (ventricular premature complexes, ventricular tachycardia, supraventricular tachycardia, atrial fibrillation) were occasionally observed in these otherwise normal foals; however, all arrhythmias disappeared within 15 minutes post partum. Because sustained accelerated idioventricular rhythms and ventricular tachycardia generally are characterized by regular rhythms on auscultation, electrocardiography is necessary to determine if such arrhythmias are present. The clinical significance of any unusual or abnormal arrhythmias should take into consideration clinical, metabolic, and hemodynamic findings.

Murmurs

Because of the foal's thin chest, the apex beat is quite prominent and heart sounds and flow murmurs are louder than in the adult horse. Valve areas in the foal are similar to those described for the adult horse. Holosystolic ejection-type murmurs are common in foals and are most likely physiologic in nature (innocent flow murmurs) rather than due to a patent ductus arteriosus (PDA). Innocent murmurs may acquire unusual tones if the foal is in lateral recumbency or is hemodynamically compromised. Functional closure of the ductus arteriosus occurs shortly after birth in most foals. In the authors' experience, a murmur indicative of left-to-right ductus arteriosus is absent immediately after birth in most foals, suggesting that functional closure has occurred.

Table 4. Foal serum enzyme activities

Age (days)	ALP u/L	GGT u/L	SDH u/L	AST u/L	ALT u/L	CK u/L
1	861–2671	18–43	0.6–4.6	146–340	0–49	40–909
3	283–1462	9–40	0.6–3.7	80–580	0–52	21–97
5	156–1294	8–89	0.8–5.3	–	–	29–208
7	137–1169	14–164	0.8–8.2	237–620	4–50	52–143
14	182–859	16–169	0.6–4.3	240–540	1–9	46–208
21	146–752	16–132	1.0–8.4	226–540	0–45	44–210
28	210–866	17–99	1.2–5.9	252–440	5–47	81–585
60	201–741	8–38	1.1–4.6	282–484	7–57	50–170
90	206–458	0–27	1.1–3.9	282–480	8–65	57–204

Source: Bauer, J.E., Normal blood chemistries, In: *Equine Clinical Neonatology*, A.M. Koterba, W.H. Drummond, P.C. Kosch (Eds.), Lea & Febiger, Philadelphia, PA, p. 604, 1990.

In a few cases, a left-to-right PDA murmur may become apparent within the first 24–48 hours after birth. Most of these foals have concurrent systemic disease (e.g., diarrhea, septicemia). A PDA (left-to-right) should not be considered abnormal if it persists for up to a few days post partum and the foal is otherwise healthy. *Table 5* assists in the clinical differentiation of PDA and flow murmurs. The definitive differentiation is made noninvasively with Doppler echocardiography.

If the foal is compromised (e.g., respiratory disease, prematurity, septicemia), the presence of a PDA may be of more concern. Hypoxemia, septicemia, endotoxemia, and/or severe respiratory disease can result in pulmonary hypertension, which may result in reverse flow through the ductus arteriosus. Until the ductus arteriosus is permanently occluded by fibrosis (approximately 1 week post partum or post functional closure), a functionally closed ductus may regain patency in the face of pulmonary hypertension, resulting in right-to-left shunting. Reversion to fetal circulation (right-to-left shunting through the foramen ovale and/or the ductus arteriosus) results in hypoxemia and this further exacerbates pulmonary vasoconstriction and hypertension. This creates a vicious cycle of hypoxemia, pulmonary hypertension, systemic hypotension, and increased right-to-left shunting. Pharmacologic closure of a PDA can be achieved with nonsteroidal anti-inflammatory drugs (NSAIDs) in premature infants. The efficacy of NSAIDs in pharmacologic closure of PDA in foals has not yet been demonstrated.

Table 5. Differentiation of flow murmurs from left-to-right patent ductus arteriosus in the foal

Parameter	Flow murmur	Patent ductus arteriosus (left-to-right)
Pulse quality	Normal	Bounding
Systolic murmur	Ejection quality	Continuous into early diastole, or typical machinery
Diastolic murmur	Absent	Early diastole to continuous
Precordial thrill	Rarely present	May be absent or present
Location (point of maximal intensity)	Aortic valve	Slightly dorsal to and caudal to aortic valve

Table 6. Cyanotic congenital heart defects

Defect	Features
Tetralogy of Fallot	Hemodynamically significant pulmonic stenosis, large VSD
Truncus arteriosus	Common trunk from both ventricular outlets; VSD must be present
Transposition of the great arteries	Aorta and pulmonary artery transposed; must have an ASD, VSD, or PDA to survive after birth
Tricuspid atresia	Atretic tricuspid valve, patent atrial septum, VSD
Hypoplastic left heart syndrome	Diminutive left ventricle, atretic mitral and/or aortic valve, enlarged right ventricle; PDA must be present to survive

ASD = atrial septal defect; VSD = ventricular septal defect; PDA = patent ductus arteriosus.

Cyanosis

Cyanosis, or hypoxemia unresponsive to oxygen administration, should prompt a thorough evaluation of the cardiovascular system. Murmurs may be absent or may range in intensity from very soft to very loud, with precordial thrills in foals with cyanotic congenital heart disease. Some of the more common cyanotic (right-to-left) congenital cardiac defects and corresponding features are listed in *Table 6*. The clinician should be aware that there are anatomic variations of each of these defects, therefore the defects listed in *Table 6* may be further subclassified. For an animal with a cyanotic congenital heart defect to survive after birth, shunting between the systemic and pulmonary circulations (i.e., through a PDA, patent foramen ovale, atrial septal defect [ASD], or ventricular septal defect [VSD]) must be present. In addition to congenital defects, reversion to fetal circulation should be considered in any critically ill neonatal foal with hypoxemia unresponsive to oxygen insufflation. Although severe respiratory disease alone may result in cyanosis, it may also lead to reversion to fetal circulation.

Echocardiographic studies can be used to document any cardiac causes of cyanosis. Congenital defects can be identified. Right-to-left shunting through the foramen ovale can be documented with bubble studies (rapid intravenous injection of agitated saline during echocardiography). This procedure is less rewarding for documenting cases of reverse PDA because of the difficulty in imaging the ductus arteriosus; however, the abdominal aorta may be imaged for bubbles instead. Bubble studies should be performed with caution in right-to-left shunts, as air embolism to the central nervous system (CNS) may occur. Saline may be agitated in a closed system, using a three-way stopcock and two "primed" syringes to agitate saline back and forth prior to injection. Dilation of the pulmonary artery (as compared with the aorta), hypertrophy of the right ventricle (which is not necessarily abnormal in the neonate), and paradoxical septal motion are compatible with pulmonary hypertension and supportive of a diagnosis of reversion to fetal circulation. Pulmonary hypertension can be more conclusively documented with Doppler echocardiography and cardiac catheterization.

Blood pressure

Monitoring systemic arterial pressure in critically ill foals is beneficial in determining the hemodynamic significance of any arrhythmias and in tailoring pharmacologic treatment of systemic hypotension. Systemic arterial hypotension can exacerbate right-to-left cardiovascular shunts and should therefore be monitored and addressed in foals at risk for reversion to fetal circulation. Noninvasive measurement of blood pressure (BP) can be performed fairly consistently with commercially available products. Published normal values for arterial BP depend on the measurement technique. Direct mean arterial BP is 70–90 mmHg; however, normal values for noninvasive measurements are variable depending on the technique, and they are often lower than direct measurements. Indirect arterial BP monitoring is performed using Doppler or oscillometric techniques.

Cardiac output

Cardiac output can be monitored noninvasively in the neonatal foal with Doppler echocardiography. Special equipment and training and patient cooperation are required for accurate employment of this technique.

RESPIRATORY SYSTEM

The respiratory rate in the neonatal foal is approximately 60–80 breaths per minute in the immediate neonatal period and declines to 30 breaths per minute within 1 hour after birth. Lung sounds are very moist immediately post partum. Transient large airway sounds and/or crackles may be detected quite easily in the dependent lung in recumbent foals without respiratory disease when they are placed in a sternal position. Thoracic auscultation is not a reliable indicator of lower respiratory disease in the foal, as often only subtle abnormalities are appreciable on auscultation, even in the presence of very severe pulmonary disease.

An elevation in respiratory rate, increased effort, and abnormalities of breathing pattern (e.g., nostril flaring, an abdominal component to the respiratory pattern, respiratory stridor) are more appreciable than auscultable changes in foals with respiratory disease. The thorax should be palpated to determine if fractured ribs are present. Brown-tinged nasal secretions may suggest meconium aspiration. Other diseases affecting the lower respiratory tract include pneumonia (viral, bacterial, and fungal), surfactant deficiency, and diaphragmatic hernia.

Arterial blood gas analysis enables characterization and elucidation of the cause of lower respiratory disorders and dictates the most appropriate course of therapy. Arterial oxygen pressures <70 mmHg are best managed with intranasal insufflation of oxygen, although positive pressure ventilation may be required if there is an inadequate response to oxygen administration (providing right-to-left cardiovascular shunting, including reversion to fetal circulation, has been ruled out). Cyanosis is not apparent until the PaO_2 is <40 mmHg. Ventilatory support is also required if the arterial carbon dioxide tension is >70 mmHg. Noninvasive measurements of blood gas concentrations include pulse oximetry and capnography. Pulse oximetry enables measurement of peripheral tissue oxygen saturation; however, the equipment is expensive, and if peripheral perfusion is poor, results do not reflect systemic arterial oxygen saturation. Capnography measures arterial carbon dioxide concentrations. Both pulse oximetry and capnography greatly facilitate ventilatory management of foals by reducing the frequency of arterial blood sampling.

Thoracic radiography, ultrasonography (which should be performed with the foal in either sternal recumbency or standing), and transtracheal aspirates are used to document and diagnose various pulmonary diseases/conditions. Radiography, although not specific, may provide information regarding the type and extent of pulmonary disease (1). Both bacterial and viral pneumonias may be characterized by alveolar and/or interstitial patterns. Ventral distribution of pathologic changes may be indicative of bacterial or aspiration pneumonia (bacterial or meconium). A somewhat wispy pattern in the mid to dorsal thorax may be seen in foals with fungal pneumonia. Premature or immature foals with surfactant disorders may not exhibit signs of respiratory distress for 24–48 hours post partum. Radiography in such cases often reveals a characteristic ground-glass appearance to the lungs. However, radiographic changes may not be evident in premature foals in the preclinical stages of the disorder.

Ultrasonography of the thorax is advisable in foals with a suspected diaphragmatic hernia or with hemothorax due to rib fracture. If possible, ultrasonography should be performed prior to radiography, as it can be performed with portable equipment at the stall. If a diagnosis of either disorder is confirmed, radiography is usually unnecessary. Because air-filled lung will float above intrathoracic intestinal contents (diaphragmatic hernia) or pleural fluid (hemothorax), the examination must be performed with the foal standing or in sternal recumbency. Rib fractures can often be identified on a gap or alteration in the contour of the cortical surface of the rib. Fractures most often occur immediately above to several centimeters above the costochondral junction. Hypoechoic regions may be identified in the adjacent lung surface and likely represent contused lung. Homogenous, slightly echogenic (cellular) fluid within the thorax is consistent with hemothorax. Occasionally, numerous gas echoes may be seen floating throughout the fluid, presumably as a result of lung laceration. Serial thoracic sonograms can be used to assess resolution or deterioration of the hemothorax, prompting thoracocentesis or surgical intervention if necessary.

Ultrasonography, like radiography, is not specific in the identification of pulmonary parenchymal disease in the foal. Sonography of the thorax of young foals with pulmonary disease, regardless of etiology, often reveals the nonspecific finding of a loss of the normal reverberation artifact pattern.

GASTROINTESTINAL SYSTEM

Examination of the gastrointestinal (GI) tract in the foal follows the same procedures as in the adult horse; the main difference is size. Small size limits the ability to perform a rectal examination, but it does offer an advantage during ultrasonographic and radiographic examination of the abdomen.

Visual examination of the abdomen may provide information regarding the location of abdominal distension and the underlying cause. External abdominal palpation is of limited value. In small foals, some abdominal structures may be identified. The inguinal rings and ventral abdomen should be palpated routinely for hernias. Bowel herniation can result in strangulation and vascular compromise. If hernias are easily reduced, then careful monitoring and frequent reduction may be adequate.

Auscultation of the abdomen provides an assessment of GI motility and should be performed from the paralumbar fossa to the ventral abdomen, on both the right and left sides. GI activity produces peristaltic and borborygmal sounds that should be heard approximately every 10–20 seconds. Tinkling or splashing sounds may be heard over the right dorsal quadrant as fluid enters the cecum. Simultaneous abdominal auscultation/percussion of a tympanitic or pinging sound identifies a gas-distended viscus adjacent to the body wall. Abdominal sounds can be classified as normal, increased, decreased, or absent. Decreases in motility suggest an ileus, which may be due to inflammatory, ischemic, or obstructive lesions. Increased motility occurs during the early stages of enteritis or intestinal obstruction.

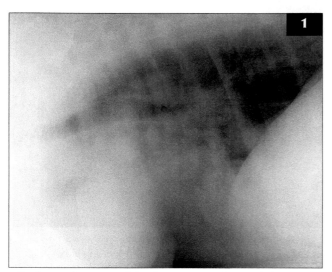

1 Radiographic view of the thorax: ventral consolidation. Note the increased opacity between the caudal border of the heart and the diaphragm.

In the neonate, evaluation of the quantity and quality of meconium is an important part of the physical examination. Meconium is an accumulation of swallowed allantoic fluid, GI secretions, and cellular debris that collects in the small colon and rectum and is passed shortly after birth. Meconium generally is black to dark brown in color and firm to pasty in consistency. Once meconium has been passed, the feces change to a softer, lighter brown consistency. The amount of meconium varies between foals, and reported passage of meconium does not rule out the possibility of meconium retention.

Nasogastric intubation helps identify a gas- or fluid-filled stomach. As large a stomach tube as can be passed through the nasal passages should be used. Fenestrations at the end of the tube help prevent obstruction of the tube with feed material. In neonates, a small, flexible tube such as a Harris flush or enema tube is ideal. A stomach pump and gravity flow or gentle aspiration with a 60 ml syringe may be used to check for reflux. With severe gastric distension, it may be difficult to pass a nasogastric tube through the cardia. Lidocaine applied to the tube or injected down the tube may be useful in relaxing the esophagus.

Abdominocentesis provides useful information about GI lesions. Ultrasonography can be used to identify areas of peritoneal fluid, particularly if abdominal distension is present. If taut loops of small intestine are identified sonographically, abdominocentesis should be avoided or performed with extreme caution owing to the increased risk of lacerating distended bowel. Abdominocentesis is performed on or to the right of the midline following aseptic preparation of the site. Sedation or local anesthetic may be required. In a foal that is struggling or in too much pain to remain standing, the tap can be performed with the foal in lateral recumbency. Normal peritoneal fluid should be clear or slightly yellow in color, with a protein concentration <25 g/L (2.5 g/dL) and a WBC count <5,000/μL.

Laboratory tests, although not diagnostic, aid in formulating the list of differential diagnoses for foals with GI disease. Changes in the total peripheral WBC count and electrolyte concentrations help differentiate early enteritis from colic requiring surgery. Marked leukopenia is suggestive of enteritis and is not a common finding with a surgical abdomen. Enteritis can induce secretory mechanisms, including bicarbonate loss from pancreatic secretions and/or failure of absorption from the large colon, resulting in loss of electrolytes and hyponatremia, hypochloremia, and/or acidosis. Serum potassium concentrations are more variable and depend on fluid losses, acid–base status, and renal function. Electrolyte abnormalities in foals with colic requiring surgery are frequently related to acid–base changes. Hypochloremia may develop in long-standing acidosis subsequent to renal changes of chloride ion for bicarbonate.

Abdominal radiography helps to determine the location, but not necessarily the cause, of gas or fluid distension. Adequate radiographs can be obtained in foals up to 230 kg (500 lb) if the available radiographic equipment includes a grid, rare earth screens, and sufficient mAs (5–28) and kVp (75–95). Gaseous distension of the small intestine, characterized radiographically by intraluminal gas–fluid interfaces, can be seen in foals with enteritis, peritonitis, or small intestinal obstruction. Multiple intraluminal gas–fluid interfaces or vertical U-shaped loops of distended small intestine are compatible with small intestinal obstructive disease. With enteritis, the small intestinal loops are smaller and concomitant large bowel distension may be seen. During large bowel obstruction, the large intestine is more distended and the colon may appear displaced within the abdomen. Contrast studies using gravity barium enemas (1–2 liters of barium mixed with warm water) are useful in identifying meconium impactions.

Abdominal ultrasonography permits characterization of small intestinal motility (absent, normal, hyper), distension (minimal, moderate, marked), and wall thickness. In older foals (>4 months of age), sonographic visualization of the small intestine is often limited to the caudal abdomen (inguinal region). Flaccid, minimally fluid-filled loops of small intestine are seen in the healthy foal. If these loops become rounded and larger, an ileus, enteritis, or small bowel obstructive disease is likely to exist. Small intestinal intussusception appears as target- or doughnut-shaped patterns, with the telescoping of one segment of bowel into another. Large intestinal gaseous distension causes reflection of sound waves, resulting in a poor ultrasonographic view of the abdomen. Abdominal fluid can be identified, quantified, and characterized. If excessive peritoneal fluid is detected, peritonitis, a ruptured viscus, or uroperitoneum may be present. Increased peritoneal fluid echogenicity is associated with increased cellularity or hemorrhage (hemoperitoneum [2]).

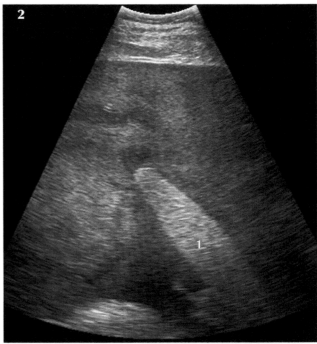

2 Ultrasound image of the abdomen of a horse with intra-abdominal hemorrhage. Note the swirling echogenic or 'smokey' appearance (1), typical of hemoperitoneum.

Examination of the foal with abdominal pain

When presented with a foal with abdominal pain, the main objective is to determine whether a surgical lesion exists. The neonatal foal does not respond as rapidly or as effectively to systemic compromise as the adult. Therefore, rapid diagnosis and resolution of a strangulating lesion is imperative. A complete physical examination in combination with ancillary tests helps distinguish between many surgical and nonsurgical causes of colic. Abdominal pain is a frequent manifestation of enteritis, but if diarrhea is infrequent or absent, then the painful foal with enteritis may be difficult to differentiate from the foal requiring abdominal surgery.

Vital signs may not always distinguish between surgical and nonsurgical colic. Changes in mucous membrane color, resulting from distributive shock (endotoxemia, septicemia, splanchnic ischemia) can be present in a variety of GI diseases. Severe toxic changes in the mucous membranes are more typical of a strangulating lesion, but they can be seen with severe, acute bacterial enteritis or with peritonitis.

The foal is less tolerant of abdominal pain than the adult horse. Therefore, the degree of pain (rolling, looking at the side) is not a sensitive indicator of the severity of abdominal disease, nor is it specific for the cause of colic. Although pain characterized by rolling up on the back and teeth grinding is usually associated with gastric ulceration, other causes of abdominal pain (e.g., intussusception) should be considered until a definitive diagnosis is made. Persistent pain that is nonresponsive to analgesics is more consistent with a surgical (usually strangulating) lesion. Mild abdominal pain, which persists or progresses to more severe colic, is compatible with enteritis, GI ulceration, or simple obstruction. Tachycardia and/or tachypnea is invariably present with severe abdominal pain. Marked, persistent tachycardia (>120 bpm) suggests a surgical lesion.

Intestinal strangulation of any duration is associated with an elevated nucleated cell count and protein concentration in the peritoneal fluid. Peritoneal fluid analysis is usually normal in enteritis and simple early obstruction. As these diseases progress, increases in peritoneal fluid cell count and protein concentration can occur, but they are not as dramatic as those seen with strangulating obstructions. Cytologic examination of peritoneal fluid does not distinguish between inflammation associated with enteritis and ischemia. Intracellular bacteria, plant material, and degenerated neutrophils may be identified in patients with a ruptured viscus.

A large quantity of gastric reflux is most typical of a strangulating small intestinal lesion, although moderate quantities of reflux can be obtained with other abdominal diseases, including enteritis. Persistent reflux suggests severe small intestinal obstruction due to a volvulus, stricture, or intussusception.

Impacted meconium is the most frequent cause of abdominal pain in the neonate. The pain may vary from mild to severe. Foals may continue to nurse and frequently strain to defecate. The absence of palpable meconium does not rule out the possibility of an impaction over the brim of the pelvis or involving the proximal small colon (high meconium impactions). Radiographs, including contrast studies, help identify retained meconium.

Examination of the foal with a nonpainful, distended abdomen

The primary cause of abdominal pain and distension in the foal is gas or fluid accumulation within the GI tract. Causes of nonpainful abdominal distension include intra-abdominal masses and excess intraperitoneal fluid. Abdominal masses include neoplasia (rare) and abscesses. Accumulation of fluid in the peritoneal space may be a result of uroperitoneum, hemoperitoneum, or excessive production of peritoneal fluid. Abdominal fluid can be identified by ballottement of a fluid wave and be confirmed on radiography or ultrasonography. Free-flowing peritoneal fluid obtained via abdominocentesis suggests increased peritoneal fluid. Peritoneal fluid analysis helps characterize the type of fluid. An elevated white cell count is indicative of peritonitis, although with peracute septic peritonitis (e.g., GI rupture), the white cell count may be normal. Degenerated neutrophils and intra- or extracellular bacteria indicate a septic process.

Peritonitis that is not secondary to primary GI disease is usually a result of abdominal abscessation or umbilical remnant infection. Some cases may be idiopathic. Ultrasonography is useful in identifying both conditions. The typical presentation of the foal with an abdominal abscess includes weight loss due to a failure to thrive and a distended or pendulous abdomen. These foals may or may not be depressed and are only intermittently febrile. A history of abdominal pain is uncommon. If acute peritonitis develops, however, these foals may present with septic/endotoxic shock.

UROGENITAL SYSTEM

Physical examination of the urogenital system includes evaluation of the external genitalia (i.e., palpation of the scrotum, prepuce, and penis in the colt, or examination of the vulva and perineum in the filly). The umbilicus can be palpated externally. Occasionally, the umbilical remnants can be palpated through the body wall. The neonate should be observed for the onset, frequency, and quantity of urine output. The mean time for first urination in the foal is 5.97 hours in the colt and 10.77 hours for fillies; however, these times can be quite variable. Mean urine production in the neonatal foal is 148 mL/kg/day.

Clinical signs of urogenital disease include depression, straining to urinate, pigmenturia, and/or decreased urine output (oliguria). With chronic renal disease or long-standing uroperitoneum resulting in persistent uremia, uremic ulceration of mucous membranes may be evident (3). When the clinical signs of urinary tract disease exist, the foal's urine production should be monitored carefully and serum chemistries evaluated for azotemia and electrolyte disturbances. Oliguria may result from prerenal, renal, or postrenal conditions. Prerenal causes include hypovolemia associated with shock, decreased fluid intake, or increased fluid loss. Fluid loss includes third-space loss into the GI tract or overt diarrhea and dehydration. Decreased fluid intake results from decreased milk consumption secondary to depression or systemic disease. Azotemia of renal origin can be caused by a variety of conditions including

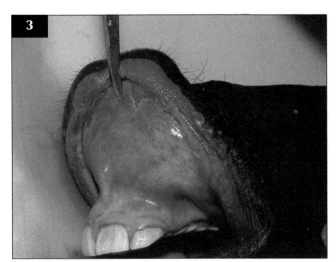

3 Uremic ulcers in the mucous membranes of a foal in which a long-standing uroperitoneum has resulted in persistent uremia.

acute tubular necrosis, nephritis, and congenital diseases. Postrenal conditions are related to obstruction or disruption of the urinary tract.

Gross or microscopic hematuria/hemoglobulinuria may be due to urogenital disease. Gross pink-red urine or a positive urine dipstick reaction for Hb can be seen with intact RBCs, Hb, or myoglobin in the urine. Differentiation between myoglobinuria and hemoglobinuria can be made by observing the color of the plasma. Pink, discolored plasma is suggestive of hemoglobinemia. Myoglobin is a smaller molecule and passes rapidly through the glomerulus, leaving the plasma clear during myoglobinemia. The definitive test to differentiate Hb from myoglobin is a protein precipitation test. Hematuria is best documented by direct microscopic examination of the urine sediment to identify intact RBCs. Hemoglobinuria is a result of intravascular hemolysis. If the PCV is normal in the face of discolored urine, then hemoglobinuria is unlikely. When hematuria is identified, renal, ureteral, bladder, or

urethral disease should be considered. A renal cause for hematuria can be confirmed by using endoscopy to visualize discolored urine passing from ureteral openings.

Sonographic evaluation of the kidneys is easily performed in foals. The left kidney can be found in the left paralumbar fossa. The right kidney is located cranial to the left kidney and can be found by scanning between the last few rib spaces cranial to the right paralumbar fossa. The kidneys should be observed for size, texture of the interstitium, dilation of the calyces, masses, and perirenal edema. Renal agenesis and cystic kidneys have been reported in the foal. Occasionally, the ureters can be observed leaving the kidneys. Dilation of one or both ureters suggests distal obstruction. Usually, the bladder can be identified in the neonate or young foal. If the bladder cannot be found, the sonographic examination should be repeated in case the bladder was empty during the examination. In the older foal the bladder can be difficult to visualize due to the presence of bowel between the bladder and the body wall. If uroperitoneum exists and a full bladder can still be visualized, a fenestration or leak in the bladder should be considered. The urachal remnant should be examined sonographically for tears secondary to infection.

Prerenal oliguria is the result of decreased blood flow to the kidneys and a subsequent decrease in glomerular filtration. Azotemia is not always present and depends on the severity and duration of the hypovolemia. Urinalysis is useful in differentiating prerenal from other causes of azotemia (*Table 7*). During dehydration, the kidneys should be concentrating urine in an attempt to conserve fluid volume. The maximum concentrating abilities of the foal's kidneys have not been determined. It has been reported that a SG of greater than 1.028 is rarely seen in foals less than 7 days of age, even during dehydration. Prerenal azotemia should respond rapidly to volume replacement and diuresis. Dopamine infusions may be required to restore renal blood flow. If untreated, hypovolemia can result in progressive renal disease.

Renal causes of azotemia or oliguria may be due to prolonged hypovolemia, acute tubular necrosis, pyelonephritis, or congenital anomalies. The presence of casts, RBCs and WBCs, and isosthenuria on urinalysis is indicative of renal disease.

Table 7. Normal ranges for standard urinalysis in the neonatal foals

SG	pH	Protein	Glucose	Crystals	Casts	Hemo-protein	Bacteria	Epithelial cells	RBCs	WBCs	Mucus
1.00–1.027	5.5–8.0	Negative to +30	Negative	Usually none; calcium oxalate rare, amorphous urate rare	Negative	Negative to +2	Negative (except free catch)	Squamous or caudate	Negative	+3/HPF	Negative to abundant

Urine SG varies with the state of hydration. During renal disease, the kidney loses its ability to alter the concentration of urine, resulting in isosthenuria. Electrolyte disturbances occur frequently in foals with renal disease. Electrolyte abnormalities associated with, but not diagnostic of, renal disease include hyponatremia, hypochloremia, hyperkalemia, and a variable acid–base status.

Postrenal azotemia is a result of obstructive or disruptive disease of the urinary tract. Obstructive urinary disease is rare in the foal. Disruption of the urinary tract is usually the result of a ruptured bladder, although injury to ureters, urachus, and urethra can occur. Bladder ruptures usually occur at birth, but can be seen in older foals secondary to trauma or to infection of the bladder or urachal remnant. Clinical signs may not be noted for several days after birth. As uroperitoneum progresses, the abdomen becomes distended, the azotemia worsens, and the foal becomes depressed. Stranguria is observed infrequently, but failure to urinate may be noted. Foals with uroperitoneum may continue to urinate; however, the volume is usually decreased.

A presumptive diagnosis of uroperitoneum can be made if typical blood work abnormalities (azotemia, hyponatremia, hypochloremia, and hyperkalemia) exist and large volumes of peritoneal fluid are identified via ultrasonography. Blood work is not diagnostic because other conditions, including renal disease and GI disease, can produce similar electrolyte abnormalities. The diagnosis of uroperitoneum is confirmed via abdominocentesis. If peritoneal fluid creatinine is at least twice the serum creatinine concentration, uroperitoneum is likely. Creatinine is a larger molecule than urea nitrogen or electrolytes and therefore it diffuses from peritoneal fluid into the systemic circulation more slowly than the other urine components.

Umbilical remnant infections (omphalophlebitis) are a common problem in older foals of all ages. In older foals, infections obtained at or shortly after birth can become clinically apparent later in life. Umbilical infection should not be ruled out if palpation of the external umbilicus is normal. The internal structures can be difficult to palpate and small areas of infection can result in serious problems. Omphalophlebitis should be included as a differential for the foal with fever of unknown origin. Typical leukogram changes suggesting infection may or may not be present.

Sonography of the umbilical remnants includes visualization of the umbilical vein as it courses cranially along the ventral midline toward the liver. In the young foal the diameter of the umbilical vein is not larger than 10 mm. The sonographic appearance may be diffusely echogenic or may contain a small continuous hypoechoic to anechoic core. If the vein is enlarged, inflammation or infection should be suspected. In the older foal the umbilical vein becomes smaller to inapparent as it develops into the round ligament of the liver. In the young foal the urachus can be identified as it leaves the umbilical stump and travels to the tip of the bladder. The umbilical arteries course along either side of the urachus and branch to run laterally and dorsally to the bladder. The normal diameter of the urachus and arteries combined is <1.8 cm, and the individual

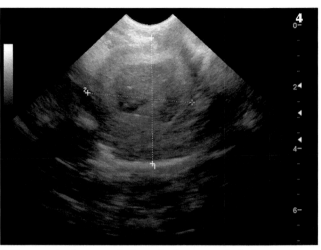

4 Short-axis ultrasound view of a large urachal abscess in a foal. Note the thickened wall that surrounds a central lumen of echogenic fluid (pus).

arteries alongside the bladder normally each measure <8 mm on diameter. A fluid core may be present in an umbilical artery as a result of coagulated blood. If the umbilical remnants are enlarged and/or if fluid cores are seen, infection should be suspected (4). In the older foal the arteries become inapparent as they develop into the round ligament of the bladder.

NERVOUS SYSTEM

The neurologic examination begins with the signalment and a thorough history including information regarding age, sex, breed, previous medical history, age at onset of neurologic signs, and any treatments administered. The examination should include a complete physical examination, because systemic diseases that involve the CNS are common in the foal.

A systematic approach to the neurologic examination might begin with assessment of the mental state and progress to evaluation of head position and the cranial nerves (CNs). A lesion of either the cerebrum or, occasionally, the brainstem results in some degree of depression. If the foal is bright and alert, then it is unlikely that a central lesion exists; however, critically ill neonates are often weak, depressed, or recumbent. These foals must be differentiated from those with primary neurologic disease. The young foal often keeps its head in a flexed position and responds to stimuli with quick, jerky movements. Evaluation of the head for position in relation to the body will determine the presence or absence of a lesion in the vestibular system, which includes the inner ear and its efferents, brainstem nuclei, and cerebellar tracts. A lesion of the vestibular system results in a head tilt, with the poll deviated laterally and the muzzle and caudal neck on a median plane. Severe lesions can produce a deviation of the entire neck to one side and a tendency to lean or circle in one direction. Asymmetric cerebral lesions also can result in a head tilt and circling in one direction. Foals with cerebral lesions are often severely depressed, and their circling is continuous and progressive.

Evaluation of the CNs is performed as in the adult horse. However, a few normal variations should be kept in mind. The palpebral reflex is present shortly after birth. Although the menace response (blinking subsequent to a menacing gesture) does not develop until several weeks of age, the foal should withdraw its head from a menacing gesture. The pupillary light reflex can be slow in the excited foal. The ability to swallow can be evaluated by observing the foal's ability to nurse. Lip and tongue tone and recognition of the udder are necessary for adequate nursing. If large amounts of milk are seen coming from the mouth or nostrils, then a swallowing deficit should be considered.

Examination of the eye should be a routine part of the basic physical and neurologic examination. Vision can be evaluated by observation of the foal's behavior, navigation through obstacles, and response to a menacing gesture. Direct and consensual light reflexes should be present. The normal cornea is clear and oval. Foals commonly have persistent papillary membrane tags that may extend freely into the aqueous or span the circumference of the iris collarette. Persistent hyaloid structures are common in foals up to four months of age. The foal's fundus is similar to that of the adult.

An advantage of performing a neurologic examination in the neonatal foal is the relative ease of testing reflexes when trying to localize a spinal cord lesion. Neonates and young foals are often hyperreflexic until they are several weeks of age. In the hindlimb, the patellar, flexor, gastrocnemius, and cranial tibial reflexes can be tested. The patellar reflex is tested with the foal in lateral recumbency and the limb to be tested supported in relaxed flexion. A brisk extension of the limb (stifle) is expected when the patellar ligaments are struck with the side of the hand. This reflex involves spinal segments L4 and L5 and is mediated through the femoral nerve. The hindlimb flexor or withdrawal reflex involves spinal segments L3–S3 and is mediated through the sciatic nerve. Pinching the skin of the distal limb, the coronary band, or the bulbs of the heel should elicit a withdrawal of the limb and/or central recognition of pain. The gastrocnemius reflex is performed by bluntly striking the gastrocnemius tendon and observing for extension of the hock. This reflex involves spinal cord segments L5–S3 and is mediated through the tibial branch of the sciatic nerve. The cranial tibial reflex is performed by holding the limb in relaxed extension and balloting the cranial tibial muscle. The expected response is hock flexion.

Reflex testing in the forelimbs includes evaluation of the flexor and triceps reflexes. The triceps reflex is tested by holding the limb in relaxed flexion and tapping the biceps tendon above its insertion at the olecranon. This reflex is mediated by the radial nerve through the cervical intumescence (C6–T1). The flexor or withdrawal reflex of the forelimb is mediated through the last three cervical and first two thoracic spinal cord segments. The expected response is flexion of the digit, carpus, elbow, and shoulder. A central response to pain should be observed.

Thoracolumbar lesions can be localized by evaluating the cutaneous reflex along the lateral body wall. Gentle pinching or poking of the skin along the lateral thorax elicits a twitching of the cutaneous trunci muscle. The sensory output is carried to the spinal cord at the level of the stimulation. It then travels cranially in spinal cord white matter to the last cervical and first thoracic segments and synapses with the lower motor neurons of the lateral thoracic nerve. The lateral thoracic nerve innervates the cutaneous trunci muscle. Damage to any portion of this pathway results in an absence of the cutaneous trunci reflex. The perineal reflex evaluates the last sacral segments and the caudal spinal cord segments. Stimulation of the perineal area results in flexion of the tail and closure of the anus.

The gait of the foal should be examined for weakness or ataxia. The newborn foal often has a choppy, springy, dysmetric gait. Signs of weakness include stumbling, knuckling, dragging a toe, or trembling. Further evaluation of weakness is performed by pushing or pulling from side to side and/or backing. Ataxia or incoordination suggests the presence of proprioceptive deficits (lack of recognition of limb position), which are most easily identified at slower gaits. Circling, turning, backing, and traveling up and down slopes in a straight line and with the head held elevated should be used to detect ataxia. In a straight line, the patient may weave or sway. Circling may elicit limb circumduction, delayed protraction, and crossing over and/or stepping on the opposite foot. Holding the head in an elevated position while walking may elicit or worsen a dysmetric forelimb gait.

Additional ancillary testing of the neurologic patient includes blood work, radiography, cerebrospinal fluid (CSF) analysis, and electrodiagnostics. Blood work is generally nonspecific, but an inflammatory leukogram suggests infection. Abnormal concentrations of serum enzymes and electrolytes help identify hepatic, muscle, or metabolic diseases. When indicated, radiographs of the skull and cervical spine can be performed. In the neonate or young foal, radiographs of the entire spine are possible. A CSF tap can be performed in either the atlanto-occipital or lumbosacral space. A minimal CSF analysis should include determination of total protein content, WBC and RBC counts, and a white cell count differential. Additional determinations include glucose, CK, pH, and electrolytes (*Table 8*).

The lumbosacral tap can be performed in a quiet or sedated, standing or recumbent foal. The lumbosacral space is identified as a depression on the midline caudal to the spinous process of the last lumbar vertebra and cranial to the spine of the sacrum. This depression is bordered laterally by the cranial edge of the tuber sacrale. A 8.75 cm (3.5 in) needle with a stylet is adequate for foals as large as 180 kg (400 lb). The area is clipped and surgically prepared. Following a local block, the needle is advanced perpendicular to the spinal cord. Frequent, gentle aspiration with a small syringe will determine when the subarachnoid space has been entered. A sudden flicking of the tail or kicking with the hindlimbs also marks entry into the space.

The atlanto-occipital tap is performed with the foal anesthetized or heavily sedated in lateral recumbency. A 3.75–8.75 cm (1.5–3.5 in), 20 gauge needle with a stylet is used. The site is

Table 8. Normal range of CSF measurements in the neonatal foal

Parameter	Value
Color	Clear
Total protein	100 mg/dL (biuret method); trace to +2 (quantitative reagent stick); 1.3347–1.3350 refractive index
Glucose	80% of blood glucose value
pH	7.34–7.40
WBC count	<5 cells/µL
RBC count	0–500 cells/µL
Creatine kinase	15.2 ± 9.2 units/L
Sodium	142.6 ± 2.8 mmol/L
Potassium	3.6 ± 2.1 mmol/L
Chloride	109 ± 3.4 mmol/L

Source: Rossdale, P.D. et al., *Equine Vet. J.*, 14, 134–138, 1982.

aseptically prepared. The tap is performed on the midline, on a line drawn across the cranial edges of the wings of the atlas. While the head is held in a flexed position, the needle is directed toward the lower lip. A slight "pop" or decrease in resistance is felt when the subarachnoid space has been entered. However, it is prudent to remove the stylet from the needle frequently to determine if the subarachnoid space has been entered.

Examination of the seizuring foal

The initial approach to the seizuring foal should be to prevent self-inflicted trauma by controlling seizures and providing a safe environment. Once this has been accomplished and venous access has been obtained, the neurologic examination, including a complete physical examination, can proceed.

Seizures are not always generalized. Tonic–clonic convulsions can include signs such as facial grimacing, twitching, chomping or smacking of the lips, head and neck rigidity, paddling, abnormal breathing, or repetitive blinking and rapid eye movements.

The most common cause of seizures in the neonate is "neonatal maladjustment syndrome" (NMS) or birth asphyxia. The onset of clinical signs is dependent on the severity of asphyxia and subsequent brain cell damage. If asphyxia is severe, clinical signs may be seen immediately after birth or progress more slowly over 24–48 hours as cerebral edema develops subsequent

to milder bouts of asphyxia. The diagnosis of NMS is made by the exclusion of other diseases and by obtaining a history that includes periparturient problems that may have resulted in hypoxemia before, during, or shortly after birth. Radiographs are normal in cases of NMS. Although not diagnostic, elevated serum creatinine is suggestive of prepartum placental compromise.

Other causes of seizures include congenital malformations (hydrocephalus), viral and bacterial infections, trauma, metabolic derangements, hepatic encephalopathy, and idiopathic epilepsy. Serum chemistry and electrolyte measurements provide information regarding metabolic abnormalities and liver disease. Hypoglycemia, a common problem in neonates, rarely results in seizures. Elevated cell counts and/or protein levels in the CSF are compatible with an infectious process.

Idiopathic epilepsy (benign epilepsy) of foals is most common in Arabian horses. Seizures are usually intermittent, and depression may be seen in the interictal period. Other causes of seizures should be excluded.

MUSCULOSKELETAL SYSTEM

A systematic examination of the musculoskeletal system begins with a visual examination to evaluate appropriate form and function, and palpation to evaluate size and shape. In the newborn foal, examination of the musculoskeletal system evaluates maturity and/or gestational age. Floppy ears, joint laxity, and a silky hair coat suggest immaturity, prematurity, or dysmaturity. The skull and vertebral column should be evaluated for curvature and the calvarium for its shape. A domed appearance to the skull indicates possible hydrocephalus, although slight doming of the skull can be present without underlying cerebral defects and may indicate growth retardation during gestation. Lateral deviation of the rostral face (wry nose) and deviations of the vertebrae (scoliosis = curvature; lordosis = extension; kyphosis = flexion) may be seen individually or in concert with other musculoskeletal defects.

The newborn foal should be evaluated for evidence of trauma. Fractures or dislocations of joints are uncommon, but can be seen secondary to dystocia and trauma after birth. Fractured ribs are one of the more frequent injuries in the newborn foal and can result in life-threatening secondary complications. Fractured ribs may be bilateral, but usually involve only one side of the rib cage. Multiple ribs are usually involved. Dislocations at the costochondral junctions may occur and are of less concern, as surrounding structures are usually left undamaged. Signs associated with multiple dislocated rib fractures (5) include tachypnea, pain, swelling, and/or a flail chest. Careful thoracic palpation helps identify individual or nondisplaced fractures. Swelling or crepitus may be present. Thoracic auscultation may identify a rubbing sound. Fractured ribs can be difficult to identify radiographically. Ultrasonography is useful for identifying whether fractures are displaced and to monitor progress of healing.

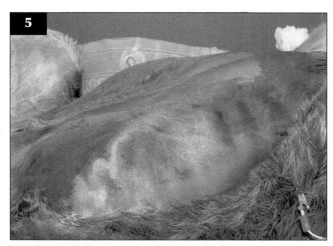

5 Multiple rib fractures in a foal. The foal is anesthetized and in dorsal recumbency.

Although less common than rib fractures, brachial plexus injuries and a ruptured gastrocnemius tendon/muscle (**6, 7**) or peroneus tertius tendon (**8**) can be seen post partum or as an injury. Clinical signs of brachial plexus injuries vary with the severity of the trauma, but usually result in some degree of radial nerve paralysis. The foal is unable to bear weight on the limb and is unable to extend the carpus or digit. Rupture of the gastrocnemius muscle can occur during foaling and is identified as a swelling above the hock in the area of the gastrocnemius muscle. Complete disruption allows flexion of the hock when the stifle is in an extended position; ultrasonography identifies muscle tearing.

All joints and physes should be palpated for heat, swelling, or edema. The foal's gait should be observed for lameness. Until proven otherwise, joint effusions (with or without heat or lameness) should be presumed infected. Arthrocentesis showing a total white cell count of >10,000 cells/µL supports a diagnosis of infection.

Angular limb deformities (ALDs) occur in the hind- and/or forelimbs. These deformities may occur individually, bilaterally, or in conjunction with other skeletal defects. Deviations in the frontal plane result in varus or valgus deformities. Deviations in the sagittal plane result in abnormal degrees of extension or flexion. Most mild to moderate deformities will self-correct with limited exercise, but they should be monitored carefully for progressive improvement. Severe flexural or angular deformities require rapid intervention before tendon and ligamentous changes prohibit adequate correction.

Patellar luxations may be identified unilaterally or bilaterally in newborn foals. Congenital luxation results from varying degrees of hypoplasia of the lateral femoral trochlear ridge. With patellar

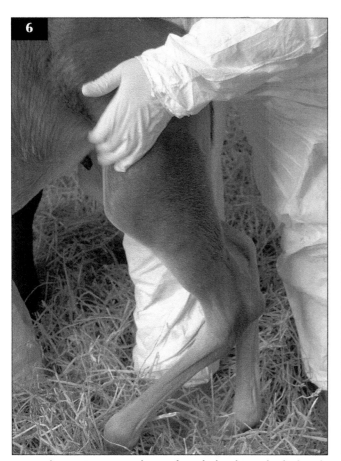

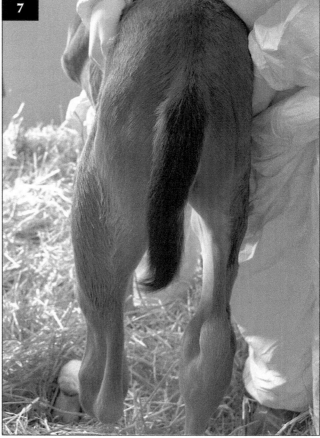

6, 7 Side on view (**6**) and view from behind (**7**) of a foal with a ruptured gastrocnemius origin.

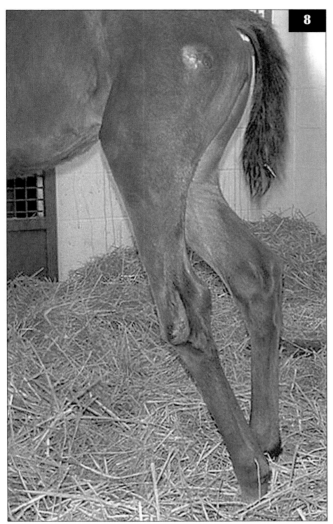

8 Ruptured peroneus tertius tendon in a foal.

luxations, examination of the stifle may identify periarticular swelling. If the abnormality is bilateral, a squatting stance may be identified.

SUMMARY

Recent advances in diagnostics have improved our ability to diagnose and treat diseases of the foal. However, these advances do not replace the physical examination as the most valuable diagnostic aid available to the equine practitioner. The basic physical examination provides the majority of information needed to make

a presumptive diagnosis, indicate the direction for ancillary tests, and formulate a plan for emergency therapy if needed.

FURTHER READING

Adams R (1990) The urogenital system. In: *Equine Clinical Neonatology* (Koterba AM, Drummond WH, Kosch PC, Eds.). Lea & Febiger, Philadelphia, PA, pp. 443–495.

Cudd TA (1988) The use of clinical findings, abdominocentesis, and abdominal radiography to assess surgical versus nonsurgical abdominal disease in the foal. In: *Proceedings of the Meeting of the American Association of Equine Practitioners*, pp. 4153–4158.

Embertson RE (1990) Gastrointestinal disorders, small intestinal and colonic obstruction in foals. In: *Current Practice of Equine Surgery* (White NA, Moore JM, Eds.). JB Lippincott, Philadelphia, PA, pp. 311–321.

Friedman WF (1992) Congenital heart disease in infancy and childhood. In: *Heart Disease: A Textbook of Cardiovascular Medicine*, 4th ed. (Braunwald E, Ed.). WB Saunders, Philadelphia, PA, pp. 887–902.

Green SL, Mayhew IG (1990) Neurologic disorders. In: *Equine Clinical Neonatology* (Koterba AM, Drummond WH, Kosch PC, Eds.). Lea & Febiger, Philadelphia, PA, pp. 496–530.

Hoffman KL, Wood AKW, McCarthy PH (1993) A protocol for the sonographic examination of the equine neonatal kidney. In: *Proceedings of the Third Conference of the International Society of Veterinary Perinatology*, pp. 80–83.

Marr CM (2015) The equine neonatal cardiovascular system in health and disease. *Veterinary Clinics of North America: Equine Practice* 8: 545.

Reed SM (1990) Neurologic examination of the neonatal foal and diagnostic testing useful to evaluate newborn foals with neurologic problems. In: *Proceedings of the Eighth Annual Veterinary Medical Forum*, pp. 601–608.

Sertich P (1993) Clinical anatomy and evaluation of equine fetal membranes. In: *Proceedings of the Annual Meeting of the Society of Theriogenology*, pp. 178–184.

Sprayberry KA (2015) Ultrasonographic examination of the equine neonate. *Veterinary Clinics of North America: Equine Practice* 8: 515.

Toribio RE, Mudge MC (2013) Diseases of the foal, musculoskeletal system. *Equine Medicine Surgery and Reproduction* 2: 439.

Vaala WE, Webb AI (1990) Cardiovascular monitoring of the critically foal. In: *Equine Clinical Neonatology* (Koterba AM, Drummond WH, Kosch PC, Eds.). Lea & Febiger, Philadelphia, PA, pp. 262–272.

Shock, Resuscitation, Fluid and Electrolyte Therapy 2

Kevin T.T. Corley and Bonnie S. Barr

SHOCK

KEY POINTS

- Shock evolves very quickly in foals, as they have poor adaptive mechanisms.
- There can be marked differences in individual organ responses to shock and the drugs used to treat it.
- In hypovolemic foals, a 1–4 L bolus of crystalloid fluids should be given acutely.
- 10–20 mL of 50% dextrose should be added to fluids to treat hypoglycemia, rather than choosing 5% dextrose for resuscitation.
- Cardiopulmonary resuscitation (CPR), using 10–20 breaths and 90–120 thoracic compressions per minute (cpm), can be successful and worthwhile in newly born foals.

INTRODUCTION

Shock describes the clinical state resulting from an inadequate supply of oxygen to the tissues. It can also occur when the tissues are unable properly to utilize the delivered oxygen. There are a number of adaptive physiologic mechanisms in place to maintain tissue oxygenation and, therefore, prevent the onset of shock. However, these adaptive mechanisms seem to be poorly developed in the foal. This is important clinically, as it means that shock evolves much more rapidly in neonatal foals than in adult horses. The key to the successful treatment of shock in foals is early, aggressive intervention.

CAUSES OF SHOCK

The main cause of shock in the foal is hypovolemia. Loss of fluid from diarrhea, inadequate nursing, and other causes results in dehydration and then hypovolemia. The reduced circulating volume results in decreased venous return to the heart, reduced cardiac filling, and decreased cardiac stroke volume. In adult horses the heart rate is increased to compensate for the decreased stroke volume. This maintains the amount of blood pumped per minute (cardiac output), at least partially protecting the horse from the effects of the hypovolemia. Neonatal foals do not appear to be able universally to mount this protective response, and approximately 40% of foals do not increase their heart rate in response to hypovolemia. This results in a decreased cardiac output, inadequate blood

flow to the tissues, and, therefore, insufficient oxygen delivered to the tissues for normal function.

Distributive shock is also common in foals with severe disease such as sepsis or marked perinatal asphyxia syndrome. Distributive shock occurs where there is dilation of the blood vessels (vasodilation), which can occur as a result of the cytokine response to bacterial infection or to hypoxia or ischemia. On a very local scale in the body, vasodilation is a protective response as it promotes increased blood flow through the affected area. However, when large parts of the body are affected and there is generalized vasodilation, it results in falling blood pressure (BP) and pooling of blood. This, in turn, results in decreased venous return to the heart and, therefore, reduced cardiac filling and a decreased cardiac output, similar to hypovolemia. This is the reason that distributive shock is initially treated in the same way as hypovolemic shock (i.e., with aggressive fluid therapy).

Hypoxic shock can occur when the blood's oxygen-carrying capacity is reduced (e.g., in neonatal isoerythrolysis [NI]) and when oxygen exchange in the lungs is impaired (e.g., in pneumonia). In NI, destruction of the foal's red blood cells (RBCs) by antibodies absorbed from the colostrum leads to a greatly decreased hemoglobin (Hb) concentration and, therefore, oxygen-carrying capacity of the blood. In pneumonia, impairment of oxygen exchange in the lungs leads to decreased Hb oxygen saturation and, therefore, the amount of oxygen carried to the tissues and organs by the blood.

Inadequate local blood flow

Local tissue blood flow can also be reduced by blockage of the capillaries. There are three main causes of capillary blockage in the foal:

1. Blockage due to external pressure causing the capillary to narrow or collapse. The most common reason is tissue edema. Edema appears to be a particular feature of perinatal asphyxia syndrome and it can occur with sepsis.
2. Blood clot formation (microthrombi) within the capillaries. Altered coagulation, leading to microthrombi formation, is again a feature of septicemia and severe perinatal asphyxia syndrome.
3. Swelling of the endothelial cells. The capillaries are sufficiently narrow that erythrocytes need to deform to pass through them. Swelling of the endothelial cells can narrow the capillaries sufficiently to completely exclude RBC flow. Endothelial cell swelling can occur in any form of shock, but appears to be a particular feature of low-flow ischemia.

* The authors acknowledge and appreciate the original contributors of this author whose work has been incorporated into this chapter.

Differences in response between tissues and organs

One of the greatest challenges for the clinician is that different tissues and organs can have quite opposite responses to physiologic and pathophysiologic stimuli. The classic example of this is the response to increased circulating epinephrine during the fight-or-flight reaction. The blood vessels of the muscles dilate, whereas those of the skin and gastrointestinal (GI) tract constrict. These differences mean that blood flow may be adequate to some tissues but not others during early shock. They also mean that interventions that are beneficial to one tissue bed may be harmful to another.

This challenge is compounded by the fact that clinical tools are generally focused on measuring whole body parameters, rather than individual organs. For example, blood for lactate concentration is generally collected from the jugular vein. The lactate concentration in this vein reflects (1) average whole body lactate production and metabolism, and (2) what is occurring in tissues of the head. One severely compromised organ may only lead to moderate increases in blood lactate, and the blood lactate concentration can decrease as whole body circulation improves, despite worsening of the one compromised organ. Pulse quality, arterial BP, and heart rate also mainly reflect whole body status. However, a few indications of individual organ perfusion are readily available to the clinician. For example, urine output, in the absence of renal failure or metabolic disturbances such as hyperglycemia, reflects the kidney perfusion.

RECOGNIZING SHOCK

Clinical signs of shock

In contrast to mature horses, shock can be difficult to detect in neonatal foals as the clinical signs may not be present or may not reflect the severity of the shock.

Mentation

The brain has a high oxygen demand and is therefore affected early when oxygen supply is insufficient. The initial clinical sign is a depressed demeanor. As the shock evolves, the foal will stop nursing, stop following the mare, and then become recumbent. It will lose its suckle reflex (**9**), stop responding to stimuli such as a finger in the ear, and eventually become comatose. Some foals seize, although this is more common following reperfusion. This sequence of events can evolve rapidly, and many foals are recumbent by the time veterinary help is sought.

Heart rate

The "correct" physiologic response to decreased cardiac stroke volume (as found in hypovolemia) or to decreased tissue perfusion is to increase heart rate. Increasing heart rate can maintain cardiac output and, therefore, tissue oxygen delivery. However, as stated above, this physiologic response does not appear to be universally present in foals. Foals with arterial hypotension ($\leq$60 mmHg) can have heart rates within the normal range and there does not seem to be a relationship between heart rate and blood lactate (a marker of tissue hypoxia, see below). This lack of compensatory tachycardia is likely to be one cause of the rapid decline seen in foals with hypovolemia and sepsis.

Pulse pressure and cold extremities

Weak pulses and cold extremities are often, but not always, a feature of shock. The hoof capsules and ear tips are frequently cold in hypovolemic animals, but they may (rarely) be warm in septic shock (so-called "warm" shock) due to peripheral vasodilation. Poor pulse quality does not necessarily indicate decreased mean arterial pressure. The pulse pressure is the difference between systolic and diastolic arterial pressure, and is independent of their absolute value and that of the mean pressure. Therefore, in hypotensive foals with markedly decreased diastolic pressure but a reasonable stroke volume, the pulse pressure can feel normal.

Mucous membranes

Mucous membrane color can be misleading in neonatal foals. Traditionally, red mucous membranes with a fast capillary refill time (CRT) have been associated with peripheral vasodilation accompanied by adequate cardiac output (**10**). Pale or blanched mucous membranes are considered indicative of peripheral vasoconstriction or anemia. Purple mucous membranes with a prolonged CRT have been associated with a low cardiac output or poor peripheral perfusion (**11**). Prolonged CRTs are an indicator of hypovolemia, but their absence does not rule it out. Dry mucous membranes have been reported to indicate dehydration. However, these changes are inconsistent and often not present in foals. Although mucous membrane color changes are frequently seen in neonatal foals, they only have a weak association with specific circulatory disturbances.

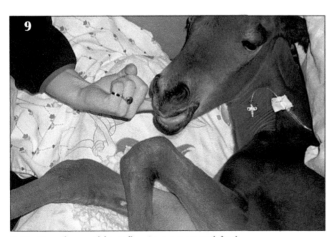

9 Testing the suckle reflex in a neonatal foal.

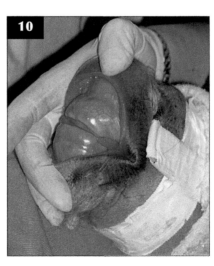

10 Red, injected mucous membranes in a foal with sepsis.

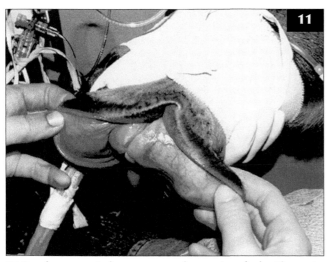

11 Purple, congested mucous membranes in a foal with sepsis.

Other physical signs

Increased respiratory rates may be seen with tissue hypoperfusion as a result of respiratory compensation for metabolic acidosis. Again, this compensation often fails in foals, and foals with normal or reduced respiratory rates may be profoundly acidotic. Increased respiratory rates may also reflect impaired gas exchange in the lungs. Foals with moderate to severe hypovolemia or hypotension will have reduced urine output, although this may often be missed when urine output is not formally monitored or there is concomitant hyperglycemia. Increased skin tenting and sunken eyes are signs of dehydration, which often accompanies hypovolemia.

<small>LABORATORY SIGNS OF SHOCK</small>
Packed cell volume and total solids concentration

Packed cell volume (PCV) (**12**) is a poor indicator of circulatory status in the neonatal foal. It is uncommon to find an increased PCV in severely hypovolemic foals, in contrast to their adult counterparts. This is probably because adults release stored erythrocytes into the circulation by splenic contraction during hypovolemia,

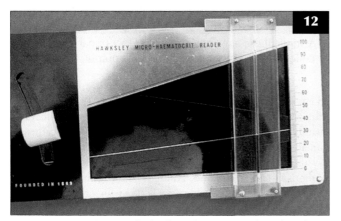

12 Measuring PCV in a foal. The tube is moved so that the bottom of the red cell column is lined up with the zero line and the top of the plasma is lined up with the 100% line. The sliding silver line is adjusted until it is level with the top of the red cell column. The intersection of the sliding silver line with the scale on the right gives the PCV.

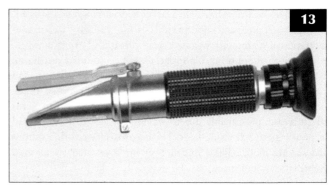

13 Refractometer for measuring total solids concentration.

markedly increasing the PCV, and this physiologic response is poorly developed in the foal. The normal range for PCV in foals in the first week of life (0.28–0.46 L/L [28%–46%]) is slightly lower than in adult horses. It is common for critically ill foals to have a PCV of 0.22–0.26 L/L (22%–26%), possibly as a result of a combination of fluid therapy and bone marrow suppression with illness. A very low PCV (<0.12 L/L [12%]), as found in severe NI, results in decreased blood oxygen-carrying capacity and tissue hypoxia.

Total solids concentration (total protein measured by a refractometer) (**13**) is also an unreliable guide to hypovolemia in the foal. Total solids may be decreased by failure of passive transfer (FPT) or by loss through the GI tract or kidney, and there is no correlation between total solids concentration and either PCV or other signs of circulatory status such as lactate concentration in the foal. The normal range for total solids in the foal (51–80 g/L [5.1–8.0 g/dL]) is also lower than that for adult horses.

Creatinine concentration

Decreased renal perfusion leads to increased creatinine concentrations in the absence of intrinsic renal dysfunction. Creatinine concentration may therefore be a useful sign of hypovolemia. In foals less than 48 hours old, however, very high creatinine concentrations can be seen independent of renal function or circulatory status. In these foals, placental function was compromised *in utero*, leading to a buildup of waste metabolites. This accumulated creatinine is excreted by the foal over the first 24–48 hours of life. Perinatal asphyxia syndrome should be considered as a differential in foals of less than 24 hours of age with increased plasma creatinine concentrations because of their association with placental insufficiency. Foals with ruptured bladders may also have increased plasma creatinine concentrations.

Blood lactate concentration

Lactate is an end-product of anaerobic metabolism and accumulates in the tissues when there is insufficient oxygen for aerobic respiration. Monitoring lactate can therefore be an extremely useful indicator of whether tissue perfusion is adequate. However, in addition to inadequate tissue perfusion, lactate concentrations may also be increased by muscle activity (e.g., in seizures) and increased circulating epinephrine concentrations and where there is sepsis and inappropriate anaerobic respiration despite adequate tissue oxygenation.

In one study of foals treated in an intensive care unit (ICU), an admission arterial blood lactate concentration of <4 mmol/L was associated with a hospital survival rate of >90%. Conversely, if the admission lactate was 4 mmol/L or greater, the survival rate was 45%.

At 18–36 hours after admission, a lactate concentration of 4 mmol/L or greater still predicted poor survival (<40%), whereas a lactate concentration of <4 mmol/L was associated with 100% hospital survival.

Although monitoring blood lactate concentrations can be an extremely useful guide to therapy, decreases in plasma lactate can lag behind improved cardiovascular status. During initial resuscitation following shock, blood lactate concentration can actually increase, presumably due to washout of lactate accumulated in poorly perfused tissue beds. During this phase, urine output and BP are more reliable measures of cardiovascular status than blood lactate concentrations. However, after the initial resuscitation phase (first 2–4 hours), treatments that result in increased blood lactate concentrations are unlikely to be beneficial to the foal and should be urgently reviewed.

MEASURING AND MONITORING SHOCK

In foals that do not respond to initial bolus fluid therapy, physiologic monitoring can be extremely useful for determining and optimizing treatment options and doses. In the hospital situation it is possible to titrate continuous infusions of drugs to measures of circulatory status such as BP and urine output. Continuous monitoring of shock is clearly not possible in the field. This, in turn, means that good outcomes are much less likely for foals in prolonged shock that cannot be referred to a hospital facility. In one group of referred hospitalized foals, those that arrived in severe shock had far fewer good outcomes than those that developed severe shock during hospital treatment. This was probably due to the fact that shock is immediately recognized and aggressively treated in already hospitalized foals, greatly shortening the time that the organs are without sufficient blood flow and oxygen.

Urine output

Urine output is an extremely useful indicator of end-organ perfusion in critically ill foals, except where renal function is compromised by intrinsic renal failure.

Urine output is measured by attaching a closed collection system to an indwelling urinary catheter (**14–16**). 12Fr Foley catheters

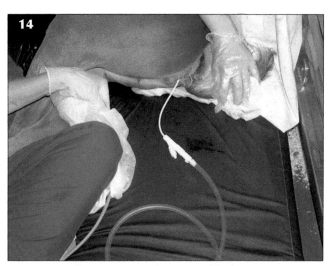

14 An indwelling urinary catheter in a filly foal. The Foley catheter is retained by inflation of the balloon with sterile saline (see **15**).

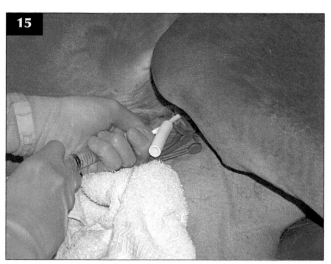

15 Inflation of the balloon of a Foley catheter in a colt foal using saline. Filling the balloon with a liquid ensures that it does not float on top of the urine, and leads to better bladder drainage.

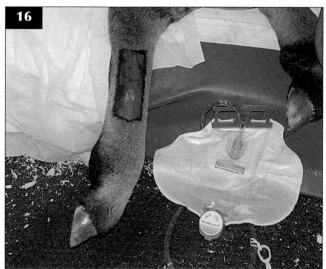

16 A surgical drainage bag connected to a urinary catheter for collection and measurement of urine output.

(33 cm long for fillies and 55–64 cm for colts) make good urinary catheters and avoid the need to suture the catheter to the foal for retention. For fillies, a stylet can make it easier to pass the catheter. Human infant feeding tubes (8–10Fr, 14.5–16.8 cm [36–42 in]) may also be used. Urinary catheters should always be placed using appropriate sterile techniques. A surgical drainage bag or standard fluid set and empty fluid bag can be used for urine collection. The surgical drainage bag has the advantages of having valves to prevent backflow and being easy to empty. Ascending infection is a risk of urinary catheterization. This risk needs to be weighed against the benefits of accurate determination of urine output and the avoidance of urine scalding, particularly in recumbent foals. Attempts to reduce the risk of infection with antibacterial impregnated catheters have not been successful in human medicine.

Therapies aimed at improving cardiovascular status that result in decreased urine output are highly unlikely to be beneficial and should be urgently reviewed. Conversely, improved urine output is one of the earliest signs of successful therapy. Falling urine output is an early indicator of hypovolemia.

Hemodynamics are not the only factors that can affect urine output. Acute renal failure may result in oliguria, anuria or, uncommonly in foals, polyuria. Other causes of decreased urine output include blocked urinary catheters and defects in bladder wall integrity. Therefore, any investigation of low urine output should include an ultrasonographic examination of the peritoneal space and confirmation of an empty bladder. Hyperglycemia is relatively common in critically ill foals and may result in an osmotic diuresis when the blood glucose concentration is above the renal threshold for resorption. This diuresis may result in increased urine output, except in cases where there is severe circulatory collapse. If an osmotic diuresis is occurring, glucose will be present in the urine. Some foals produce small amounts of urine despite having apparently adequate hemodynamics. These foals may respond to furosemide therapy. However, because of the potential detrimental effects of furosemide on a failing circulation, it is vital to rule out hemodynamic causes of oliguria before its use.

Arterial blood pressure

Arterial BP measurements are extremely useful both to identify foals in shock and to titrate therapy aimed at reversing shock and supporting the cardiovascular system.

The most accurate way to measure arterial pressure is directly through a catheter placed in an artery connected to an electronic pressure transducer at the level of the sternal manubrium. In most foals it is relatively easy to place a 20 gauge, 3.8 cm (1.5 in) catheter in the dorsal metatarsal artery. The facial, radial, and caudal auricular arteries may also be catheterized. In hypotensive or edematous foals, using an over-the-wire catheter and the Seldinger technique can make catheterization easier. The main problem with direct monitoring of BP is maintenance of the catheter, especially in struggling or seizuring foals. The authors' preferred technique is to place a rolled, half 4 × 4 gauze (swab) on either side of the catheter and then wrap it with self-adhesive bandage. An injection cap is placed on the end of the catheter. All connections to the catheter are via a needle placed into this injection cap (17–25). This allows the needle to come out of the injection cap if the foal struggles, without accidentally pulling out the arterial catheter.

Indirect measurement of arterial pressure has the advantage of being noninvasive and quicker to set up than direct measurement. This is particularly important at admission in hospitalized foals, as measurements can be made quickly after admission while other procedures such as jugular catheterization are performed. Oscillometry is the technique of choice, with the cuff placed over the coccygeal, dorsal metatarsal, median, or posterior digital arteries. Careful placement of a cuff around the base of the tail probably results in the most consistent and accurate measurements (26). The cuff should encircle at least 80% of the part's circumference and the width should be at least 40% of the part's circumference. For accuracy the same cuff should be used consistently on the same part. Another method of indirect measurement involves the use of a Doppler transducer over a peripheral artery along with a cuff

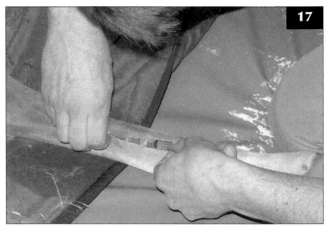

17 Infiltration of local anesthetic subcutaneously over the dorsal metatarsal artery prior to catheterization.

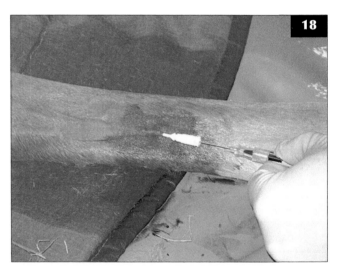

18 Placing a 20 gauge, 1.5 in catheter in the dorsal metatarsal artery using the Seldinger technique.

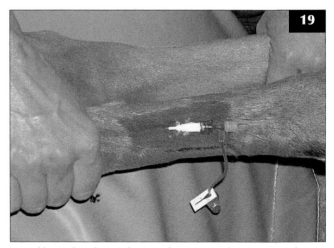

19 Infiltrate local anesthetic subcutaneously over dorsal metatarsal artery then place a 20 gauge, 1.5 in catheter.

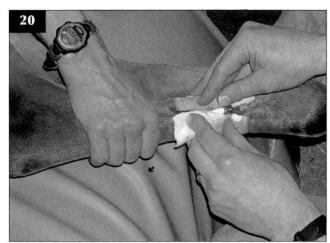

20 Using two rolled 4 × 4 gauze (swabs) either side of the arterial catheter to stabilize it in position, prior to wrapping.

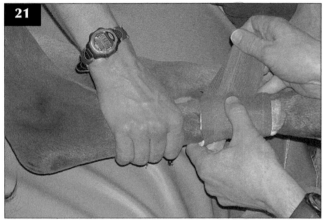

21 Fix catheter to the skin with bonding glue then wrap the catheter with a self-adhesive bandage.

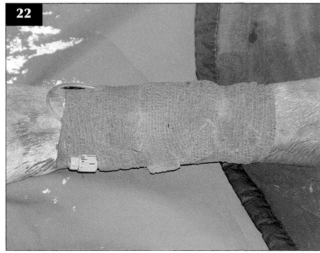

22 Wrapped catheter ready to be connected.

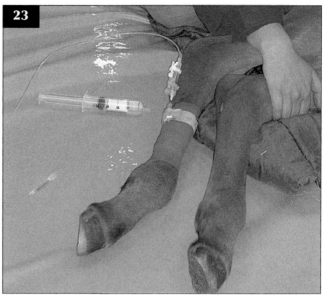

23 Using narrow bore, saline-filled, extension tubing connected to an electronic pressure transducer to directly measure arterial blood pressure in a foal. The extension tubing is connected to the arterial catheter by means of a needle, through an injection cap.

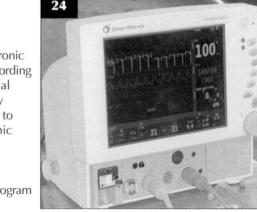

24 An electronic monitor recording direct arterial pressure (by connection to the electronic pressure transducer) and an electrocardiogram of a foal.

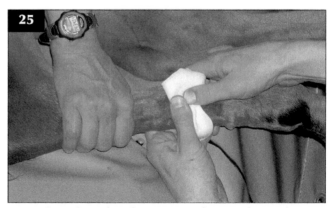

25 Applying firm, digital pressure to the site of arterial puncture after the catheter has been removed. This should be done for two minutes.

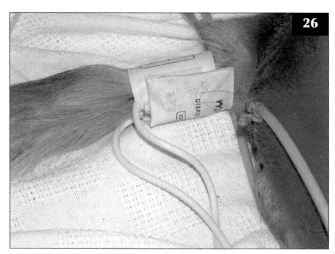

26 Correct placement of a tail cuff for indirect (oscillometric) measurement of arterial blood pressure.

placed proximal to the transducer. This method only measures systolic arterial pressure and the accuracy in the neonatal foal is unknown. With either indirect method it is advisable to take three measurements to ensure consistent results before making any therapeutic decisions based on them.

In general, mean arterial pressure should be maintained above 60 mmHg. In order to achieve this, the cardiovascular system should be reviewed, and therapy considered, if the mean arterial pressure is <69 mmHg. In very premature foals, a target of 50–60 mmHg may be more appropriate. However, the aim of therapy is to increase tissue perfusion, and not to increase BP per se. It is important, therefore, to assess the effectiveness of therapy in the context of other indicators of tissue perfusion such as blood lactate concentration, urine output, and mentation. Directing all therapy at maintaining a target BP, while ignoring other indicators of cardiovascular status, is not appropriate.

Cardiac output monitoring

Cardiac output (CO) is the product of stroke volume (SV) and heart rate (HR). CO monitoring can be extremely useful in foals that fail to show the predicted response to treatment. As well as providing a direct measurement of cardiac function, it also allows calculation of SV and systemic vascular resistance (SVR). These three factors can help determine whether the hemodynamic disturbances are due to cardiac dysfunction (reflected by CO and SV) or changes in the vasculature (reflected by SVR). Furthermore, if SV is decreased and does not increase in response to a fluid challenge, decreased CO is likely to be due to intrinsic myocardial dysfunction rather than hypovolemia.

Lithium dilution is one method of measuring cardiac output of a neonatal foal in an ICU (**27–30**). Transthoracic echocardiography has been used to measure CO in people, small animals, and the adult horse. Volumetric echocardiography using the Bullet method has been documented to provide an accurate and noninvasive estimate of CO in neonatal foals. An ultrasound with basic cardiology functionality is needed. Views for the measurement can easily be accessed from the right parasternal window and include long-axis four-chambered view (modified to

include the apex of the left ventricle) and short-axis view of the left ventricle at the level of the papillary muscle just below the mitral value. In the long-axis four-chambered view the length of the ventricle is measured in systole and diastole, whereas in the short-axis view the area of the ventricle is measured. The values are put into a formula to obtain SV and HR is determined by measurement of R-R interval on the ECG.

REVERSING SHOCK

It is imperative in foals in shock to restore tissue perfusion as quickly as possible. To do this efficiently and without detriment to the foal requires an ordered approach (i.e., treat the hypovolemia aggressively, support cardiac output with inotropes, and support blood vessel tone with vasopressors).

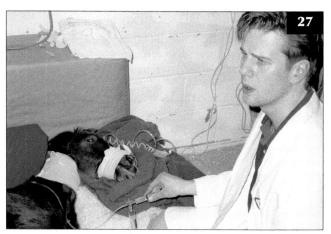

27 Lithium dilution cardiac output measurement. 0.45 mmol of lithium chloride (3 mL) is placed into the extension set shown, which is connected to the jugular catheter. Saline is then injected rapidly through the extension set, delivering a bolus of exactly 3 mL lithium chloride into the jugular vein.

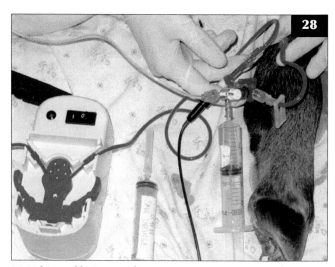

28 Lithium dilution cardiac output measurement. Lithium sensor connected with one side to a catheter in the dorsal metatarsal artery, and the other side to a peristaltic pump, drawing blood at 4 mL/min.

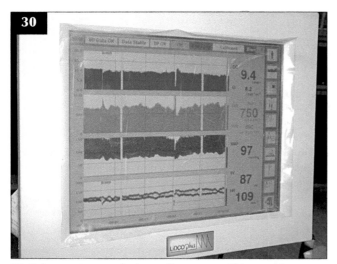

29 Lithium dilution cardiac output measurement. The time–concentration curve of the lithium (green curve) passing the sensor is related to cardiac output. A dedicated computer automatically calculates cardiac output.

30 Pulse contour analysis cardiac output. This machine continuously measures cardiac output based on the contour of the pulse waveform from the direct arterial blood pressure measurement. The lithium dilution cardiac output is used to calibrate the machine. Although potentially a very useful technique, at the time of writing pulse contour analysis has not been validated in the neonatal foal.

Treating hypovolemia

Early identification and treatment of hypovolemia markedly improves outcome. Foals are very vulnerable to developing hypovolemia over a very short time span. Unfortunately, neonatal foals appear to compensate poorly for hypovolemia, which not only makes the effects more severe than in mature horses, but also makes hypovolemia harder to identify.

In mature horses the signs of hypovolemia are tachycardia, cold extremities, tachypnea, decreased pulse pressure, and reduced jugular pulse. Unfortunately, none of these signs are consistently present in hypovolemic foals. In a series of referred cases, 20 foals had

a mean arterial pressure of <60 mmHg on admission. Eight (40%) of these 20 foals had a normal heart rate (70–105 beats per minute [bpm]), and in six of these foals the hypotension was reversed with intravenous fluids alone. Therefore, tachycardia is not a consistent finding of hypovolemia in foals. For these reasons, it is necessary to have a high index of suspicion for hypovolemia in neonatal foals. Foals with any of the clinical signs associated with hypovolemia in adult horses, and foals that have not nursed for 4–6 hours, are likely to be hypovolemic.

Volume of fluid to administer

Two concepts can be considered when treating hypovolemia in foals, both of which result in similar treatment patterns. Hypovolemic foals typically require 20–80 mL/kg of crystalloid fluids acutely.

Shock dose

The "shock dose" concept is borrowed from small animal medicine and so is familiar to many. The shock dose for a neonatal foal is 50–80 mL/kg of crystalloid fluids. Depending on the perceived degree of hypovolemia, a quarter to one half of the shock dose is given as rapidly as possible (over less than 20 minutes) and the foal is reassessed. If the foal requires further fluid, another quarter of the shock dose is given and again the foal is reassessed. The final quarter of the shock dose is only given to severely hypovolemic foals.

Fluid boluses

The incremental "fluid bolus" concept is borrowed from human medicine. It is a much more practical method, except when an electronic infusion pump is available. The caveat is that it assumes a similar bodyweight between all patients and, for this reason, it has not been adopted in small animal medicine.

The bolus method involves giving a bolus of 1 L of crystalloids (i.e., approximately 20 mL/kg bodyweight for a 50 kg [110 lb] foal) and then reassessing. Up to three further boluses may be given, reassessing the foal after each one. Foals that are most obviously hypovolemic require at least two boluses. In foals whose bodyweight is not close to 50 kg, the method needs to be adjusted so that the bolus is approximately 20 mL/kg. In pony foals and very premature Thoroughbred foals, boluses of 500 mL are usually appropriate. In large draft foals the first bolus should be 2 L.

How much to give

Whether using the shock dose method or the fluid bolus method, the animal must be reassessed during acute fluid therapy to judge if further fluids are required. Foals with a strong pulse and improved mentation and that are urinating probably do not require any further resuscitation fluids. These foals are likely to still require fluids to correct dehydration and electrolyte imbalances and to provide for maintenance and ongoing losses (see below). Foals with a continued weak pulse (or low BP) and depressed mentation and that have not urinated may require further acute fluids, up to the maximum of 80 mL/kg or 4 L.

It is advisable to auscultate the lungs and trachea before and during aggressive fluid therapy, because pulmonary edema is an important theoretical complication. Fortunately, pulmonary edema appears to be extremely rare in critically ill foals aggressively resuscitated with crystalloids. Crackles in foals, classically associated with pulmonary edema, are more likely to represent opening and closing of collapsed alveoli rather than edema. Severe pulmonary edema will result in wet sounds in the trachea and a frothy pink fluid from the nares or mouth. If edema does occur, furosemide (0.25–1 mg/kg i/v) should be administered and further fluid therapy carefully titrated, preferably by means of central venous pressure (CVP) or pulmonary pressures.

Treatment of hypovolemia takes precedence over any concerns about the possibility of causing cerebral edema and thus worsening perinatal asphyxia syndrome. Inadequate cerebral perfusion due to hypovolemia is extremely detrimental to these foals, prolonging the ischemic event. This is far more important than theoretical concerns over cerebral edema.

Choice of fluid
Electrolytes
Balanced electrolyte formulas specifically designed for resuscitation (e.g., Hartmann's solution, lactated Ringer's solution [LRS], or Normosol-R) are the best fluids to use.

Colloids
The role of colloids such as hetastarch and pentastarch in resuscitation of foals is still unclear. They have two theoretical advantages over crystalloid fluids: (1) they persist in the circulation longer, and (2) they raise, rather than lower, oncotic pressure. However, studies in human critical care have not demonstrated any advantage of colloids over crystalloids for resuscitation. The dose is much lower than for crystalloids. The shock dose is 10 mL/kg of 6% hetastarch and 10% pentastarch or 15 mL/kg of 6% tetrastarch. If using the bolus method, each bolus should be of 200–300 mL. The total daily dose of hetastarch should not exceed 10 mL/kg and for pentastarch and tetrastarch should not exceed 15 mL/kg. At higher doses, hydroxyethyl starches interfere with coagulation and may cause clinical bleeding. There is also evidence that the use of hydroxyethyl starches increases the risk of acute renal failure in human patients. This risk is worst for hetastarch and least for tetrastarch.

Sodium chloride
Sodium chloride has traditionally been used as a resuscitation fluid in human medicine. It is an acidifying fluid and therefore may not be the best choice for acute resuscitation in foals, as most of these foals are acidotic. Some foals with ruptured bladders can be very hyperkalemic. In these foals, 0.9%–1.8% sodium chloride is a good choice for resuscitation and is theoretically preferable to balanced electrolyte solutions, which contain potassium. If electrolytes cannot be measured, sodium chloride is probably the fluid of choice in foals known to have a ruptured bladder. When treating a hypovolemic foal where a ruptured bladder is just one of the differentials, balanced electrolyte solutions may be more indicated.

Hypertonic saline
Hypertonic saline (7%–7.5% sodium chloride) has no role in the resuscitation of neonates. It may cause a rapid change in plasma osmolarity, resulting in brain shrinkage and subsequent vascular rupture with cerebral bleeding, subarachnoid hemorrhage, and permanent neurologic damage or death. Neonates are particularly susceptible. The change in plasma osmolarity is more severe in animals with renal insufficiency, a common finding in critically ill foals.

Sodium bicarbonate
Sodium bicarbonate has no role in the resuscitation of neonates. Although many hypovolemic foals are acidotic, virtually all these foals have lactic acidosis. Restoration of vascular volume and tissue perfusion with a balanced polyionic fluid should be the primary objective. The administration of sodium bicarbonate prior to the restoration of normovolemia increases plasma pH, but it has the opposite effect on cerebrospinal fluid (CSF) and intracellular fluid, which may be extremely detrimental to acidotic foals. Thus, alkalinizing therapy is not indicated in foals unless severe acidosis persists after volume resuscitation. At that time if the pH is less than 7.1 or the blood bicarbonate concentration is less than 15 mmol/L, bicarbonate can be added to the maintenance fluid therapy.

Glucose-containing fluids
Administration of intravenous glucose is often part of resuscitation therapy in foals. This is because the glycogen stores at birth are only sufficient for approximately 2 hours' energy requirements in the unfed foal and because fat stores are also very low at birth. Therefore, foals that are not nursing are very prone to hypoglycemia. However, foals may also be hyperglycemic at hospital admission, presumably as part of the physiologic response to cortisol release. In a series of 178 referred hospitalized foals, 66 (37%) were hypoglycemic (blood glucose <4.4 mmol/L [80 mg/dL] at admission) and 33 (18.5%) were severely hypoglycemic (<2.8 mmol/L [50 mg/dL]). Seventy-nine foals (44.5%) were hyperglycemic (>6.1 mmol/L [110 mg/dL]), but only 17 (9.5%) were severely hyperglycemic (>10 mmol/L [180 mg/dL]).

Both hypoglycemia and hyperglycemia may be harmful. Following cerebral hypoperfusion (a feature both of shock and of perinatal asphyxia syndrome), hyperglycemia may be more detrimental than hypoglycemia. For this reason, it is advisable to monitor the blood glucose frequently in foals. It is common to find that foals with marginal blood glucose concentrations on admission (3.9–5.0 mmol/L [70–90 mg/dL]), have normal blood glucose concentrations following (non-glucose-containing) acute fluid resuscitation. The authors' policy is to administer glucose during acute resuscitation only if the blood glucose is <3.4 mmol/L (60 mg/dL), except in premature foals. Premature foals have decreased glycogen reserves compared with mature foals and therefore are supplemented with glucose if their blood glucose is <5.0 mmol/L (90 mg/dL).

There is good evidence from human critical care that keeping blood glucose concentrations within a narrow range (4.4–6.1 mmol/L [80–110 mg/dL]) is associated with better outcomes. For this reason, it may be advisable to measure glucose hourly in the initial stages of foal care and use insulin to control blood glucose concentrations if necessary. However, these data were generated in human adult patients and, to date, no equivalent information exists for the foal.

5% dextrose and 5% glucose solutions are not good choices for resuscitation in the foal. After 30 minutes, only 10% of the volume given is left in the circulation, and each liter will drop the plasma sodium concentration by 4–5 mmol/L in the foal. They are also not a great source of nutrition. To meet the resting energy requirements (44 kcal/kg/day) of a 50 kg foal, 11–13 L per day would need to given. This is more than double a foal's maintenance fluid requirements and would cause considerable electrolyte disturbances.

50% dextrose or 50% glucose solutions may be preferable to the 5% solutions. Each milliliter of 50% dextrose is equivalent to 1.7 kcal and each milliliter of 50% glucose is equivalent to 1.9 kcal. It may be used in two ways. In the hospital setting, the 50% solution should be administered via an electronic pump, separately from the resuscitation fluids. The starting rate will depend on the degree of hypoglycemia. As a rule of thumb, a starting rate of 20 mL/h is appropriate for mild hypoglycemia and 50 mL/h for severe hypoglycemia. In the field, it is probably best to add the 50% solution to the resuscitation fluids. In this situation, 10–20 mL of 50% dextrose or glucose solution should be added per liter of resuscitation fluid. If blood glucose can be measured, the amount of 50% dextrose added to the resuscitation fluids should be varied based on the measured blood glucose, aiming to deliver approximately 20 mL/h for mild hypoglycemia and 50 mL/h for severe hypoglycemia.

Inotrope and vasopressor therapy

Inotropes and vasopressors should only be considered following acute fluid resuscitation. Using inotropes before sufficient fluid therapy can result in tachycardia and increased myocardial oxygen consumption. If oxygen delivery to the heart is marginal, this can result in cardiac arrhythmias.

The heterogeneity of responses to therapy and the inability effectively to monitor individual tissue perfusion means that it is extremely difficult to predict accurately the response to a given treatment. Therefore, the response to treatment should always be monitored and treatments adjusted as necessary. For this reason, drugs with a very short onset of action and rapid metabolism are preferred. This allows titration to effect and helps prevent harm by prolonged inappropriate treatment. However, the rapid metabolism also means that it is necessary to administer these drugs as a constant rate infusion (CRI). The consequences of inaccurate dosing may be severe and therefore an electronic infusion pump is recommended for the administration of all vasoactive drug infusions (**31, 32**).

Inotropes

Inotropes act to increase cardiac stroke volume. Stroke volume is the difference between the end-diastolic volume and the end-systolic volume of the ventricle. Fluid therapy acts to increase stroke volume by increasing end-diastolic volume. Inotropes, on the other hand, decrease end-systolic volume by increasing myocardial contraction. In foals that do not respond to fluid therapy, inotropes represent a further way of increasing cardiac output and, therefore, blood flow. However, inotropes increase cardiac work and thus oxygen consumption, which may be important when oxygen delivery is marginal.

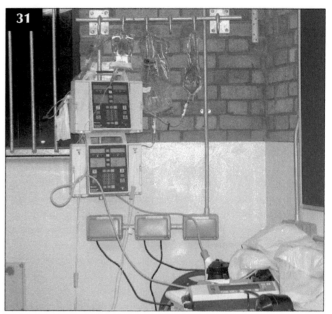

31 Electronic infusion pumps for accurate delivery of fluids and vasoactive drugs.

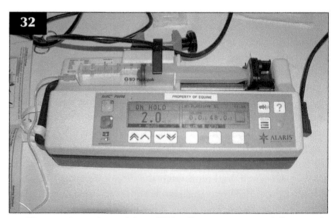

32 Electronic syringe driver. This allows accurate delivery of slow continuous infusions. A particular advantage of using this device is that a small amount of drug may be prepared initially to assess whether it achieves the desired effect.

Dobutamine

Dobutamine is a catecholamine with a strong affinity for the beta-1 adrenoceptor and weak affinity for the beta-2 and alpha-adrenergic receptors. The main clinical use of dobutamine is as an inotrope to increase oxygen delivery to the tissues. For this reason, specific indications for dobutamine therapy are low cardiac output or decreased central venous oxygen tension despite adequate fluid therapy.

In a canine model of endotoxemia, dobutamine (5–10 µg/kg/min) had a beneficial effect on splanchnic perfusion and urine output when compared with fluid therapy alone. In a rat model of endotoxemia, dobutamine maintained intestinal villi blood flow at pre-endotoxic levels. This beneficial effect on splanchnic perfusion is also seen with dobutamine therapy in human septic patients, but not with dopamine therapy. Maintenance of splanchnic perfusion may be important in foals, as it may prevent bacterial translocation across the intestinal wall and establishment or worsening of septicemia. Dobutamine may also have a role in improving splanchnic perfusion when vasopressors such as norepinephrine or epinephrine are used, presumably through its action on beta-2 receptors. Therefore, low-dose dobutamine (up to 5 µg/kg/min) is probably indicated during vasopressor therapy.

It may also be advisable to assess the response to dobutamine before starting vasopressor therapy in order to ensure adequate cardiac output when it cannot be measured. However, dobutamine can decrease SVR and mean arterial pressure, probably through its action on beta-2 adrenergic receptors, and is therefore rarely suitable as monotherapy in hyperdynamic shock.

Dobutamine should be diluted in isotonic saline, 5% dextrose, or LRS. The dose should be carefully titrated from a starting point of 1–3 µg/kg/min in foals.

Isoproterenol

Isoproterenol is a beta-1 and beta-2 adrenergic agonist. In normal horses, administration of the drug results in significant tachycardia and decreased arterial pressure. This tachycardia and vasodilation limits its clinical utility.

Vasopressors

Vasopressor agents act to increase vascular smooth muscle tone, principally in the arterioles. This increases the pressure gradient across a tissue capillary bed, allowing perfusion. However, resistance to flow is also increased. For this reason, it is important to titrate vasopressor agents carefully in order to achieve an optimum balance between perfusion pressure and flow.

Norepinephrine

Norepinephrine (noradrenaline) is a strong alpha-adrenergic agonist with affinity for beta-1 receptors and no demonstrable beta-2 activity. Norepinephrine is used clinically to restore adequate organ perfusion pressure in vasodilatory shock. The specific clinical indications for norepinephrine are markedly decreased SVR or decreased mean arterial pressure that responds to neither fluids nor an inotrope such as dobutamine. The beta-2 adrenergic effects of norepinephrine help to offset the negative effects on cardiac output of the increased cardiac afterload associated with vasoconstriction. Indeed, cardiac output may be increased by 10%–20% as a result of increased stroke volume. However, inappropriately high doses of norepinephrine may result in decreased stroke volume due to increased afterload and reduced end-organ perfusion. BP, urine output, and other cardiovascular parameters should therefore be carefully monitored during norepinephrine infusion.

In human septic shock, norepinephrine is a more effective vasopressor than dopamine. Furthermore, in septic humans requiring >5 µg/kg/min dopamine, addition of norepinephrine results in significantly higher hospital survival (38%) than increasing the dopamine infusion rate (18%). Previous concerns that norepinephrine might have adverse effects on renal function, based on work in normal subjects, have been shown not to be the case in sepsis and endotoxemia. In sheep with experimental hyperdynamic sepsis, infusion of 0.4 µg/kg/min norepinephrine resulted in significantly increased mean arterial pressure, myocardial performance, stroke volume, and creatinine clearance, and no change in renal and mesenteric blood flow, which were already significantly increased by the onset of sepsis.

The addition of low-dose dobutamine (5 µg/kg/min) to norepinephrine has been demonstrated to result in better splanchnic perfusion in human septic patients, possibly due to splanchnic vasodilation mediated by beta-2 adrenergic agonism by dobutamine. In a sheep model of peritonitis, a combination of norepinephrine and dobutamine was superior to norepinephrine in terms of survival time, measures of splanchnic perfusion, urine output, and histologic alterations in pulmonary and intestinal tissue. A combination of dopamine and norepinephrine was also superior to norepinephrine alone, but with some parameters (e.g., urine output and intestinal pathology) it was inferior to the norepinephrine/dobutamine combination.

Concurrent norepinephrine and low-dose dobutamine infusion was investigated in seven critically ill foals that remained hypotensive despite dobutamine or dopamine therapy. There was an increase in mean arterial pressure in six of the seven foals and an increase in urine output in all the foals, coincident with the start of the norepinephrine infusion. Three out of the seven foals survived to compete as racehorses.

Norepinephrine should be diluted in 5% dextrose. The dose should be carefully titrated from a starting dose of 0.1 µg/kg/min. Effects may be seen in some patients at doses as low as 0.01 µg/kg/min. The highest dose of norepinephrine the authors have used in a foal that ultimately survived is 1.5 µg/kg/min.

Epinephrine

Epinephrine is a strong agonist for both alpha- and beta-adrenergic receptors, with no dopaminergic activity. Although epinephrine is an effective vasopressor, its negative effects on the splanchnic circulation may limit its clinical usefulness. In contrast to norepinephrine, epinephrine decreased mesenteric blood flow relative to aortic blood flow in a rat model of endotoxemia. In human patients with severe sepsis, the splanchnic blood flow was found to be lower with epinephrine than with norepinephrine. The clinical relevance of these observations regarding the splanchnic circulation is debated.

In human medicine the main clinical use of epinephrine is as a "rescue" vasopressor agent when the dose of dopamine or norepinephrine is not sufficient to restore adequate organ perfusion pressure. Survival is very poor when epinephrine is used for this purpose. Patients may be refractory to norepinephrine because of alteration in the binding capacity of alpha-adrenergic receptors. The vasopressor action of epinephrine is also mediated by alpha-adrenergic receptors. For this reason, V1 agonists such as vasopressin (see p. 28) may be a more logical choice than epinephrine for norepinephrine refractory shock because they act on a totally different class of receptors.

Epinephrine should be diluted in isotonic saline, 5% dextrose, or LRS. The dose should be carefully titrated from a starting dose of 0.1 µg/kg/min.

Phenylephrine

Phenylephrine is an alpha-agonist with little or no agonism at beta-adrenergic and dopaminergic receptors. The short half-life of phenylephrine means that, like the other catecholamines, it needs to be administered as a CRI. However, clinical experience and available data suggest that the half-life of phenylephrine is longer than that of norepinephrine in the horse, and clinical effects may last for up to 30 minutes after the infusion is stopped.

In human septic patients, infusion of phenylephrine was associated with increases in mean arterial pressure and SVR, with no change in cardiac output. In normal adult horses, phenylephrine infusion resulted in increased SVR and mean arterial pressure, but decreased cardiac output. The decrease in cardiac output was a result of decreased heart rate, and cardiac stroke volume was unchanged. Similar findings were found in anesthetized normal neonatal foals; however, these were normal horses, and findings in septic or endotoxic animals may differ. These findings may suggest that norepinephrine, which is also an agonist for beta-1 receptors and, therefore, a positive inotrope, may have advantages over phenylephrine as a vasopressor. If phenylephrine is used as a vasopressor, it should be used in conjunction with a beta agonist such as dobutamine.

Dopamine

Dopamine is an alpha-, beta-1-, and beta-2-adrenergic receptor agonist and an agonist for dopaminergic receptors. This results in a complicated drug profile, where different effects predominate at different doses. At high doses, the alpha-adrenergic effects predominate and dopamine is principally a vasopressor. At lower doses, the beta-adrenergic effects predominate and dopamine is principally an inotrope. Some clinicians recommend dopamine as the first choice vasopressor because they believe that the action on beta-2 and dopaminergic receptors may prevent excessive vasoconstriction in vulnerable vascular beds such as the splanchnic circulation. However, available evidence from humans and experimental animals suggests that dopamine may actually impair rather than improve GI perfusion. Furthermore, the plasma concentration of dopamine with a given infusion rate is extremely variable between individual human subjects and, therefore, the effects of a given infusion rate of dopamine are unpredictable.

Dopamine has other potentially adverse effects. Infusion of dopamine results in suppression of all anterior pituitary-dependent hormones, with the exception of cortisol, in adult human patients. Furthermore, cessation of dopamine infusion results in rebound hypersecretion of some of these hormones. Dopamine also may suppress chemoreflex sensitivity to hypoxia, resulting in a decreased ventilatory response, which may have relevance in foals that are marginal for requiring mechanical ventilation.

Low-dose dopamine does not increase creatinine clearance in normal adult horses and low-dose (or "renal-dose") dopamine has no benefit in the prevention or treatment of renal failure in human patients. High-dose dopamine is not as effective as norepinephrine for restoring hemodynamics in human hyperdynamic shock. Based on a single case, this may also be true in foals. Norepinephrine successfully reversed hypotension in a foal that had failed to respond to high-dose dopamine (24 µg/kg/min).

If used, dopamine should be diluted in isotonic saline, 5% dextrose, or LRS. If being used as an inotrope, the starting dose should be 2–5 µg/kg/min. If being used as a vasopressor, the starting dose should be 5–10 µg/kg/min.

Vasopressin and terlipressin

Arginine vasopressin and terlipressin are non-catecholamine vasopressors that have recently been the subject of intense research in human patients and animal models. Vasopressin acts on V1a receptors in the periphery to cause vasoconstriction and on V2 receptors in the collecting tubule of the nephron to cause water resorption.

Interestingly, vasopressin is approximately five times more potent a vasopressor in endotoxemia and septic shock than in normal subjects. This may be explained, at least in part, by indirect actions to counteract the vasodilation of shock. Vasopressin restores some of the vasoconstrictor effect of circulating catecholamines, which is reduced in septic shock, even though plasma concentrations of catecholamines are increased. Vasopressin also acts to inactivate adenosine triphosphate (ATP)-dependent potassium channels, restoring the ability of smooth muscle to contract. Vasopressin also acts to reduce the amount of cyclic guanosine monophosphate (cGMP) induced by nitric oxide, and therefore the amount of myosin phosphatase produced.

Data from human medicine have shown that vasopressin is equivalent to norepinephrine in terms of hospital outcome. Some authors have expressed concern that V1 agonists may decrease blood flow in the GI tract. Recent evidence in a rat endotoxemia model demonstrated that terlipressin improved ileal microcirculation in aggressively fluid resuscitated animals, but was detrimental in animals receiving only 10 mL/kg/h of crystalloid fluids. This evidence suggests that V1 agonists may be unsuitable for use in foals that are under fluid resuscitated or are maintained on conservative fluid therapy regimes.

Anecdotal evidence suggests that vasopressin is useful as a pressor agent in foal septic shock and that it has similar properties to those seen in human patients. The suggested starting dose is 0.25–0.5 mU/kg/min for vasopressin. Terlipressin has been administered to humans as a bolus of 1–2 mg; this resulted in a progressive increase in mean arterial pressure, which was maintained for at least 5 hours. It is vital to ensure adequate fluid resuscitation prior to administration of these drugs.

FLUID THERAPY FOR DEHYDRATION, ELECTROLYTE REPLACEMENT, AND MAINTENANCE IN THE FOAL

Early, aggressive, and appropriate fluid therapy is one of the most important factors in determining outcome in critically ill foals. Neonatal foals are particularly susceptible to dehydration and hypovolemia, and may show signs of dehydration after only 2.5 hours of inadequate fluid intake (33).

There are four goals of fluid therapy: (1) reverse the hypovolemia; (2) treat the dehydration; (3) correct electrolyte and acid–base imbalances; and (4) provide fluid for maintenance and to counter ongoing losses.

DEHYDRATION

Dehydration should be addressed once the hypovolemia has been treated. The rehydration phase aims to replace extravascular fluid losses. Crystalloid fluids are a logical choice for rehydration as they readily diffuse into the interstitial fluid from the vasculature. Rehydration should take place over the first 12–24 hours

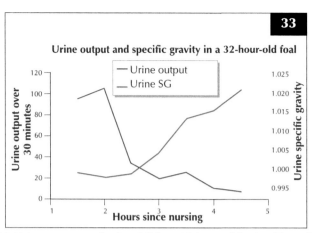

33

Urine output and specific gravity in a 32-hour-old foal

33 Urine output and urine SG in a 32-hour-old mixed breed foal. The foal was separated from the mare at time zero. A jugular catheter was placed and, from 60 minutes, the foal was infused with 2.5 mL/kg/h of an isotonic balanced electrolyte solution (lactated Ringer's solution). At 2.5 hours after separation from the mare, despite infusion of the fluids, the urine output decreased and the urine SG increased, indicating dehydration.

of therapy. The amount given should be based on the clinical estimate of the degree of dehydration (*Table 9*) after treatment for hypovolemia and the response to fluid therapy. Most septic foals with venodilation and ongoing capillary leak will require continuing aggressive fluid resuscitation during the first 24 hours of management. During this period, input is typically much greater than output, and the ratio of input to output is of no use in judging fluid resuscitation needs during this time period.

Typically, horses with obvious clinical signs of dehydration will require 50–100 mL/kg (2.5–5.0 L for a 50 kg [110 lb] foal) of fluid to replace their deficits. Following treatment of hypovolemia, a fluid plan should be made for the first 24 hours that includes fluids for rehydration, maintenance, and ongoing losses. Clinical signs

are not an accurate way of estimating fluid requirements, and so frequent monitoring is required to ensure that adequate fluids are being delivered. When fluid losses have been adequately replaced, the urine SG should be <1.010, except in foals with renal failure. Ensuring adequate fluid therapy in foals with renal failure is difficult and is probably best achieved by measurement of the response of CVP to fluid therapy.

MAINTENANCE RATES

For the neonatal foal maintenance fluid therapy is challenging because every critically ill neonatal foal has unique fluid requirements. These requirements are dependent on metabolic rate, gestational age, environmental temperature, breed, surface area, growth rate and underlying disease process. Foals with gastrointestinal losses have a higher fluid requirement than those without excessive fluid loses or those at risk for the development of tissue edema or fluid overloading. The most commonly used maintenance fluid rate for neonates is 4–6 mL/kg/h. This rate is for a neonate receiving no enteral fluid and without excessive fluid losses. Another maintenance rate is 2 mL/kg/h. This rate is similar to the Holliday-Segar formula used for human neonates, which estimates fluid rate based on basal metabolism, and is a "dryer" fluid rate when compared to the other rate. It is important to establish a starting rate that suits most cases but be willing to modify this rate when needed due to certain circumstances. In a foal that is receiving multiple IV infusions it is important to take into account all volumes in order to avoid fluid overload.

Physiologically for the foal a constant rate infusion (CRI) is more appropriate but at times not practical. If bolus administration is used, smaller more frequently administered boluses are better tolerated in the neonatal foal. To determine adequate bolus volume, the 24-hour maintenance volume is divided by the number of boluses to be administered that day. Polyionic fluids are best to bolus because they are unlikely to result in electrolyte abnormalities. Additional electrolyte supplementation to the fluid bolus is not advised. Close monitoring is crucial for determining if the

Table 9. Clinical signs associated with different degrees of dehydration and hypovolemia in the neonatal foal

Degree of dehydration	Skin tenting	Mucous membranes	Capillary refill time	Heart rate	Other signs
Moderate (approx. 5%)	1–2 seconds	Moist or slightly tacky	Normal (<2 seconds)	Normal (70–110 bpm)	Decreased urine output
Marked (approx. 8%–10%)	1–5 seconds	Tacky	Variable Often 2–3 seconds	Normal or increased (70–140 bpm)	Decreased arterial blood pressure
Severe (>10%)	1–5 or more seconds	Dry	Variable Often >4 seconds	Normal or increased (70–180 bpm)	Reduced jugular fill Barely detectable peripheral pulse Sunken eyes

Note that signs are not consistently present in foals.

fluid plan is adequate. Urine output is an excellent response to fluid therapy. Serial measurements of urine specific gravity (SG) are a good indicator of fluid status in foals with normal renal function. SG rises prior to other signs of insufficient fluid therapy (**33**). The normal urine SG of a foal is in the range 1.001 to 1.008.

Electrolytes in neonatal foals
Sodium
Normal neonatal foals have a low requirement for sodium because they are efficient at conserving sodium. Critically ill neonatal foals appear unable to regulate plasma sodium concentration properly because perinatal disease affects renal sodium handling ability. Sodium overload is a common sequel to fluid therapy with sodium-containing fluids.

Resuscitation formulas are sodium rich and administering them for maintenance or treatment of dehydration frequently results in hypernatremia (sodium concentration of greater than 150 mmol/L). Conversely, using sodium-poor solutions such as 5% dextrose often causes hyponatremia.

One solution is to use Plasmalyte-M or Plasmalyte-56 (Baxter) for maintenance. The composition of these fluids is given in *Table 10*. They appear to contain approximately the right amount of sodium for neonatal foals and make managing the sodium concentration during maintenance therapy far easier. These fluids do contain glucose, which must be taken into account when formulating nutrition plans. Another option is to administer two types of fluids, 5% dextrose in water and sodium-containing fluids, which allows sodium and fluids requirements to be met independently. It is best to administer these fluids as a CRI.

Depending on the disease process, some neonatal foals have a higher sodium requirement. Those with gastrointestinal disorders or certain renal disorders may require more because of increased loss of sodium. Like an adult, the older foal is able to tolerate the sodium in balanced electrolyte formulas.

Hyponatremia and hypernatremia should be corrected slowly. Hyponatremia should be corrected at a rate not exceeding 0.5 mEq/L/h unless seizure activity secondary to the hyponatremia is present. In this case increasing the sodium concentration more rapidly (not to exceed the value of 120 mEq/L) may stop seizure activity. Hypernatremia should also be corrected at a slow rate of 0.5 mEq/L/h.

Chloride
Foals treated with furosemide repeatedly or as a CRI almost always develop hypochloremia, which, in some cases, can be profound. Depending on their potassium status, these foals are best treated with potassium chloride or sodium chloride. It is the authors' usual practice to start a potassium chloride infusion at the same time as furosemide therapy, at a rate of 0.3–0.5 mEq/kg/h, in foals with a potassium concentration of less than 4.5 mmol/L. Hydrochloric acid is used to treat hypochloremia in man, but the authors have not yet been brave enough to try this in foals.

Hyperchloremia is rare, but can occur secondary to renal tubular acidosis. Renal tubular acidosis is diagnosed by blood acidosis with a paradoxical normal or alkaline urine. If hyperchloremia without hypernatremia is a feature, it is treated with judicious administration of sodium bicarbonate.

Potassium
Hypokalemia is a relatively common finding in hospitalized foals, and almost all critically ill foals require supplementation with potassium chloride at some point during their fluid therapy. As with adult horses, potassium should not be supplemented intravenously at rates higher than 0.5 mmol/kg/h. Empirical supplementation is usually around 10–40 mEq/L of KCL.

Hyperkalemia usually only occurs with ruptured bladders. Possible treatments for symptomatic or severe (>7 mmol/L) hyperkalemia include calcium gluconate (1 mL/kg i/v over 10 minutes), sodium bicarbonate (1–2 mEq/L i/v over 15 minutes), and 50% dextrose solution (2 mL/kg i/v over 5 minutes).

Calcium
Ionized calcium is the active form of calcium in plasma and the value can be affected by inappetence, sepsis, gastrointestinal disorders, or renal disease. If the foal is showing clinical signs, or the ionized calcium concentration is <0.85 mmol/L, calcium should be administered (approximately 10–30 mL of 23% calcium gluconate i/v as the initial dose). The most prominent clinical signs tend to be ataxia and weakness, rather than the synchronous diaphragmatic flutter seen in adult horses. Foals seem to be particularly susceptible to hypocalcemia if maintained on parenteral nutrition with no enteral nutrition. In addition to calcium therapy, vitamin D_3 should be considered in these foals.

Magnesium
Magnesium is an important cofactor for many enzymatic reactions, and ionized magnesium is the physiologically active form. Conditions associated with hypomagnesemia include sepsis, gastrointestinal disorders, respiratory and metabolic alkalosis, acute renal failure, hyperlipemia, and parenteral nutrition. Severe hypomagnesemia in the horse can result in ventricular arrhythmias and also muscle tremors, ataxia, seizures, and calcification of elastic tissue. In some experimental studies magnesium has been shown to prevent or reduce hypoxic brain injury, thus it can also be given as a therapy for hypoxic ischemic encephalopathy (HIE).

If the ionized magnesium concentration is <0.35 mmol/L, magnesium should be supplemented with 16–64 mmol/kg (4–16 mg/kg) magnesium sulfate over 4–6 hours. The magnesium concentration should then be remeasured to determine if a higher or lower rate of continued supplementation is required.

Hypermagnesemia is rare in neonatal foals. The most likely cause is inadvertent overadministration of magnesium, especially in a foal with renal insufficiency. Clinical signs reported in mature horses include flaccid paralysis with recumbency, tachycardia, tachypnea, and nondetectable peripheral pulses. Treatment in a neonatal foal is by administration of 10 mL of 40% calcium gluconate, repeated after an hour, and increased intravenous fluids to promote diuresis.

Phosphate
Clinical signs of hypophosphatemia reported in small animals and humans include hemolysis, skeletal muscle weakness and rhabdomyolysis, leukocyte dysfunction, ventricular arrhythmias, and reduced cardiac output. These clinical signs occur in neonatal foals, but it is often hard to be sure whether they are related to low blood phosphate concentrations.

Table 10. Composition of fluids commonly used in neonatal foals

Fluid	Na (mmol/L)	K (mmol/L)	Cl (mmol/L)	Ca (mmol/L)	Mg (mmol/L)	Lactate (mmol/L)	Acetate (mmol/L)	Gluconate	Dextrose	kcal/mL	mOsm/L	COP
Resuscitation formulas												
Hartmann's solution	131	5	111	2	–	29	–	–	–	0.009	305	–
Plasmalyte-148	140	5	98	–	3	–	27	23	–	0.015	294	–
Plasmalyte-R	140	10	103	5	3	8	47	–	–	–	312	–
Normosol-R	140	5	98	–	3	–	27	23	–	–	–	–
Lactated Ringer's solution	130	4	109	3	–	28	–	–	–	0.015	294	–
Maintenance formulas												
Plasmalyte-56	40	13	40	–	3	–	16	–	–	–	111	–
Plasmalyte-56 and 5% Dextrose	40	13	40	–	3	–	16	–	5	0.17	363	–
Plasmalyte-M	40	16	40	5	3	12	12	–	5	0.2	377	–
Colloids												
Hespan	154	–	154	–	–	–	–	–	–	–	308	31
Hextend	143	–	124	2.5	0.45	28	–	–	5	0.179	307	31
HAES-Steril 6%	154	–	154	–	–	–	–	–	–	–	308	36
Other fluids												
50% Dextrose	–	–	–	–	–	–	–	–	50	1.7	2526	–
50% Glucose	–	–	–	–	–	–	–	–	50	1.9	2770	–
5% Dextrose (D5W)	–	–	–	–	–	–	–	–	5	0.17	253	–
10% Dextrose (D10W)	–	–	–	–	–	–	–	–	10	0.34	505	–
2.5% Dextrose/0.45% Saline	77	–	77	–	–	–	–	–	2.5	0.085	280	–
0.9% Saline	154	–	154	–	–	–	–	–	–	–	290	–

Complied from product data sheets and a variety of other resources. It is recommended to check the data sheet of the product to be used before administration.
COP = colloid osmotic pressure.

The authors have not supplemented phosphate in neonatal foals. In mature horses, Addiphos® (sodium potassium phosphate, Fresenius-Kabi), administered at between 0.01 and 0.03 mmol/kg/h of phosphate and making sure that potassium supplementation does not exceed 0.5 mmol/kg/h, appears to be effective.

Hyperphosphatemia appears to be very rare in neonatal foals. Clinical findings reported in small animals include diarrhea, hypocalcemia, hypernatremia, and an increased propensity to metastatic soft tissue calcification. Treatment recommended in small animals includes intravenous fluids to correct any acidosis and promote renal phosphorus excretion, and dextrose-containing fluids to promote translocation of phosphorus into cells.

Bicarbonate

Bicarbonate supplementation may be necessary in foals that are actively losing bicarbonate from diarrhea or severely and persistently acidotic. It is important to establish normovolemia prior to administration of bicarbonate. Sodium bicarbonate is the most commonly administered form added to fluids. The bicarbonate deficit may be estimated as follows: bicarbonate estimate (mEq) = 0.5 × body weight (kg) × (25-patient HCO3).

It is often suggested that one half of the calculated deficit be given over 1 hour, then blood electrolyte values repeated. The remainder of the deficit can be replaced over the next 12–24 hours. Bicarbonate should not be administered to a foal with impaired ventilation as carbon dioxide excretion is limited and bicarbonate administration can potentiate carbon dioxide production. Bicarbonate administration may induce hypokalemia as potassium ions enter the cells in exchange for hydrogen ions, therefore potassium concentrations should be closely monitored. Sodium concentration should also be monitored due to the large sodium load that is provided with this therapy.

SUCCESSFUL FLUID THERAPY

The key to successful management of fluid and electrolyte status in critically ill foals is monitoring. The disease process in these foals is very dynamic, and what was adequate an hour ago can suddenly become inadequate. Frequent physical examination and repeated measuring of acid–base status and electrolytes are essential for optimum treatment.

CARDIOPULMONARY RESUSCITATION

Although there are many reasons for cardiopulmonary arrest (CPA) in the foal, respiratory arrest almost always precedes cardiac arrest in the newborn foal. Newborn foals can arrest as a result of the birthing process without any specific underlying pathophysiology or CPA can result secondary to systemic disease. Veterinarians require a thorough understanding of CPR in advance of these skills being required. An arrest is often a tense situation, in which the veterinarian needs calmly to direct other people who may have no or only rudimentary knowledge of CPR. Sometimes this direction will be by telephone, as veterinarians are not present at many foalings. Veterinarians can also improve CPR by arranging training sessions for staff of larger breeding operations prior to the foaling season.

RECOGNITION OF RESPIRATORY OR CARDIAC ARREST

Normal stage two labor should take less than 20 minutes. Regular breathing should start within 30 seconds of birth. The heart rate should be regular and around 70 bpm. Foals have pain and sensory awareness at birth and develop a righting reflex within 5 minutes. Respiratory rather than cardiac arrest is virtually always primary in the newborn foal. The arrest is usually a result of asphyxia, itself caused by premature placental separation, early severance or twisting of the umbilical cord, prolonged dystocia, or airway obstruction by fetal membranes. Some foals will not start breathing spontaneously without any apparent birthing misadventure.

Foals requiring resuscitation are those that gasp for longer than 30 seconds, foals with no respiratory movements or no heart beat, those with a heart rate of <40 bpm, and foals with obvious dyspnea. Foals at risk of arresting should be identified prior to foaling, so that a veterinarian can be present. Risk factors include vaginal discharge during pregnancy, placental thickening, any illness of the dam during pregnancy, and delivery by cesarean section.

EQUIPMENT FOR CARDIOPULMONARY RESUSCITATION

Foals can occasionally be successfully resuscitated with little or no equipment, but a small amount of equipment greatly increases the chance of success. The basic list of equipment is clean towels; 8 mm and 10 mm internal diameter 55 cm long nasotracheal tubes; a 5 mL syringe for nasotracheal tube cuff inflation; a self-inflating resuscitation bag; a bulb syringe; a small flashlight; and a bottle of epinephrine, five 2 mL sterile syringes, and 20 gauge 1 in and steel 14 gauge 1–1.5 in needles. Disposable resuscitation bags, which can be reused after thorough cleaning, are considerably less expensive to purchase than reusable bags.

Additional equipment includes an oxygen cylinder and flow meter, three 1 L bags of LRS, a fluid administration set, a 14 gauge i/v catheter, a 6 Fr dog urinary catheter, and an electrical defibrillator (*Table 11*). Stud farms without resident veterinarians should consider purchase of a suitable facemask, together with a resuscitation bag or pump (**34**). The equipment for CPR should be placed in a dedicated, single, easily carried container (**35**). Equipment should be thoroughly checked prior to the foaling season.

AN ORDERED PLAN FOR CARDIOPULMONARY RESUSCITATION
The first 20 seconds—preparing for cardiopulmonary resuscitation

The first 20 seconds after birth are devoted to assessing the foal and preparing for CPR. The extent of action at this point depends on the likelihood that the foal will require resuscitation. In the foal born by cesarean section, these 20 seconds are spent vigorously drying the foal with clean towels, manually clearing the mouth of secretions, and positioning the foal in lateral recumbency on a firm, dry surface. In a meconium-stained foal, these 20 seconds should be devoted to suctioning the airway. Airway suctioning should ideally start as soon as a meconium-stained head appears at the vulva, prior to the foal taking its first breath. If the foal is covered in thick meconium, suctioning of the trachea should also be attempted using a 60 mL syringe and rubber tubing. Suctioning of fluids from the oropharynx can induce bradycardia or even cardiac arrest via vagal reflexes, and for this reason, suctioning with a bulb

Table 11. Suggested equipment for cardiopulmonary resuscitation of the newborn foal

Essential equipment

	Preferred option 1	Preferred option 2	Acceptable option
Tactile stimulation	Clean, dry towels		Paper towels
Suction equipment	Bulb syringe	60 mL syringe and soft rubber tubing	
Airway management	Nasotracheal tube (8 and 10 mm ID, 55 cm long)		Foal mask
Lung inflation	Self-inflating resuscitation bag	Resuscitation pump	Anesthetic machine with 1 L reserve bag
Drugs	Epinephrine (1:1000) in preloaded syringes		Epinephrine (1:1000) in glass vials

Useful equipment

Airway management	Nasotracheal tube (7 and 12 mm ID, 55 cm long)
Oxygenation	Oxygen cylinder
Drugs	Lactated Ringer's solution and 14 gauge i/v catheter
Defibrillator	Capable of delivering 400 joules
Monitoring	End-tidal CO_2 monitor, electrocardiogram, small flashlight

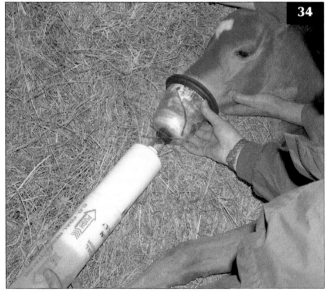

34 Pump and mask resuscitation of a foal. The pump delivers a set volume, thereby avoiding volutrauma. The pump and mask are made by McCulloch Medical, Auckland, New Zealand.

syringe may be safer than using a mechanical unit. It is safest to only suction for 5 seconds at a time. In foals that are born normally within 20 minutes, these 20 seconds should consist of quiet observation in order to ensure that the foal's airway is clear and that it is breathing spontaneous.

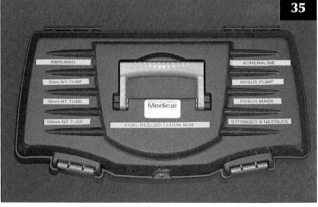

35 Equipment box for resuscitation of foals. The box is easily carried and labeled with its contents.

Airway

The best way to ensure an adequate airway is to intubate the foal. Intubation via the nose is preferred to intubation via the mouth, as there is less risk of tube damage as the foal regains consciousness. If two brief attempts at nasotracheal intubation are unsuccessful, further attempts should be via the mouth. Ideally, intubation should be completed within less than 30 seconds.

For intubation, the foal can be in lateral or sternal recumbency. The head should be in a straight line with the neck. To pass a tube via the nose, one hand should be used to push the tip of the tube medially and ventrally in the nares into the ventral meatus.

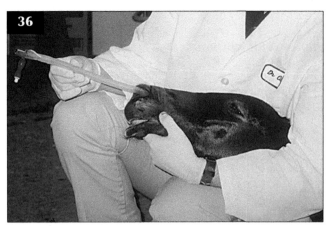

36 Nasotracheal intubation of a foal. The tube is placed ventrally and medially in the nares to pass through the ventral meatus into the nasopharynx. The head is extended to allow passage of the tube through the larynx and into the trachea. Intubation is best achieved with the foal held in sternal recumbency (pictured) or with the foal in lateral recumbency.

The other hand is used to advance the tube smoothly (**36**). To pass a tube via the mouth, the tongue should be gently pulled forward and to the side with one hand to help stabilize the larynx. The tube is advanced smoothly over the tongue, in a midline position. In both cases, rotation of the tube when the end is in the pharynx can be helpful. Once the tube is in place, the cuff should be gently inflated.

It is vital to check that the tube has successfully passed into the trachea by compressing the thorax and simultaneously feeling the expired air at the proximal tube end. The thoracic wall should also be seen to rise when the first breath is given. If the tube has entered the esophagus, it can often be felt in the cranial neck just left and dorsal to the larynx or proximal trachea.

Breathing

The optimum rate of ventilation is not known, but experience suggests that rates of between 10 and 20 bpm are appropriate. If available, 100% oxygen should be used for resuscitation. However, studies of human neonate CPR suggest that resuscitation with room air is equally as effective. The best method of providing artificial respiration is a self-inflating resuscitation bag connected to a nasotracheal or endotracheal tube. This allows controlled ventilation and avoids the risk of aerophagia or forcing material (e.g., meconium or mucus) into the airways. Aerophagia can significantly constrain ventilation, because filling the stomach with gas can put pressure on the diaphragm and prevent the lungs fully expanding.

When using a resuscitation bag, the optimum method is to place the bag on the floor and to kneel next to the bag with the shoulders over the bag. The hands should be placed flat and together on the bag. This allows controlled use of body weight to help compression of the bag (**37**). Many resuscitation bags have a valve to limit the pressure to 30–40 cmH$_2$O. This is the maximum pressure that should be applied for the first breath. Subsequent breaths should only require a pressure of 15–20 cmH$_2$O.

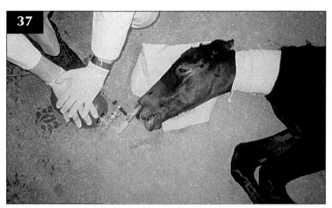

37 Artificial respiration in a foal using a self-inflating resuscitation bag connected to a nasotracheal tube. The bag can optionally be connected to an oxygen source. The bag should be depressed 10–20 times per minute.

An alternative to a self-inflating resuscitation bag is a resuscitation pump (**34**). The commercially available model delivers a tidal volume of 780 mL and can be connected to a nasotracheal tube or to a mask. Anesthetic machines with a minimum reserve bag of 1 L and oxygen demand valves may also be used for resuscitation, but they carry a significant risk of volutrauma. Masks, rather than tracheal tubes, probably represent the best option for CPR by laypeople. Aerophagia, a significant risk with masks, can be reduced by gentle occlusion of the esophagus over the larynx. However, this may require an extra person.

Mouth-to-nose resuscitation can occasionally be successful. With the foal in lateral recumbency, one hand should be used to cup the chin and occlude the down nostril. The other hand should support the back of the head. The head should be dorsiflexed as far as possible to straighten the airway, but the head should not be lifted (**38**). The esophagus should be occluded, if possible.

Doxapram was historically recommended for stimulating respiration at birth. The drug has been shown to reduce cerebral blood flow and to increase myocardial oxygen demands in

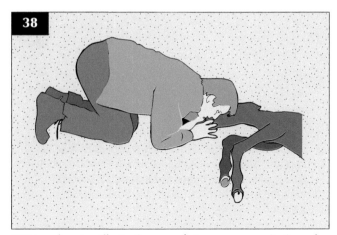

38 Line drawing illustrating mouth-to-nose resuscitation of a foal. The head should be dorsiflexed as far as possible in order to straighten the airway, but the head should not be lifted.

experimental animals. This class of drug is also ineffective in secondary apnea. Doxapram is therefore no longer recommended.

Circulation

Most human infants who require artificial ventilation at birth do not need chest compressions, and the same is probably true of foals. Thirty seconds after starting ventilation the foal should be assessed to decide whether circulatory support is required. Thoracic compressions should be started if the heart beat is absent, <40 bpm, or <60 bpm and not increasing.

The optimum rate for thoracic compressions in the foal is not known. A rate of 80 cpm has been shown to result in significantly better circulation than 40 or 60 cpm in adult horses. Rates between 80 and 120 cpm are therefore likely to be appropriate for foals. However, rates this high rapidly fatigue the resuscitator. Therefore, it is recommended to switch the person doing the thoracic compressions every 2–5 minutes. Ventilation must continue during thoracic compressions. The recommended ratio is 2 breaths/15 thoracic compressions. It is not necessary to stop thoracic compressions during breaths.

The foal should be in lateral recumbency and moved to a firm dry surface, if not already done. The foal's rib cage should be quickly palpated and, if fractured ribs are suspected, the foal should be turned so these are on the underneath side. The person doing the thoracic compressions should kneel by the foal's spine and place his/her hands on top of each other just caudal to the foal's triceps, in the highest point of the thorax. Resuscitators should have their shoulders directly above their hands, enabling them to use their body weight to help compress the thorax. This helps reduce resuscitator fatigue (**39**).

DRUGS

Drugs should be considered if the heart rate remains below 40 bpm and is not increasing after 30 seconds of thoracic compressions and adequate ventilation. Thoracic compressions must continue after a drug has been given, as all drugs require a circulation to reach

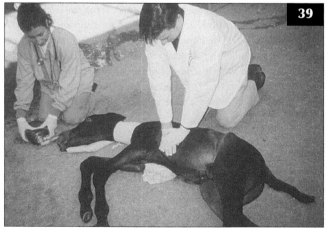

39

39 Thoracic compressions and artificial respiration in a foal. The person doing the thoracic compressions should kneel by the foal's spine and place his/her hands on top of each other, just caudal to the foal's triceps, in the highest point of the thorax.

the point of action, no matter what route they are delivered. The preferred route for drugs is intravenous. The jugular vein is usually obvious in foals and can be injected relatively easily, even when there is no circulation. If intravenous injection is not possible, drugs may either be delivered via the trachea or by intraosseous injection. For intratracheal administration, the needle of the syringe should be placed in the midline of the neck and through the skin and the ligament between two tracheal rings, below the level of balloon of the nasotracheal tube, if present. An alternative method is to attach a dog urinary catheter to the syringe and pass the urinary catheter down the center of the nasotracheal tube so that the end is in the trachea. For intraosseous injection, a 14 gauge needle should be in the proximal medial one-third aspect of the tibia or the radius. The needle is harder to place in the radius. The intratracheal dose of drugs may be higher than the intravenous dose, whereas the intraosseous dose is probably the same. Intracardiac injection should never be used because of the risk of laceration of a coronary artery or deposition of the drug in the myocardium resulting in fibrillation. If drugs are required for resuscitation, the prognosis is poor.

The primary drug for resuscitation is epinephrine. The intravenous dose is 0.01–0.02 mg/kg (0.5–1 mL of the 1 mg/mL [1:1000] solution for a 50 kg foal). Because it has a short half-life, epinephrine should be given every 3 minutes until the return of spontaneous circulation. The dose for intratracheal epinephrine is 0.1–0.2 mg/kg (*Table 12*). Epinephrine increases vascular tone through alpha adrenoreceptors. This results in an increased aortic diastolic pressure, which increases blood flow through the coronary arteries and myocardium during the relaxation phase of thoracic compressions. Vasopressin is a nonadrenergic endogenous stress hormone which has marked peripheral vasoconstrictor activity during cardiac arrest. A single dose (0.6 U/kg/IV) can be given as an adjunct to epinephrine.

Volume expansion is recommended for foals that have a poor response to resuscitative efforts, have weak pulses with a good heart rate, or remain pale or cyanotic after oxygenation. The initial dose is 10 ml/kg of balanced electrolyte solution (LRS or Normosol-R) or 2 mL/kg hydroxyethyl starch (hetastarch, pentastarch, or tetrastarch). Fluids may be administered intravenously or intraosseously, but not via the trachea. The use of sodium bicarbonate is highly controversial. There is conflicting data on its effectiveness in experimental cardiac arrest and it may be counterproductive by initially decreasing intracellular pH.

Drugs other than epinephrine and fluids should only be used in the case of documented cardiac dysrhythmias. This requires an electrocardiogram (ECG) machine, which is unlikely to be readily available in the field. Moreover, most human infants with serious dysrhythmias have sustained overwhelming cerebral as well as cardiac injury, suggesting that newborn foals that develop a dysrhythmia may be unlikely to survive. However, many normal foals may have arrhythmias for up to 15 minutes following birth, including wandering pacemaker, atrial premature contractions, and ventricular premature contractions. These dysrhythmias do not require specific treatment.

Asystole, recognized by the absence of cardiac electrical activity, should be treated with epinephrine as described above. Ventricular fibrillation, recognized by rapidly undulating

Table 12. Epinephrine doses in neonatal cardiopulmonary resuscitation

Drug	mL/50 kg	Drug concentration	Dose/kg	mL/kg
Epinephrine (i/v)	0.5–1 mL every 3 min	1 mg/mL	0.01–0.02 mg	0.01–0.02
Epinephrine (intratracheal)	5–10 mL every 3 min	Up to 1 mg/mL	Up to 0.1–0.2 mg	Up to 0.1–0.2

electrical activity with no discernable complexes, is most effectively treated with an electrical defibrillator. The dose is 1–4 J/kg (50–200 J for a 50 kg foal), increasing the energy by 50% at each defibrillation attempt.

Atropine and calcium should not be used in CPR of newborn foals. Atropine has little effect if the bradycardia is not vagally mediated; it increases myocardial oxygen consumption and may precipitate tachycardias. The recommended treatment for brady-dysrhythmias is artificial ventilation and thoracic compressions. Although calcium improves the contractility of the normal heart, during cardiac arrest it leads to an increased cytosolic calcium concentration, which results in disruption of myocardial function.

MONITORING THE EFFECTIVENESS OF CARDIOPULMONARY RESUSCITATION

During CPR, monitoring the effectiveness of the resuscitative efforts can help adjust the technique to the individual patient. For example, the rate of ventilation and the rate and pressure of thoracic compressions can be varied. The pulse, if palpable, is the best way of monitoring thoracic compressions. The progress of CPR can be monitored by the heart beat, if present, which is used to decide when to stop thoracic compressions. Although an ECG is useful for monitoring the heart rhythm, it is not adequate for monitoring CPR because electrical activity in the heart can continue without effective contractions (pulseless electrical activity). CPR can also be monitored by the pupillary light reflex. If the person doing the thoracic compressions keeps a flashlight in their mouth, they can then lean across and assess the pupil response and size without interrupting the resuscitation efforts. The pupil is widely dilated and fixed with inadequate resuscitation, whereas an adequate circulation results in a more normal pupil, which responds to light.

If the equipment is available, an end-tidal carbon dioxide monitor (capnograph) is extremely useful for assessing the effectiveness of CPR. The higher the expired carbon dioxide tension, the more effective the resuscitation efforts, because more carbon dioxide is being transported to the lungs and ventilated. End-tidal carbon dioxide tensions >15 mmHg indicate good perfusion and portend a good prognosis, whereas tensions persistently lower than 10 mmHg indicate ineffective CPR and a poor prognosis.

WHEN TO STOP

Ventilation should be stopped when the heart rate is above 60 bpm and spontaneous breathing is well established. This can be tested by stopping ventilation and disconnecting the bag or pump for 30 seconds and checking for a respiratory rate above 16 breaths per minute, a regular respiratory pattern, and normal respiratory effort. The first few breaths may be gasping, but they should be followed by a normal respiratory rate and pattern. Premature withdrawal of ventilation is reported to be the most common mistake in human neonatal CPR.

If started, thoracic compressions should be continued until a regular heartbeat of over 60 bpm has been established. There should be no lag period between the stopping of support and the onset of a spontaneous heartbeat. Therefore, CPR should not be stopped for longer than 10 seconds to assess the circulation. Clinical experience suggests that if spontaneous circulation and respiration are not present after 15 minutes, then survival is unlikely.

CARE FOR FOALS AFTER RESUSCITATION

Foals that have been resuscitated continue to require support and should be intensively monitored for at least 30 minutes. Supplemental oxygen should be provided, either by facemask or by nasal cannula. A careful physical examination should be performed and, if available, the heart should be monitored with an ECG.

The consequences of the period of asphyxia during arrest and resuscitation can be serious and may not be apparent for 24–48 hours after the arrest. Perinatal asphyxia can result in a syndrome of altered neurologic status, seizuring, and impaired GI and cardiovascular function (previously called HIE or neonatal maladjustment syndrome). There is no way to prevent the effects of asphyxia. Vitamin E, selenium, and dimethyl sulfoxide may possibly reduce oxidative damage. Fluid therapy is indicated to support cardiac output and correct electrolyte abnormalities. The administration of inotropes may be helpful in supporting cardiac output. Glucose therapy is helpful for general metabolic support. The decision whether to refer a foal for intensive care is based on many factors including availability and the costs versus the economic worth of the foal. Success rates also vary, but are in the order of 70%–80% for most ICUs. Foals that have been successfully resuscitated are at high risk of complications, and referral should be strongly considered if circumstances allow.

FURTHER READING

Corley KTT (2002) Monitoring and treating haemodynamic disturbances in critically ill neonatal foals. Part I—Haemodynamic monitoring. *Equine Veterinary Education* 14: 270–279.

Corley KTT (2002) Monitoring and treating haemodynamic disturbances in critically ill neonatal foals. Part II—Assessment and treatment. *Equine Veterinary Education* 14: 328–336.

Corley KTT (2004) Fluid therapy. In: *Equine Clinical Pharmacology* (Bertone JJ, Horspool LL, Eds.). WB Saunders, London, UK, pp. 327–364.

Corley KTT, Furr MO (2000) Cardiopulmonary resuscitation in newborn foals. *Compendium on Continuing Education for the Practicing Veterinarian* 20: 957–967.

Fielding CL (2014) Crystalloid and colloid therapy. *Veterinary Clinics of North America: Equine Practice* 30: 415–425.

Fielding CL, Magdesian KG (2015) Sepsis and septic shock in the equine neonate. *Veterinary Clinics of North America: Equine Practice* 31: 483–496.

Giguere S, Bucki E, Adin DB, Valverde A, Estrada AH, Young L (2005) Cardiac output measurement by partial carbon dioxide rebreathing, 2-dimensional echocardiography, and lithium-dilution method in anesthetized neonatal foals. *Journal of Veterinary Internal Medicine* 19: 737–743.

Jokisalo JM, Corley KTT (2014) CPR in the neonatal foal: Has recover changed our approach? *Veterinary Clinics of North America: Equine Practice* 30: 301–316.

Magdesian KG (2004) Monitoring the critically ill equine patient. *Veterinary Clinics of North America:Equine Practice* 20: 11–39.

Magdesian KG, Madigan JE (2003) Volume replacement in the neonatal ICU: Crystalloids and colloids. *Clinical Techniques in Equine Practice* 2: 20–30.

Palmer J (2007) Neonatal foal resuscitation. *Veterinary Clinics of North America: Equine Practice* 23: 159–182.

Slovis N (2014) Field techniques for resuscitation of foals. In: *AAEP Focus on the First Year of Life Proceeding*, pp. 6–9.

Infectious Diseases

3

Bonnie S. Barr

INTRODUCTION

Infectious diseases have been recognized as posing a threat to the health and well-being of horses for thousands of years. Equine populations have been devastated on occasion by epidemics of specific diseases. The constant movement of horses within countries and from continent to continent makes it harder to combat and eradicate some of these diseases. Also, overcrowding, misuse of antibiotics, and poor management practices have resulted in the emergence of resistant strains of some of these organisms. Fortunately, recent advances have made our ability to detect, define, and treat these diseases much easier. Working out the best way to prevent and control infectious diseases has resulted from knowledge gained following outbreaks. The goal of this chapter is to provide an overview of each disease discussed and to provide information on its etiology/pathophysiology, clinical signs, diagnostic techniques, and treatment options. Infectious diseases not covered in this chapter will be cross-referenced to the appropriate chapter where relevant.

SEPSIS

KEY POINTS

- Sepsis is the leading cause of morbidity and mortality in equine neonates.
- Events prior to, during, or after parturition may predispose a neonate to infection.
- Historical information and physical examination findings are important in diagnosis.
- Infection may be localized or generalized.
- Treatment intensity depends on the severity of the disease.
- Preventive measures may include good management practices.

DEFINITION/OVERVIEW

Sepsis is the most important cause of morbidity and mortality in the neonatal foal. Often the neonate survives the initial insult, but secondary complications occur and result in a devastating and unfavorable long-term outcome. Sepsis was originally defined as a systemic disease caused by microorganisms and their by-products. This definition is partially correct, but microorganisms and their by-products are just the tip of the iceberg. A more appropriate definition identifies sepsis as a response caused by a cascade of intrinsic mediators released in response to the presence of bacterial toxins, resulting in reactions mediating the host's attempt to destroy the bacteria and tissues infected by the bacteria. The body's response with pro-inflammatory mediators is termed systemic inflammatory response syndrome (SIRS), which is normally counterbalanced with a compensatory anti-inflammatory response syndrome (CARS). If this system gets out of control, multiple organ dysfunction can occur and eventually death can result. Early recognition of the risk factors that can predispose the neonate to infection and eventual septicemia is as important as treating the disease. The predisposing risk factors (*Table 13*) may be events

---

Table 13. Risk factors that may predispose the neonate to infectious diseases

Foal

- Prematurity
- Hypoxic ischemic disease (neonatal maladjustment, "dummy foal" syndrome)
- Hypothermia
- Failure of passive transfer
- Immature or suppressed immune response
- Stress
- Poor nutrition
- Poor husbandry
- Delayed time to stand
- Delayed time to nurse
- Rejection by the dam

Mare

- Premature lactation
- Vaginal discharge
- Premature placental separation
- Placentitis
- Prenatal illness in the dam
- Dystocia
- Poor nutrition
- Poor husbandry
- Stress

that occurred prior to parturition (e.g., illness of the dam or premature lactation) or after parturition (e.g., FPT or hypothermia). Early recognition of signs of sepsis and intervention are key to the successful outcome for the individual. As with other infectious diseases, prevention is very important.

ETIOLOGY/PATHOPHYSIOLOGY

In addition to common bacterial causes (*Table 14*), viral infections (equine viral arteritis [EVA], equine herpesvirus [EHV]-1 and -4) and systemic fungal infections (*Candida albicans*) can result in sepsis.

Infections can be acquired *in utero*, during birth, or after birth. Portals of entry of pathogens include the gastrointestinal (GI) tract, respiratory tract, placenta (secondary to *in-utero* infection) and umbilicus. Often the route of infection can be difficult to identify exactly.

CLINICAL PRESENTATION

It is important to remember that a septic neonate may show no localizing signs of illness and that severe disease may be present before any clinical signs are observed. Early in the disease, subtle nonspecific signs include slight lethargy, weakening suckle reflex, diminished appetite, and excessive time spent in lateral recumbency or sleeping (**40, 41**). Other clinical signs of sepsis include abnormal mucous membranes, abnormal capillary refill time (CRT) associated with the peripheral vasodilation and increased cardiac output, tachycardia, tachypnea, bounding peripheral pulses, extremities that are still warm, and variable body temperature (**42, 43**). Late in the disease process the foal may be recumbent, dehydrated, and almost moribund, have cold extremities, be hypotensive, have weak peripheral pulses, be tachycardic, have dry injected mucous membranes with a

prolonged CRT, and show evidence of respiratory compromise. Once the pathogen enters the neonate's body, the infection may localize in a body system or may remain generalized. A localizing infection may result in pneumonia, enteritis, septic arthritis, meningitis, or omphalitis (*Table 15*).

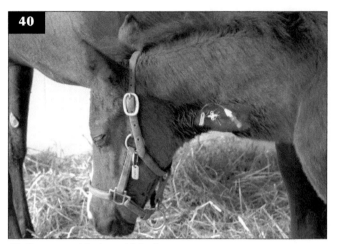

40 Depressed 2-day-old foal.

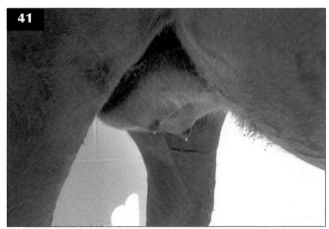

41 Distended udder in a mare. An indication that the foal is not nursing and a cause for concern.

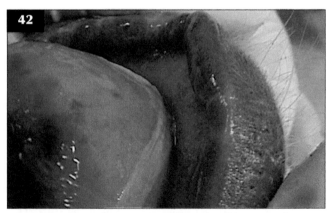

42 Hyperemic oral mucous membranes with areas of petechiation in a 1-day-old septic neonate.

Table 14. Bacterial causes of septicemia in the neonatal foal

Escherichia coli

Klebsiella spp.

Salmonella spp.

Enterobacter spp.

Actinobacillus spp.

Pseudomonas spp.

Enterococcus spp.

Acinetobacter spp.

Streptococcus spp.

Staphylococcus spp.

Clostridium spp.

Pasturella spp.

Bacillus spp.

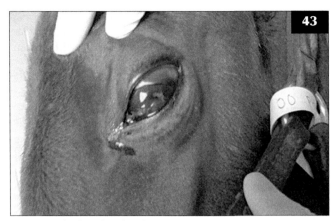

43

43 Septic foal with scleral injection.

DIFFERENTIAL DIAGNOSIS

Sometimes it is difficult to differentiate between hypoxic ischemic disease (neonatal maladjustment syndrome) and sepsis. Occasionally, the newborn foal will succumb to sepsis as a secondary complication of hypoxic ischemic disease. Other differentials include metabolic/endocrine derangements and head trauma.

DIAGNOSIS

A definitive diagnosis is based on a positive blood culture, but there are limitations to this diagnostic modality. First, results are usually not available for at least 48 hours. Second, a large number of foals with histologic evidence of sepsis have a negative blood culture. This may be due to the fact that the foal had been previously treated with antimicrobials or had a low circulating population of bacteria at the time the blood culture was obtained. Therefore, other factors need to be considered in the diagnosis of sepsis in the newborn foal. Often, history and physical examination findings are sufficient for a working diagnosis of sepsis. This should include days of gestation (last breeding date) and any maternal (premature lactation, vulvular discharge), foaling (dystocia, premature placental separation), or postfoaling problems (hypothermia, failure of passive transfer [FPT]). Any abnormalities (see *Table 13*) should raise the suspicion for sepsis. Initially, changes in the physical examination may only be subtle and may consist of changes in the foal's behavior such as depression and lethargy. A careful physical examination of the mare may indicate that her udder is distended and leaking milk, indicating that the foal is not nursing well. In other cases the foal may present recumbent, obtunded, hypotensive, and dehydrated, indicating septic shock.

Leukopenia, characterized by neutropenia, is the most common hematologic abnormality noted in an acutely septic foal. Hypoglycemia (glucose <3.3 mmol/L [<60 mg/dL]) is often noted in foals <24 hours old with sepsis and results from bacterial consumption, failure to nurse, and lack of glycogen reserves. Common biochemical abnormalities include an azotemia and hyperbilirubinemia. Low immunoglobulin G (IgG) levels have a strong correlation with the presence of sepsis. Fibrinogen can be useful in identifying those individuals that have been infected or exposed to inflammatory placental disease *in utero*, because these individuals have higher than normal fibrinogen at birth. In cases of acute sepsis, fibrinogen values are usually only mildly increased. Other abnormalities noted are acid–base derangements and abnormalities of the coagulation cascade.

Table 15. Organ systems involved in septicemia

System	Disease	Diagnostics	Therapy
Respiratory	Pneumonia Pleuritis	Thoracic radiographs Thoracic ultrasound Percutaneous transtracheal aspirate (if foal is stable) Thoracocentesis	Antimicrobials Intranasal oxygen Mechanical ventilation
Gastrointestinal	Enteritis Ileus Intussusception Volvulus Colitis	Nasogastric refluxing Abdominal ultrasound Abdominal radiographs Exploratory laparotomy	Antimicrobials Fluids Analgesics Prokinetics Parenteral nutrition
Musculoskeletal	Septic arthritis Osteoarthritis	Arthrocentesis (with culture/sensitivity) Radiographs	Antimicrobials joint lavage Regional limb perfusion
Neurologic	Meningitis	Cerebrospinal tap	Antimicrobials Anti-inflammatories Anti-convulsants
Umbilical	Omphalitis Patent urachus	Ultrasound of umbilical structures	Antimicrobials

An additional diagnostic aid, which was initially developed by human neonatologists and has been adapted for the equine, is the sepsis score. Twelve items based on the perinatal information, physical examination, and laboratory data are used to determine the sepsis score. Values for each variable are converted to a score on a scale of 0–4; the higher the score for each individual item, the greater the relationship to sepsis. Perinatal data that are analyzed include problems during pregnancy and gestational age of the neonate. Physical examination findings include temperature, signs suggestive of a local infection, mentation, and the presence of nontraumatic petechiation or scleral injection. Important laboratory data include neutrophil count, band neutrophil count and presence of toxic change within the neutrophil, glucose level, fibrinogen level, and IgG results. Once the score is tallied, a total score of 11 or higher is considered to be septic. The higher the score the more likely the neonate is septic. The sepsis score is a useful clinical tool, but not 100% reliable. A strong clinical suspicion of sepsis should lead one to treat the foal despite a low sepsis score. In this instance a recalculation of the sepsis score 24 hours later may be prudent, especially if the neonate was evaluated in the very early stages of the disease process.

MANAGEMENT

Antimicrobial therapy is the key to a successful outcome when confronted with the possibility of a septic foal and it should be administered as soon as sepsis is suspected. Appropriate antimicrobial therapy should include broad-spectrum antimicrobials that are effective against Gram-positive and Gram-negative organisms. An appropriate choice would be a beta-lactam (e.g., penicillin) and an aminoglycoside (e.g., amikacin). When treating a compromised neonate with an aminoglycoside, therapeutic drug monitoring is recommended to ensure appropriate dosing. In addition, serial creatinine levels or urinalyses are recommended to monitor for potential renal side effects. If the neonate's renal function is questionable, another choice would be a third-generation cephalosporin alone or in combination with penicillin. Once the result of the blood culture is available, antimicrobial therapy may need to be modified. Unfortunately, the range of oral antibiotics is limited. Possible oral antimicrobials to consider include chloramphenicol and trimethoprim–sulfa combinations. Amoxicillin, cefalexin, and cefadoxil have limited bioavailability in older foals. Cefpodoxime proxetil, a third-generation cephalosporin, is available for oral administration, has good bioavailability, and has a reasonable spectrum of coverage. Antimicrobial treatment is usually continued for 2 weeks; longer if a localized infection has developed. If a fungal infection is suspected, the neonate should be treated with antifungals in addition to the antimicrobials.

Providing appropriate nutritional support is critical to the care of a septic neonate. A foal that is still able to nurse on its own should be closely monitored to make sure that it is nursing well, but one that is recumbent and weak should be supplemented with a feeding tube or parenteral feedings of dextrose solution or total parenteral nutrition.

Maintenance or restoration of effective circulating volume is a top priority in cases of sepsis. Aggressive intravenous fluid therapy is the mainstay of cardiovascular support, but in some instances pharmacologic intervention is necessary. An in-depth discussion on fluid therapy and inotropes and vasopressors can be found in Chapter 2 (Shock, Resuscitation, Fluid and Electrolyte Therapy).

Nutritional support is important. If the foal is not nursing supplemental nutrition should be provided either enterally or parenterally. Nutritional options and guidelines are discussed in Chapter 18.

If there is evidence of complete or partial FPT, the neonate should be treated appropriately. Treatment options are discussed in Chapter 4.

Septic foals, especially those that are recumbent, are susceptible to pulmonary dysfunction because of a variety of factors including dependent lung atelectasis, pneumonia, pulmonary edema, and surfactant dysfunction. In these foals it is important to minimize ventilation and perfusion mismatching by maintaining the foal in sternal recumbency and providing humidified intranasal oxygen.

The degree of nursing care required depends on the individual neonate. General nursing care includes monitoring the color and appearance of the mucus membranes and the temperature, pulse, and respiration, keeping the environment clean and dry, and administering medications. Some neonates require intensive care such as frequent turning from side to side, maintaining in sternal recumbency, oxygen therapy, and parenteral nutrition (**44, 45**).

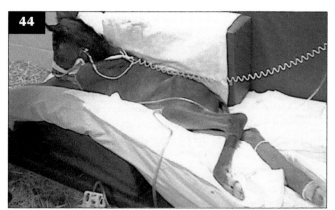

44 Septic neonate receiving supportive care. Note the clean bed. The foal is propped in sternal recumbency and has an intravenous catheter and a urinary catheter.

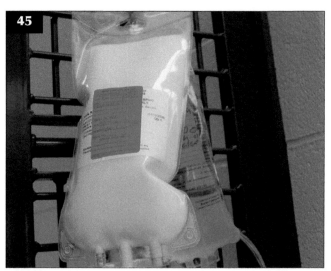

45 Total parenteral nutrition for a septic compromised neonate.

Table 16. Good management practices to reduce the incidence of sick newborn foals

Environment

- Ensure that the foaling stall is clean.

- After foaling, put fresh bedding in the stall.

- Clean/disinfect foaling stall between mares.

- Each stall should have the manure removed daily or twice daily and fresh bedding provided.

Handlers

- Ensure each handler has clean hands prior to handling the newborn foal, especially when working with a foal to encourage it to nurse.

Udder cleanliness

- Clean udder, perineum, and hindquarters *prior* to allowing the newborn foal to nurse.

- Use soap and water and *dry* the area after washing.

- Perform this washing/drying outside the stall to prevent contamination of the stall.

Colostral intake

- Ensure that the mare has good quality colostrum either by testing or visual inspection.

- Make sure the foal nurses adequately prior to 12 hours of age.

- If any concern about the quality or quantity of colostrum, provide another source.

- If any concern about the foal's ability to nurse, tube feed with colostrum.

- Ensure adequate passive transfer of IgG. If failure of passive transfer, treat with plasma.

Umbilical care

- Ensure proper umbilical care with 4% chlorohexidine solution or povidone–iodine solution.

- Treat twice a day for 2–3 days.

- Wash hands before and after treatment.

Other organ systems (e.g., respiratory, GI) may be initially involved or become secondarily infected. *Table 15* summarizes the disease manifestations, diagnostics procedures, and therapies involved in dealing with these systems.

The long-term prognosis in foals with several organ systems involved is guarded. Those without multiple organs system sequelae have a good prognosis. The key to prevention is good management (*Table 16*).

VIRAL INFECTIONS

EQUINE VIRAL ARTERITIS

KEY POINTS

- Persistently infected stallions are reservoirs.
- EVA is a cause of abortion.
- Rare cause of respiratory distress, interstitial pneumonia, and enteritis in foals.
- Passive immunity is important.
- Causes nonspecific clinical signs in the foal.

DEFINITION/OVERVIEW

EVA is a contagious viral disease that is distributed worldwide. Seroprevalence is higher in Standardbreds and Warmbloods. Persistently infected stallions are critical reservoirs in the equine population. Infection early in gestation results in abortion (**46**). Although it is rare, EVA causes a severe fulminating interstitial pneumonia and fibrinonecrotic enteritis in foals.

ETIOLOGY/PATHOPHYSIOLOGY

EVA is caused by equine arteritis virus (EAV), which is an arteriovirus (an RNA virus). The two most important modes of transmission of EVA are via the respiratory route, involving infective aerosolized respiratory tract secretions of an acutely infected horse, and venereally by an acute or chronically infected stallion.

A congenitally acquired infection results from transplacental transmission of EAV when a pregnant mare is exposed to the virus very late in gestation. Often the signs of maternal infection are mild and overlooked. Initial multiplication of virus takes place in bronchial macrophages in the lungs.

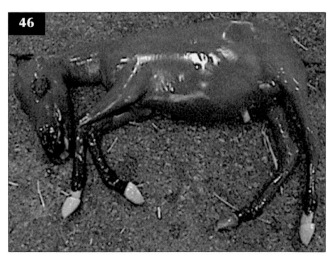

46 Aborted fetus.

Within 48 hours of infection, EAV can be found in the regional lymph nodes, especially the bronchial nodes. By the third day after challenge, viremia has developed and virus is widely distributed in various body tissues and fluids. The virus causes a panvasculitis, with initial lesions in the blood vessels of the lungs and then throughout the body. The virus also localizes in various epithelial sites.

CLINICAL PRESENTATION
Affected foals may be born weak or they may be born healthy and develop respiratory signs within the first 48 hours of life. Clinical signs of EVA include fever, weakness, depression, anorexia, cough, epiphora, nasal discharge, dependent limb edema, colic, and diarrhea. The foal may present in respiratory distress or it may be found dead. The severity of clinical signs observed in these cases may be attributed either to the route of infection, the strain of the virus and the size of the virus challenge, or the immune status of the foal.

DIFFERENTIAL DIAGNOSIS
Without histologic evaluation of tissues and virus isolation, EVA is difficult to distinguish from other causes of respiratory distress (see *Table 45*), fever (see *Table 19*), or pneumonia (EHV-1/4, influenza, see *Table 49*) in the foal.

DIAGNOSIS
Antemortem diagnosis can be difficult to make. A history of endemic disease or recent abortions on the farm can aid in the diagnosis. Clinical pathologic findings in affected individuals include hypoxia, hypercapnia, respiratory acidosis sometimes complicated by metabolic acidosis, neutropenia/neutrophilia, lymphopenia/lymphocytosis, thrombocytopenia, and hyperfibrinogenemia. However, these clinical pathologic findings are not exclusively indicative of EVA.

Positive serology tests for EVA suggest *in-utero* infection, although only a pre-suckle sample is reliable due to the passive transfer of maternal immunity in seroconverted mares. Specimens for virus isolation from the live animal include nasopharyngeal swabs or washings, conjunctival swabs, and citrated ethylenediamine tetra-acetic acid (EDTA) or heparinized blood samples. The organism can also be isolated from amniotic fluids. Specimens must be sent to an appropriate laboratory.

MANAGEMENT
Appropriate nursing care, nutritional support, respiratory support, and antimicrobial therapy should be included in the management of these cases. Foals with EVA are generally born to seronegative mares, therefore treatment with intravenous plasma with a high titer against EVA may be beneficial. Passive immunity seems to play a large role in protection against this disease in neonates, therefore ingestion of good quality colostrum from a vaccinated mare is protective for the foal. Foals that are suspected of having EVA should be isolated because they are generally shedding large quantities of virus and pose a threat to other neonates and pregnant mares.

Overall, the prognosis is grave.

EQUINE HERPESVIRUS

KEY POINTS
- Equine herpesvirus is ubiquitous in the equine population.
- Most often has a fatal outcome in neonates.
- Older foals usually succumb to a secondary bacterial infection.
- Neonates often icteric with neutropenia and lymphopenia.
- Diagnostics include detection of viral particles via polymerase chain reaction.

DEFINITION/OVERVIEW
The horse is the host to several herpesviruses. EHV-1 causes respiratory disease, abortions, and equine herpesvirus encephalomyelitis. EHV-1 has been documented to cause fatal interstitial pneumonia in the neonate. In the older foal, EHV-1 and EHV-4 commonly cause infection of the upper respiratory tract, but may also disrupt the normal defense mechanism of the airway, allowing the establishment of secondary bacterial infections. EHV-2 is ubiquitous in horses and may cause keratoconjunctivitis and pharyngeal lymphoid hyperplasia in young horses (**47**).

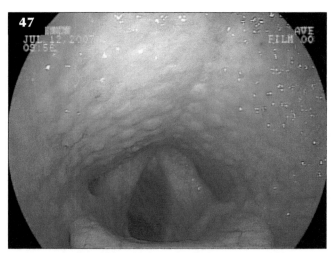

47 Pharyngeal lymphoid hyperplasia in a 2-year-old horse.

ETIOLOGY/PATHOPHYSIOLOGY

EHV-1 and -4 are alpha herpesviruses, whereas EHV-2 and EHV-5 are gamma herpesviruses. EHVs are ubiquitous in the equine population because of their ability to establish a latent infection. Severe neonatal illness can result when the mare is infected with EHV-1 during late gestation. Infection in the older foal is from exposure to another infected animal.

The virus attaches and replicates in the mucosal epithelial cells of the nasal passage, pharynx, and tonsillar tissue. The virus is then transported to other organs by mononuclear cells. The incubation period is 2–10 days.

CLINICAL PRESENTATION

The neonate may be born weak or normal, although clinical signs will appear within 48 hours of birth. Clinical signs include respiratory distress, weakness, icterus, fever, tachycardia, petechial hemorrhages, and, in some cases, diarrhea. The older foal may only have mild signs including biphasic fever, depression, and serous nasal discharge. Often, clinical signs of a secondary bacterial infection are evident.

DIFFERENTIAL DIAGNOSIS

It is difficult to differentiate a herpesvirus infection from other causes of a weak newborn such as septicemia, hypoxic ischemic disease (neonatal maladjustment syndrome), metabolic/electrolyte abnormalities, and neonatal isoerythrolysis (NI). Additional differentials would include causes of fever (see *Table 19*) and causes of respiratory distress (see *Table 45*).

DIAGNOSIS

A complete farm history of respiratory disease or recent abortions may aid in the diagnosis. Physical examination usually does not help differentiate EHV-1 from other infectious diseases, although icteric mucous membranes is a common physical examination finding.

Clinical pathologic changes such as leukopenia characterized by a left shift, neutropenia, and severe lymphopenia are suggestive, but not definitive, of perinatal EHV-1 infection. In some cases, liver enzymes are increased.

Serologic testing of acute and convalescent sera will demonstrate a fourfold rise in antibody titers in those foals with recent infections. However, the results of serologic testing may be difficult to interpret because some do not seroconvert and maternal antibodies may give a false-positive result. Virus isolation can be performed on samples obtained from a nasal swab (**48**), heparinized whole blood sample and tissue, although these results may take a few days. Polymerase chain reaction (PCR) is a rapid diagnostic aid and can be performed on nasal swabs and whole blood collected in EDTA samples. Recently quantitative ("real-time") PCR techniques have been devised that allow estimation of virus load in samples, which is helpful for diagnosis of latently infected horses.

MANAGEMENT

Treatment for neonatal EHV-1 infection usually includes intensive nursing care, respiratory support, antimicrobial therapy, nutritional support, and NSAIDs. Antiviral medications such as acyclovir and valacyclovir have been used in the treatment of EHV-1 infections.

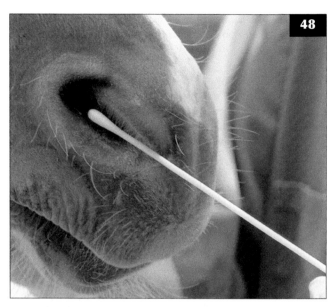

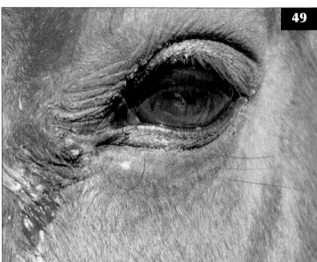

48 Swabbing the nasal passage with a polyester-tipped swab to test for viral diseases. **49** Ocular discharge in a 2-month-old foal with viral infection.

Little information exists on the pharmacokinetics and activity of these medications in foals. Hyperimmunized plasma may be beneficial. Foals that are suspected of having EHV-1 should be isolated because they are generally shedding large quantities of virus and pose a threat to other neonates and any pregnant mare. In the older foal with mild clinical signs, treatment should include rest, monitoring for secondary complications, and isolation.

The majority of foals infected with EHV-1 in the perinatal period die, and those that survive require intensive care.

EQUINE INFLUENZA

KEY POINTS
- Highly contagious.
- Transmission primarily through nose-to-nose contact.
- May cause mild clinical signs or fatal interstitial pneumonia.

- Most often sets the individual up for a secondary bacterial infection.
- Diagnosis based on immunoassay testing for viral antigen or virus isolation.

DEFINITION/OVERVIEW

Equine influenza causes respiratory outbreaks worldwide in horses of all ages. The pediatric patient is susceptible, especially when stressed or in situations of overcrowding and in areas with poor ventilation. Infection can result in mild clinical signs to a fatal interstitial pneumonia.

ETIOLOGY/PATHOPHYSIOLOGY

Equine influenza is caused by an orthomyxovirus that has many variants. This virus is classified into subtypes based on hemagglutinin and neuraminidase surface antigens.

Transmission is primarily through direct nose-to-nose contact and the virus is highly contagious. The aerosolized virus is inhaled and attaches to the N-acetylneuraminic acid receptors on respiratory cells by hemagglutinin spikes on the organism. The neuraminidase alters the efficiency of the mucocilliary apparatus. Replication of the virus occurs after endocytosis of the organism into the cell and release into the cytoplasm of the cell. The virus spreads throughout the respiratory tract within 1–3 days, damaging the epithelial cell and cilia in the trachea and bronchial trees.

CLINICAL PRESENTATION

Clinical signs of an equine influenza infection can sometimes be mild (e.g., fever, lethargy, anorexia, serous nasal discharge, and occasionally a dry deep cough). Severe signs include respiratory distress with nostril flare, labored breathing, and an anxious appearance.

DIFFERENTIAL DIAGNOSIS

Influenza infections can be difficult to differentiate from other bacterial, fungal, or viral causes of pneumonia. If there is no evidence of a pulmonary cause for the fever or respiratory distress, other body systems need to be investigated (see *Tables 19* and *45*).

DIAGNOSIS

As with other viral infections, a complete farm history should be obtained and a thorough physical examination of the individual should be performed. Abnormal lung sounds may be auscultated, especially if secondary bacterial infections are present.

Hematologic changes initially include leukopenia characterized by a moderate to marked lymphopenia, and later a monocytosis. These changes are transient and are only seen early in the course of the disease. Later, a neutrophilia and hyperfibrinogenemia may be documented, especially if a secondary bacterial infection is established. Arterial blood gas may display hypoxemia, depending on the severity of the infection. However, none of these hematologic changes are diagnostic for influenza.

Virus isolation can be performed using nasopharyngeal swabs, nasopharyngeal lavage, or tracheal aspiration within the first 24–48 hours of infection. After this time, success in isolating the virus diminishes. Immunoassays for detection of viral antigen, can be run on nasal discharge or a nasal swab that has been placed in virus isolation media. Reverse transcription PCR on nasopharyngeal swabs and nasal or tracheal wash samples is the test of choice as it is highly sensitive and provides rapid diagnosis. Serum antibody titer is usually not very useful because maternal antibodies will make interpreting the results difficult. Diagnosis based on titer levels requires comparison of acute and convalescent samples.

MANAGEMENT

In those individuals suspected of having mild infections, therapy should include monitoring for secondary complications, rest, and isolation from susceptible animals. Therapy in individuals that present in respiratory distress should include broad-spectrum antimicrobials and anti-inflammatories. Depending on the case, intranasal oxygen and appropriate nutritional support may be beneficial. Prevention includes vaccinating mares at appropriate times prior to foaling and vaccinating foals around 3 months of age (*Tables 17* and *18*).

Table 17. Recommended vaccination schedule for foals

Recommendations are for foals that have received adequate colostrum from mares or plasma from donors that have been vaccinated for tetanus, influenza, rhinopneumonitis, Eastern and Western encephalomyelitis, rabies, and West Nile virus (± rotavirus and botulism).

Age	Protocol
5–6 months	EHV-1 and -4, Eastern and Western encephalomyelitis, tetanus, West Nile virus, rabies
6–7 months	EHV-1 and -4, Eastern and Western encephalomyelitis, tetanus, West Nile virus, rabies, influenza (i/m or intranasal)
8–9 months	EHV-1 and -4, Eastern and Western encephalomyelitis, tetanus, influenza (i/m or intranasal)
10–11 months	Influenza (i/m only)

If in an area endemic for botulism, administer Bot-Tox at 3, 4, and 5 months of age.

Refer to the American Association of Equine Practitioners website.

Table 18. Guidelines for vaccinating broodmares

• Tetanus toxoid, influenza: 1 month prior to foaling

• Eastern/Western encephalomyelitis, West Nile virus: 4–6 weeks prior to foaling

• Rabies: 4–6 weeks prior to foaling

• Rhinopneumonitis: months 3, 5, 7, and 9 of pregnancy

Note: These are general guidelines. Some may vary depending on location.

Additional vaccinations that can be administered depending on location:

• 8th, 9th, 10th month of pregnancy: botulism (if previously had botulism series, only one booster is needed 30 days before foaling)

• 8th, 9th, 10th month of pregnancy: rotavirus (mare needs three vaccinations each year)

Note: Avoid vaccinating during the first trimester.

Refer to the American Association of Equine Practitioners website.

EQUINE ADENOVIRUS

KEY POINTS
- Most often causes subclinical infection.
- Fatal to Arabian foals with severe combined immunodeficiency (SCID).
- Immunocompetent foals recover, immunocompromised foals do not.
- Can predispose to secondary bacterial infections.

DEFINITION/OVERVIEW
Adenovirus as a cause of disease is reported sporadically, and fatal adenoviral infections occur only in immunocompromised foals. Nonfatal infections have been diagnosed in both immunocompetent and immunocompromised foals. Adenovirus may predispose foals to secondary bacterial infection, resulting in foal pneumonia.

ETIOLOGY/PATHOPHYSIOLOGY
Equine adenovirus infection is caused by an adenovirus, which is widespread in the equine population. Equine adenovirus type 1 (EAdV1) has been isolated from horses with respiratory signs and equine adenovirus type 2 has been isolated from the feces of foals with diarrhea. The virus persists in the upper respiratory tract (URT) of adult horses. It attacks the respiratory epithelium, resulting in swollen epithelial cells that slough into the bronchioles and alveoli, leading to pulmonary atelectasis and bronchopneumonia. Adenovirus may also infect gastrointestinal cells and is shed in feces.

CLINICAL PRESENTATION
Clinical signs in foals with equine adenovirus infection include depression, weakness, fever, cough, abnormal lung sounds, and ocular (**49**) and nasal discharge. Diarrhea has been reported in 25% of the documented cases. Usually, the infection is subclinical.

DIFFERENTIAL DIAGNOSIS
Differentials include other causes of fever (*Table 19*) and coughing (see *Table 48*).

Table 19. Causes of fever in the pediatric patient

Viral disease (upper respiratory tract)

Strangles (*Streptococcus equi*)

Pneumonia (bacterial, viral, or fungal)

Pleuropneumonia/pleuritis

Gastrointestinal disorder—enteritis, salmonellosis, *Rotavirus*

Colitis—salmonellosis, *Rotavirus*, clostridiosis

Septicemia

Septic arthritis

Urachal abscess

Peritonitis

Abscess—thoracic, abdominal, hepatic

Tyzzer's disease

Pericarditis

Bacterial endocarditis

Pneumocystis carinii pneumonia

Neoplasia

Immune-mediated hemolytic anemia

Immune-mediated thrombocytopenia

Neonatal isoerythrolysis

Combined immunodeficiency of foals

Hepatitis

Hypoxic ischemic disease/encephalopathy

DIAGNOSIS

Polymerase chain reaction is the most readily available test for detection of EAdV-1 from a nasal pharyngeal swab, wash, or transtracheal aspirate. Serologic testing by hemagglutination inhibition can detect a rise in antibody titers in samples taken 10–14 days apart. Other diagnostics tests include virus isolation or electron microscopy. The Arabian breed is more susceptible, especially if diagnosed with SCID. Lymphopenia is a constant finding in all fatal cases. In nonfatal cases, a transient lymphopenia is observed and is followed by lymphocytosis.

MANAGEMENT

Treatment includes broad-spectrum antimicrobials and appropriate supportive care. Hyperimmunized plasma is beneficial if the foal has FPT.

Immunocompetent foals usually make a full recovery, whereas immunocompromised foals often do not recover.

BACTERIAL INFECTIONS

STREPTOCOCCUS EQUI

KEY POINTS

- If fever, purulent nasal discharge, and submandibular lymphadenopathy, consider *S. equi* until proven otherwise.
- Organism requires equid for survival, therefore carrier animal can harbor organism for years.
- Transmission is by nose-to-nose contact or indirectly via fomites.
- Treatment varies depending on the severity of clinical signs.
- Best means of prevention is good management practice including isolating and testing new arrivals.

DEFINITION/OVERVIEW

Streptococcus equi, the causative agent of equine strangles, typically causes a disease of the URT and lymph nodes, although disease of the lower respiratory tract (LRT) can occur. Strangles can infect foals, especially in cases of a herd outbreak. Good farm management is important in protecting foals from infection.

ETIOLOGY/PATHOPHYSIOLOGY

S. equi is a Gram-positive organism that requires an equid for its survival. Infection can occur by direct nose-to-nose contact with a diseased animal, indirectly by contact with a contaminated fomite, or, rarely, through aerosolization of secretions from a carrier animal that is shedding the organism. Carrier animals can harbor the organism in the guttural pouches and may shed the organism intermittently for many months to years. The incubation period varies from 3 to 14 days after exposure.

The organism enters the nose or mouth and attaches to the lingual and palatine tonsils, forming microabscesses. Within hours, the organism travels to the lymph nodes in the pharyngeal or tonsillar region and multiplies. Spread to other lymph nodes or organs may be hematogenous or by lymphatic channels. The organism evades phagocytosis through a combination of the SeM protein and the hyaluronic acid capsule. The SeM protein may also be responsible for adherence to (or penetration of) the nasopharyngeal mucosa. Pyrogenic mitogens SePE-H and SePE-I are involved in the acute-phase reaction and local edema by triggering release of

proinflammatory cytokines from mononuclear cells. Variations in the virulence of the organism are a result of the level of expression of the SeM protein and hyaluronic acid capsule.

CLINICAL PRESENTATION

S. equi infection is typically a disease of the URT, although LRT disease and bastard strangles have been reported. The onset of disease is marked by depression, fever, mucoid nasal discharge, slight cough, loss of appetite, difficulty swallowing, and slight swelling and tenderness in the intermandibular area. Eventually, the nasal discharge becomes purulent and the abscesses in the submandibular, submaxillary, or retropharyngeal lymph nodes enlarge and become hard and painful (**50, 51**). Most animals recover quickly after rupture and drainage of the lymph nodes. Abscessation of the retropharyngeal lymph nodes can result in compression of the trachea or larynx and acute respiratory obstruction. Guttural pouch empyema may result if the abscessed retropharyngeal lymph nodes rupture into the pouch (**52**). Bronchopneumonia can result from aspiration of pus

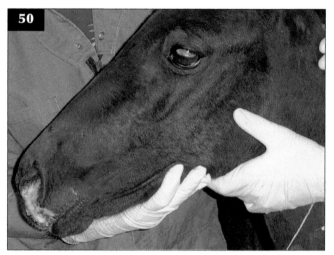

50 Purulent nasal discharge in a 1-month-old foal.

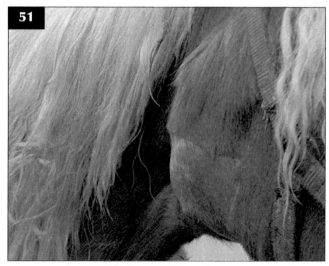

51 A retropharyngeal abscess due to *Streptococcus equi* infection.

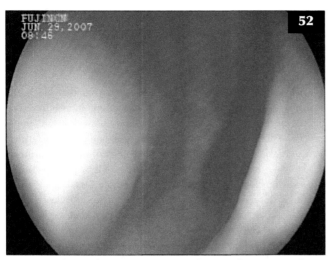

52 Guttural pouch empyema. Note the purulent material on the floor of the guttural pouch.

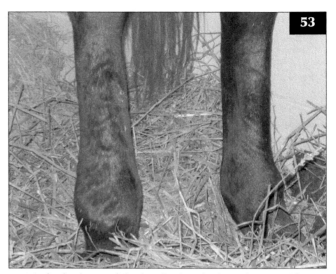

53 Marked edema of the hindlimbs of a broodmare with purpura hemorrhagica secondary to a recent *S. equi* infection.

or metastatic spread of the organism to the lungs. Bastard strangles occurs when the organism metastasizes and abscesses occur in other organs, with clinical signs noted months after the initial infection. Purpura hemorrhagica is an aseptic necrotizing vasculitis associated with *S. equi* infections and it is believed to be due to immune complex deposition in blood vessel walls. Nasal shedding does not begin until a day or two after the onset of the fever and persists for 2–3 weeks.

DIFFERENTIAL DIAGNOSIS
See *Tables 19, 45*, and *47*.

DIAGNOSIS
A complete farm history is a helpful aid in diagnosing *S. equi* infection. Physical examination findings of swelling and tenderness in the intermandibular area on a foal from a farm with an endemic problem should raise red flags.

Hematologic changes include a neutrophilia and hyperfibrinogenemia, although these are nonspecific for *S. equi*.

Bacterial culture of purulent material from an abscessed lymph node, a nasal swab, or a pharyngeal lavage or guttural pouch lavage is the gold standard for detection of *S. equi*. Fluid obtained from a pharyngeal lavage or guttural pouch lavage can be submitted to an appropriate laboratory for PCR identification. PCR does not differentiate between dead and live organisms; therefore, a positive test should be confirmed by culture. PCR is useful for detecting asymptomatic carriers and in determining the success of elimination of the organism from the guttural pouches. Serum can be submitted for SeM-specific antibodies and is useful in diagnosing recent infection, but not necessarily current infection. The SeM-specific antibodies can also be used to support a diagnosis of *S. equi*-associated purpura hemorrhagica (**53**) or bastard strangles.

See also bacterial and viral pneumonia in Chapter 8 (Respiratory Disorders).

MANAGEMENT
S. equi is sensitive to many antimicrobials including penicillin, chloramphenicol, erythromycin, and tetracycline, although an appropriate sensitivity pattern should be obtained at the time of

culture. Treatment with systemic antimicrobials in cases with mild signs and no evidence of respiratory compromise or systemic involvement is controversial. Ideally, systemic antimicrobial therapy should be reserved for individuals that are in respiratory distress from obstruction of the airway by enlarged retropharyngeal lymph nodes, have had high fevers for a prolonged period of time, have prolonged depression, or show involvement of other organ systems. A tracheostomy and additional nursing care may be required in foals with severe respiratory compromise. Foals with guttural pouch empyema are treated with daily lavage of the guttural pouch until most of the exudate is removed (**54**). In addition, penicillin mixed with gelatin is instilled into the pouch. The gelatin–penicillin mix is more effective in remaining in the pouches than a straight aqueous solution. If purulent material persists in the guttural pouches, inspissation occurs resulting in discrete masses known as chondroids.

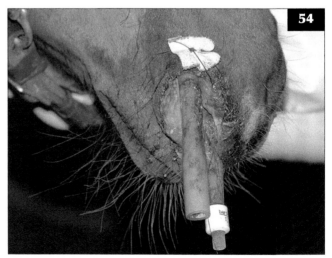

54 An indwelling Foley catheter for topical treatment and lavage of the guttural pouch due to a *S. equi* infection in a 2-month-old foal.

55 Chondroids in the guttural pouch of a 4-month-old foal. An attempt is being made to remove the chondroids using a polyp retrieval basket. (Courtesy of B. Waldridge.)

Nonsurgical removal of chondroids can be achieved by using a polyp retrieval basket through the biopsy channel of an endoscope (**55**).

Infected individuals should be isolated until a guttural pouch lavage sample tested by PCR and culture is negative or until three consecutive weekly nasopharyngeal lavage samples tested by PCR and culture are negative. Prevention of spread during an outbreak and prevention in general includes isolation of individuals that are clinically affected, isolation of foals known or suspected to be infected, and isolation of foals exposed to clinically affected horses. New animals should be isolated for 21 days and screened for *S. equi* by repeated nasopharyngeal swabs or lavages. Another screening procedure is PCR and culture of a guttural pouch lavage because the guttural pouches are where the vast majority of subclinical infections (carriers) occur. Several intramuscular vaccines are available, but the level of immunity stimulated by these vaccines is low because of failure to induce local protection. An intranasal vaccine is available, which produces an appropriate mucosal response along with an appropriate serum response. In the case of an outbreak, the best management practice is to isolate, segregate, and treat as needed and eventually identify and treat carrier animals.

The prognosis is good if there is no systemic involvement or respiratory compromise.

RHODOCOCCUS EQUI

KEY POINTS
- *R. equi* is endemic in some areas.
- Causes bronchopneumonia, although 50% of the time extra-pulmonary lesions are present.
- Diagnosis is confirmed by culture or PCR amplification of virulence associated protein A.
- Treatment is with a macrolide and rifampin for 4–6 weeks.
- Prognosis is poor with multiple organ systems infected.
- Prevention and early identification of affected foals is important.

DEFINITION/OVERVIEW
Rhodococcus equi is a soil saprophyte that is also found commonly in herbivore feces. It is an important cause of subacute to chronic

bronchopneumonia in foals up to 6 months of age. Infection usually manifests itself as a bronchopneumonia with abscessation, although extrapulmonary lesions are frequently reported.

ETIOLOGY/PATHOPHYSIOLOGY
R. equi is a pleomorphic Gram-positive organism that has been frequently isolated from soil samples throughout the world, even in areas never inhabited by horses. Despite this widespread environmental distribution, *R. equi* infection is endemic to some farms, occurs occasionally on others, or may never be found on a farm.

The major route of exposure is inhalation of dust particles laden with virulent *R. equi* organisms. Virulent strains express a 15–17 kDa virulence associated protein (vapA) and have a large virulence plasmid of 85–90 kb containing the vapA gene. The pathogenesis of the organism is related to its ability to survive and replicate within alveolar macrophages by inhibiting phagosome–lysosome fusion and altering the normal phagocyte maturation process. Only vapA-positive bacteria are capable of inhibiting this fusion. Ultimately, the replication of *R. equi* within macrophages results in the death of the host cell.

CLINICAL PRESENTATION
The clinical signs of bronchopneumonia due to *R. equi* infection are variable. Early clinical signs of bronchopneumonia are vague and include mild fever or a slight increase in respiratory rate. As the pneumonia progresses, the clinical signs include inappetence, lethargy, fever, and tachypnea. An increased effort, a nostril flare, and an increased abdominal component characterize the tachypnea. Occasionally, a foal will present in acute respiratory distress. Extrapulmonary lesions can be associated with pneumonia or be independent of pneumonia. The most common extrapulmonary manifestations, which include the GI, musculoskeletal, optic, neurologic, hematologic, cardiovascular, and hepatic systems (**56–58** and **59–62**) are summarized in *Table 20*. Infection of the liver, kidneys, heart, and integument rarely occurs.

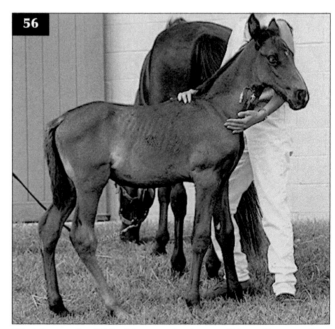

56 A 2-month-old foal in poor body condition, diagnosed with a *R. equi* abdominal abscess.

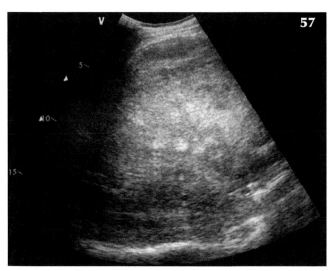

57 *R. equi* infection. Ultrasonographic view of a large abdominal abscess.

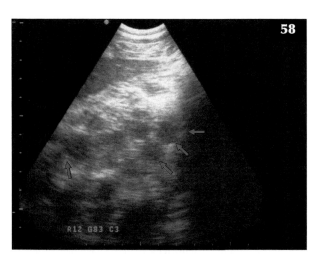

58 *R. equi* infection. Ultrasonographic view of multiple small mesenteric abscesses (arrows).

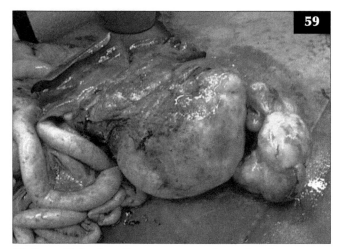

59 *R. equi* infection. Postmortem specimen showing an abdominal abscess.

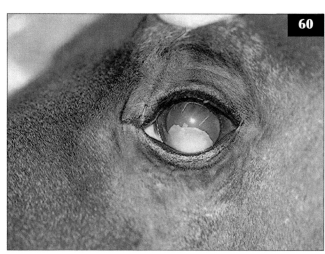

60 Anterior uveitis secondary to *R. equi* infection.

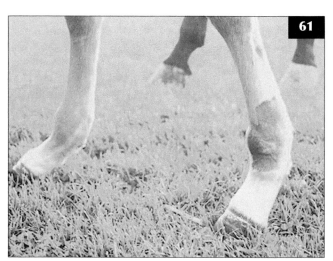

61 Immune-mediated polysynovitis secondary to *R. equi* infection.

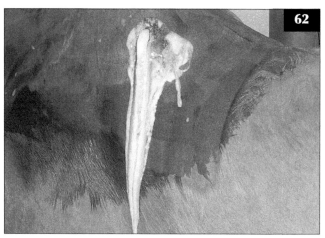

62 A subcutaneous abscess along the neck of a 4-month-old foal. Culture identified *R. equi* as the source of the infection.

Table 20. Extrapulmonary manifestations of *R. equi* infection

Organ system	Disease	Clinical signs	Diagnostics	Treatment
Gastrointestinal	Ulcerative colitis Abdominal lymphadenitis Typhlitis Single, large abdominal abscess	Colic Diarrhea Weight loss Poor growth	Abdominal ultrasound Abdominocentesis (culture/sensitivity) Exploratory laparotomy	Antimicrobials Fluids Analgesics Anti-inflammatories
Musculoskeletal	Polysynovitis Septic arthritis Osteomyelitis	Joint distension Lameness (rarely apparent with polysynovitis)	Arthrocentesis Cytology and culture Radiographs	Antimicrobials Anti-inflammatories Lavage of joint (if septic) Arthrotomy
Ophthalmologic	Anterior uveitis Panophthalmitis	Blepharospasm Fibrin in anterior chamber	Ophthalmologic examination History of *R. equi* Stain cornea	Antimicrobials for *R. equi* Systemic anti-inflammatories Topical NSAIDs
Hematologic	Anemia Thrombocytopenia	Weakness Pale mucous membranes Pigmenturia Petechiation	CBC Platelet count	Maintain antimicrobial therapy for *R. equi* Corticosteroids Blood transfusion
Neurologic	Vertebral body abscess Vertebral body osteomyelitis	Ataxia Paresis	Radiographs Ultrasound CSF tap (often unrewarding)	Antimicrobials Anti-inflammatories

DIFFERENTIAL DIAGNOSIS

Bacterial culture results are needed to differentiate *R. equi* from other causes of bacterial pneumonia (see *Table 49*), other causes of fever (see *Table 19*), and respiratory distress (see *Table 45*).

DIAGNOSIS

History of previous *R. equi* pneumonia on a farm may help to identify an at-risk individual. Initial auscultation of the thorax reveals a diffuse increase in bronchial sounds, which progresses to localized cranioventral wheezes and, eventually, to diffuse crackles with marked tracheal sounds.

Radiographs of the thorax will reveal changes that vary from a prominent interstitial pattern to dense patchy alveolar opacities, lung consolidation, and abscesses (**63**). Radiographs can help to establish the severity of the lesions and the response to therapy.

Thoracic ultrasound can be helpful if the lesions extend to the periphery, but radiographs are generally more useful. Ultrasound changes can range from pulmonary consolidation to discrete nodular densities (**64–66**).

Common hematologic changes include hyperfibrinogenemia and neutrophilic leukocytosis, with or without a monocytosis, although these changes are nonspecific for *R. equi*. Anemia or thrombocytopenia would indicate immune-mediated destruction of the RBCs or platelets.

Cytologic evaluation and aerobic bacterial culture of a transtracheal aspirate is the best way to make a diagnosis and can distinguish *R. equi* pneumonia from other forms of pneumonia and also aid in establishing a sensitivity pattern. Cytologic evaluation

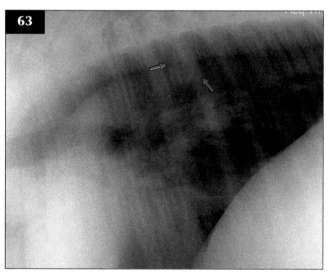

63 Radiograph of a 3-month-old foal with *R. equi* pneumonia. Note the opacities (arrows), which have a "cotton ball" appearance.

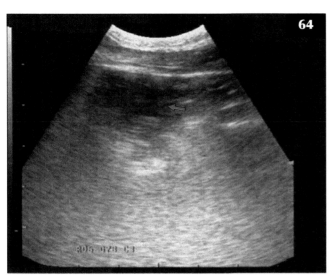

64 Ultrasound of the thorax of a 2-month-old foal with *R. equi* pneumonia. Note the pulmonary abscess (arrow).

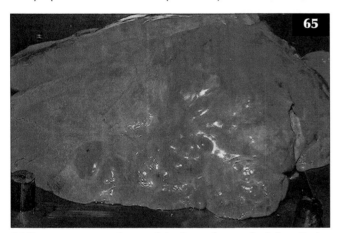

65 Postmortem specimen of the lungs from a foal that died of *R. equi* pneumonia. Note the numerous abscesses.

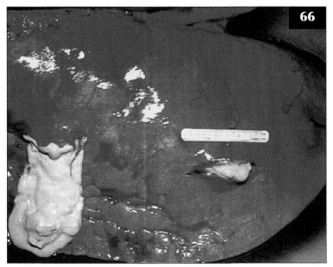

66 Postmortem specimen of the lungs from a foal that died of *R. equi* pneumonia. Note the purulent material within the abscess.

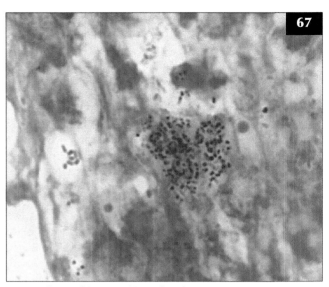

67 Cytology of *R. equi*. Note the characteristic Gram-positive pleomorphic rods, which also have a "Chinese figure" or "watermelon seed" appearance. (Courtesy of S. Reed)

reveals Gram-positive pleomorphic rods, which are suggestive of *R. equi* (67). If a transtracheal wash cannot be performed because of the severity of the disease, a presumptive diagnosis can be made from clinical signs, hematologic changes, the age of the foal, and a history of an endemic problem on the farm.

Serologic tests have low sensitivity and specificity. A positive diagnosis can be made by amplification of the vapA gene using PCR from transtracheal aspirate, but bacterial culture offers the advantage of antimicrobial susceptibility testing and identification of other bacteria.

MANAGEMENT

The most common antimicrobial combination used to treat *R. equi* infection is a macrolide (erythromycin, azithromycin, or clarithromycin) with rifampin. These drugs are bacteriostatic and synergistic against *R. equi* and the combination is lipophilic in nature and penetrates abscesses and cells. The advantages of azithromycin and clarithromycin include enhanced oral bioavailability, prolonged half-lives, and higher concentrations in pulmonary epithelial lining fluid (PELF) and bronchoalveolar cells. Gamithromycin, a long-acting macrolide approved to treat respiratory disease in cattle, is active against *R. equi*. Intramuscular administration maintains adequate levels in PELF and phagocytic cells for about 7 days but increased adverse reactions are noted. An additional antimicrobial may need to be added to the treatment regimen if the transtracheal aspirate culture results reveal the presence of another pathogenic organism that is not susceptible the macrolide or rifampin. Response to treatment is noted with resolution of clinical signs, normalization of hematologic values, and resolution of radiographic lesions. Usually, treatment ranges from between 2 and 9 weeks. Strains resistant to macrolides and rifampin have been documented. Possible alternatives include doxycycline, chloramphenicol, or high doses of trimethoprim-sulfonamide. Adverse reactions associated with macrolide and rifampin administration include diarrhea and an idiosyncratic reaction characterized by hyperthermia and tachypnea. Enterocolitis in mares of treated foals has been rarely reported.

The administration of hyperimmunized plasma obtained from donors vaccinated with *R. equi* antigens has become a mainstay of prevention in foals on endemically affected farms. Studies have yielded conflicting results regarding the efficacy of plasma administration; however, most evidence indicates that plasma administration decreases the incidence of disease and death from *R. equi*. Unfortunately, this procedure is cost prohibitive for many horse owners, labor intensive, and not without risk of a possible anaphylactic reaction. The universally accepted protocol for plasma administration is 1 L within the first few days of life, followed by a second administration at between 30 and 50 days of age. The protocol is based on the suspected time of exposure to *R. equi*, the neonate's naïve immune system, and the length of time anti-*R. equi* antibody is maintained at a high concentration. Studies have indicated that the administration of azithromycin to neonates reduces the incidence of *R. equi* pneumonia on farms with endemic *R. equi*. However, chemoprophylactic use of azithromycin is controversial due to the concern of selecting for antibiotic-resistant bacteria. *Table 21* lists several recommendations for prevention of *R. equi* infection.

Table 21. Recommendations for the prevention of *R. equi* infection

- Decreasing the size of the infective challenge
  - Avoid overcrowding
  - Decrease the amount of dirt or sandy areas in paddocks
  - Rotate pastures
  - House in well-ventilated and dust-free areas
  - Isolate animals with clinical signs (shed more virulent form in feces)
  - Remove manure frequently from stalls, paddocks, and pastures
  - Do not spread manure on pastures
- Early recognition of disease
  - Daily rectal temperatures
  - Frequent physical examinations with auscultation of the thorax
  - Serial monitoring of WBC counts and blood fibrinogen
  - Ultrasound of the thorax (every 2 weeks or more often)
- Passive immunization
  - Administration of hyperimmune plasma (1 L) at birth and 30 days of age

---

The prognosis for survival was reported in one study to be around 70%–80%, with death more likely in those foals that had severe respiratory signs, severe thoracic radiographic changes, lameness, and joint effusion. Fifty-four percent of the foals survived to race once, and their overall racing performance was average. These findings suggest that appropriate therapy needs to be instituted but, more importantly, preventive and control measures must be taken to prevent the disease, especially on farms where the disease is endemic.

LEPTOSPIROSIS

KEY POINTS
- Worldwide distribution.
- Affects many species (humans, domestic animals, and wildlife).
- Caused by a spirochete, with multiple serovars.
- Non-host-adapted infection differs from host-adapted infections.
- Associated with abortions, premature births, renal disease, respiratory distress.
- Diagnosis based on serologic tests or detection of organism in the urine.
- Treatment supportive plus penicillin and tetracyclines.

DEFINITION/OVERVIEW
Leptospirosis is a common disease of many warm-blooded species with over 250 serovars identified. It causes disease in the adult horse and has also been associated with abortions, neonatal deaths, suspected premature births, and clinical disease in foals. Leptospirosis is a zoonotic disease with the source of infection being direct or indirect contact with the urine of an infected animal.

ETIOLOGY/PATHOPHYSIOLOGY
Mobile, unicellular, spiral-shaped organisms called spirochetes cause leptospirosis. There are several species of *Leptospira* that are divided into serogroups and serovars based on DNA sequencing. The most common serovars to cause problems in equids include *pomona*, *grippotyphosa*, *harjo*, *bratislavia*, and *icterohaemorrhagiae*.

Leptospires can enter through the mucous membranes of the conjunctiva, nasopharynx, oral cavity, esophagus, small intestine, and genital tract. Abraded or soft, moist skin may also be a portal of entry. Bacteremia occurs 4–10 days after the initial infection and invasion of internal organs occurs during bacteremia. The severity of organ involvement depends on the presence of a humoral immune response or the ability and rapidity of the host to mount one. Opsonization by circulatory antibodies can rapidly eliminate bacteremia. If the antibody response is not adequate, severe tissue invasion and damage may occur. Once tissue invasion occurs, infection can persist despite the presence of circulating antibodies. Localized infection may involve tissues and fluids of areas such as the eyes, proximal kidney tubules, genital tract, and central nervous system. The persistence of the infection is dependent on host serovar adaptation. If the infection is by a non-host-adapted organism, infection is short and urinary shedding brief to nonexistent. If the serovar is a host-adapted organism, colonization is often persistent and may continue for the life of the host. Fetal infection occurs subsequent to localization in the pregnant uterus. Fetal infection (dependent on the stage of gestation) results in abortion, still birth, or weak neonates.

CLINICAL PRESENTATION

Leptospirosis infection in the neonate and older foal is characterized by respiratory distress, pyrexia, jaundice, and depression. The neonate may be small in size, weak, and unable to stand. Renal disease with hematuria has also been documented.

DIFFERENTIAL DIAGNOSIS

Differentials for hematuria include trauma, acute renal tubular necrosis, drug toxicosis, hemolysis as a result of hypertonic solutions, septicemia, congenital malformations, and intravascular hemolysis (see *Tables 19* and *45*).

DIAGNOSIS

A history of previous leptospiral abortions/outbreaks and rising leptospiral titers in the mares is important. Physical examination may reveal a weak foal with hematuria and a severe leukocytosis. Diagnosis of leptospirosis is based primarily on the results of serologic tests or detection of leptospires in the urine. The best serological test is the microscopic agglutination test (MAT). A titer >/= 1:800 is suggestive of recent exposure; if the titer is low and leptospirosis is suspected, another sample should be submitted in 10–14 days. Care should be taken in interpretation of a foal with a high titer that has ingested colostrum; in this case the mare's titer should be taken into consideration. Urine obtained from a mare or neonatal foal suspected of being infected with leptospires is often the specimen of choice for the diagnosis of leptospirosis and for culturing of the organism. Immunofluorescence (fluorescent antibody test [FAT]) and dark-field examination of the urine are the most reliable tests for identifying leptospires. The proper collection and handling of the samples are critical to culture success, so the diagnostic laboratory should be contacted for specific instructions on handling of the urine sample. If possible, the urine should be collected prior to antimicrobial treatment.

MANAGEMENT

The antimicrobials of choice for the treatment of leptospiral infection in a foal are penicillin and ampicillin. Oxytetracycline, doxycycline, and streptomycin have been used in adults. Additional supportive care such as oral feeding, respiratory care, appropriate nursing care, and intravenous fluids may also be needed. Often, the foal is azotemic, so careful monitoring of kidney function must not be overlooked. A vaccine specifically for horses is available for prevention of abortion and uveitis caused by *L. pomona*.

OTHER INFECTIOUS DISEASES

A discussion of salmonellosis, clostridiosis, *Rotavirus* spp. infection, *Lawsonia intracellularis* infection, and cryptosporidiosis can be found in Chapter 5 (Alimentary Tract Disorders).

PREVENTION OF INFECTIOUS DISEASES

The best method of prevention of infectious disease on an equine farm, especially a breeding farm, is through proper management. Farms should focus on preventing entry of an infectious agent onto the premise and controlling the spread of an infectious agent, should it enter the establishment (*Table 22*). Lack of good management may result in introduction of an infectious disease to a naïve population, which can result in serious emotional and financial consequences.

Table 22. Guidelines for the prevention of infectious disease on the farm

- Appropriate vaccination and deworming program
- Isolate all new arrivals including those that have returned from competitions, breeding facilities, sales, and the veterinary hospital
  - Monitor temperatures twice a day
  - Monitor for any nasal discharge or coughing
  - Consider testing for *Streptococcus equi*, EHV–1, or *Salmonella* spp. (if there is a problem in the area or individual has come from an endemic area)
- Require medical history on *all* new arrivals
- Minimize traffic to and from the facility
- House animals according to age
- Keep facility clean
- Do not spread manure on the pastures
- Remove manure from paddocks and pastures
- Isolate any individual that has clinical signs of an infectious disease
  - Move to a separate isolation barn or isolate in the stall with appropriate barrier precautions
  - Do not move any animals into or out of the barn for several weeks
- Establish protocol for handling/treating the individual with the suspected infectious disease
  - Include hand hygiene, protective clothing, disinfectant foot dips, manure disposal
  - Appropriate cleaning and disinfecting protocol
- Establish a protocol for diagnosing the cause of the infectious disease (what samples to send and where to send them)

FURTHER READING

AAEP (American Association of Equine Practitioners) infectious disease control (www.aaep.org/info/infectious-disease-control).

AAEP (American Association of Equine Practitioners) vaccination guidelines (www.aaep.org/info/vaccination-guidelines).

Allen GP, Murray MJ (2004) Equid herpesvirus 2 and equid herpesvirus 5 infections. In: *Infectious Diseases of Livestock*, 2nd ed. (Coetzer JAW, Tustin RC, Eds.). Oxford University Press, Oxford, UK, pp. 860–868.

Balasuriya UBR (2014) Equine viral arteritis. *Veterinary Clinics of North America: Equine Practice* 30: 543–560.

Bell SA, Leclere M, Gardner IA, Maclachlan NJ (2006) Equine adenovirus 1 infection of hospitalized and healthy foals and horses. *Equine Veterinary Journal* 38: 379–381.

Bernard WV (1993) Leptospirosis. *Veterinary Clinics of North America: Equine Practice* 9: 435–444.

Brewer BD, Koterba AM (1988) Development of a scoring system for the early diagnosis of equine neonatal sepsis. *Equine Veterinary Journal* 20: 18–22.

Cavanagh HM, Mahony TJ, Vanniasinkam T (2012) Genetic characterization of equine adenovirus type 1. *Veterinary Microbiology* 155: 33–37.

Cohen ND (2014) *Rhodococcus equi* foal pneumonia. *Veterinary Clinics of North America: Equine Practice* 30: 609–622.

Del Piero F, Wilkins PA, Lopez JW, Glaser AL, Dubovi EK, Schlafer DH, Lein DH (1997) Equine viral arteritis in newborn foals: Clinical, pathological, serological, mircrobiological and immunohistochemical observations. *Equine Veterinary Journal* 29: 178–185.

Dunkel B, Corley KTT (2015) Pathophysiology, diagnosis and treatment of neonatal sepsis. *Equine Veterinary Education* 27: 92–98.

Frellstedt L, Slovis NM (2009) Acute renal disease from *Leptospira interrogans* in three yearlings from the same farm. *Equine Veterinary Education* 21: 478–484.

Giguere S, Cohen ND, Chaffin MK, Slovis NM, Hondalus MK, Hines SA, Prescott JF (2011) Diagnosis, treatment, control, and prevention of infections caused by *Rhodococcus equi* in foals. *Journal of Veterinary Internal Medicine* 25: 1209–1220.

Landolt GA (2014) Equine influenza virus. *Veterinary Clinics of North America: Equine Practice* 30: 507–522.

Mallicote M (2015) Update *on Streptococcus equi subsp equi* infections. *Veterinary Clinics of North America: Equine Practice* 31: 27–42.

Marsh PS, Palmer JE (2001) Bacterial isolates from blood and their susceptibility patterns in critically ill foals: 543 cases (1991–1998). *Journal of the American Veterinary Medical Association* 218: 1608–1610.

Palmer J (2014) Update on the management of neonatal sepsis in horses. *Veterinary Clinics of North America: Equine Practice* 30: 317–336.

Reed SM, Toribio R (2004) Equine herpesvirus 1 and 4. *Veterinary Clinics of North America: Equine Practice* 20: 631–642.

Sellon D, Long M (Eds.) (2014) *Equine Infectious Diseases*, 2nd ed. Elsevier, Philadelphia, PA.

Immunologic and Hematologic Disorders

4

William V. Bernard

IMMUNOLOGIC DISORDERS

KEY POINTS

- The pre-suckle newborn foal is basically considered agammaglobulinemic; however, antibody production to specific antigens can occur in the fetus in the last third of gestation.
- The newborn foal has a functioning but immature cellular immune system; cellular immune response does not reach adult status until approximately 1–2 months of age.
- The pre-suckle foal is limited in its response to pathogens until post-suckle transfer of immunity has occurred.
- Ig-rich colostrum is produced in the last month of gestation.
- Colostral Ig is concentrated from the general circulation.
- Colostrum (antibody-rich milk) is short lived: 12–24 hours post suckle.
- Colostrum contains other factors that enhance immunity.
- Intermammary production of IgA continues throughout lactation.
- Ingested Ig is transferred into the general circulation through the process of pinocytosis.
- The process of pinocytosis is limited in duration to approximately 24 hours, with a peak between 6 and 12 hours.
- A measurable peak of serum Ig occurs by 24–48 hours of age, with a subsequent decline resulting from catabolism and expanding plasma volume.

INTRODUCTION

The newborn foal is immunologically competent (i.e., can immunologically respond to pathogens or foreign antigens); however, the response is slow in comparison with that of the mature, adult immune system. The equine fetus has lymphocytes (both T and B lymphocytes) present by the mid-second trimester of gestation. However, total lymphocyte numbers do not increase to adult numbers until approximately 1 month of age, therefore this branch of the immune system (cell-mediated immunity) is immature at birth. Antibody production to specific antigens (humoral immunity) can occur in the fetus by the early third trimester. *In-utero* transfer of immunoglobulins does not occur in the foal. The diffuse epitheliochorial placenta of the mare does not allow for *in-utero* transfer of large molecules such as immunoglobulins. The newborn foal is agammaglobulinemic at birth. Colostrum-deprived foals do not have detectable Ig at birth or until they are several days of age (67). The presuckle foal possesses an immature but functioning cellular immune system and lacks autogenous Ig at birth, therefore its immune defense against pathogens is limited until post-suckle transfer of immunity has occurred.

Ig-rich colostrum (high antibody content mammary secretions) is produced by the mare in the last month of gestation. The major concentration of Ig likely occurs in the last few weeks of gestation. Ig is not manufactured in the mammary gland, but is concentrated from circulating Ig. This secretion of circulating Ig is mediated hormonally. The majority of immunoglobulin (Ig) contained in colostrum is of the IgG/IgG(T) class. The duration of colostrum (antibody-rich milk) production is brief, with normal milk secretions replacing colostrum by 12–24 hours post foaling (68). Colostrum also contains other properties (e.g., local protectants, lactoferrin, and complement) that enhance immune function. Phagocytic and serum opsonic activity is dependent on adequate intake and absorption of colostrum (69). Opsonization is dependent on Ig, or complement, binding to the surface of bacteria. Opsonization in foals with partial FPT is significantly lower than that of adults (70). Anti-trypsins in colostrum prevent the breakdown of Ig by the digestive process of the GI tract.

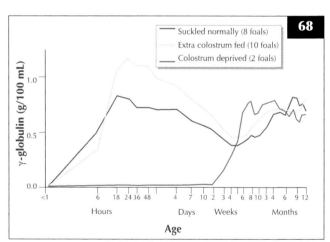

68 Gamma globulin levels in colostrum-fed and colostrum-deprived foals. (From Jeffcott, L.B., *J. Comp. Pathol.*, 84, 93, 1974.)

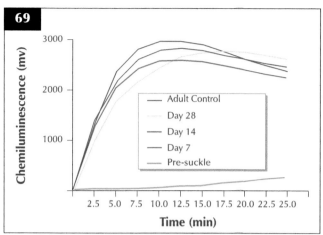

69 Chemiluminescence response of adult neutrophils using pre- and post-suckle foal serum as the opsonin. Post-suckle serum had >6 g/L (600 mg/dL) IgG. Chemiluminescence generated with pre-suckle serum as the opsonin was less than that generated at other times (*p* < 0.05). (From LeBlanc, M.M., *Proceedings of the 33rd Annual Meeting of the American Association of Equine Practitioners*, 755, 1987.)

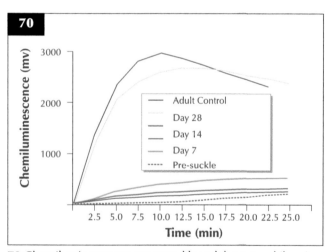

70 Chemiluminescence generated by adult neutrophils using serum of foals with <3.5 g/L (350 mg/dL) IgG as the opsonin. Chemiluminescence generated by adult neutrophils using serum of foals with >6 g/L (600 mg/dL) IgG as the opsonin (D-D) is included as comparison. Opsonic activity of foal serum containing <3.5 g/L (350 mg/dL) of IgG was less than control and less than foal serum with >6 g/L (600 mg/dL) of IgG (*p* < 0.05). (From LeBlanc, M.M., *Proceedings of the 33rd Annual Meeting of the American Association of Equine Practitioners*, p. 755.)

Although the Ig content of milk secretions characteristically decreases after birth, intramammary production of IgA continues throughout lactation.

Absorption of colostrum is accomplished via specialized epithelial cells within the small intestine (pinocytosis). The process of pinocytosis is nonselective. Large macromolecules such as Ig are engulfed and transferred into the general circulation

through lymphatics. The life span of the specialized pinocytotic cells is limited. The maximum capacity for absorption is in the first 12–16 hours of life, followed by a linear decline in absorptive capacity up to 24 hours after birth. The specialized cells of pinocytosis are replaced by more mature cells. The replacement of pinocytic cells is not a function of colostrum absorption and occurs whether or not colostrum has been ingested. The mature epithelial cells are not capable of large macromolecule absorption. Subsequent to the ingestion of colostrum, which occurs shortly after birth, Ig will appear in the serum by 6 hours of age and generally peaks at 24–48 hours of age, with a subsequent decline as a result of catabolism and expanding plasma volume (**68**).

FAILURE OF PASSIVE TRANSFER OF IMMUNITY

KEY POINTS
- Failure of passive transfer (FPT) is the failure to achieve adequate circulating Ig (antibody) levels.
- The accepted definition of FPT is a serum IgG of <2 g/L (200 mg/dL) and partial failure as a serum IgG of 2–4 g/L (200–400 mg/dL).
- FPT is caused by inadequate production, ingestion, or absorption of colostrum.
- Colostral IgG concentration of 30 g/L (3,000 mg/dL) is considered adequate.
- Prevention of FPT should be based on good management and ensuring ingestion of adequate colostrum.
- Treatment of FPT or partial FPT using plasma products should be a decision based on management practices, historical and current disease problems, and environmental cleanliness.

DEFINITION/OVERVIEW
FPT of immunity can be defined simply as the failure of the newborn foal to achieve adequate circulating Ig concentrations after birth; however, using a number (of hours) to define FPT is problematic, as numerous other factors are involved. The post-suckle Ig concentration is also influenced by the sampling time. The literature describes FPT as a serum IgG concentration of <2 g/L (200 mg/dL), and partial FPT as a concentration of <4 g/L (400 mg/dL). Healthy foals in a clean, well-managed environment are generally well protected by IgG values of 4 g/L (400 mg/dL). Newborn foals in an unhealthy environment or exhibiting complications may require higher values of IgG for protection. Another important factor to consider is the specificity of colostral Ig to specific pathogens in the foal's environment. An adequate IgG level does not guarantee complete protection against all pathogens.

ETIOLOGY/PATHOPHYSIOLOGY
The causes of FPT can be classified into three groups (*Table 23*): inadequate maternal production of Ig-rich colostrum, inadequate intake of colostrum by the newborn foal, and inadequate absorption of colostral Ig.

Inadequate maternal production of Ig-rich colostrum
Premature delivery can result in FPT because of inadequate colostral production or inadequate fetal maturity. Inadequate

Table 23. Possible causes of failure of passive transfer

- Inadequate maternal production of immunoglobulin-rich colostrum:
  - Premature delivery
  - Premature lactation
  - Agalactica
  - Failure of production of high-quality colostrum
- Inadequate colostral intake by the newborn foal:
  - Complete rejection of the foal
  - Partial acceptance of the foal
  - Any factor in the foal that prevents adequate suckling of the mare
- Inadequate absorption:
  - Limited sites for pinocytosis
  - Early gastrointestinal closure
  - Inadequate transfer of immunoglobulin to systemic circulation
  - Catabolism as a source of calories

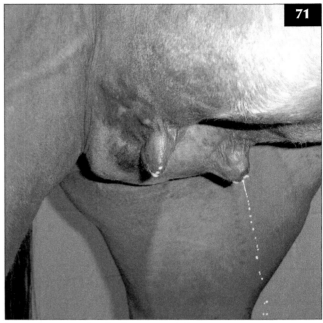

71 Mammary gland of a mare exhibiting premature lactation.

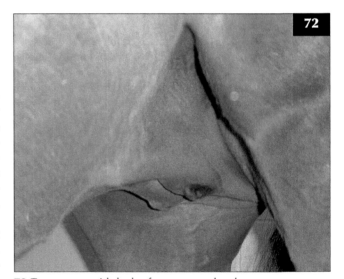

72 Term mare with lack of mammary development.

fetal maturity may result in deficient pinocytosis of macromolecules, although specialized pinocytotic cells are present early in fetal development. Another potential cause of inadequate colostrum production is premature lactation (**71**). In a normal progression toward foaling, an individual mare may "drip milk" for several days before foaling. Premature lactation at the date of expected foaling is not necessarily the result of a fetal–placental abnormality; however, premature lactation earlier in gestation does usually indicate a fetal–placental abnormality. Premature lactation at the expected time of foaling does not absolutely result in inadequate colostrum production; however, it does suggest the need for evaluation of colostrum or of post-suckle Ig levels.

Agalactia (lack of milk production) (**72**) can be a result of various disease states in the mare (including inadequate nutrition) or be due to oral toxin ingestion. Toxicities influencing mammary development and milk production include the ingestion of endophyte-infected fescue grass (or hay) in the third trimester.

Individual mares may inherently produce small volumes of milk and inadequate amounts of colostrum. Mare colostrum production is likely to be genetically controlled, therefore the mare that produces poor colostrum may do so repeatedly. Colostral Ig concentrations can vary between breeds and between individuals. A colostral Ig concentration of 30 g/L (3,000 mg/dL) is considered adequate for successful passive transfer of Ig.

Inadequate ingestion of colostrum by the newborn foal

Inadequate ingestion of colostrum can occur when mares initially lactate poorly, are nervous, do not allow the foal to suckle (which can include complete rejection of the foal), or do not "let down" milk adequately to allow for Ig absorption during the critical period. Foal factors include disease processes, weakness, or delayed time to standing and suckling. Malabsorption of Ig has been suggested as a cause of FPT; however, scientific explanation or documentation of such a factor does not exist.

Inadequate absorption of colostral Ig

Factors causing inadequate absorption of colostrum are not well defined, but may include limited sites for pinocytosis, early closure of these sites, inadequate transfer of Ig to the systemic circulation, and, possibly, catabolism as a source of needed calories.

DIAGNOSIS

Diagnosis of FPT is based on measuring the concentration of Ig in foal serum. The timing of when blood samples are drawn for IgG evaluation is important. The foal that suckles Ig-rich colostrum shortly after birth may have adequate detectable IgG levels at 6–12 hours. However, the foal that does not ingest large volumes of colostrum early in life may not have adequate detectable IgG levels until 12–24 hours after birth.

Single radial immunodiffusion (SRID) is the "gold standard" of IgG interpretation. This test uses antiserum to equine IgG and compares precipitation patterns produced in agar gel with known standards. The test is quantitative and specific for IgG. The drawbacks of the SRID test are expense and time (the test takes 24 hours to produce results).

Rapid and inexpensive turbidity tests have been developed for interpretation of Ig content. The zinc sulfate turbidity test is the standard. Zinc sulfate is added to foal serum, which makes the globulins insoluble. The insolubility results in a visible cloudiness or a measurable change in the optical density, which can be detected spectrophotometrically. The Ig content of the sample can then be determined based on a standard curve. A glutaraldehyde clot test and a sodium sulfite turbidity test can also be used.

Additional tests developed for the determination of Ig include latex agglutination and enzyme-linked immunosorbent assay (ELISA). The latex agglutination test uses latex particles coated with anti-equine IgG. These particles agglutinate in the presence of Ig. The test is rapid (10 minutes) and can be performed on foal serum or whole blood. The test is reliable when performed correctly. The ELISA test uses a semiquantitative membrane filter to measure Ig in foal serum. Color calibration spots are compared with the intensity of the color reaction on the test filter. When using any of these "stall-side kits," it is recommended that there are comparisons to known standards or to the SRID test.

MANAGEMENT

As discussed earlier, the currently accepted definition of FPT is that total FPT is when there is an IgG concentration of <2 g/L (200 mg/dL) and partial FPT when the IgG concentration is 2–4 g/L (200–400 mg/dL). Most clinicians would consider an IgG value of <2 g/L (200 mg/dL) as necessitating therapy; however, many foals with IgG levels of 2–4 g/L (200–400 mg/dL) will remain healthy. Therapy of partial FPT should be considered on a case-by-case basis. The management practices and history of current and/or previous diseases on the premises must be considered. It is advisable that a foal with partial FPT should be monitored closely for signs of infection.

The primary approach to the management of FPT is prevention, with treatment being the choice when prevention fails. The basis for prevention is to ensure that there is ingestion of quality colostrum in a timely manner. The mare's colostrum should be evaluated and the foal monitored carefully for adequate postfoaling

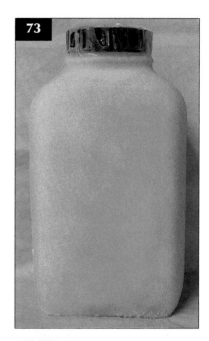

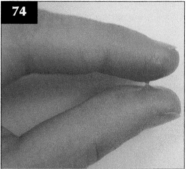

73, 74 Colostrum should be yellow-gold in color (**73**) and sticky to the touch (**74**).

responses. The normal foal should stand and nurse within 2 hours of parturition. Good-quality colostrum should be sticky to the touch, yellow-gold in color (**73**), and appear thick (**74**). The use of these subjective, visual, and tactile criteria may be misleading. Colostrum can be more accurately evaluated by use of a hydrometer that determines specific gravity (SG). There is a very good correlation between the SG and IgG content of colostrum (**75**) and between the SG of the dam's colostrum and the foal's serum IgG concentration (**76**). Adequate colostrum has a SG of 1.060 or greater, which correlates to an IgG concentration of 30 g/L (3,000 mg/dL). A Brix refractometer can also be used to evaluate colostral quality; a level of 23 or higher correlates with adequate colostral IgG content.

When the mare's colostrum is adequate (i.e., 30 g/L [3,000 mg/dL] IgG), but the foal does not or cannot suckle, then the mare's colostrum should be provided for the foal via a nasogastric tube or bottle. If the mare's colostrum is of poor quality, then supplemental colostrum should be provided. Colostrum can be purchased or a supply can be obtained from mares that have previously foaled. If a mare has very good-quality colostrum, subsequent to her foal sucking, 200–250 mL of colostrum can be saved, tested (IgG content and antibodies to red cell antigens), and frozen for future use. Using this method, a colostrum bank can be established. Stored colostrum can be frozen for up to 1 year without losing quality.

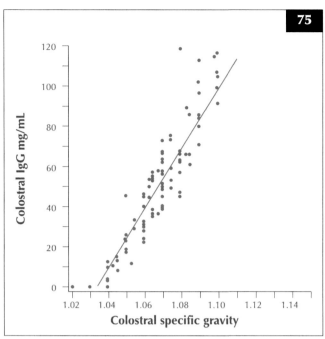

75 Relationship of IgG concentration to specific gravity in colostrum ($r^2 = 0.81$). (From LeBlanc, M.M. et al., *J. Am. Vet. Med. Assoc.*, 189, 57, 1986.)

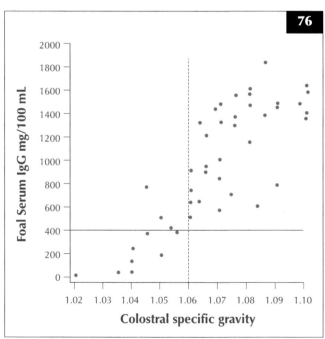

76 Scattergram of serum immunoglobulin G (IgG) concentrations in foals 24 hours after birth compared with colostral specific gravities of their dams. The solid line represents the foal serum IgG concentrations below which partial or complete failure of passive transfer occurs. The dashed line represents a colostral specific gravity of 1.060. (From LeBlanc, M.M. and Tran, T.Q., *J. Reprod. Fertil.*, 35, 735, 1987.)

The IgG content can last for more than 1 year, but prolonged freezing can destroy other protective components of colostrum. The amount of colostrum necessary to provide adequate transfer of immunity is variable and dependent on foal size and colostral quality. A general rule is that at least 1–2 liters of good-quality colostrum should be administered in the first 12 hours of life. It is preferable to divide the colostrum into several feedings. Colostral supplements are available and can produce IgG levels in the normal range. These products are generally serum based and do not contain other protective factors of colostrum.

Foals >12 hours of age are unlikely to absorb adequate amounts of ingested colostrum, therefore FPT in these individuals is addressed with systemic administration of plasma or serum products. Sources include locally collected plasma, commercial plasma, or concentrated serum products. Locally collected products may have an advantage, as immunity to local pathogens should be present. A disadvantage to plasma therapy is the constant, but infrequent, possibility of an anaphylactic reaction. Foals with FPT should receive 200–500 mg IgG/kg bodyweight. IgG measurements should be repeated after plasma administration.

COMBINED IMMUNE DEFICIENCY

KEY POINTS

- Combined immune deficiency (CID) is a heritable, congenital disease of the Arabian foal.
- The immunodeficiency is a lack of lymphoid precursors resulting in a lack of both T and B lymphocytes.
- Typical clinical signs are unresponsive or recurrent infection.
- Diagnosis is based on lymphopenia, an absence of circulating IgM, and hypoplasia of lymphoid tissue.

DEFINITION/OVERVIEW

CID is a congenital, heritable disease of Arabian foals. To the author's knowledge, there is only one reported case of CID in a non-Arabian foal (an Appaloosa). The condition is inherited as an autosomal recessive trait, which identifies both the dam and sire as carriers (heterozygotes) for CID. It has been determined that about 25% of the Arabian mares and foals in the United States are heterozygotes and that the incidence of the disease is approximately 2%. The breeding of heterozygote horses perpetuates the CID disease in the Arabian population.

ETIOLOGY/PATHOPHYSIOLOGY

The immunodeficiency is a result of a genetically determined lack of lymphoid precursors resulting in a lack of both T and B lymphocytes, hence the name "combined immune deficiency." As a result of the absence of T and B cells, these foals are unable to produce an antigen-specific immune response. The immune deficiency is limited to the lymphatic system. Normal numbers of effective neutrophils, macrophages, and an intact complement system are present in affected individuals. Even though CID foals fail to produce mature T and B lymphocytes, they produce lymphoid "killer" cells (large granular lymphocytes) with inducible cytotoxic activity. These cells can produce nonspecific protection against some viral pathogens. Affected foals do not produce gamma interferon.

CLINICAL PRESENTATION

The typical presentation is of an overwhelming, unresponsive, or recurrent infection. If adequate colostral transfer of antibodies has occurred, affected CID foals usually appear normal and free of infection until maternal antibodies begin to wane. This time period is variable and dependent on the passive transfer of Ig. Clinical signs may be seen as early as 3–4 weeks of age. Subsequent to the loss of maternal immunity, bacterial, viral, and other opportunists such as *Cryptosporidium* spp. and *Pneumocystis carinii* result in the demise of the foal before 6 months of age. The respiratory tract is the most frequently affected body system, although the liver or GI tract may also be involved. Affected foals may initially respond to antibiotics only to develop additional infection from other pathogens or opportunists.

DIAGNOSIS

Diagnosis of CID is based on three criteria: lymphopenia (<1,000/µL), hypoplasia of lymphoid tissue, and absence of IgM. At least two of these factors should be present to confirm a diagnosis. A simple and early test that can exclude the diagnosis of CID is a pre-suckle test for the presence of IgM. The normal equine fetus produces IgM *in utero* and maternal–colostral IgM is present in the foal blood post suckle. Therefore, an IgM-positive blood sample from a pre-suckle foal suggests normal functioning lymphoid tissue.

Normal newborn pre-suckle foals will, however, have low lymphocyte counts (<1,000/µL of blood) for the first 24–48 hours of life. By 24–48 hours of age, lymphocytes increase to >1,000/µL. Pre-suckle CID foals will have no detectable IgM and lymphocyte counts do not increase in the first few days of life.

Normal post-suckle foals will have lymphocyte counts >1,000 cells/µL and IgM derived from endogenous production or colostral absorption. Post-suckle CID foals will have maternal–colostral-derived IgM and lymphocyte counts <1,000 cells/µL. Maternally derived IgM usually wanes by 30 days of age. By 30–40 days of age, the absence of IgM and lymphocyte counts of <1,000 cells/µL are suspicious of CID. The recognition that transplanted histocompatible lymphocytes (bone marrow transplant) produce normal immune function suggests that the genetic defect is at the level of the lymphoid precursor cell. Recently, a defect in DNA-dependent protein kinase required for immune system development has been recognized. The gene encoding for the DNA kinase has been cloned and sequenced. When the normal genetic sequence is compared with the mutant sequence, a 5-base pair deletion is identified. A commercial test is now available that can determine whether an Arabian horse is heterozygous for CID.

Necropsy or biopsy identifies lymphoid tissue hypoplasia and confirms the diagnosis. Necropsy may reveal the primary disease process (immunodeficiency) or the secondary complications caused by the infectious agents. The lymphoid lesions of hypoplasia are seen in lymph nodes, spleen, and thymus. Thymus may contain a few lymphocytes and hypoplastic epithelial cells. The spleen and lymph nodes are virtually devoid of lymphocytes. The lymph nodes lack plasma cells and lymphoid follicles.

MANAGEMENT

Although a bone marrow transplant has been reported to have successfully treated a CID foal, it would be unwise to use these individuals in a breeding program. Bone marrow transplantation is expensive, difficult, and requires a histocompatible full sibling donor. The patient's thymic and bone marrow environment can support the differentiation of normal stem cells from the bone marrow donor. Plasma administration and/or continuous antibiotic therapy can prolong the life of a foal with CID. The majority of affected individuals, unless the immune system is reconstructed, die within 6 months of age. Client education and an explanation of the genetic basis of the disease is imperative. An understanding of the significance of a heterozygote in a breeding program can benefit future breeding decisions.

AGAMMAGLOBULINEMIA

DEFINITION/OVERVIEW

Agammaglobulinemia is an uncommon condition that results in a lack of gamma globulin production. Breeds represented are the Thoroughbred, Standardbred, and Quarter Horse. Affected foals have thus far been males. They lack B lymphocytes and therefore cannot produce Ig. Functional T lymphocytes in normal numbers are present. The presence of cellular immunity provides defense against many viruses and other opportunists. The presence of T lymphocytes in agammaglobulinemic foals results in a longer life expectancy than in a CID-affected foal, and a few of these foals have lived beyond 1 year of age.

ETIOLOGY/PATHOPHYSIOLOGY

It is suggested that agammaglobulinemia is a genetic disorder that may be X-linked in inheritance. It is an X-linked disorder in humans. Dams of affected animals would be carriers and transmit the condition to one-half of their male offspring; one-half of their female offspring would then be carriers. The genetic basis has not been proven; however, additional immune function testing is advisable in any future foals of these mares. Affected individuals are unable to produce an antigen-specific immune response.

CLINICAL PRESENTATION

Affected individuals show signs of recurrent/unresponsive infection as maternal immunity declines. These infections may be seen as early as 2 months of age. As with CID, infections typically involve the respiratory and gastrointestinal (GI) tracts. Affected foals survive longer than CID-affected foals because of their intact T lymphocytic function.

DIFFERENTIAL DIAGNOSIS

The differential diagnosis would include CID.

DIAGNOSIS

Affected foals will have normal T lymphocyte function and normal numbers of circulating lymphocytes. Circulating Ig levels will vary with age as a result of maternally derived immunity. Subsequent to the decline of maternal immunity, an absence of gamma globulin is identified. Lymphocyte evaluation will reveal an absence of B lymphocytes expressing surface IgM. Microscopic evaluation reveals a lack of lymphoid follicles and circulating plasma cells.

MANAGEMENT
Antibiotic therapy and intravenous plasma administration can be used to prolong the life of affected individuals.

HEMATOLOGIC DISORDERS

KEY POINTS
- The primary hematologic disorder of the neonate is anemia.
- Clinical signs are dependent on the rapidity of blood loss.
- Anemia can be considered in categories of decreased production, increased destruction, or increased loss of red blood cells (RBCs).
- The primary causes of anemia are blood loss, neonatal iso-erythrolysis (NI), or anemia of chronic disease.

INTRODUCTION
Hematologic disorders in the neonate and pediatric patient consist primarily of anemia. Polycythemia (increased RBC numbers) is a rare condition occasionally seen in adult horses. Clinical signs of anemia are variable and dependent on the rapidity of loss of RBCs (oxygen-carrying capacity). Signs of anemia can be gradual and include lethargy (77), exercise intolerance, inappetence,

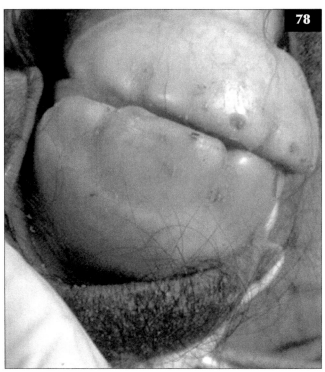

78 Pale oral mucous membranes in a foal as a result of severe anemia.

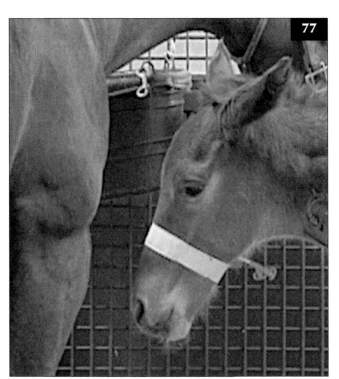

77 Anemia can cause clinical signs of lethargy/depression, as demonstrated in this foal.

pallor (78), and hypotension. If blood loss is rapid, signs may include recumbency, tachypnea, and tachycardia. Hypovolemic shock can develop when there is loss of more than one-third of the blood volume. When investigating anemia, it is helpful to consider if the cause can be categorized as either decreased production, increased destruction, or loss of RBCs. The primary causes of anemia are blood loss, immune-mediated hemolytic anemia (IMHA) of NI, and anemia of chronic disease. Other less common causes will not be discussed in detail, but are mentioned under differential diagnoses or in the relevant tables.

DECREASED ERYTHROCYTE PRODUCTION

KEY POINTS
- Decreased RBC production as a cause of anemia in the foal is uncommon.
- Anemia of chronic disease would be the most common cause of decreased RBC production.
- Pale mucous membranes may be observed.

DEFINITION/OVERVIEW
Decreased RBC production is an occasional cause of anemia in the foal. Factors that can influence the production of red cells include the micronutrients required for their production, decreased erythropoiesis, or alterations in iron metabolism. The major cause of decreased RBC production is the anemia that is seen secondary to chronic disease.

Table 24. Causes of anemia

- Decreased erythrocyte production:
  - Nutritional deficiencies (iron, copper, folate, B_{12}, cobalt)
  - Anemia of chronic disease
- Increased erythrocyte destruction (hemolysis):
  - Infection
  - Immune-mediated:
    - Neonatal isoerythrolysis
    - Autoimmune hemolytic anemia
  - Red blood cell defects:
    - Glutathione reductase deficiency recognized in a familial disease in Standardbred horses
- Increased loss of erythrocytes:
  - External loss
  - Internal loss

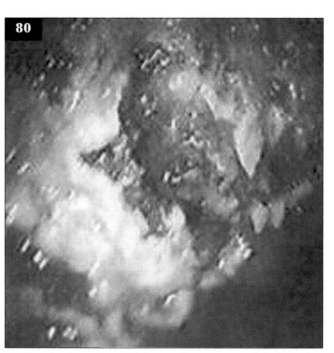

80 Gastric ulceration with hemorrhage can result in blood loss, as shown in this foal.

ETIOLOGY/PATHOPHYSIOLOGY

Decreased erythrocyte production can occasionally be caused by nutritional deficiencies (*Table 24*). Multiple nutrients, minerals, and vitamins are required for adequate red cell production. Nutritional deficiencies are unusual, but may be seen when artificial diets are used in growing foals. Iron would be considered the most common nutrient deficiency resulting in anemia. GI disease can result in nutrient malabsorption, potentially leading to deficiencies of necessary micronutrients. Significant external blood loss (**79**),

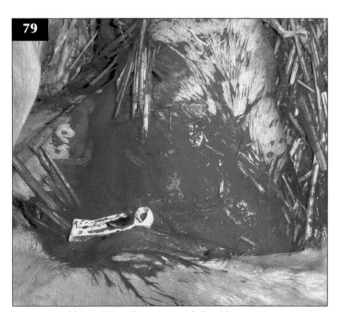

79 External blood loss from an umbilical hemorrhage.

particularly if chronic, can result in iron deficiency anemias. The milk diet is deficient in iron. Chronic gastric ulceration with hemorrhage (**80**) is a potential cause of chronic external hemorrhage.

Anemia of chronic disease is a more common cause of decreased erythrocyte production in the foal. Chronic infections such as pneumonia (**81**), omphalophlebitis (**82**), osteomyelitis (**83**), abscesses (**84**), or GI disease are fairly common in the foal. The alteration in red cell numbers is generally not dramatic, usually does not result in clinical signs of anemia, and is generally noted (and treated) as a secondary complication. Chronic infection results in a defect of iron mobilization in the face of adequate iron stores, decreased RBC survival, decreased erythropoiesis secondary to cytokine release, and reduced iron availability as a result of sequestration in macrophages.

CLINICAL PRESENTATION

Clinical signs of anemia secondary to decreased red cell production are often nonspecific and can include lethargy, depression, exercise intolerance, and pale mucous membranes. The patient with anemia of chronic disease is unlikely to present with anemia as the primary complaint; however, mucous membrane color may be pale (**78**). The patient may present with signs of chronic disease (i.e., fever, failure to thrive/unthrifty/poor doer, or weight loss [**85**]).

Abdominal abscesses are not uncommon in the foal and these foals may present with weight loss in the face of abdominal distension (**86**). Chronic respiratory disease may present with fever, cough, and tachypnea, or may be more occult with depression and unthriftiness as the only signs.

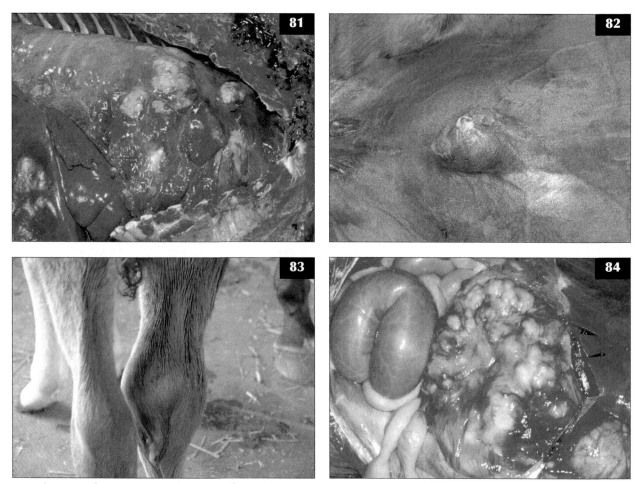

81–84 Chronic infection. (81) Pulmonary abscess. (82) Pus from the umbilicus. (83) Osteomyelitis. (84) Abdominal abscess.

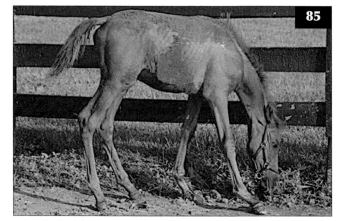

85 A foal with chronic infection (pneumonia) showing signs of being unthrifty, not doing very well, and failing to thrive.

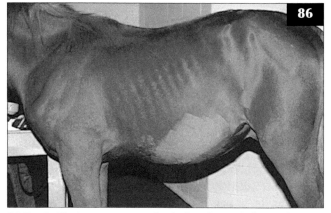

86 Pot-bellied appearance of a foal with an abdominal abscess.

DIFFERENTIAL DIAGNOSIS

The differential diagnosis of an anemia of decreased production includes the anemias of increased loss and destruction of RBCs. The differentials for the nonspecific signs of chronic anemia include a variety of conditions that would result in lethargy, depression, and exercise intolerance. The identification of pale mucous membranes should aid the differentiation from these conditions.

DIAGNOSIS

Iron deficiency anemia in the foal is typically the result of chronic or acute (massive) blood loss in combination with a lack of dietary iron. The most common source of chronic hemorrhage is the GI tract, and gastric ulceration is the most common cause of GI hemorrhage. Acute blood loss can occur from the umbilicus at foaling, from hemoperitoneum, or from traumatic injury. As the milk diet is deficient in iron, young foals with significant red cell loss may not regenerate significant red cell numbers. Older foals with food sources other than milk generally have enough iron to overcome the potential for iron deficiency anemia. The microcytic, hypochromic changes in red cells seen in humans and dogs are not usually seen in the horse because equine erythrocytes are of a smaller size. Indices that may be used to document the disorder include increased iron-binding capacity, decreased serum iron concentration, and marrow stores of iron. Anemia of chronic disease is typically associated with an inflammatory leukocytosis (increased white blood cell [WBC] count, total protein, and fibrinogen) suggestive of infection. Further evaluation of the patient for the source of infection is generally rewarding. Hematologic indices may indicate a monocytic normochronic anemia. Bone marrow biopsies will indicate reduced amounts of iron in RBC precursors, with increased reticuloendothelial storage of iron.

MANAGEMENT

Treatment for anemia of chronic disease should be directed at the underlying cause. Therapy for deficiency anemia should include identification of a potential underlying cause. Oral administration of iron supplements is preferred over intravenous preparations. Anaphylactic reactions have been reported with parenteral preparation of iron.

INCREASED ERYTHROCYTE DESTRUCTION/IMMUNE-MEDIATED HEMOLYTIC ANEMIA

KEY POINTS

- Immune-mediated anemia may be autoimmune or alloimmune.
- NI is dramatically more common than autoimmune anemias in the foal.
- Hemolysis is initiated by antibody recognition of RBC antigens.
- Hemolysis may be intra- or extravascular.
- Clinical signs of anemia depend on the degree of anemia and the rapidity of onset.
- Definitive diagnosis is based on identification of antibody attached to the RBC surface.

DEFINITION/OVERVIEW

IMHA is a result of a cytotoxic response. Autoantibodies directed against red cell surface antigens result in immune-mediated destruction of the RBC. The RBCs are destroyed via erythrophagocytosis or by lysis. This antibody-mediated destruction may include either intravascular or extravascular hemolysis. Affected patients often show clinical signs of anemia. Total protein values are normal. Icterus may accompany the anemia, as the liver's ability to metabolize and excrete bilirubin is exceeded. Signs of intravascular hemolysis may be present. Nonimmune-mediated hemolytic anemia may be seen secondary to infection. Bacterial toxins of *Clostridium staphylococcus*, *Salmonella* spp., and, potentially, other organisms can cause direct damage to the RBC membrane, resulting in hemolysis. The most common immune-mediated anemia seen in the foal is NI.

ETIOLOGY/PATHOPHYSIOLOGY

Antibodies involved in IMHA are classified as alloimmune or autoimmune. An autoimmune antibody is an antibody directed against self, while alloimmunity is a process of isoimmunization against an antigen of others of the same species. Primary IMHA is a process in which normally suppressed B lymphocytes produce antibodies against normal red cell surface antigens. Secondary IMHA is significantly more common than primary IMHA. Secondary IMHA is a result of alterations that occur on the red cell surface antigens and resulting opsonization and lysis or removal by the reticuloendothelial system. Alterations in the surface RBC proteins that result in IMHA can be induced by drug interactions, neoplasia, viruses or bacteria, or antigen–antibody complex deposition on the surface of RBCs. The alloimmune hemolytic anemia, NI, that occurs secondary to the mare's production of red cell antibodies is discussed in the next section.

The primary antibodies involved are IgG (warm agglutinin disease) and IgM (cold agglutinin disease). Surface RBC antigens are recognized by antibodies and initiate cytotoxic events. Complement activation results in either cell lysis or phagocytosis. If lysis occurs, then the process is an intravascular hemolysis. Phagocytosis is initiated when the reticuloendothelial cells recognize the Fc fragment of IgG on the C3b component of complement. The reticuloendothelial removal of RBCs occurs in the liver or spleen and is therefore extravascular.

CLINICAL PRESENTATION

Clinical signs are dependent on the degree of anemia and the rapidity of onset. Physical examination includes pale mucous membranes (**78**), tachycardia, tachypnea, and lethargy (**77**). A systolic heart murmur may be heard in the presence of hypovolemia. An anemia of rapid onset can result in signs of shock. Patients usually adapt to slower onset anemia. Clinical signs other than pallor or icterus may not be noted until red cell numbers are very low. Intravascular hemolysis often results in pigmenturia.

DIFFERENTIAL DIAGNOSIS

The differential diagnosis includes haptens such as drugs, diseases that induce antigen–antibody deposition on the RBC surface, infections (viral or bacterial) that induce a secondary autoimmune hemolytic anemia (AIHA), excessive rapid administration of hypertonic solutions, and NI. Primary IMHA is uncommonly identified in the foal.

DIAGNOSIS

Clinical signs other than pallor and icterus are often nonspecific. Icterus can occur with liver disease. The anemia may be moderate to severe; clinical signs will correspond. Urinalysis or observation of serum may identify pigmentation/discoloration. Red cell agglutination may be present; however, this must be differentiated from rouleaux formation. The Coombs test (anti-erythrocyte antibody) is the test of choice to detect the presence of IMHA (*Table 25*). The direct Coombs test detects antibodies attached to the red cell surface. Blood is collected in EDTA tubes, the reagent added is a species-specific antiserum, and red cell agglutination is the end result.

> **Table 25. Frequently used tests when evaluating immunologic or hematologic disorders**
>
> - Coombs test: Identifies antibodies attached to the red cell surface
> - Hemolytic crossmatch: Detects mare serum antibodies to foal red blood cells
> - Agglutination crossmatch: Detects mare serum antibodies to foal red blood cells
> - Jaundiced foal agglutination test (JFAT): Detects colostral (milk) antibodies to foal red blood cells
> - Jaundiced foal test or NI screen: Crossmatch

MANAGEMENT

Treatment of NI will be discussed in the next section. Treatment of IMHA includes managing the underlying disease process (e.g., resolution of infection or removal of drug therapy). Corticosteroid therapy can be useful: dexamethasone (0.1–0.2 mg/kg i/v q12–24h) or prednisolone (0.05–0.1 mg/kg p/o q12–24h). Oral prednisolone therapy may follow intravenous dexamethasone therapy. Treatment duration is dependent on disease severity and response to therapy. A tapering or low alternative drug dose may be necessary.

NEONATAL ISOERYTHROLYSIS

KEY POINTS

- NI is an antibody-mediated (immune-mediated) destruction of foal RBCs.
- The mare produces offending antibodies in response to foreign RBC antigens.
- NI is a preventable disease; a test in late gestation can identify mare RBC antibodies.
- The RBC antigen that the mare responds to is from *in utero* or periparturient exposure to fetal RBCs.
- The mare produces an antibody to the foals RBC antigens (obtained from the stallion) if they are different than hers.
- The foal absorbs these RBC antibodies from colostrum.
- The absorbed circulatory antibodies agglutinate or result in hemolysis of the foal's RBCs.

DEFINITION/OVERVIEW

NI is an immunologic disease that results in RBC destruction in the neonate. The condition can be defined as an immune-mediated anemia. The anemia is considered an alloimmune disease, as the offending antibody is produced by the mare. The mare produces antibodies to foreign red cell antigens that "leak" across the placental unit during gestation or at parturition. Therefore, the condition is usually seen in the multiparous mare; however, it can be seen in the primaparous mare. These antibodies to foreign red cell antigens enter the colostrum in late gestation. Ingestion of colostrum containing antibodies to foal red cell antigens results in agglutination or hemolysis of RBCs and subsequent anemia. All breeds are potentially susceptible to the condition. Analysis of frequently involved blood types suggests that 14% of all foals could have erythrocyte incompatibilities with the dam. However, alloimmunization does not occur with every incompatible pregnancy, therefore the actual incidence is less than 14%. There is also a breed variation in the production of alloantibodies. Thoroughbred mares and Standardbred mares produce 10% and 20% rates of detectable serum anti-RBC antibody, respectively. The incidence of clinical NI is reported to be approximately 2% and 4% in Thoroughbreds and Standardbreds, respectively.

ETIOLOGY/PATHOPHYSIOLOGY

The antibodies responsible for NI are produced when the mare produces an antibody response to a foreign antigen. The foreign antigen is a foal RBC surface antigen that the mare does not possess on her own RBCs. These antigens are a result of the stallion's red cell antigen type being passed to the foal. The stallion and the foal have an immunologically different red cell type to that of the mare. The mare may become exposed (sensitized) to foreign cell antigens in a few different ways. The most common exposure is likely during gestation or parturition. Hemorrhage at parturition or placental leakage during gestation results in mare exposure to foal RBCs. It is considered that repeat exposure in multiparous mares results in antibody values that are significant enough to cause red cell destruction in the foal. Mares may rarely become sensitized to red cell antigens secondary to blood transfusions.

The red cell surface antigens are known as "factors," and over 30 factors are recognized. These factors (surface molecules) are produced by six different red blood cell groups. These groups have been labeled A, C, D, K, P, and U. The factors are then labeled according to the group that produced them. For example, if group A produces two factors, they would be Aa and Ab. The red cell antigens (factors) that are most commonly associated with NI (90%) are Qa and Aa. These two antigens are common in the genetic makeup of the horse and are immunogenic. Mares that lack these factors are at a risk of producing foals with NI. Other antigens (factors) that less commonly produce NI include Ab, Da, Db, Dc, Ua, Ka, Pa, Qrs, Qb, Qc, R, S, and T. Ca antibodies are also frequently identified in pre-term mares, but these antibodies do not cause isoerythrolysis. Ca antibodies bound to the surface of red cell antigens do not result in lysis or agglutination.

The red cell antibodies that are absorbed in colostrum can result in rapid intravascular hemolysis. This reaction is mediated with other components of the immune system such as complement. Some foals that ingest red cell antibodies do not show evidence of red cell destruction for days after birth, suggesting a more gradual removal of RBCs (extravascular hemolysis). It is also thought that variation in onset of hemolysis may be dependent on the immune system of the foal. As the immune system of the foal matures, the pathways of hemolysis, agglutination, and/or reticuloendothelial system removal of red cells progresses.

CLINICAL PRESENTATION

Affected foals are normal at birth. Clinical signs of NI typically appear in the first few days of life; however, as previously mentioned, the disease can be seen in foals up to 5–7 days of age.

Clinical signs of NI are referable to a decrease in oxygen-carrying capacity that results from the anemia (lack of sufficient hemoglobin to carry oxygen). Severely affected foals may die before other clinical signs are noted. The classic clinical sign of NI in the foal is jaundice or icterus (**87–89**). Other clinical signs (*Table 26*) may include a continuation of weakness, depression, poor suckle, tachycardia, tachypnea, pigmenturia, and/or pale mucous membranes. Hemoglobinemia and/or hemoglobinuria are usually present. Secondary and less common signs may include renal or liver failure

and kernicterus or bilirubin encephalopathy. The icterus is a result of tissues stained with unconjugated or conjugated bilirubin resulting from red cell breakdown products. Weakness, depression, and tachycardia are a result of the anemia influencing oxygen delivery. The more uncommonly seen liver/renal disease may be related to the anoxia and/or direct cellular change as a result of high levels of bilirubin. Kernicterus is a descriptive term for the discoloration (jaundice) of cranial structures. Bilirubin encephalopathy describes the clinical signs that are seen when the central nervous system

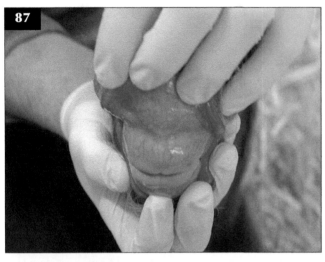

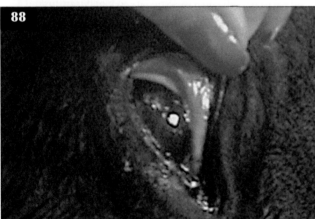

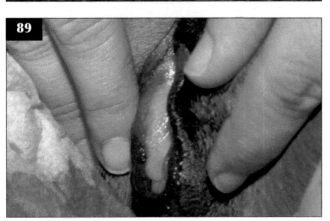

87–89 Icteric oral mucous membranes (**87**), icteric sclera (**88**), and icteric vulvar membranes (**89**).

Table 26. Typical clinical signs of neonatal isoerythrolysis

- Icterus/jaundice
- Weakness
- Depression
- Tachypnea
- Tachycardia
- Pale oral mucous membranes
- Hemoglobinemia
- Hemoglobinuria

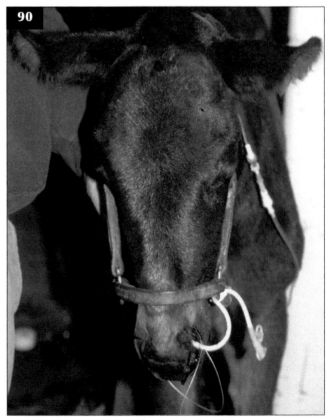

90 Bilirubin encephalopathy in a foal with neonatal isoerythrolysis.

(CNS) becomes saturated with bilirubin (**90**). Bilirubin encephalopathy is an infrequent sequela of NI, but it can be seen when bilirubin levels are excessive. The condition is usually lethal.

DIFFERENTIAL DIAGNOSIS

Differential diagnoses include other conditions resulting in anemia and icterus. These would include other immune-mediated anemias, organ system disease, sepsis, and hemorrhage (*Tables 24* and *27*). However, hemorrhage only results in icterus if the blood loss is internal.

DIAGNOSIS

Diagnosis of NI is based on history, signalment, typical clinical signs, and appropriate laboratory confirmation. Numerous tests will identify the presence of maternal alloantibodies. These tests use agglutination or hemolysis as the test end-point.

The hemolytic crossmatch using an addition of exogenous complement is considered the test of choice. Mare serum mixed with foal RBCs in the presence of complement will hemolyze the foal's RBCs if alloantibodies are present. A mare is considered positive if dilutions >1:16 produce complete hemolysis.

A crossmatch between mare and foal can also be used. This test crosses mare serum with foal RBCs; agglutination is the end-point. The test can have false positives; rouleaux formation can confuse the interpretation of agglutination. The mare/foal crossmatch can also produce false negatives; if complement is not included in the test, then hemolysis will not occur.

The primary reaction caused by mare alloantibodies is hemolysis, not agglutination. Demonstration of hemolysis is a more accurate test. A Coombs test can be used to identify antibodies bound to foal RBCs; however, it is not specific. An additional useful test is the jaundice foal agglutination test (JFAT). Foal RBCs are centrifuged with dilutions of mare colostrum. The formation of clumps at the bottom of the tube in dilutions of 1:16 or greater is considered positive.

MANAGEMENT

NI should be considered a disease of prevention. Although the incidence is not high and the outcome can be positive, complications and death do occur. Prevention can be achieved by not allowing those mares that are producing colostral red cell antibodies to nurse their foal until colostrum is no longer being produced and/or until foal absorption of antibodies is no longer occurring. This can be accomplished by blood typing the mare and stallion or, more

efficiently, by screening the mare for antibodies to red cells (JFAT or NI screen). This test looks for mare alloantibodies and is performed in the last month of gestation. If an incompatibility is present or the mare is producing red cell antibodies, the foal is typically muzzled (or prevented access to the mare's colostrum) (**91**) while being supplemented with stored colostrum and fed milk via an indwelling nasogastric tube or bottle) (**92, 93**) for 24–48 hours. The fed milk can be a commercial milk-replacer or milk from a donor mare. The mare should be hand milked frequently and the colostrum discarded. An agglutination test (mare colostrum/foal RBCs) can be

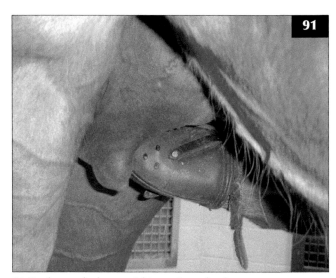

91 Foal muzzled to avoid ingestion of colostrum.

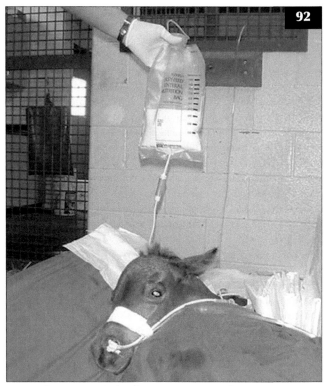

92 Feeding via an indwelling nasogastric tube.

Table 27. Differential diagnoses of icterus in the foal

- Hepatic disease
- Intravascular/extravascular hemolysis
- Physiologic disorders
- Sepsis
- Anorexia

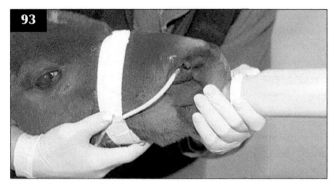

93 Feeding via a bottle.

used to determine when there are no longer antibodies remaining in the mare's milk; subsequently, the foal can be allowed to nurse. If there is concern regarding muzzling of a suspect foal (mare serum positive), the JFAT or hemolytic test can be performed before a newborn foal is allowed to nurse. An alternative to the mare screening test (JFAT or NI screen) is to blood type the mare. Mares that are Aa or Qa negative can be selectively bred to stallions that are also Aa or Qa negative; however, this method is impractical as it limits stallion selection. Additionally, it does not completely eliminate the possibility of other factors resulting in alloimmunization of the mare. Approximately 1 in 2,000 pregnancies may result in NI foals from red cell factors other than Aa or Qa.

TREATMENT OF ANEMIC FOALS

KEY POINTS
- Treatment of an anemic foal is based on the clinician's judgment of hypovolemic shock.
- Blood transfusions may be necessary.
- Blood transfusion is not without complications..

Treatment of a foal that has become anemic is necessary when the oxygen-carrying capacity of the RBCs decreases to a level where clinical signs of hypovolemic shock are present. Monitoring red cell numbers (count, PCV, or hematocrit) is an initial approach; however, there is not a level (cut-off point) at which blood transfusions should be administered. The decision should be made from the clinical examination and the degree of hypovolemia. The foal with a packed cell volume (PCV) of <0.2 L/L (20%) must be monitored carefully. The clinician should combine blood work with clinical signs in order to make the decision as to when a transfusion is necessary. Clinical signs of hypovolemia should include attitude, degree of strength, respiratory rate, and heart rate. The clinical signs in foals with a PCV of <0.2 L/L (20%) can vary considerably; this may be a result of the rapidity with which the anemia has occurred.

The decision for a transfusion should be made carefully, as complications, including transfusion reactions and the large bilirubin load that the addition of RBCs provides, exist. The foal that becomes weak, depressed, and develops a persistent tachycardia is likely to need a blood transfusion. Hemoglobin replacement products can be used as an alternative to transfusion or as a means to increase oxygen-carrying capacity until a transfusion is available. Hemoglobin products are safe; however, their half-life is of short duration.

Before administration of a transfusion, an appropriate donor must be chosen. The most accurate method to determine compatibility is a crossmatch between the donor and the patient. This includes both a major crossmatch (patient's plasma with donor red cells) and a minor crossmatch (donor's plasma with patient red cells). When the availability of a crossmatch is limited, or time does not allow the clinician to await results, then choices must be made based on the most likely compatibilities. The best donor has no anti-red-cell antibodies in its serum and has a blood type that will not react with the ingested antibody of the foal. Advanced screening can identify potential donors. The ideal donor is Qa and Aa antigen positive, as the majority of anti-red-cell antibodies are anti-Qa or anti-Aa. This blood type does not guarantee compatibility, as other red cell antigens can elicit red cell antibody production. The dam is also a potential source of red cells. The mare's whole blood must be washed free of serum antibodies; the remaining red cells will be compatible as the dam does not produce antibodies to her own RBCs. Washing of the mare's red cells requires repeated centrifugation after mixing with saline. This method is impractical unless the practitioner has access to a large refrigerated centrifuge.

Administration of the transfusion should be done with caution and with the use of a blood administration set (**94**). Transfusion

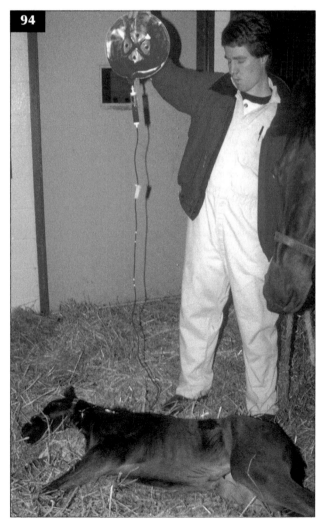

94 Transfusion of an anemic foal.

reactions can result in tachycardia, tachypnea, and/or other signs of anaphylaxis. The blood volume of the foal is approximately 7.5% of its body weight (e.g., 3.5 L in a 50 kg foal). Generally, administration of 1–2 liters of blood or washed red cells is adequate. Monitoring red cell numbers and/or transfusion response (clinical signs) is advisable. A rule of thumb would be to raise the PCV by 0.1 L/L (10%). The PCV typically, but gradually, decreases over the next few days as further red cell destruction occurs and transfused red cells are removed. The goal of therapy is to provide the patient with time to produce more red cells than are being destroyed. Individual or, more frequently, multiple transfusions can result in a significant life-threatening hyperbilirubinemia. When large amounts of RBCs are transfused, the reticuloendothelial and/or hepatic mechanisms of bilirubin excretion can be overwhelmed. This results in excessively elevated bilirubin levels. With extensive hyperbilirubinemia, bilirubin diffuses into tissues and disrupts cellular processes. Encephalopathy and liver or renal failure may ensue.

The therapy for bilirubin encephalopathy is limited and generally unsuccessful. A low dose of phenobarbital (0.5–1.0 mg/kg) may increase the microsomal enzyme metabolism of bilirubin.

THROMBOCYTOPENIA

KEY POINTS
- Thrombocytopenia is not a problem frequently identified in the foal.
- The most common cause is an alloimmune condition related to platelet antibodies in the dam.

DEFINITION/OVERVIEW
Thrombocytopenia is generally considered to be a platelet count of <100,000 platelets/μL. In the horse, platelets can be decreased through decreased production, injury, destruction, or increased consumption or utilization. Thrombocytopenia is not a commonly identified condition of the foal. Thrombocytopenia in foals has been seen in situations of repeat administration of plasma or secondary to administration of plasma intended for the prevention of *Rhodococcus equi* pneumonia. This is likely an initiation of an immune-mediated event; however, it has not been documented as such. The most commonly recognized cause of thrombocytopenia in the foal is the alloimmune-mediated destruction of platelets in the neonate.

ALLOIMMUNE THROMBOCYTOPENIA AND ULCERATIVE DERMATITIS

KEY POINTS
- A condition of thrombocytopenia often associated with dermatitis occurs in the foal.
- The condition is an alloimmune process, with foal ingestion and absorption of colostral antiplatelet antibodies.
- Thrombocytopenia results in petechiation and possibly hemorrhage.
- Dermatitis is most frequently seen around the eyes, mouth, and perineal region.

DEFINITION/OVERVIEW
The condition of thrombocytopenia and ulcerative dermatitis has been reported in a few foals and has been seen by several clinicians who treat large numbers of equines. The condition is more commonly noted in mule foals. The syndrome is seen in the neonatal age period. Neutropenia has occasionally been seen in association with the thrombocytopenia. Affected foals generally have a good prognosis for recovery.

ETIOLOGY/PATHOPHYSIOLOGY
This condition is an alloimmune process, with foal ingestion and absorption of mare antiplatelet colostral antibodies. It is as yet undetermined why the mare produces antiplatelet antibodies. Mares bred to different sires have produced sequential foals developing thrombocytopenia. Antiplatelet antibodies attach to the surface of the foal's platelets, leading to reticuloendothelial removal from circulation. Histopathology of the skin lesions identifies multiple vesicle formation (dermoepidermal), which may progress to separation, with fibrin, cellular debris, and RBCs filling the cleft.

CLINICAL PRESENTATION
Signs of thrombocytopenia include petechiation (95, 96), ecchymosis, and prolonged bleeding from venipuncture sites (97).

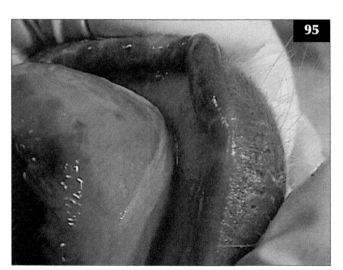
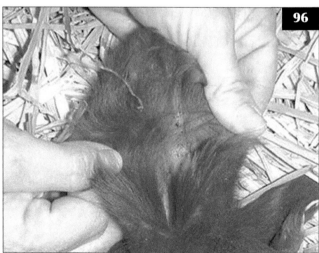

95, 96 Oral mucus membrane petechiation (**95**) and aural petechiation (**96**) in a foal with alloimmune thrombocytopenia.

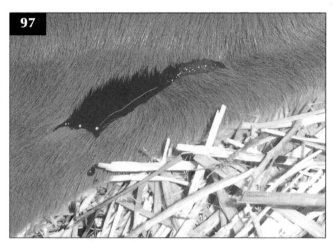

97 Prolonged bleeding from a venipuncture site.

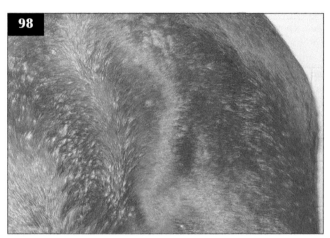

98 Crusting dermatitis in a foal with alloimmune thrombocytopenia and ulcerative dermatitis.

Skin lesions are variable and may include oral/lingual ulcers and a crusting dermatitis found most frequently around the eyes, muzzle, or perineal regions (**98**). The dermatitis can also be seen in the inguinal, axillary, or trunk regions. Affected foals have been seen with associated hemolytic anemia and they may be icteric. The thrombocytopenia may be severe. Affected foals may be depressed, weak, and/or nurse poorly to not at all. A neutropenia may be seen in conjunction with the dermatitis and thrombocytopenia.

DIFFERENTIAL DIAGNOSIS

The differential diagnosis includes other causes of thrombocytopenia (sepsis or possibly viral diseases). Pemphigus would be the primary skin lesion to consider. The combination of a skin lesion with a thrombocytopenia is suggestive of the condition.

DIAGNOSIS

Diagnosis is based on age and signalment and, if feasible, the diagnosis is confirmed with demonstration of platelet-associated antibodies. Laboratory findings are restricted to a thrombocytopenia, with an occasional neutropenia. Identifying mare serum antibodies to the foal's platelets confirms the condition to be alloimmune and not autoimmune. Histopathology of the skin lesions has revealed dermal hemorrhage, epidermal clefting, and superficial papillary necrosis.

MANAGEMENT

Whole blood transfusion may be necessary if significant blood loss has occurred. Administration of platelet-rich plasma collected in plastic containers from an appropriate donor (minor crossmatch) is necessary in circumstances where clinical signs progress. Glucocorticoids may be considered, but they have not been routinely required. Platelet counts generally increase in 5–10 days. Skin lesions resolve with time.

FURTHER READING

Giguere S, Polkes A (2005) Immunologic disorders in neonatal foals. *Veterinary Clinics of North America: Equine Practice* 21: 241–272.

LeBlanc M (1990) Immunologic conditions. In: *Equine Clinical Neonatology*, 1st ed. (Koterba AM, Drummond WH, Kosch PC, Eds.). Lea and Febiger, Philadelphia, PA, pp. 275–296.

McClure J (1997) Neonatal isoerythrolysis. In: *Current Therapy in Equine Medicine 4* (Robinson NE, Ed.). WB Saunders, Philadelphia, PA, pp. 592–594.

Toribio RE, Mudge MC (2013) Disease of the foal. In: *Equine Medicine Surgery and Reproduction,* 2nd ed. (Mair TS, Love S, Schumacher J, Smith RKW, Frazer G, Eds.). Saunders/Elsevier, Philadelphia, PA, pp. 423–450.

Trogdon-Hines M (1997) Immunodeficiency of foals. In: *Current Therapy in Equine Medicine 4* (Robinson NE, Ed.). WB Saunders, Philadelphia, PA, pp. 581–585.

Alimentary Tract Disorders 5

William V. Bernard

INTRODUCTION

Diseases of the alimentary tract are relatively common in the foal. Abdominal pain (colic), weight loss/failure to thrive, and enterocolitis are the primary clinical categories of gastrointestinal (GI) disease encountered. The investigation of alimentary disease includes a thorough history and physical examination. The age of the patient can be useful in determining the initial differential diagnoses. Radiography, ultrasonography, gastroscopy, and laboratory testing further enhance the clinician's ability to diagnose the disease process. Breed predilections exist.

HISTORY

The history can prove useful in establishing a list of differential diagnoses for alimentary disease. For example: What is the past medical history and current or historical problems with other animals on the farm (fever, diarrhea, weight loss); has the patient in question had problems or therapies that might predispose them to GI disease (antibiotic therapy can frequently cause GI upsets); have there been changes in management, including feeding practices; is the complaint is abdominal pain, if so, the duration of the problem is significant; when was the last time the foal was observed; does the foal present in a state of severe depression to stupor, which may mean severe prolonged pain; what are the signs of pain; were any other signs noted (many other conditions can initially appear as abdominal pain)?

SIGNALMENT

Other than scrotal/inguinal herniation or ovarian torsion, the gender of the patient is unlikely to influence GI disease. Males have been reported to be more prone to bladder rupture and meconium impaction, but the author's experience has shown no difference in sex predilection for these two conditions. Meconium is generally passed within the first 24 hours after birth. Congenital defects can be breed related. The lethal white syndrome is observed in specific Paint Horse crosses.

PHYSICAL EXAMINATION

The physical examination of the GI tract starts with a routine yet thorough physical examination of all the body systems. This will identify abnormalities in associated body systems and avoid overlooking related disease processes that may present as GI disease. Examination of the GI tract in the foal follows the same procedures as in the adult horse, the main difference being size. Small size limits the ability to perform a rectal examination, but it offers an advantage during ultrasonographic and radiographic examination of the abdomen. Small intestinal disease is more common in foals; therefore, these procedures are more rewarding.

Visual examination of the abdomen may provide information regarding the location of abdominal distension and the underlying cause. External abdominal palpation is of limited value. In small foals, some abdominal structures may be identified. The inguinal rings, umbilical region, and ventral abdomen should be palpated routinely for hernias. Bowel herniation can result in strangulation and vascular compromise. If hernias are easily reduced, careful monitoring and frequent reduction may be adequate.

Auscultation of the abdomen provides an assessment of GI motility and should be performed from the paralumbar fossa to the ventral abdomen on both the right and left sides. GI activity produces peristaltic and borborygmal sounds that should be heard approximately every 10–20 seconds. Tinkling or splashing sounds may be heard over the right dorsal quadrant as fluid enters the cecum; however, in young foals the lack of development of the cecum and large bowel influences the presence of borborygmal sounds. Simultaneous abdominal auscultation–percussion of a tympanitic or pinging sound identifies a gas-distended viscus adjacent to the body wall. Abdominal sounds can be classified as normal, increased, decreased, or absent. Decreases in motility suggest an ileus, which may be due to inflammatory, ischemic, or obstructive lesions. Increased motility occurs during the early stages of enteritis or intestinal obstruction.

In the neonate, evaluation of the quantity and quality of meconium is an important part of the physical examination. Meconium is an accumulation of swallowed amniotic fluid, GI secretions, and cellular debris that collects in the small colon and rectum and is passed shortly after birth. Meconium is generally black to dark brown in color and firm to pasty in consistency. Once meconium has been passed, the feces change to a softer, lighter brown quality. The amount of meconium varies between foals and reported passage of meconium does not rule out the possibility of meconium retention.

DIAGNOSIS

ABDOMINAL RADIOGRAPHY

Abdominal radiography helps to determine the location, but not necessarily the cause, of gas or fluid distension. Adequate radiographs can be obtained in foals up to 230 kg (500 lb) if the available radiographic equipment includes a grid, rare earth screens, and sufficient mAs (5–28) and kVp (75–95). Gaseous distension in foals with enteritis, peritonitis, or small intestinal obstruction is characterized radiographically by intraluminal gas–fluid interfaces (**99**). Multiple intraluminal gas–fluid interfaces or vertical U-shaped loops of distended small intestine are compatible with small intestinal obstructive disease (**100**). With enteritis, the small intestinal loops are smaller and concomitant large bowel distension may be seen. During large bowel obstruction, the large intestine is more distended and the colon may appear displaced within the abdomen (**101**). Contrast studies using gravity barium enemas (100–200 mL barium mixed with warm water) are useful in identifying meconium impactions (**102**).

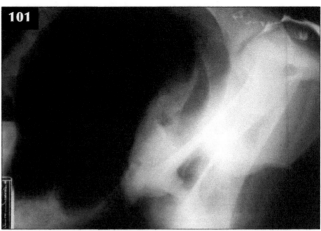

101 Radiograph showing large bowel obstruction. The large bowel is distended with displacement within the abdomen.

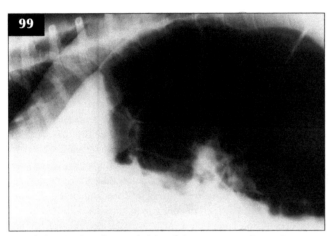

99 Abdominal radiograph identfying gaseous distension characterized by gas–fluid interfaces.

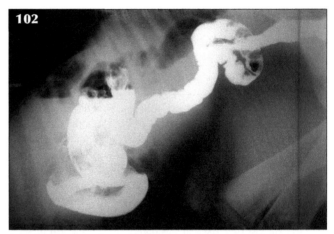

102 Contrast studies using barium, as illustrated here, are useful in identifying meconium impactions.

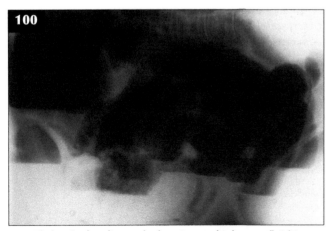

100 Abdominal radiograph showing multiple gas–fluid interfaces (vertical U-shaped loops) of distended small intestine compatible with small intestinal obstruction disease.

ABDOMINAL ULTRASONOGRAPHY

Abdominal ultrasonography permits characterization of small intestinal motility (absent, normal, hyper), distension (minimal, moderate, marked), and wall thickness. In older foals (>4 months of age), sonographic visualization of the small intestine is often limited to the caudal abdomen (inguinal region). Flaccid, nearly empty loops of small intestine are seen in the healthy foal (**103**). As intraluminal contents increase, ileus, enteritis, or small bowel obstructive disease may be present. Absence of motility may be seen in all these instances. The presence of motility does not exclude an obstruction, but makes it less likely. As an obstructive lesion progresses over time, the size of the small bowel increases, bowel walls are not discernible, and motility is lacking (**104**). Small intestinal intussusception appears as target- or doughnut-shaped patterns with the telescoping of one segment of bowel into another (**105**). Large intestinal gaseous distension causes reflection of sound waves, resulting in a poor ultrasonographic view of the abdomen. Abdominal fluid can be identified, quantified, and characterized. If excessive peritoneal

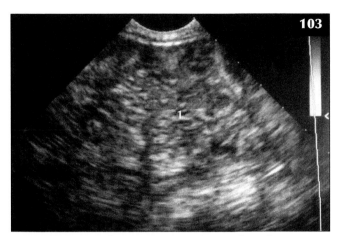

103 Ultrasonographic appearance of normal small intestine. Note the flaccid, nearly empty loops of small intestine. 1: small intestine.

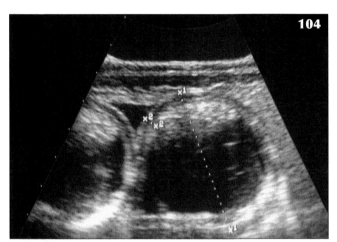

104 Distended fluid-filled bowel with increasing size and a lack of motility suggestive of obstruction.

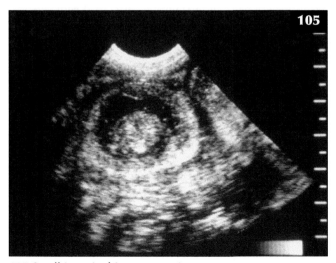

105 Small intestinal intussusception can appear as target- or doughnut-shaped patterns.

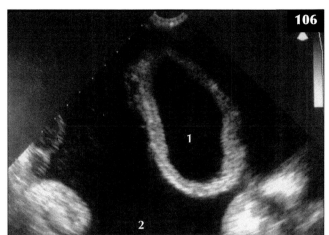

106 Excessive peritoneal fluid accumulation. Note the anechoic fluid surrounding intestinal contents. 1: bladder; 2: uroperitoneum.

fluid is detected (**106**), peritonitis, a ruptured viscus, or uroperitoneum may be present. Increased peritoneal fluid echogenicity is associated with increased cellularity. Gas echoes suggest the presence of a ruptured viscus.

OTHER DIAGNOSTIC AIDS
Nasogastric intubation
Nasogastric intubation may help identify a gas- or fluid-filled stomach. As large a stomach tube as can be passed through the nasal passages should be used. Fenestrations at the end of the tube help prevent obstruction of the tube with feed material. In neonates, a small, flexible tube such as a Harris Flush or enema tube is ideal.

A stomach pump and gravity flow or gentle aspiration with a 60 mL syringe may be used to check for reflux. With severe gastric distension, it may be difficult to pass a nasogastric tube through the cardia. Lidocaine applied to the tube or injected down the tube may be useful in relaxing the esophagus. Ultrasonography can be used to confirm the presence or absence of gastric distension.

Abdominocentesis
Abdominocentesis provides useful information about GI lesions. It is helpful to use ultrasonography to identify areas of peritoneal fluid, particularly if abdominal distension is present. If taut loops of small intestine are identified sonographically, abdominocentesis should be avoided or performed with extreme caution because of the increased risk of lacerating distended bowel. Abdominocentesis is performed on, or to the right of, the midline following aseptic preparation of the site. Sedation or local anesthetic may be required. In a foal that is struggling or too painful to remain standing, the tap can be performed with the foal in lateral recumbency. If fluid is not "free flowing," gentle aspiration with a small syringe may be helpful. Normal peritoneal fluid should be clear or slightly yellow in color, with a protein count <25 g/L (2.5 g/dL) and a WBC count <5,000/μL. A peritoneal fluid cell count of between 5,000 and 10,000 cells/μL may be within normal limits; counts of >10,000 cells/μL are considered abnormal.

Laboratory tests

Laboratory tests, although not diagnostic, aid in formulating a differential diagnosis list for foals with GI disease. Changes in the total peripheral WBC count and electrolyte concentrations may help differentiate early enteritis from surgical colic. Marked leukopenia is suggestive of enteritis and is not a common finding with a surgical abdomen. Enteritis can induce secretory mechanisms, including bicarbonate loss from pancreatic secretions and/or failure of absorption from the large colon, resulting in loss of electrolytes, hyponatremia, hypochloremia, and/or acidosis. Serum potassium concentrations are more variable and depend on fluid losses, acid–base status, and renal function. Electrolyte abnormalities in cases of surgical colic are frequently related to acid–base changes; hypochloremia may develop in long-standing acidosis subsequent to renal exchange of chloride ion for bicarbonate. However, occasionally, patients with a ruptured stomach may have hypochloremia, hyponatremia, and acidosis.

EXAMINATION OF FOALS WITH ABDOMINAL PAIN

When presented with a foal with abdominal pain, the main objective is to determine whether a surgical or nonsurgical lesion exists. The neonatal foal does not respond as rapidly or as effectively to systemic compromise as the adult. Rapid diagnosis and resolution of a strangulating lesion is imperative. The causes of abdominal pain in the foal range from volvulus to skin irritation from excessive iodine treatment of the umbilicus. A complete physical examination in combination with ancillary tests helps distinguish between many surgical and nonsurgical causes of colic. Abdominal pain is a frequent manifestation of enteritis, but if diarrhea is infrequent or absent, then the painful foal with enteritis may be difficult to differentiate from the foal requiring abdominal surgery, regardless of the results of extensive diagnostic testing (*Table 28*).

Vital signs may not always distinguish between surgical and nonsurgical colic. Changes in mucous membrane color resulting from distributive shock (endotoxemia, septicemia, splanchnic ischemia) can be present in a variety of GI diseases; therefore, changes in mucous membrane color are an unreliable indication of the surgical versus the nonsurgical patient. Severe toxic changes in mucous membranes are more typical of a strangulating lesion, but they can be seen with severe, acute bacterial enteritis or with peritonitis.

Foals are less tolerant of abdominal pain than adult horses. The degree of pain is not a sensitive indicator of the severity of abdominal disease in the foal. Pain characterized by rolling up on the back and teeth grinding has historically been associated with gastric ulceration; however, it is not uncommon for other causes of pain to show similar clinical signs. Other causes of abdominal pain (e.g., intussusception) are more common. Persistent pain that is nonresponsive to analgesics is more consistent with a surgical (usually strangulating) lesion. Mild abdominal pain, which persists or progresses to more severe colic, is compatible with enteritis, GI ulceration, or simple obstruction. Tachycardia and/or tachypnea is invariably present with severe abdominal pain or toxemia due to a ruptured viscus. Marked, persistent tachycardia (>120 bpm) suggests a surgical lesion.

Table 28. Differentiating the foal with painful enteritis from the surgical abdomen

	Surgical	Nonsurgical
Severe toxic changes in mucous membranes	More typical of a strangulating lesion	Can be seen with severe bacterial enterocolitis or peritonitis
Persistent nonresponsive abdominal pain	More consistent with a surgical lesion	Pain frequently present, not usually as persistent/severe
Marked, persistent tachycardia	Suggestive of a surgical lesion	
Elevated peritoneal fluid nucleated cell count	Most consistent with a strangulating lesion	
Large quantity of gastrointestinal reflux	Most consistent with a small intestinal strangulating lesion	Can be present with enterocolitis
Fever		Most consistent with enterocolitis

Intestinal strangulation of any duration is "usually" associated with an elevated nucleated cell count and protein concentration in the peritoneal fluid. Peritoneal fluid analysis is commonly normal in enteritis and simple early obstruction. As these diseases progress, increases in peritoneal fluid cell count and protein can occur, but they are not as dramatic as those seen with strangulating obstructions. Cytologic examination of peritoneal fluid does not distinguish between inflammation associated with enteritis and ischemia. Intracellular bacteria, plant material, and degenerated neutrophils may be identified in patients with a ruptured viscus.

A large quantity of gastric reflux is most typical of a strangulating small intestinal lesion, although moderate quantities of reflux can be obtained with other abdominal diseases, including enteritis. Persistent progressive reflux suggests, but is not diagnostic of, a small intestinal obstruction due to a volvulus, stricture, intussusception, or other small bowel disease.

Impacted meconium is the most frequent cause of abdominal pain in the neonate. The pain may vary from mild to severe. Foals may continue to nurse and frequently strain to defecate. The absence of palpable meconium does not rule out the possibility of an impaction over the brim of the pelvis or involving the proximal small colon (high meconium impactions). Radiographs, including contrast studies, help to identify retained meconium.

EXAMINATION OF FOALS WITH A NONPAINFUL DISTENDED ABDOMEN

Causes of nonpainful abdominal distension include intra-abdominal masses and excess intraperitoneal fluid. Abdominal masses include neoplasia (rare) and abscess formation. Accumulation of fluid in the peritoneal space may be a result of uroperitoneum, hemoperitoneum, or excessive production of peritoneal fluid. Abdominal fluid can be identified by ballottement of a fluid wave and be confirmed with ultrasonography. Peritoneal fluid analysis characterizes the type of fluid. An elevated white cell count is indicative of peritonitis, although with peracute septic peritonitis (e.g., GI rupture) the white cell count may be normal due to dilution. Degenerated neutrophils and intra- or extracellular bacteria indicate a septic process.

Causes of peritonitis other than primary GI disease are abdominal abscessation, umbilical remnant infection, or hematogenous in origin. The typical presentation of a foal with an abdominal abscess includes weight loss or failure to thrive and a distended or pendulous abdomen. These foals may or may not be depressed and are only intermittently febrile. A history of abdominal pain is not common. If acute peritonitis develops secondary to abscessation, these foals may present with septic/endotoxic shock.

Uroperitoneum is another common cause of abdominal distension in the foal and may present with or without signs of pain. Uroperitoneum is generally secondary to a ruptured bladder or leaking urachal remnant. Ultrasonographic evaluation identifies an anechoic peritoneal effusion. Abdominocentesis can increase the suspicion of a uroperitoneum (see Chapter 9, Urinary and Umbilical Disorders).

DISORDERS OF THE ORAL CAVITY AND SOFT PALATE

CLEFT PALATE

KEY POINTS

- Defects are an abnormality of embryogenesis.
- Defects in the primary palate result in difficulties suckling or prehending.
- Defects in the secondary palate result in dysphagia.
- Diagnosis of secondary palate abnormalities can be made conclusively via endoscopy.
- Pneumonia is a frequent secondary complication of cleft palate.
- The success of surgical repair is dependent on the extent of the palate defect.

DEFINITION/OVERVIEW

Cleft palate is a congenital abnormality with defects of either the primary or secondary palate. Defects of the primary palate (external nares and lips) result in visible abnormalities of the lips or external nares. Defects of the secondary palate (hard and soft palate) are more common and usually include the caudal one-half to three-quarters of the soft palate.

ETIOLOGY/PATHOPHYSIOLOGY

Defects occur as a result of an abnormality during embryogenesis described as failure of fusion of the lateral palatine processes. It is not known whether cleft palate is a heritable condition. Defects in the soft palate affect the ability to swallow. Defects in the primary palate result in difficulties in suckling or prehension.

CLINICAL PRESENTATION

Foals with abnormalities of the primary palate will have visible difficulties in suckling or prehending. Foals with secondary cleft palate often present with bilateral nasal discharge. The degree of palatal defect will dictate whether nasal discharge is present. The discharge consists of (or contains) milk (after suckling) (107) or feed material (after eating). Foals with palatal defects may cough frequently. These foals may also present with pneumonia subsequent to aspiration of feed material. Respiratory disease (if present) is typically represented by consolidation ventrally, which may or may not result in obvious clinical respiratory disease. Foals with pneumonia secondary to cleft palate may present with weight loss or failure to thrive.

DIFFERENTIAL DIAGNOSIS

Causes of dysphagia (see Chapter 10, Neurologic Disorders), nasal discharge (see Chapter 8, Respiratory Disorders), chronic cough, or failure to thrive.

DIAGNOSIS

A suspicion of cleft palate is gained from the signalment, history, and clinical examination. Palpation of the palate through the mouth can identify defects of the palate. Endoscopic evaluation of the pharynx is the most reliable method of diagnosing a cleft palate. Endoscopy will identify variable absence of soft palate, with a lack of palatal tissue in contact with the ventral aspect of the epiglottis. Auscultation, radiographs, and/or ultrasonographic evaluation of the lungs should be performed to look for the presence of aspiration pneumonia.

MANAGEMENT

Treatment of cleft palate includes surgical repair of the palatal defect and therapy of respiratory disease if present. Surgical prognosis is dependent on the extent of the defect; adequate palatal

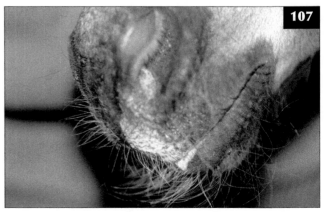

107 Foal with a cleft palate. Note the milky nasal discharge.

tissue must be present to perform adequate surgical apposition. The overall prognosis for full recovery is poor and postoperative care is extensive. Postsurgical care includes resting the surgical site, which may include an indwelling nasogastric tube, esophagostomy, or parenteral nutrition. The prognosis for correction of soft palatal lesions is considered to be better than that for hard palatal involvement.

MAXILLARY AND MANDIBULAR PROGNATHISM

KEY POINTS
- Prognathism is likely an embryogenic abnormality.
- Maxillary prognathism is an overbite.
- Mandibular prognathism is an underbite.
- The abnormality is in the lack of opposing tooth occlusion and/or prehension, and mastication.
- Surgical correction is dependent on the degree of malocclusion.
- Frequent dental attention may be adequate for premolar abnormalities.

DEFINITION/OVERVIEW
Maxillary prognathism is a congenital abnormality also known as overbite, parrot mouth, or brachygnathism. Mandibular prognathism (underbite, monkey-mouth) is much less common (**108**). Occasionally, normal individuals can develop this abnormality after birth.

ETIOLOGY/PATHOPHYSIOLOGY
Maxillary prognathism likely results from an abnormality during embryogenesis. The heritability of the condition has not been proven.

Maxillary prognathism results in an abnormality in the occlusion of the incisors and/or premolars. The degree of malocclusion dictates the difficulty with which the patient will be able to masticate properly. The various forms of prognathism include abnormal occlusion of the incisors (typically the upper incisors projecting beyond the lower) or normal occlusion of the incisors with abnormal occlusion of the premolars. Many horses may have some degree of overbite and, unless the condition is severe, the majority can eat normally. Premolar malocclusion is often more of a problem, as the lack of apposition allows unopposed growth of the opposing teeth and the development of hooks.

CLINICAL PRESENTATION
When the condition is severe, individuals may present with obvious visible overbite. These individuals may have difficulty with prehension of food material. Foals with parrot mouth can usually suckle without problems. Abnormal premolar alignment may result in the formation of hooks, which can result in mouth pain and quiddor.

DIFFERENTIAL DIAGNOSIS
Differential diagnosis may include maxillary or mandibular fractures, infected teeth, foreign bodies, or other dental abnormalities.

DIAGNOSIS
Diagnosis is made via visual examination of the mouth, looking for appropriate occlusion of the incisors and molars. This should include observation of the ability to masticate properly and without pain. When examining for occlusion, the horse's head should be maintained in the normal position during the examination, as raising the head can shift the mandible caudally. Radiographs of the dental arcade can be useful.

MANAGEMENT
Many individuals with varying degrees of prognathism may function normally. Treatment of prognathism is considered controversial, as the hereditability of the condition remains in question. Premolar abnormalities can be addressed with frequent dental attention. Surgery can be attempted in foals if the degree of malocclusion is not greater than 2–5 cm. The surgical procedure consists of placing a wire on either side of the maxilla at the level of the second and third premolar. The implanted wires can be left in place until the arcade discrepancies are corrected.

DISORDERS OF THE ESOPHAGUS

The esophagus is a muscular tube that connects the oropharynx with the stomach. The esophagus functions to transport material to the stomach and to prevent retrograde movement of material from the stomach. The muscular layer of the esophagus contains both striated and smooth muscle. The cranial two-thirds and distal one-third consist of striated muscle and smooth muscle, respectively. Innervation of the esophagus is a combination of motor, sympathetic, and parasympathetic input. The proximal two-thirds (striated muscle) is under neurogenic control of the pharyngeal and esophageal branches of the vagus nerve. The esophageal branch of the vagus nerve also supplies the parasympathetic innervation of the distal esophagus. Sympathetic innervation of the esophagus is minimal. The esophagus travels dorsally on the midline above the trachea until approximately the cranial one-third of the neck, where it passes to the left (rarely to the right) and more superficially. The esophageal mucosa consists of a stratified squamous epithelium. The esophageal phase of swallowing is initiated when the upper esophageal sphincter is relaxed; esophageal peristalsis propels a bolus through the lower esophageal sphincter and into the stomach.

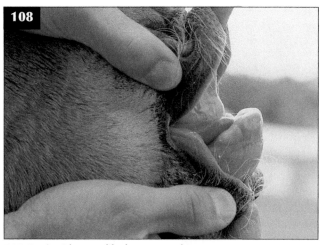

108 Foal with mandibular prognathism.

Congenital and acquired disorders can result in esophageal disease. Congenital disorders are uncommon, but may include cysts or varying types of diverticulum, or megaesophagus. The more common causes of esophageal disease are acquired disorders (e.g., impaction or obstructions) and ulceration with esophagitis. Ectasia (dilation of unknown origin), achalasia (neuronal dysfunction resulting in failure of relaxation of the distal esophagus with dilation proximally), and megaesophagus secondary to vascular ring abnormalities are rarely reported. Megaesophagus may also be seen in conjunction with ulcerative esophagitis. In this circumstance it is difficult to determine whether the ulceration is primary or secondary to reflux of acid contents from the stomach.

As the hallmark of esophageal disease is dysphagia, the differential diagnosis list is extensive. Causes of dysphagia (*Table 29*) include systemic disease, central nervous system (CNS) disorders or brainstem lesions, obstructions from the mouth to the stomach, congenital disorders of the oropharynx or esophagus, peripheral neural disorders, or gastric outflow obstruction.

The diagnosis of esophageal disorders includes physical examination, plain and contrast radiography, and endoscopy. The primary physical abnormality is dysphagia as noted by ptyalism (salivation), feed material dropping from the mouth, and/ or discharge at the nostrils. Horses with choke may repeatedly attempt to swallow and retch subsequent to these attempts. A complete examination of the mouth, looking for other causes of dysphagia, is of primary importance. Palpation of the neck in

the region of the jugular furrow may identify an area of enlargement. Diffuse swelling with crepitance may indicate rupture of the esophageal wall. Passage of a nasogastric tube can confirm the presence of obstruction. The presence of a cough may indicate aspiration. Thorough auscultation of the thorax, ± thoracic radiography and/or ultrasonography, should be performed with any esophageal disease to ensure there is no significant pneumonia.

Radiographic evaluation includes survey films and a contrast esophagram when necessary. A survey film determines the appropriate radiographic settings for the best esophageal images and can identify impactions or foreign bodies. Contrast studies using barium paste or liquid barium can identify obstructions, a dilated esophagus, strictures, and mucosal defects. Barium paste outlines longitudinal esophageal folds and localizes obstructions and mucosal defects when barium is noted in surrounding soft tissues. Liquid barium, administered into the proximal esophagus, can be useful particularly when the lesion is not an obstruction. Liquid barium administered under pressure with a cuffed nasogastric tube can identify displacements of the esophagus (extraluminal masses), strictures, and dilations of the esophagus. Double contrast studies (air insufflation subsequent to liquid barium) permits examination of mucosal folds with the esophagus distended. Air insufflation can be provided through a cuffed tube or through the air port of an endoscope.

Endoscopic evaluation (esophagoscopy) provides visualization of obstructive lesions, mucosal abnormalities, and strictures. The nature and severity of radiographic abnormalities can be further investigated. Air insufflation during evaluation is necessary to distend the normally collapsed muscular tube of the esophagus. The normal appearance of the mucosa is a pale white color with longitudinal folds that may undergo peristalsis and will collapse over the endoscope if air insufflation is not maintained. Transverse folding of the esophagus may be present as the endoscope is passed toward the stomach. Transverse folds should not be considered abnormal unless they persist with esophageal dilation. The presence of saliva mixed with ingesta may obscure vision of an obstruction or stricture.

The management of esophageal disorders is dependent on the etiology.

ESOPHAGEAL OBSTRUCTION (CHOKE)

KEY POINTS
- Esophageal obstruction is the most common esophageal abnormality of the foal.
- Diagnosis can be based on endoscopy.
- Pharmacologic intervention may resolve the obstruction.

DEFINITION/OVERVIEW
Esophageal obstruction is defined as obstruction of the esophagus with either feed material or a foreign body. The diet of the foal (primarily milk) makes esophageal obstruction less common in the foal than in the adult; however, choke remains the most common esophageal disorder encountered in the foal. Esophageal obstruction should be included in the differential of any age foal with dysphagia.

Table 29. Causes of dysphagia
- Prematurity
- Congenital oral/pharyngeal abnormalities:
  - Cleft palate
  - Subepiglottic cyst
- Congenital laryngeal abnormalities
- Dorsal displacement of the soft palate or rostral displacement of the palatopharyngeal arch
- Pharyngitis
- Hypoxic ischemic encephalopathy
- Encephalopathy, hepatic or other encephalopathy
- Meningitis
- Brainstem lesion
- Tetanus
- Equine herpesvirus
- Equine protozoal myelitis
- Botulism
- Hyperkalemic periodic paralysis
- Nutritional myodegeneration
- Hypocalcemia
- Megaesophagus or other esophageal disorders
- Retropharyngeal abscessation of the oral or pharyngeal region
- Tumors of the oral or pharyngeal region
- Foreign bodies

ETIOLOGY/PATHOPHYSIOLOGY

The most common cause of esophageal obstruction is gluttonous behavior, although ingestion of foreign bodies occasionally obstructs the esophagus. Rapid feedstuff ingestion results in larger than normal, dry, difficult to swallow boluses of feed. Impactions may consist of concentrates, roughage, foreign objects, or sometimes bedding.

CLINICAL PRESENTATION

The foal presenting with esophageal obstruction may act depressed or agitated. Affected animals may spend inordinate amounts of time at a water source, either attempting to drink or "playing" with the water. Ptyalism and dysphagia are prominent features of presentation. Regurgitation of food material and saliva from the mouth or nostrils may be noted (**109**). Affected horses may cough secondary to aspiration of material into the trachea. Odynophagia (painful swallowing) and retching may be noted.

DIFFERENTIAL DIAGNOSIS

See *Table 29*.

DIAGNOSIS

See Disorders of the Esophagus, pp. 78–79.

MANAGEMENT

Ideally, the location and type of the obstruction should be ascertained before commencing treatment of choke, as this can have a bearing on the type of therapy instituted. Smooth muscle relaxants are frequently successful in an initial approach to the choked horse. Oxytocin (1 IU/kg i/v or i/m) and butylscopolamine (0.3 mg/kg i/v) have been used. These two drugs produce relaxation of the striated muscle of the proximal esophagus and smooth muscle of the distal esophagus, respectively. If the pharmacologic approach to obstruction is not successful, gentle passage of a nasogastric tube, with or without flushing of water under pressure, should be undertaken. The combination of gentle lavage and pharmacologic relaxation of the esophageal musculature is frequently successful. If this approach is not successful, a more aggressive approach of lavage should be pursued. With more aggressive lavage, it is necessary to prevent aspiration into the trachea. This can be achieved by using a cuffed endotracheal tube and/or a cuffed nasotracheal tube. The cuffed endotracheal tube can be passed and inflated before initiating lavage and removed with the cuff inflated in an attempt to remove any material that has entered the trachea. Heavy sedation facilitates the procedure and keeps the head lowered, thus aiding in the prevention of aspiration. If aggressive lavage and smooth muscle relaxants are still not successful, surgery can be considered as a last option. Surgery remains a last resort as the procedure is difficult to perform and stricture secondary to esophagostomy is a potential sequela.

ESOPHAGEAL ULCERATION/ESOPHAGITIS

KEY POINTS

- Gastric esophageal reflux is the most common cause of esophageal ulceration.
- The most common cause of gastroesophageal reflux is gastric outflow obstruction.
- Clinical signs may include anorexia, ptyalism, and bruxism.
- Endoscopy is the basis of diagnosis.
- Management requires removal of the inciting cause.

DEFINITION/OVERVIEW

Gastric esophageal reflux is the most common cause of esophageal ulceration. Reflux of acidic gastric contents ulcerates the esophageal mucosa. This type of ulceration is often influenced by the folds of the esophagus and is linear in appearance. Ingested contact irritants or pressure necrosis secondary to esophageal obstruction can occasionally result in ulceration.

ETIOLOGY/PATHOPHYSIOLOGY

Exposure of the esophageal mucosa to caustic chemicals can result in mucosal irritation and ulceration. Reflux of gastric acid secondary to gastric outflow obstruction results in a linear reflux esophagitis of the distal esophagus (**110**). The degree of esophageal damage is related to the nature of the fluid and duration of exposure. Gastric acid, bile salts, and pepsin may all be irritating to the squamous mucosa of the esophagus. The most common cause of reflux esophagitis in foals is gastric outflow obstruction. Persistent distal esophagitis/ulceration can result in decreased esophageal sphincter tone and a self-perpetuation of gastric reflux. Severe cases can develop motility disorders, chronic inflammation, and fibrosis, with persistent esophageal dilation. Protracted esophageal obstructions applying excessive local pressure to the in-contact esophagus can result in local ischemia and subsequent necrosis of the mucosal wall. These ulcerations can be partial or circumferential.

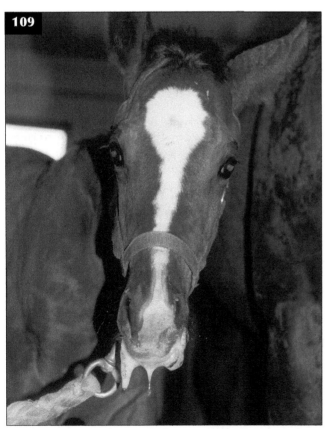

109 Frothy salivation in a foal with esophageal obstruction or choke.

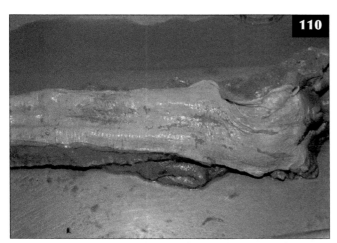

110 Necropsy specimen showing linear ulceration of the esophagus.

CLINICAL PRESENTATION

A foal with esophagitis presents differently from a foal with an esophageal obstruction. Esophagitis results in pain that can be persistent or appear worse when swallowing. Pain can result in anorexia, ptyalism, and bruxism. However, similar to esophageal obstruction, patients with esophageal ulceration may present with dysphagia, nasal discharge, depression, agitation, and regurgitation of food material from the mouth or nostrils.

DIFFERENTIAL DIAGNOSIS

See *Table 29*.

DIAGNOSIS

Endoscopic evaluation of the esophagus is the preferred method of diagnosis. Radiographic contrast studies can be used if endoscopic examination is not available. Contrast studies may identify retention of contrast material and mucosal irregularities. Endoscopy allows direct visualization of the ulcerated mucosa (**111**); a linear pattern is suggestive of gastric reflux esophagitis (**110**).

MANAGEMENT

The primary aim in the management of esophagitis is removal of the inciting cause. Medical treatment will fail unless the primary cause is corrected. Gastric decompression via a nasogastric tube can be sufficient for a functional gastric outflow or proximal enteritis/ileus. Anatomic gastric outflow obstruction must be resolved surgically. Medical control of gastric acid (see Management of gastric ulceration, p. 86) should be used in cases of reflux esophagitis. Coating agents such as sucralfate may provide temporary relief.

ESOPHAGEAL STRICTURE

KEY POINTS

- Strictures are classified with regard to the involvement of the layers of the esophageal wall.
- Congenital strictures are rare.
- Acquired strictures are caused by trauma to the esophageal wall.
- Diagnosis is based on endoscopic examination.
- Dietary management can be useful.
- Esophageal surgery can have complications.

DEFINITION/OVERVIEW

Strictures are defined as narrowing of the esophageal lumen (**112, 113**). They can be classified as to their involvement of the esophageal layers: (1) mural lesions that involve the adventitia and muscularis; (2) esophageal rings or webs that involve only the mucosa or submucosa; and (3) annular stenosis that involves all layers of the esophageal wall. The prognosis will vary with the nature of the strictures.

ETIOLOGY/PATHOPHYSIOLOGY

Esophageal strictures can be congenital or acquired. Congenital lesions are rare. Those reported are a result of congenital anomalies of the aortic arch. Acquired lesions can be the result of exogenous or endogenous traumatic injury. The most common causes of trauma include external blows or lacerations of the neck, longstanding esophageal obstruction, esophageal ulceration (**113**), and corrosive or internal foreign body injury.

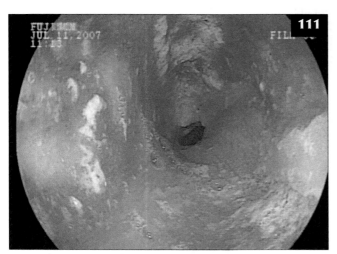

111 Endoscopy revealing severe esophageal ulcers as a result of reflux esophagitis secondary to outflow obstruction.

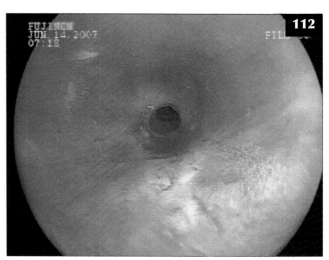

112 Endoscopic visualization of an esophageal stricture.

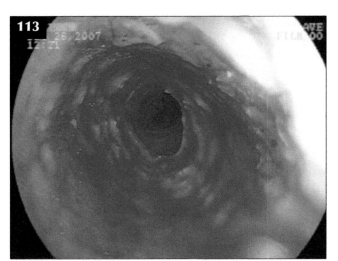

113 Endoscopy showing stricture of the esophagus with circumferential ulceration secondary to obstruction.

The mucosa of the esophagus responds rapidly (regeneration) to injury. If the injury is superficial (mucosal), the healing response is generally benign, which may produce a mild narrowing of the esophageal lumen secondary to the primary inflammatory response. Deeper (esophageal wall) injury can result in repair that results in cicatrix formation (fibrinous tissue synthesis, wound contraction, annular stenosis) or partial narrowing of the lumen.

CLINICAL PRESENTATION
As with foals with obstruction of the esophagus (see Esophageal Obstruction), the characteristic presentation of esophageal stricture is of recurrent feed impaction. The clinical signs are described under esophageal obstruction (p. 80).

DIFFERENTIAL DIAGNOSIS
The differential diagnoses are the same as for esophageal obstruction (p. 79–80) (*See Table 29*).

DIAGNOSIS
See Esophageal Obstruction. Endoscopic observation is most useful (**112**).

MANAGEMENT
Medical therapy of esophageal stricture is often unrewarding. Dietary management is the primary goal. Provision of moistened feeds or slurries, complete feeds, pellets, or grass as the only roughage can be successful on a long-term basis in a limited number of cases. Bougienage (passage of a slender cylinder through the stricture with the purpose of stretching or enlarging the opening) can be attempted. This technique meets with variable success in the horse and may be dependent on the duration and severity of the stricture. Esophageal surgery is fraught with complications, but is necessary if conservative approaches are unsuccessful. Extensive descriptions of the surgical approach to esophageal stricture can be found elsewhere. Surgical repair will require esophageal rest, which will necessitate alternative sources of nutrition. Alternative feed sources include total or partial parenteral nutrition or extraoral alimentation using an esophagotomy tube.

ESOPHAGEAL RUPTURE/PERFORATION

KEY POINTS
- Esophageal rupture is potentially a life-threatening event.
- Local necrosis secondary to chronic obstruction is the most common cause.
- Cellulitis is a usual complication.
- Local/external swelling is frequently noted.
- Radiographic contrast studies may be useful.

DEFINITION/OVERVIEW
Rupture or perforation of the esophagus may involve any portion of the esophagus including the cranial esophageal sphincter. Esophageal rupture is a potentially life-threatening event. Leakage of feed material or salivary secretions subcutaneously results in cellulitis.

ETIOLOGY/PATHOPHYSIOLOGY
Perforation of the esophagus can result from sharp object lacerations, penetrating objects, focal pressure necrosis, or ulceration secondary to protracted obstruction. Rupture of the cranial esophageal sphincter is an occasional occurrence and is generally the result of repeated or overzealous nasogastric intubation.

Subsequent to perforation, subcutaneous leakage of saliva, secretions, and feed material often occurs. Subcutaneous tissue contamination results in a cellulitis. The cellulitis can become progressive, dissecting along facial planes. Progression of cellulitis can result in sloughing of overlying skin, mediastinitis, and pleuritis. Subcutaneous emphysema may be present. Emphysema may be a result of air entering through the esophageal injury or anaerobic gas production.

CLINICAL PRESENTATION
Clinical signs of esophageal rupture include signs of obstruction and often include considerable cervical swelling (**114**). This swelling is often warm and painful, indicative of infection. Subcutaneous emphysema may be present. Progressive cellulitis

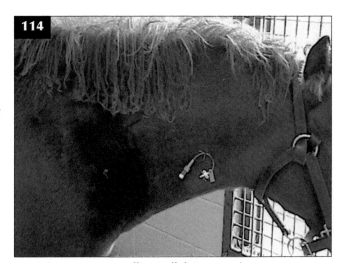

114 Subcutaneous swelling/cellulitis secondary to an esophageal rupture.

may dissect along fascial planes, leading to mediastinitis and possibly peritonitis. Overlying skin may be sloughed.

DIFFERENTIAL DIAGNOSIS

Other conditions causing signs of esophageal disease should be considered (see previous sections). If and when ventral cervical swelling becomes evident, other conditions that could result in cervical swelling must be considered. These would include penetrating wounds, abscesses, trauma resulting in hematomas, or vertebral fractures.

DIAGNOSIS

Esophageal rupture can be identified via endoscopy. Radiographs may identify subcutaneous emphysema (115). Significant swelling/inflammation at the injury site or adjacent structures can make endoscopic visualization more difficult. Cranial esophageal sphincter rupture may be difficult to observe visually. Contrast studies using water-soluble contrast material will identify extravasated material. Paste and liquid contrast materials are available in human medicine. Pastes can be applied orally or top-dressed on feed. The placement of liquid barium in the cranial esophagus via a nasogastric tube typically provides the best contrast for radiographic interpretation.

MANAGEMENT

Esophageal perforations can be allowed to heal via second intention. Surgical exploratory may be necessary to provide adequate drainage and possibly to debride necrotic tissue at the site of the perforation. Broad-spectrum antibiotic therapy is imperative. Excessive loss of salivary secretions can result in a metabolic acidosis. Nutritional support often becomes a limiting factor, as the esophagus must be rested as wound contraction occurs. An esophagostomy tube (or nasogastric tube) can be placed for nutritional support.

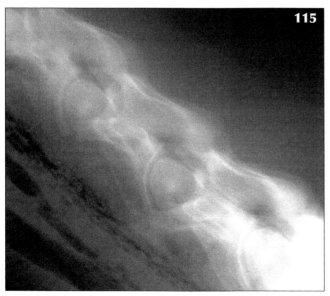

115

115 Radiographic evidence of subcutaneous emphysema secondary to an esophageal rupture.

ESOPHAGEAL DIVERTICULUM

KEY POINTS
- Esophageal diverticulum is a herniation of intact mucosa through a defect in the muscular wall.
- Acquired esophageal diverticulum as a result of trauma is most common.
- Large diverticula may result in clinical signs of obstruction.
- Obstruction may be recurrent.
- Small diverticula may be managed with soft/moist feeds.

DEFINITION/OVERVIEW

An esophageal diverticulum is a herniation of the mucosa through a defect in the esophageal wall. The diverticulum can be described as "pulsion" or "traction" based on the etiology.

ETIOLOGY/PATHOPHYSIOLOGY

Diverticula can be congenital or acquired. Acquired diverticula are significantly more common. Acquired diverticula can occur when the muscular layer of the esophagus is damaged. Traction diverticula develop during the healing process of injury or surgical intervention. A pulsion diverticulum is produced by intraluminal pressure and abnormal local peristalsis.

Small diverticula, particularly traction diverticula, are of little significance. Large pulsion diverticula may result in obstruction.

CLINICAL PRESENTATION

Diverticula can result in recurrent signs of choke. Occasionally, postprandial cervical esophageal enlargement may be noted.

DIFFERENTIAL DIAGNOSIS

See Esophageal Rupture/Perforation, pp. 82–83 (*Table 29*).

DIAGNOSIS

Diagnosis involves endoscopy or contrast radiography (see Esophageal Rupture/Perforation, p. 83).

MANAGEMENT

Large diverticula may require surgical intervention. Smaller diverticula can be managed using alternative feed sources, which may include pasture only, moistened/soaked roughage, or a more strenuous nutritional approach such as mashes or gruels. The long-term prognosis is dependent on the size of the diverticula.

MEGAESOPHAGUS

KEY POINTS
- Primary megaesophagus is rare.
- Chronic obstruction or esophagitis is the most common cause of megaesophagus.
- Megaesophagus results in difficulty in normal transfer of feed material to the stomach.
- Contrast radiography is diagnostic.

DEFINITION/OVERVIEW

Megaesophagus is the descriptive term used for esophageal dilation. Primary megaesophagus is very rare in the foal. Megaesophagus is more typically reported secondary to other esophageal diseases.

Achalasia (failure of the distal esophagus to relax with subsequent dilation of the proximal segment) has not been reported in foals. Megaesophagus is a more common cause secondary to the esophageal disorders discussed previously.

ETIOLOGY/PATHOPHYSIOLOGY

Chronic esophageal obstruction is the most frequent cause of megaesophagus in foals. Megaesophagus may also occur secondary to reflux esophagitis, with the resulting abnormal peristalsis and partial obstruction of the cardia contributing to esophageal dilation. Idiopathic megaesophagus and megaesophagus secondary to vascular ring anomalies have been reported in the foal. Other causes of megaesophagus include conditions that influence innervation. Disruption of central, afferent, or efferent pathways controlling esophageal motility could result in megaesophagus. Esophageal dilation results in inability or difficulty in the normal transfer of food material aborally to the stomach.

CLINICAL PRESENTATION

See Esophageal Obstruction (p. 80). Failure to thrive may be noted in congenital or chronic cases. Chronic pneumonia secondary to aspiration may be present.

DIFFERENTIAL DIAGNOSIS

See Esophageal Obstruction (p. 99) (*See Table 29*).

DIAGNOSIS

Esophagoscopy identifies an enlarged lumen and a lack of peristaltic waves. Fluid may pool ventrally. Ulceration of the distal esophagus may be seen if GI reflux is the cause of the esophageal dilation. Contrast radiography (liquid barium placed in the proximal esophagus via nasogastric tube) identifies pooling of contrast material ventrally and stagnation evident on repeat radiographic views.

MANAGEMENT

Conservative therapy with feed management has been used successfully to treat idiopathic dilation. Resolution of gastric outflow obstruction, and hence esophageal ulceration and functional obstruction, can resolve megaesophagus secondary to esophageal irritation.

DISORDERS OF THE STOMACH/ DUODENUM

GASTRIC ULCERATION, GASTRODUODENAL ULCERATION AND GASTROESOPHAGEAL REFLUX DISEASE

KEY POINTS
- Gastric ulceration is a common condition in foals.
- The distal esophagus or proximal duodenum may be involved.
- Ulceration occurs when protective mechanisms are overwhelmed by aggressive factors.
- Gastric ulcers can be asymptomatic.
- The classic triad of clinical signs of ulcer disease in foals is bruxism, ptyalism, and dorsal recumbency.
- Gastric ulceration can result in a variety of nonspecific clinical signs.
- Diagnosis of gastric ulceration is based on gastroscopy.

- The goal of medical therapy is to alter the acid content of the stomach.
- Acid neutralization (use of antacids) has a short duration of action.
- H_2 receptor antagonists have poor bioavailability in the horse, with only a moderate duration of action.
- Protein pump inhibitors (omeprazole) have a prolonged duration of action and are the best choice for healing of gastric ulcers.

DEFINITION/OVERVIEW

Ulceration of the proximal segments of the GI tract is common in the foal. Clinical signs can be mild to severe and sequelae can occasionally be catastrophic. Involvement of the duodenum with this condition is much more common in foals than in the adult horse. GI mucosal damage can result in inflammation, erosion, or ulceration. Erosion can be defined as disruption of the superficial layer, whereas ulceration results in deep penetration into the mucosa. The neonate is capable of significant acidification of the stomach by 2 days of age. The glandular mucosa is fully differentiated at birth and capable of maintenance of a protective mucus barrier. The squamous epithelium of the stomach (nonglandular mucosa) undergoes epithelial hyperplasia, which may be stimulated by local growth factors and/or exposure to an acid environment.

ETIOLOGY/PATHOPHYSIOLOGY

In basic terms, it can be stated that acid equals ulceration. Mucosal ulceration occurs when protective mechanisms (i.e., mucus, bicarbonate barrier, and mucosal blood flow) are overwhelmed by aggressive factors (e.g., gastric acid and pepsin). Aggressive factors can be influenced by alterations in blood flow secondary to systemic disease processes, changes in diet or interruption of regular nursing (loss of buffer capacity), high concentrate diets (which contain large amounts of soluble carbohydrates), and physiologic stress resulting in alteration in mucosal blood flow. The squamous (nonglandular) mucosa of the stomach has minimal protective ability and is therefore much more susceptible than the gastric (glandular) mucosa to acid injury (**116**).

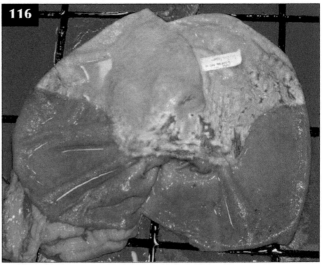

116 Gastric ulceration in the nonglandular portion of the stomach.

Exposure to mucosal injury to acid results in pain. Progressive, untreated ulcerative disease can result in gastroesophageal reflux, gastric outflow obstruction, pyloric or duodenal stricture, perforation (gastric or duodenal) with peritonitis, or hemorrhage.

CLINICAL PRESENTATION
The clinical signs of gastric ulceration vary with location and severity; ulcers can be asymptomatic ("silent"). The classic triad of clinical signs described with gastroduodenal ulceration is ptyalism, bruxism, and dorsal recumbency (**117**). Bruxism and dorsal recumbency (rolling up on the back) are nonspecific signs of GI pain. Ptyalism is a more common sign of esophagitis. Other clinical signs that may be seen include failure to thrive, depression, decreased or an absence of nursing, and possibly behavioral changes (*Table 30*). Gastric ulceration can cause acute, massive hemorrhage and sudden death. There may be no clinical signs evident before hemorrhage, suggesting a rapid onset of ulceration or the presence of silent ulcers.

DIFFERENTIAL DIAGNOSIS
Esophageal disease, GI diseases resulting in abdominal pain, and any condition causing depression and decreased appetite must be considered.

DIAGNOSIS
Diagnosis is based on endoscopic visualization of the affected area (**118, 119**). Ulceration is most common in the squamous mucosa adjacent to the margo plicatus. To provide adequate visualization of the stomach it may be necessary to fast the foal for 8–12 hours. The stomach of the suckling foal may be visualized adequately without a fasting period or with a shorter fasting time period. Influx of air into the stomach (through the endoscope) to reveal the mucosal folds and rinsing of feed material off the mucosal surface are critical to the complete gastric examination. When endoscopy is not available, response to therapy (although not definitive) can indicate the presence of disease.

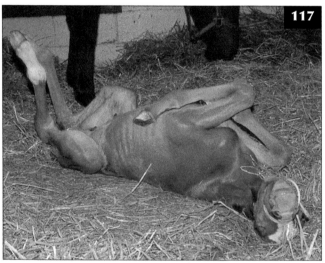

117 This foal with gastric ulceration is showing signs of abdominal pain and is in dorsal recumbency.

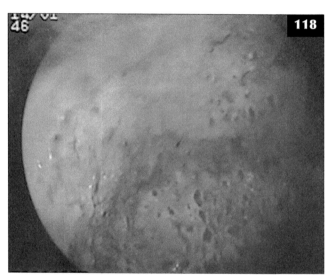

118 Gastroscopic visualization of gastric ulceration.

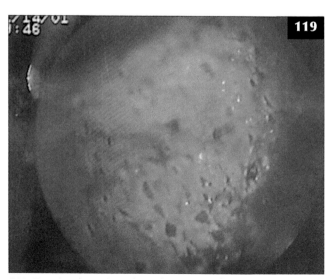

119 Gastric ulceration along the margo plicatus.

Table 30. Clinical signs of gastric ulceration

- Bruxism
- Ptyalism
- Dorsal recumbency
- Colic
- Failure to thrive
- Depression
- Inappetence
- Decreased nursing or shortened duration of nursing
- Behavioral changes

MANAGEMENT

Resolution of any underlying disease processes and undertaking management changes that can alleviate the problems that may have resulted in the ulceration (i.e., feeding too much grain, overcrowding) can be adequate to resolve gastric ulcers; however, appropriate medical therapy can alleviate clinical signs and resolve ulceration more rapidly. The goal of medical therapy is to alter the acid content of the stomach or to provide mucosal protection from acid exposure. Oral therapy is generally the route of choice (*Table 31*) unless the patient is not to be fed because of medical reasons (e.g., refluxing or dysphagic).

Protective agents include sucralfate and misoprostol. Sucralfate binds to gastric glandular mucosa, therefore promoting blood flow, prostaglandin synthesis, and mucus production. Sucralfate may also promote healing of duodenal ulcers; however, it should be noted that sucralfate does not promote healing of squamous mucosal ulcers. Misoprostol, a prostaglandin E analog, increases mucosal blood flow. Unfortunately, expense and side effects of abdominal pain, diarrhea, and inappetence have limited its use.

Alteration of the acid content of the stomach can be approached through acid neutralization, H_2 antagonists, or proton pump inhibitors. Antacids (magnesium oxide, aluminum hydroxide) provide the most rapid change in gastric acidity; however, their duration of effect is short lived. Antacids can provide symptomatic relief, but they must be given frequently (every 2–4 hours) and in large volumes to produce healing of ulcers.

The H_2 receptor antagonists block acid secretion by competitively inhibiting receptor sites on the parietal cell. The bioavailability of the H_2 antagonists used in the horse (ranitidine and cimetidine) is poor, therefore response to therapy with these compounds has been variable. The H_2 antagonists reduce gastric acidity for 1–8 hours.

Proton pump inhibitors irreversibly bind to the parietal cell proton pump that secretes hydrochloric acid. When used at appropriate doses, inhibition of acid production is present for up to 24 hours. Two or more doses of proton pump inhibitor are required for maximal inhibition (development of adequate tissue concentrations) of acid secretion. Proton pump inhibitors such as omeprazole may well be the best choice for healing of gastric ulcers. Healing will not occur in the face of repeat exposure of ulcers to an acid environment.

PYLORIC AND DUODENAL STENOSIS/STRICTURE

KEY POINTS
- Acquired pyloric stenosis is more common than congenital.
- Pyloric stenosis and duodenal stricture are typically secondary to ulceration, with narrowing or stricture as a result of the healing process.
- Clinical signs may include abdominal pain, ptyalism, bruxism, depression, anorexia, and weight loss.
- Endoscopic examination often identifies reflux esophagitis.
- Upper GI contrast study identifies lack of gastric emptying.
- Surgical bypass of the affected area is necessary.

DEFINITION/OVERVIEW

A structural resistance to gastric outflow in the region of the pylorus or gastric antrum is defined as pyloric stenosis. It may be congenital or acquired. Duodenal stricture is typically located in the proximal duodenum. The stricture may involve the common bile duct. Duodenal strictures are rarely seen in adult horses and are not common in foals.

ETIOLOGY/PATHOPHYSIOLOGY

Pyloric disease in the foal can be congenital or acquired. Congenital stenosis is typically a hypertrophy as a result of thickening of the pyloric musculature. Acquired stenosis is the healing response (fibrosis and contraction) to ulceration in the antrum and/or pylorus. Duodenal stricture is typically a sequela of mucosal ulceration; however, it may be seen secondary to hypertrophied segments of bowel wall (**120**). The definitive etiology of hypertrophy is only speculative. A diffuse duodenal inflammation (duodenitis) can be seen with, or secondary to, enteritis. Stricture or narrowing occurs subsequent to the duodenal inflammation resolving. Multiple cases of duodenitis/duodenal stricture on a single farm have suggested a possible infectious etiology.

Narrowing of the pyloric region of the stomach results in functional difficulty or complete obstruction of gastric outflow and potentially reflux esophagitis. Cicatrix formation (narrowing of the lumen secondary to healing) can occur subsequent to duodenal ulceration. Clinical signs become evident when narrowing is significant enough to obstruct a basal flow of ingesta.

Table 31. Pharmacologic choices for therapy of gastric ulcers (see Chapter 17, Pharmacology, for dosages)

- Antacids
- Sucralfate
- Ranitidine
- Cimetadine
- Omeprazole

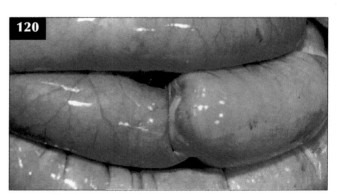

120 Small intestinal stricture *in situ.*

Table 32. Clinical signs seen with gastric outflow obstruction

- Varying degrees of abdominal pain
- Ptyalism (salivation)
- Bruxism
- Painful swallowing
- Failure to thrive/weight loss
- Anorexia
- History of diarrhea or concurrent diarrhea
- Aspiration pneumonia
- Spontaneous reflux, particularly under sedation

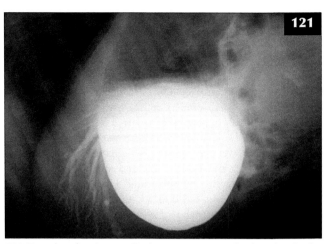

121 Duodenal stricture. Barium contrast study showing lack of gastric emptying.

CLINICAL PRESENTATION

Pyloric stenosis and duodenal stricture are very similar in their clinical presentation (*Table 32*). Both conditions can present with a wide array of clinical signs depending on the degree and duration of stenosis/stricture. Difficulty or a lack of gastric emptying will result in varying degrees of abdominal pain. In chronic disease, reflux esophagitis results in painful swallowing. Salivation (ptyalism) can be intermittent or persistent. Teeth grinding (bruxism) may be an indicator of pain. The degree of pain can be mild to severe. Depression, anorexia, inappetence, and weight loss (unthrifty, failure to thrive) may ensue. Gastric reflux will occasionally occur spontaneously, particularly if the patient is under the influence of a tranquilizer. Aspiration pneumonia is a potential sequela to gastric reflux. Peritonitis and local adhesions may be present if stenosis is secondary to ulceration with leakage of GI contents. Patients with duodenal stricture often have a history of diarrhea (chronic or intermittent).

DIFFERENTIAL DIAGNOSIS

The initial differential diagnosis is extensive and includes esophageal disease, other gastric diseases (gastric ulcers), and abdominal diseases resulting in colic. Once the diagnosis is narrowed to an outflow obstruction of the stomach, the differential includes duodenal obstruction or functional outflow obstruction.

DIAGNOSIS

The initial presumptive diagnosis is based on a physical examination that suggests outflow obstruction. Endoscopic examination of the esophagus often identifies a reflux esophagitis. The most common cause of reflux is gastric outflow obstruction. If the stomach can be emptied adequately enough to allow the antrum and pylorus to be evaluated endoscopically, a narrowing of these regions with or without ulceration and fibrosis may be visualized. Hypertrophy of the pyloric musculature is more difficult to diagnose and may only be confirmed via direct palpation during an exploratory celiotomy.

An upper GI barium contrast study can confirm the absence of gastric emptying (**121**). Subsequent to emptying the stomach of any retained fluid, 10 mL/kg of liquid barium is placed (via stomach pump or gravity flow) into the stomach via a nasogastric tube. Radiographs of the stomach are performed before barium administration, after administration, and at subsequent 15-minute intervals. The normal stomach should begin emptying immediately, with barium visible within the small intestine within 15 minutes. A lack of visible barium in the small intestine by 30–45 minutes confirms an absence of gastric emptying; however, a lack of emptying can be functional or anatomic. Exploratory surgery is often necessary to confirm the cause of gastric outflow obstruction.

Clinical chemistries are frequently nonspecific, suggesting secondary infection; however, when duodenal ulceration/stricture involves or obstructs the entrance of the common bile duct into the duodenum, elevations in biliary-specific liver enzymes (GGT) may be present.

Ultrasonographic examination may be useful. Gastric distension is a nonspecific finding associated with duodenal or pyloric stricture. Coincident small intestinal fluid distension and hyperperistalsis may support functional ileus (anterior enteritis) versus duodenal stricture, but this finding is not definitive. Rarely, a stricture may be visualized.

MANAGEMENT

Decompression of the stomach with a nasogastric tube and medical treatment of mucosal ulceration can provide symptomatic relief of abdominal pain. Surgical bypass of anatomic obstructions has been successful and is required for long-term survival. Prognosis is related to successful surgical bypass. Involvement of the common bile duct with the stricture is likely related to future growth potential. When bypass surgery is successful, the majority of these patients appear to mature to expected size/weight. The bypass chosen is dependent on the location and extent of duodenal involvement. Surgical prognosis is influenced by factors such as secondary complications (peritonitis, adhesions, aspiration pneumonia), duodenal location of the stricture, and involvement of the common bile duct. Prokinetic drugs should not be used if an anatomic obstruction is suspected.

DISORDERS OF THE SMALL INTESTINE ASSOCIATED WITH COLIC

HERNIATION

Herniation of abdominal contents can occur either externally (outside the body wall proper) or internally (through internal structures), and can be a result of acquired or congenital conditions. The clinical signs of internal GI herniation most frequently result in small bowel obstruction (strangulating or nonstrangulating), severe abdominal pain (**122**), and subsequent cardiovascular changes suggestive of splanchnic ischemic shock (**123**). External herniation can, but does not always, result in compromised bowel. When external hernias are manually reducible, the

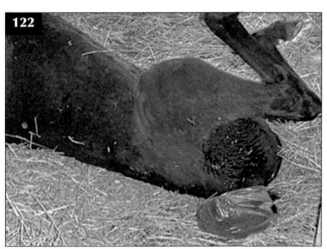

122 Foal with internal gastrointestinal herniation exhibiting signs of severe abdominal pain.

Table 33. Causes of abdominal pain
• Gastric ulceration
• Gastric outflow obstruction
• Herniation (external and internal)
• External:
○ Umbilical
○ Inguinal
○ Scrotal
• Internal:
○ Diaphragmatic
○ Epiploic foramen
○ Mesenteric defects
• Small intestinal volvulus
• Intussusception
• Small intestinal impaction
• Necrotizing enterocolitis
• Focal nonstrangulating infarction
• Large colon volvulus
• Large colon impaction
• Large colon displacement
• Atresia coli
• Ileocolonic aganglionosis
• Meconium impaction/retention
• Atresia recti/ani
• Fecaliths
• Abdominal abscessation
• Enterocolitis

123 Mucous membrane changes compatible with severe bowel compromise.

vascular supply is generally not affected. Diaphragmatic herniation, in addition to signs of abdominal pain, presents with signs of respiratory disease/distress. The differential diagnosis of herniation of abdominal contents includes other conditions resulting in abdominal pain or external body wall swelling (*Table 33*). Strangulating hernias require surgical correction. External nonstrangulating hernias may resolve spontaneously. Bandaging to support scrotal or inguinal hernias is described specifically under these conditions

EXTERNAL HERNIATION

Inguinal and umbilical hernias are commonly found examples of external herniation (**124, 125**); omphaloceles (**126**) are another example. External herniations are visible and palpable and clinical signs are referable to the location and the presence or degree of bowel compromise. Many external hernias may be manually reducible. Diagnosis of external herniation is based on the presence of an external swelling/protuberance that is referable to body wall abnormalities and extravasation of bowel through the body wall. Palpation or ultrasound of external swellings identifies the presence of GI contents.

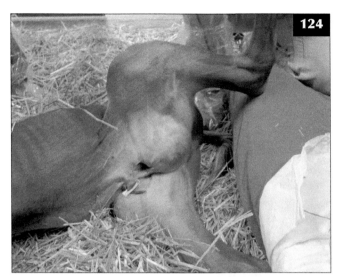

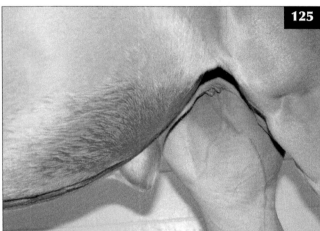

124, 125 External herniation. (**124**) Inguinal herniation of small intestine. (**125**) Umbilical herniation.

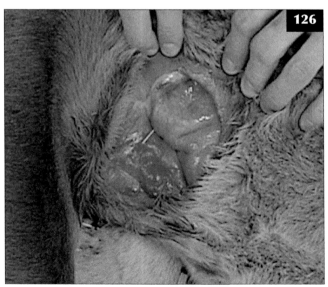

126 Omphalocele, a congenital defect in the body wall.

INGUINAL AND SCROTAL HERNIAS

Key points

- An inguinal hernia is defined as protrusion of bowel through the internal ring.
- A scrotal hernia is defined as protrusion of bowel through the internal and external inguinal ring.
- An indirect hernia lies within the vaginal tunic.
- A direct hernia is through a rent in the vaginal tunic.
- Hernias that are reducible in dorsal recumbency are frequently treated conservatively.
- Large or complicated hernias require surgical intervention.

Definition/overview

Inguinal and scrotal hernias are defined by their advancement through the internal and external ring. Protrusion of bowel through the internal inguinal ring, but not through the external inguinal ring, is termed "inguinal herniation." When the bowel extends beyond the external ring into the scrotum, the hernia is termed "scrotal" (**127**).

Etiology/pathophysiology

The majority of inguinal and scrotal herniations in foals are indirect. An indirect hernia lies within the vaginal tunic. Direct inguinal or scrotal hernias occur when a rent in the peritoneal lining or

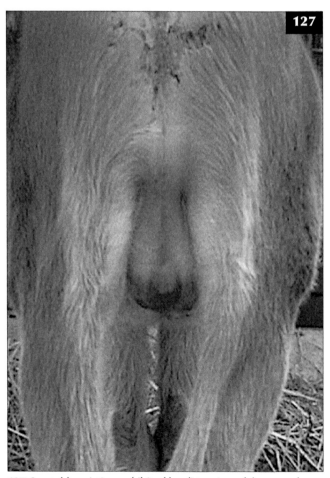

127 Scrotal herniation exhibited by distension of the scrotal sac.

vaginal tunic is present. These direct herniations are sometimes referred to as "ruptured hernias"; bowel enters the subcutaneous space of the scrotum or prepuce.

MANAGEMENT

Uncomplicated inguinal hernias generally resolve spontaneously. When the hernia is reducible with the foal in dorsal recumbency, the hernia can be treated conservatively. Surgical correction of uncomplicated hernias may be required if resolution does not occur within 3–6 months or if they become excessively large. Conservative management of uncomplicated hernias can include daily manual reduction or, in some cases, support bandages.

Complicated hernias (direct or ruptured, with escape of bowel into the subcutaneous space) are usually not reducible. Intermittent colic may be evident. Large scrotal, preputial, or periputial swellings may become severe. Surgical repair is usually required.

UMBILICAL HERNIAS/OMPHALOCELES

KEY POINTS
- Benign umbilical hernias are a common defect in the foal.
- A complicated umbilical hernia results when bowel escapes into the surrounding subcutis through a tear in the peritoneal lining.
- Complicated umbilical hernias frequently result in compromised bowel.
- Omphalocele is herniation of bowel through the entire bowel wall.
- Uncomplicated large or persistent umbilical hernias will need repair.
- Complicated umbilical hernias frequently require repair.
- Omphalocele requires emergency correction.

DEFINITION/OVERVIEW

Umbilical herniation is a common defect in young or newborn foals. These herniations, if reducible, are usually benign and resolve with time. Complicated umbilical hernias may develop, with tearing of the peritoneal lining and escape of herniated bowel into the subcutis. These hernias often result in bowel compromise (**128**).

An omphalocele (**126**) is a protrusion of GI contents through a congenital defect in the body wall adjacent to the umbilicus. If the peritoneal lining is torn, these foals are born with abdominal contents external to the abdominal cavity. The quantity of herniated bowel is dependent on the size of the congenital defect. The omphalocele may be congenital or acquired (trauma). The congenital form is significantly more common. Congenital forms can be identified prepartum during transabdominal ultrasonography.

MANAGEMENT

Hernias larger than 10 cm may need to be surgically repaired. Hernias that persist for months may need surgical repair or "banding." Banding must be cautious and can be performed with commercially available equipment or handmade clamps.

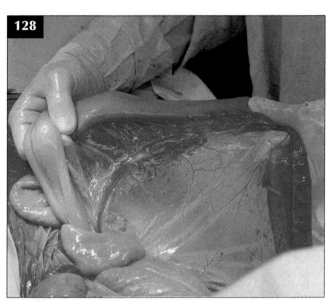

128 Bowel compromise secondary to a strangulating umbilical hernia.

Complicated umbilical hernias frequently require surgical correction. The omphalocele, whether congenital or acquired, must be corrected immediately.

INTERNAL HERNIATION

Diaphragmatic hernias are the more commonly found internal hernias. Diagnosis of internal herniation is based on identification of small bowel obstruction/distension in the patient exhibiting clinical signs of abdominal pain. Ultrasound and/or radiography can identify abnormal small intestinal conditions. The specific (definitive) diagnosis of the exact type of herniation is difficult to make (with the exception of diaphragmatic herniation) without an exploratory surgery. The decision for exploratory surgery is made based on the presence of small intestinal distension and clinical signs.

DIAPHRAGMATIC HERNIA

KEY POINTS
- Congenital diaphragmatic herniation is rare.
- Traumatic diaphragmatic herniation is secondary to fractured ribs.
- Respiratory compromise along with colic is a frequent clinical sign.
- Surgical repair is necessary.

ETIOLOGY/PATHOPHYSIOLOGY

Diaphragmatic hernias occur through congenital or acquired defects in the diaphragm. Congenital diaphragmatic herniation is a rare incomplete fusion of the pleural/peritoneal folds in the dorsal tendinous portion of the diaphragm. Traumatic diaphragmatic hernias can be the result of blunt trauma, but they are more frequently a result of laceration of the diaphragm induced by fractured ribs. Fractured ribs are a common neonatal foaling

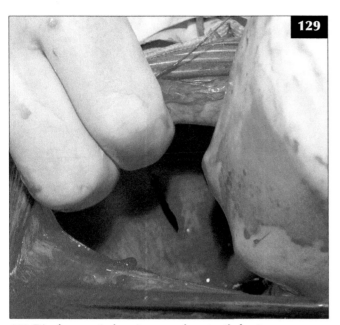

129 Diaphragmatic hernia secondary to rib fractures.

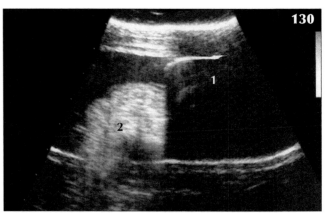

130 Ultrasonographic identificatioin of bowel within the thoracic cavity. 1: lung; 2: gut.

injury; sharp edges can result in cardiac, intercostal artery, pulmonary, or diaphragmatic injury (**129**). Typically, these occur at birth (although herniation of intestinal contents may not occur until later in life in some cases), but they can occur in the older foal with external blunt trauma. These hernias can be difficult to recognize and should be included in the differential for neonatal colic. Respiratory compromise along with colic is a frequent clinical sign.

CLINICAL PRESENTATION
Herniation of bowel into the thoracic cavity compromises respiratory efforts and affects complete aeration of the lungs. Cyanotic oral mucous membranes and/or abnormal blood gas values are frequently present.

DIAGNOSIS
Fractured ribs may be easily observed if the fractures are numerous and displaced. Careful palpation of both sides of the rib cage can identify the less obvious fracture. Fractures resulting in diaphragmatic trauma are often found in the caudal rib cage. Diaphragmatic herniation should be ruled out in newborn foals with severe rib fractures and evidence of cyanosis (respiratory compromise) and colic.

A diaphragmatic hernia can be identified pre-exploratory by observation (ultrasonographic and/or radiographic) (**130, 131**) of GI contents in the thoracic cavity. Ultrasonography of the thorax in such cases should be performed with the foal in sternal recumbency or in a standing position, because air-filled lung may obscure visualization of fluid or intestinal contents within the thoracic cavity.

MANAGEMENT
Surgical repair of the diaphragm is required. Results are dependent on the severity of the laceration, bowel compromise, and/or the degree of congenital abnormality.

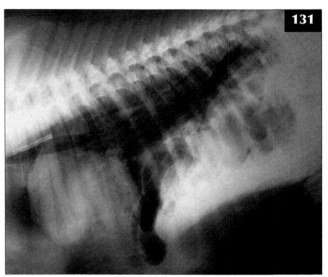

131 Radiographic visualization of a diaphragmatic hernia. Note the bowel within the thoracic cavity.

MESENTERIC DEFECTS, MECKEL'S DIVERTICULUM, MESODIVERTICULAR BAND

Mesenteric rents (defects) (**132, 133**) can be congenital or acquired and they may, rarely, result in incarceration of bowel. They are found most commonly in the small intestinal mesentery, but they can be identified in the mesentery of the large or small colon or the mesodiverticular band.

Meckel's diverticulum and the mesodiverticular band are formed by remnants of the omphalomesenteric duct and the left or right vitelline arteries, resulting in an extra sheet of mesentery that attaches to the antimesenteric surface of the jejunum. Bowel incarceration results from entrapment between these remnants and other portions of the GI tract. The mesodiverticular band is infrequently present.

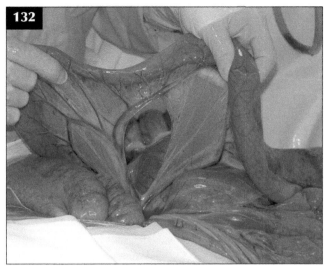

132 Mesenteric rent: small intestine.

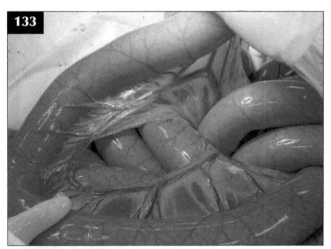

133 Mesenteric defect.

SMALL INTESTINAL VOLVULUS

KEY POINTS
- Common cause of colic in the foal.
- Compromised blood supply frequently results in splanchnic ischemic shock.
- Pain often progresses to persistent, severe, and nonresponsive.
- Diagnosis is based on clinical signs and identification of distended small bowel.

DEFINITION/OVERVIEW
Small intestinal volvulus is a common cause of colic in the foal (*Table 33*).

ETIOLOGY/PATHOPHYSIOLOGY
Dietary changes or parasitism have been suggested as underlying causes of the condition. Typically, the jejunum and/or ileum may be involved to various degrees. Volvulus of the small intestine can rapidly result in strangulation of the vascular supply. Compromised

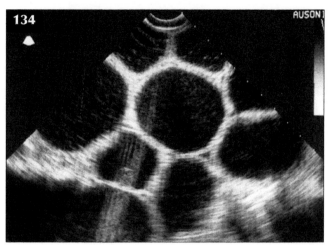

134 Distended loops of small bowel suggestive of a volvulus or other obstructive disease of the small intestine are visible on this ultrasonogram.

blood flow results in local changes, which subsequently result in systemic changes described as splanchnic ischemic shock (see Chapter 2, Shock, Resuscitation, Fluid and Electrolyte Therapy).

CLINICAL PRESENTATION
The foal with small intestinal volvulus typically presents with severe, persistent, nonresponsive pain. Tachycardia and/or tachypnea may be present. Splanchnic ischemic shock results in alterations in mucous membrane character (evidence of toxemia). Gastric distension and abdominal distension often develop. When a small intestinal volvulus is present for an extended duration of time, the foal may present in recumbency with abdominal distension and minimal evidence of pain (the foal may no longer feel pain because it has been suffering from the pain for a long time).

DIFFERENTIAL DIAGNOSIS
Conditions resulting in abdominal pain (*Table 33*).

DIAGNOSIS
Diagnosis is based on the clinical signs and the presence of small intestinal distension. Abdominal ultrasound/radiography identifies motile or nonmotile, distended loops of small bowel (134). Pain is persistent and nonresponsive.

MANAGEMENT
Management consists of controlling pain until an exploratory and surgical correction can be provided. Supportive therapy/treatment for shock may be necessary dependent on the degree of ischemic bowel (see Chapter 2, Shock, Resuscitation, Fluid and Electrolyte Therapy, p. 17).

INTUSSUSCEPTION

KEY POINTS
- Intussusception is an invagination or telescoping of one segment of bowel into another.
- Presenting signs typically involve mild to moderate intermittent pain.
- Ultrasonographic visualization is possible.

DEFINITION/OVERVIEW

Small intestinal intussusception (invagination of small intestine into itself) (135–137) is not commonly identified in the foal. Foals of any age are susceptible.

ETIOLOGY/PATHOPHYSIOLOGY

Predispositions to small intestinal intussusception include parasitism or altered motility secondary to enteritis. Initially, an intussusception may result in a simple obstruction. As the condition progresses, edema and vascular compromise may develop. These lesions are described as nonstrangulating necrosing lesions.

CLINICAL PRESENTATION

Foals with intussusception may present with varying degrees of abdominal pain. The signs of pain may be violent and severe; however, they are typically of a mild to moderate, often intermittent, insidious, low-grade nature. Gastric distension with gastric refluxing may be present.

DIFFERENTIAL DIAGNOSIS

Enterocolitis, conditions resulting in abdominal pain (*Table 33*).

DIAGNOSIS

Diagnosis of intussusception is based on ultrasonographic evaluation of the abdomen (138, 139).

MANAGEMENT

Exploratory celiotomy is necessary. Gentle retraction may relieve an intussusception; however, resection is generally required. The prognosis for recovery is related to the extent of bowel involved; however, successful resection should result in a favorable prognosis.

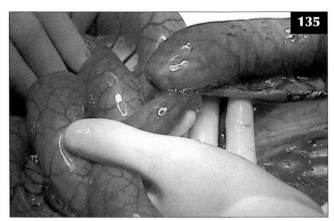

135 Small intestinal intussusception *in situ*.

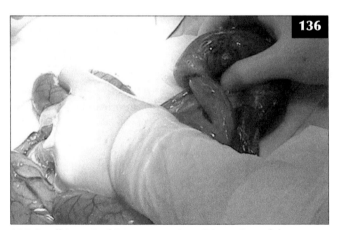

136 Small intestinal intussusception. Distension of the proximal segment results in abdominal pain.

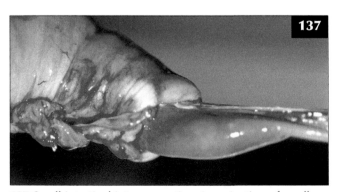

137 Small intestinal intussusception. Invagination of small intestine into itself.

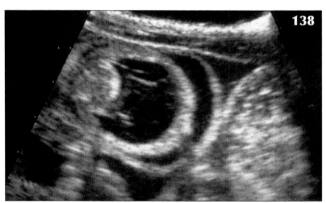

138 Target- or doughnut-shaped lesions identifying intussusception are visible on this ultrasonogram.

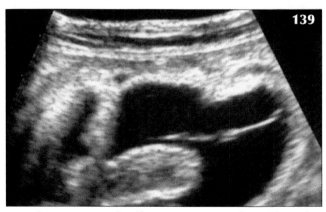

139 Ultrasonogram identifying intussuscepted small bowel.

SMALL INTESTINAL IMPACTION

KEY POINTS

- Luminal impactions of the small intestine are uncommon.
- Ascarid impactions may be seen.
- Clinical signs include varying degrees of abdominal pain.
- Bowel compromise is generally not present.

DEFINITION/OVERVIEW

Luminal obstructions of the small intestine are uncommon in foals. Simple obstructions may result in a variety of clinical syndromes. The intestinal stages of ascarids may cause obstruction (140). Anthelmintic treatment commonly precedes ascarid impactions. Affected foals may be unthrifty and appear parasitized.

ETIOLOGY/PATHOPHYSIOLOGY

Ascarid impaction typically results in a simple obstruction; however, intussusception, ulceration, devitalization of bowel wall, erosion, and peritonitis may ensue.

CLINICAL PRESENTATION

The typical presentation is that of a simple GI obstructive disease. Complicated (prolonged, untreated, severe) impactions can result in peritonitis and signs of septic shock. Affected foals may be (but not necessarily) unthrifty and poor doing.

DIFFERENTIAL DIAGNOSIS

Other conditions causing abdominal pain (*Table 33*).

DIAGNOSIS

Diagnosis can be made via visualization (ultrasonographic) of distended/fluid-filled small intestine. Occasionally, ascarids may be found in gastric reflux or visualized via ultrasound.

MANAGEMENT

Exploratory surgery (141) is necessary if pain persists or if cardiovascular compromise is present. The use of slow-acting anthelmintics can prevent the development of impactions in parasitized foals.

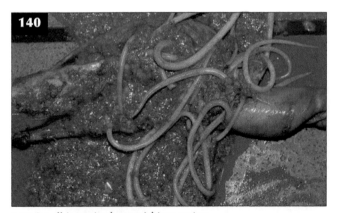

140 Small intestinal ascarid impaction.

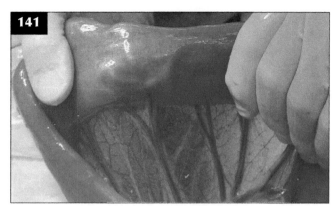

141 Ascarids in small intestine identified during exploratory surgery.

NECROTIZING ENTEROCOLITIS

KEY POINTS

- Necrotizing enterocolitis is related to a peripartum lack of oxygen delivery to portions of the GI tract.
- Bacterial colonization of necrosing bowel is a subsequent component.
- The onset of enteral feeding is often related to the initiation of clinical signs.
- Clinical signs relate to pain (colic), devitalized bowel, and sepsis/ischemic shock.
- Pneumatosis intestinalis (gas lucency) in the bowel wall may be identified.

DEFINITION/OVERVIEW

Necrotizing enterocolitis is an acquired GI disease of neonates and is most frequently identified in the premature foal (142, 143). The disease can be related to the initiation of enteral feeding.

ETIOLOGY/PATHOPHYSIOLOGY

The condition is thought to be initiated by a hypoxic ischemic insult at birth. The lack of oxygen at delivery may be related to shock, a lack of blood flow, or peripartum hypoxia. Bowel wall ischemia and bacterial colonization result in cell death and vascular compromise and necrosis, with splanchnic ischemic and endotoxic/exotoxic shock. Bacterial colonization with gas-forming anaerobes is common. Bowel perforation with peritonitis may ensue.

CLINICAL PRESENTATION

Patients are often hospitalized individuals undergoing treatment for serious illness or prematurity. The onset of the condition may be related to the initiation of milk feeding or with overfeeding, which provides a substrate for bacterial overgrowth. Varying degrees of abdominal pain and shock/sepsis are observed. Abdominal distension and melena (144) are often identified. Peritonitis may be present.

DIFFERENTIAL DIAGNOSIS

Enteritis/enterocolitis, other conditions that result in abdominal pain and melena (*Table 33*).

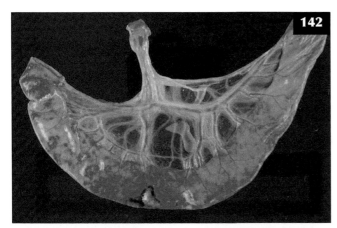

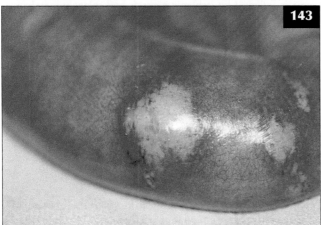

142, 143 Necrotizing enterocolitis of the small intestine.

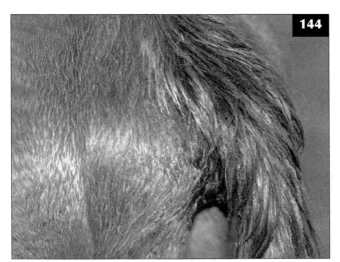

144 Melena. Note the dark brown/red stool.

DIAGNOSIS

Diagnosis is based on signalment (neonate) and clinical signs of intestinal distension and toxic shock. Pneumatosis intestinalis (gas lucency in the bowel wall) can be seen radiographically. These lucencies may be cystic, linear, or in a ring pattern, and

are a result of gas-producing bacteria within the layers of the bowel wall. Pneumatosis intestinalis can also be identified via ultrasound examination.

MANAGEMENT

Discontinuation of enteral feeding and supportive care with broad-spectrum antimicrobial therapy may be successful. Exploratory surgery with removal of devitalized bowel can be attempted. The prognosis for survival is grave.

FOCAL/NONSTRANGULATING INFARCTION

ETIOLOGY/PATHOPHYSIOLOGY

Focal intestinal infarction (**145**) can be caused by verminous arteritis (migration of *Strongylus vulgaris* within the intestine or vasculature), a focal ischemia (which may be secondary to shock), or a focal bacterial colonization of the bowel wall.

Focal infarction can result in progressive devitalization of bowel wall, septicemia, bacteremic alterations in motility, abdominal pain, and/or peritonitis.

CLINICAL PRESENTATION

The clinical presentation is variable, depending on the severity and extent of the lesion or lesions. The condition may present as a low-grade insidious GI condition with mild intermittent pain and unthriftiness, or more severe abdominal pain with toxic shock may be evident.

DIFFERENTIAL DIAGNOSIS

Other conditions resulting in abdominal pain (*Table 33*).

DIAGNOSIS

Diagnosis is difficult as all the diagnostic findings are generally nonspecific. Abdominocentesis may identify peritonitis. Exploratory surgery is definitive.

MANAGEMENT

If larval migration is suspected, then therapy for such is indicated. Surgical resection of large areas of infarction may be indicated.

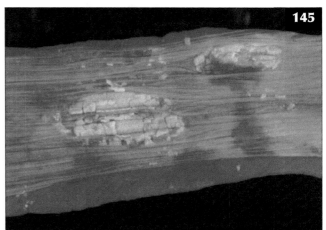

145 Small intestinal focal infarction.

DISORDERS OF THE COLON ASSOCIATED WITH COLIC

DISPLACEMENT OF THE LARGE COLON

KEY POINTS
- Colonic displacement is not common in the foal.
- The obstruction is nonstrangulating.
- Mild to moderate signs of colic are typical.
- Surgical correction is required.

DEFINITION/OVERVIEW
Normally, the large colon is fairly constantly maintained in a normal spatial relationship by positioning with other abdominal organs. Colonic displacement is not a common GI disorder in the foal, particularly the neonate or young foal; however, it becomes more prevalent as the digestive tract develops to digest solid foods.

ETIOLOGY/PATHOPHYSIOLOGY
The position of the colon may be changed by alterations in motility or digestion. Gas distension of the large colon is considered one of the major causes of colonic displacement. Colonic displacement is a nonstrangulating obstruction, therefore vascular obstruction is not present. Intermittent to persistent or moderate to severe gas accumulation and distension will occur.

CLINICAL PRESENTATION
The clinical presentation varies depending on the degree of distension. Clinical signs of colic are typically mild to moderate. Pain may be intermittent and responsive to analgesics. Gastric reflux is usually not a major component of the condition; however, tension on the ileocolic ligament can produce a moderate amount of reflux.

DIFFERENTIAL DIAGNOSIS
Conditions resulting in abdominal pain (*Table 33*), particularly nonstrangulating obstructions.

DIAGNOSIS
Clinical signs in combination with identification of large bowel distension can lead to a presumptive diagnosis. In the absence of rectal examination findings, large bowel distension may be identified via simultaneous auscultation–percussion or radiography. Ultrasound examination identifies gas-filled large bowel. Abdominocentesis is generally unremarkable.

MANAGEMENT
Management requires surgical correction.

LARGE COLON VOLVULUS

KEY POINTS
- Large colon volvulus is less commonly seen in foals as opposed to adults.
- Vascular compromise is a component of this condition.
- Severe, nonresponsive pain and clinical signs of splanchnic ischemic shock are typical.

DEFINITION/OVERVIEW
Large colon volvulus is a common cause of severe colic in the adult horse and, less commonly, a cause of colic in the foal. The neonate or young foal is rarely affected and the condition does not typically present until the diet changes to roughage and concentrates. Twists of the colon are more common at the base, but they may occur anywhere in the large colon.

ETIOLOGY/PATHOPHYSIOLOGY
The etiology of large colon volvulus is multifactorial and may include high concentrate feeding practices. Vascular obstruction with volvulus of the colon is the primary factor related to the severity of the condition. Vascular obstruction may initially involve venous supply or both venous and arterial vasculature. Colonic edema is followed by ischemic necrosis and splanchnic ischemic shock.

CLINICAL PRESENTATION
The clinical presentation varies with the amount of colonic involvement, the degree of volvulus, and the progression of splanchnic ischemic shock. Severe abdominal pain accompanied by signs of shock are typical. Signs of shock include abnormal mucous membrane color, cold extremities, weak pulses, dehydration, and poor capillary refill times (CRTs). Tachycardia and tachypnea may be evident. Abdominal distension is common (**146**).

DIFFERENTIAL DIAGNOSIS
Conditions resulting in abdominal pain (*Table 33*), particularly those suggestive of a strangulating obstruction.

DIAGNOSIS
In the absence of rectal examination findings, the diagnosis is based on clinical examination findings, severe abdominal pain, evidence of shock, and the presence of large colon distension. Radiography identifies large bowel distension in the absence of small bowel distension. Results of abdominocentesis are variable.

MANAGEMENT
Management involves therapy for shock (see Chapter 2, Shock, Resuscitation, Fluid and Electrolyte Therapy, pp. 23–32) and rapid surgical intervention (**147, 148**).

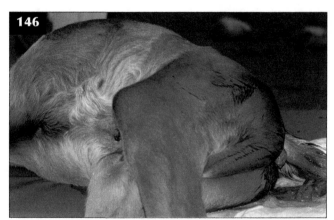

146 Severe abdominal distension in a foal.

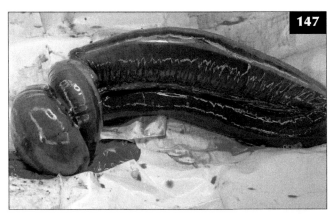

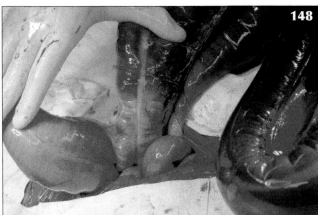

147, 148 Large colon volvulus in situ in a 4-day-old foal (**147**) and after surgical correction of the volvulus (**148**).

LARGE COLON IMPACTION

KEY POINTS
- Large colon impactions are not common in the foal.
- A large colon impaction is nonstrangulating.
- Clinical signs are of a simple obstructive GI disease.

DEFINITION/OVERVIEW
Typical feed impactions of the large colon, as seen in adult horses, are not common in the foal. Foreign body material (e.g., gravel or sand) obstructions can occasionally be seen. Meconium (high meconium retention/impaction) can obstruct the transverse or right dorsal colon.

ETIOLOGY/PATHOPHYSIOLOGY
Impactions are nonstrangulating; however, they can occasionally cause local ulceration or infarction. The primary physiologic events are obstruction of the flow of ingesta, altering motility, gas distension, and subsequent pain.

CLINICAL PRESENTATION
The clinical presentation is of a simple GI obstructive disease with variable degrees of abdominal pain. Clinical signs of shock are not typically evident.

DIFFERENTIAL DIAGNOSIS
Other causes of abdominal pain (*Table 33*), particularly those that are suggestive of a simple obstruction.

DIAGNOSIS
Diagnosis of impaction is based on evidence of a simple obstructive disease and ultrasonographic/radiographic identification of a distended large bowel. Peritoneal fluid evaluation is typically unremarkable.

MANAGEMENT
Hydration of feed impactions with double-dose maintenance intravenous fluids has been useful. The use of mineral oil or cathartics given via a nasogastric tube meets with variable success. Surgical intervention is often necessary.

ATRESIA COLI

KEY POINTS
- Atresia coli is an absence of a segment of colon.
- Clinical signs include progressive development of abdominal pain shortly after birth.
- Fecal material (meconium) is not present at the perineum.
- Radiographic contrast studies may aid the diagnosis.
- Surgical repair is generally not possible.

DEFINITION/OVERVIEW
Atresia coli is a sporadic congenital condition resulting in the absence of segments of the colon. There appears to be no particular breed or genetic predisposition.

ETIOLOGY/PATHOPHYSIOLOGY
The cause of atresia coli is unknown. A loss of blood supply to the developing colon is thought to be involved. Segmental lack of colon results in simple obstructive disease as aboral flow of fluids (milk) or meconium is obstructed.

CLINICAL PRESENTATION
Presenting signs of abdominal pain occur shortly after birth (within the first 24 hours) (**149**).

Abdominal distension is progressive (**150, 151**). Affected foals may initially nurse well, but they lose interest and become depressed as obstruction progresses. The initial intake of milk results in fluid and gas accumulation. Meconium is not passed, fecal material is not evident at the perineum, and the foals may strain. A yellow-white mucous material may be present. Gastric reflux is frequently observed as the condition progresses.

DIFFERENTIAL DIAGNOSIS
Conditions resulting in colic in the neonate (*Table 34*).

DIAGNOSIS
Definitive diagnosis is difficult without exploratory surgery. Identification of an obstructive disease with progressive distension and an absence of definitive meconium are highly suggestive. Radiographic contrast studies, either upper GI or lower GI (barium

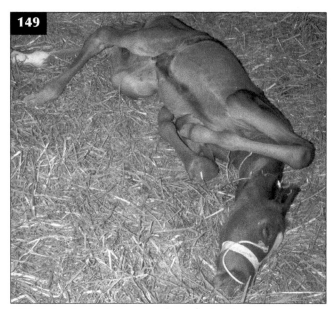

149 Abdominal pain in a newborn foal with atresia coli.

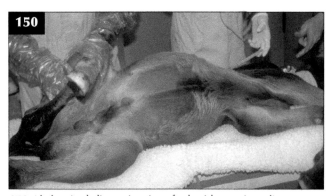

150 Abdominal distension in a foal with atresia coli.

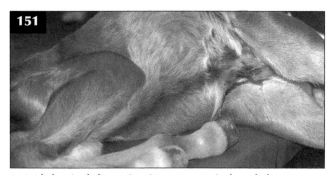

151 Abdominal distension in a progressively colicky newborn foal.

Table 34. Abdominal pain (colic) in the neonate
- Gastric ulceration
- Gastric outflow obstruction
- Meconium obstruction/retention
- Herniation
- Small intestinal volvulus
- Colonic displacement (rare)
- Intussusception
- Ileocolonic aganglionosis
- Atresia coli/recti
- Enterocolitis/enteritis

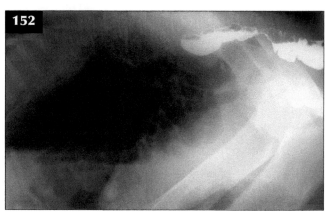

152 Radiographic contrast study of a foal with atresia coli. Note the blind-ended pouch.

MANAGEMENT
Surgical repair (anastomosis) of the remaining ends of the missing remnants of colon can be attempted. The prognosis depends on the degree of colonic absence (153), but it is generally poor. In the majority of cases it is physically impossible to re-appose the ends of the atretic colon; however, there are reports of successful repair.

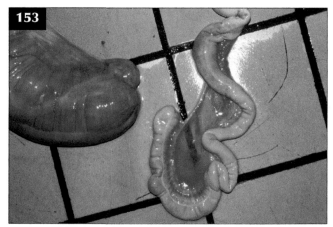

153 Segmental absence of large bowel in a foal with atresia coli.

enema), may identify failure of normal movement (upper GI) or a blind-ended pouch (152). A lower GI contrast study occasionally reveals a blind-ended pouch and more commonly identifies a congenital (atrophic) pattern to the small colon. Abdominocentesis is generally unremarkable.

ILEOCOLONIC AGANGLIONOSIS

KEY POINTS

- Ileocolonic aganglionosis is a congenital defect typically seen in white foals.
- The atrophic segment is a result of an absence of myenteric ganglia.
- Clinical signs develop within hours of birth.
- Surgical repair (anastomosis) is not usually feasible.

DEFINITION/OVERVIEW

Ileocolonic aganglionosis is a congenital defect (absence) of the myenteric ganglia of the distal ileum, cecum, large colon, and small colon. The condition is typically seen in white foals that are a result of a cross between horses of Overo color pattern lineage (**154**). The condition is also called the "lethal white" syndrome or "Overo lethal white" syndrome.

ETIOLOGY/PATHOPHYSIOLOGY

The absence of myenteric ganglia cells in the intestinal wall results in atrophic and/or atretic GI tract from the ileum through portions of the small colon. Small intestinal distension results from a failure of aboral movement of meconium and ingested milk.

CLINICAL PRESENTATION

Affected foals develop clinical signs shortly after birth, usually within 24 hours. Clinical signs include depression, colic, and abdominal distension. Affected foals are generally all white, with pink skin and blue irises.

DIFFERENTIAL DIAGNOSIS

Conditions resulting in abdominal pain in the neonate (*Table 34*), particularly those conditions resulting in colic shortly after birth (i.e., enterocolitis, atresia coli, and meconium impaction).

DIAGNOSIS

Diagnosis is based on the history of an all white foal with Overo parentage that begins evidence of abdominal pain shortly after birth. Ultrasound examination is not specific; it only indicates GI distension and ileus. Contrast radiography can identify a lack of aboral digestive movement. Exploratory celiotomy definitively identifies the atrophy/atresia of the GI tract. Histopathology confirms the absence of myenteric ganglia in the wall of the GI tract.

MANAGEMENT

Because of the extensive involvement of the GI tract, the condition is invariably fatal.

FOCAL INFARCTION/NECROSIS

(See Focal/Nonstrangulating Infarction, p. 95).

COLITIS

(See Enterocolitis, pp. 105–107).

DISORDERS OF THE SMALL COLON AND RECTUM

MECONIUM IMPACTION/RETENTION

KEY POINTS

- Meconium is produced by glandular secretions, swallowed amniotic fluid, epithelial cells, mucus, and bile.
- Meconium is the first stool passed by the foal.
- Meconium is typically passed within the first 24–48 hours of life.
- Meconium impactions are classified as high or low impaction. Low impactions (small colon/rectum) far outnumber high impactions.
- Clinical signs of impaction refer to the discomfort (pain) associated with retained meconium.
- Meconium retention is the most common cause of colic in the newborn foal.
- Contrast radiography is useful in the diagnosis.
- Cautious administration of an enema (or enemas) is usually successful.
- Control of pain may be necessary during resolution of meconium retention.
- Surgical resolution is required for high impactions.

DEFINITION/OVERVIEW

Meconium is a product of glandular secretions, swallowed amniotic fluid, epithelial cells, mucus, and bile. Through-out gestation this material is moved along the GI tract by peristalsis and stored in the colon and rectum. Meconium varies in color from a glossy black to a dark brown (**155**). The consistency and form of this first stool can be hard, grape-sized pellets or a sticky, tarry

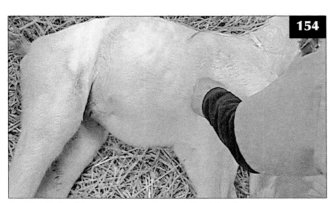

154 Lethal white syndrome in an all-white foal.

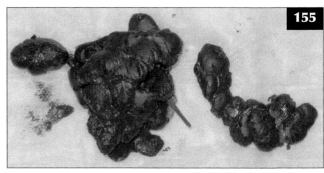

155 Normal meconium varies from glossy black to dark brown.

toothpaste-like material. The change to a less tenacious material generally indicates that the meconium has been passed.

ETIOLOGY/PATHOPHYSIOLOGY

The initial passage of meconium usually begins in the first few hours after birth. Meconium passage is generally complete within 24 hours, but can take up to 48 hours. The time spent evacuating meconium is not the critical factor when considering meconium retention. The degree of pain/discomfort/straining and alterations in the routine foal behavior are critical factors to be considered when evaluating the possibility of meconium retention. It is not atypical for newborn foals, standing or in lateral recumbency, to strain considerably when passing meconium. These attempts should be productive. Male foals (possibly as a result of a narrowed pelvic inlet) and foals born after a prolonged gestation appear to be predisposed to meconium retention. Meconium retention has been classified as either high or low impaction. A low impaction is an obstruction of the small colon/rectum at the pelvic inlet. Low impactions far outnumber the occurrence of high impactions. A high impaction is a more proximal obstruction of the GI tract, generally the transverse or right dorsal colon.

Retention of meconium results in a failure of aboral digestive movement with subsequent gas/fluid distension leading to abdominal pain.

CLINICAL PRESENTATION

Clinical signs of meconium retention may include any combination of the following: repetitive unproductive tenesmus, tail flagging/swishing, stretching, posturing as if to defecate, abdominal pain, abdominal distension, or lack of interest in suckling (**156**). Frequent efforts at defecation may be confused with attempts to urinate. Advanced signs of abdominal pain include dorsal recumbency, rolling from side to side, or violent collapse. Meconium retention is the most common cause of abdominal pain in the newborn foal. It should be noted that the clinical signs seen with meconium retention are nonspecific. Other differentials of abdominal pain should be considered.

DIFFERENTIAL DIAGNOSIS

Conditions resulting in abdominal pain in the neonate (*Table 34*).

DIAGNOSIS

Diagnosis is based on clinical signs, physical examination findings, and other diagnostic testing. Digital examination can identify fecal material at the pelvic inlet; however, absence of a positive digital finding should not rule out meconium retention. If retention is suspected, the response to a mild enema can be diagnostic. If clinical signs of abdominal pain persist, then abdominal radiography and ultrasonography should be pursued. Passage of a nasogastric tube may identify gastric reflux. Peritoneal fluid analysis may be useful in ruling out other causes of abdominal pain. Abdominal ultrasound can be used to rule out other disease processes. Abdominal ultrasound can identify meconium and associated bowel distension. Radiographs of the abdomen can identify meconium and/or gas distension of small or large intestine. Contrast radiography (barium enema) can be very useful if other diagnostics are nondefinitive (**157**). A barium enema is performed with a soft rubber catheter and gravity flow of 500–1,000 mL of liquid barium contrast material. The opaque barium material is radiographically identified surrounding a large mass of meconium.

MANAGEMENT

Treatment of meconium retention varies with severity and duration. Simple, cautious manual removal of fecal material can occasionally be all that is necessary. Mild enemas usually provide adequate softening/lubrication for passage of retained material. Enema solutions vary in quantity and contents. Commercial products are available and can be effective. A safe, nonirritating enema solution consists of 500–1,000 mL of warm water with 5–10 mL of soft soap. Repetitive enemas can be irritating to the sensitive rectal mucosa. For this reason it is preferable to use fewer large volume enemas rather than frequent small volume procedures. Soft flexible catheters are much preferred over the rigid counterparts. Gravity flow retention enemas containing 4% acetylcysteine have been recommended and can be effective.

The use of laxatives or cathartics given via a nasogastric tube may be beneficial, particularly if the impaction is suspected to be proximal. Mineral oil (200–400 mL), castor oil (30 mL), and milk of magnesia (120 mL) have been recommended. The effectiveness of these products is more likely via stimulation of GI motility rather than by a local direct effect on the meconium. Cathartics

156 Pain associated with meconium retention initially involves stretching, straining, and tail flagging.

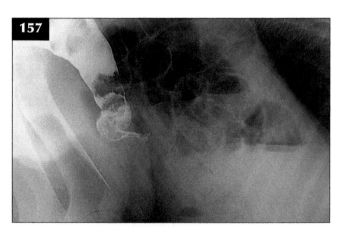

157 Contrast study showing a large mass of retained meconium.

should be used cautiously as they can be very irritating to the mucosal lining of the GI tract. Fluid therapy is unlikely to be useful in softening meconium impactions. A straining foal with a pelvic obstruction and a full bladder (as a result of fluid therapy) may be more prone to bladder rupture. Pain control is an important and analgesics are beneficial when used judiciously. A colicky foal cannot pass meconium effectively. Passage of a nasogastric tube to assess the presence of abdominal distension should be routine when treating (and diagnosing) a colicky foal. If abdominal distension becomes excessive despite therapy, then cecal trocarization and/or a exploratory surgery may become necessary. It is rare that abdominal surgery is required to resolve low impactions. Surgery may be necessary due to unrelenting, nonresponsive pain and/or severe gas distension. In these circumstances an alternative cause of abdominal pain or a proximal meconium obstruction (right ventral or transverse colon) is generally identified.

ATRESIA RECTI AND ATRESIA ANI

KEY POINTS
- Atresia of the rectum or anus is a lack of complete development.
- These conditions are rare in the foal.
- Clinical signs of abdominal pain are seen within 24 hours of birth.
- Physical examination or contrast studies are diagnostic.
- Surgical repair is dependent on the degree of atresia.

DEFINITION/OVERVIEW
Atresia recti and atresia ani are rare conditions of the neonatal foal. They are due to a lack of complete development of the anus and rectum.

ETIOLOGY/PATHOPHYSIOLOGY
The exact cause of atresia recti and atresia ani is unknown; however, it is generally considered that intestinal atresia results from a congenital loss of blood flow to the affected segments. Atresia of the rectum or anus leads to a simple obstruction and subsequent gas distension and colic.

CLINICAL PRESENTATION
Abdominal pain with progressive abdominal distension is present within 24 hours of birth. A lack of an anal orifice or a palpable blind end pouch may be observed. In the filly, rectovaginal fistulas may result in a small amount of feces passing from the vagina.

DIFFERENTIAL DIAGNOSIS
Other conditions resulting in abdominal pain in the neonate (*Table 34*).

DIAGNOSIS
Diagnosis can be based on physical examination or, if necessary, contrast studies.

MANAGEMENT
Surgical repair of atresia ani can be completed via anastomosis of the terminal rectum and the skin. Rectovaginal fistulas must

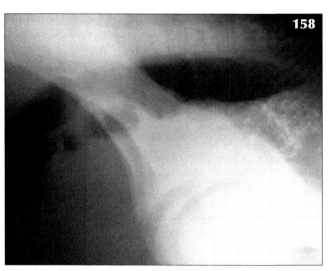

158 Gravel impaction identified via radiography.

be repaired. Surgical repair of atresia recti is complicated by a lack of surgical exposure.

FECALITHS

DEFINITION/OVERVIEW
Fecaliths are concretions of fecal and foreign material. Examples include straw, shavings, and gravel (**158**). The condition is most commonly seen in miniature and pony foals (neonatal), but it can be seen in older foals.

ETIOLOGY/PATHOPHYSIOLOGY
Obstruction of aboral flow results in simple obstruction, abdominal pain, and distension.

CLINICAL PRESENTATION
Affected foals may initially present with depression and anorexia. Straining to defecate may be seen. Abdominal pain may be mild to moderate. If the condition is untreated, abdominal distension and severe progressive colic ensues.

DIFFERENTIAL DIAGNOSIS
Other conditions resulting in abdominal pain (*Table 34*).

DIAGNOSIS
Digital examination may identify rectal impactions. Contrast radiography can be useful.

MANAGEMENT
(See Management of Meconium Impaction/Retention, pp. 100–101).

DISORDERS INVOLVING THE PERITONEAL CAVITY

ABDOMINAL ABSCESSATION

KEY POINTS
- Abdominal abscessation is typically the result of hematogenous spread of respiratory pathogens.

- *Rhodococcus equi* and *Streptococcus* spp. are commonly identified.
- Abscesses are generally located in the mesentery of the small intestine.
- Adhesions are a frequent complication.
- Weight loss/failure to thrive and abdominal distension, ± abdominal pain, are typical clinical signs.
- Inflammatory leukogram is typical.
- Ultrasonography can be diagnostic.
- Surgical removal is difficult.
- Long-term antibiotic therapy with broad-spectrum antimicrobials can occasionally be successful.

DEFINITION/OVERVIEW

Abdominal abscessation is more commonly found in older foals. The abscesses are a result of septicemia/bacteremia, with mesenteric lymph node localization of bacteria. Most abdominal abscesses are located in the mesentery of the small intestine, but they can be found in the bowel wall or parenchyma of abdominal organs such as the liver and spleen. Abscesses of umbilical remnants are common; these are discussed in Chapter 9 (Urinary and Umbilical Disorders, pp. 180–182).

ETIOLOGY/PATHOPHYSIOLOGY

The bacteremia causing the abscessation often originates from the respiratory or GI tract. Abscesses may also result from leakage of GI contents or surgical contamination. In the foal, the two most common pathogens are *Rhodococcus equi* and *Streptococcus* spp.

The position and size of an abdominal abscess result in the functional and/or toxemic changes that influence the structure involved or structures in contact with the mass. Septicemic effects can ensue dependent on the position of the abscess and bacterial involvement. Leakage of bacteria may result in diffuse, severe peritonitis. An adhesion of GI contents to the abscess is one of the major and more frequent complications.

CLINICAL PRESENTATION

The clinical presentation of a foal with an abdominal abscess is often that of weight loss or failure to thrive. A distended abdomen may be present (**159**); however, the presentation can be variable,

with nonspecific signs such as a fever of unknown origin, colic (mild-chronic to acute-severe), depression, anorexia, and diarrhea. Clinical signs vary with the position and size of the abscess and other involvement of GI structures.

DIFFERENTIAL DIAGNOSIS

Other conditions that result in failure to thrive (*Table 35*) and abdominal pain (*Table 33*).

DIAGNOSIS

Ultrasonographic examination of the abdomen is the diagnostic test of choice (**160**). Abscesses vary in size and shape. Typically, they are not formed, "round" structures. Adhesions of one or more segments of bowel can confuse the ultrasonographic interpretation. Abscesses infrequently appear homogeneously echogenic. Abdominal abscesses are more often heterogeneous and hypoechoic. Caution should be taken not to misinterpret the urinary bladder for a caudal abdominal abscess. Lymph node abscessation, characterized by grape-like hypoechoic 1–2 cm masses along the cecocolic vessels (right side of mid to caudal abdomen), is not uncommonly seen with the abdominal form of *R. equi* infection. In older foals, colon contents can obscure visualization of any abdominal abscess, therefore muzzling for 12 hours prior to examination may be helpful. Negative results do not completely rule out the presence of an abscess.

Other tests in combination with clinical signs that may indicate abdominal abscessation include hematology and serum chemistry,

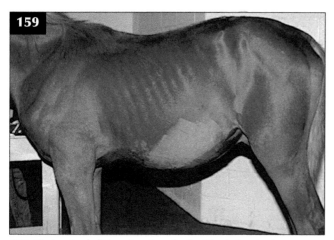

159 Abdominal distension in a foal with abdominal abscessation.

Table 35. Conditions that result in weight loss/failure to thrive

- Inadequate nutritional intake
- Chronic infection:
  - Abscessation
  - Respiratory
  - Gastrointestinal
  - Pleural
  - Peritoneal
  - Renal
  - Hepatic
- Chronic disease:
  - Liver
  - Respiratory
  - Renal
  - Gastrointestinal
- Neoplasia
- Cardiac disease
- Renal disease
- Hepatic disease
- Parasitism
- Infiltrative bowel disease
- Chronic salmonellosis or other chronic gastrointestinal infection
- Portosystemic shunt

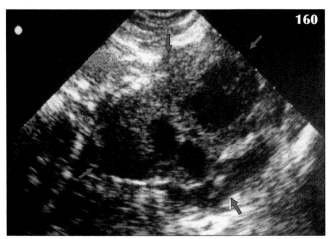

160 Ultrasonographic appearance of an abdominal abscess (arrows).

abdominocentesis, serology, and nuclear scintigraphy. Hematology and serum chemistry may reveal evidence of chronic infection. Anemia, hyperproteinemia, or hyperfibrinogenemia are variably present with chronic infection. Results of abdominocentesis are variable and can range from normal to an elevated protein content or white blood cell (WBC) count (neutrophilia). Serology identifying the presence of serum neutralizing antibodies to *S. equi* may indicate the presence of an occult infection. Serology identifying antibodies to *R. equi* are not reliable and are considered to indicate exposure and not current infection. Nuclear scintigraphy using labeled WBCs has been used with variable success.

MANAGEMENT

Therapy for abdominal abscessation consists of two approaches: exploratory celiotomy with removal or marsupialization, and/or long-term antibiotic therapy. Long-term antibiotic therapy should be based on culture results if available; otherwise, broad-spectrum antimicrobials should be used taking into account the fact that the likely organisms involved are *R. equi* and *S. equi*. Culture of abdominal fluid or direct sampling of the abscess should be performed if a celiotomy is attempted. Surgical removal of an abscess is generally difficult to impossible to achieve because of local involvement (adhesions) of adjacent structures (**161, 162**).

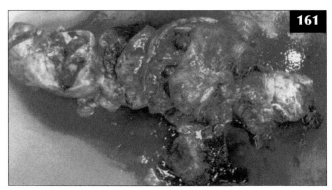

161 Abdominal abscesses are often adhered to associated structures.

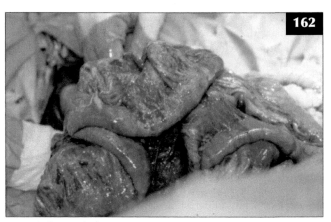

162 Abdominal abscess *in situ*.

Marsupialization is also difficult unless the abscess is ventral and close to the abdominal wall.

PERITONITIS

KEY POINTS
* Peritonitis is defined as inflammation of the peritoneal lining.
* Peritonitis can be septic or nonseptic, focal or diffuse.
* Clinical signs of peritonitis range from fever of unknown origin to septic shock.
* Abdominocentesis is the diagnostic test of choice.
* Abdominal ultrasound can guide an abdominocentesis and provide initial information regarding cellularity.

DEFINITION/OVERVIEW

Peritonitis is defined as an inflammation of the peritoneal lining. The peritoneal lining consists of a single layer of mesothelial cells, loose connective tissue, and adipose tissue. Peritonitis can be classified as peracute, acute, or chronic, indicating the onset or time course of the condition. The presence of bacteria determines septic versus nonseptic, and primary or secondary indicates whether the source of the bacteria is known. The region of the peritoneum involved is referred to as diffuse or focal.

ETIOLOGY/PATHOPHYSIOLOGY

Bacteria may enter the peritoneal cavity via the lymphatic vasculature, transmigration from bowel wall, or leakage of bowel contents or abdominal abscess. Septic peritonitis results in inflammation of the peritoneal lining, with subsequent exposure of the systemic circulation to bacterial endotoxins/exotoxins. Diffuse peritonitis of a septic nature involving bacteria that produce toxins results in severe septic shock. Local peritonitis may result in adhesion formation and subsequent GI signs.

CLINICAL PRESENTATION

The clinical presentation of peritonitis is variable and dependent on the source, severity, and pathogen. Patients may present in septic shock with cardiovascular collapse and/or fever of unknown origin. The diffuse nature of the process and the organisms involved determine the severity of the clinical signs. In moderate to mild nonoverwhelming peritonitis, the signs are nonspecific and compatible with the presence of infection and/or GI dysfunction. These nonspecific clinical signs may include any combination of signs such as fever, colic, depression, anorexia, weight loss, and/or diarrhea.

DIFFERENTIAL DIAGNOSIS

The differential diagnosis of acute, diffuse, septic peritonitis should include other conditions resulting in acute septic bacterial infection of any body cavity, splanchnic ischemia (compromised bowel with ischemic necrosis), and endotoxic/exotoxic (in combination with bacterial infection or as a product of enterocolitis) cardiovascular collapse. Differentials for a more insidious "low-grade" peritonitis include conditions that result in signs of infection and/or GI dysfunction.

DIAGNOSIS

Diagnosis of peritonitis is initially based on clinical examination findings. When septic shock is present, a rapid determination of the source of infection should be attempted subsequent to emergency therapy. Other sources of infection must be ruled out. Abdominocentesis can identify the presence of peritoneal contamination. Typically, the cell count is elevated with acute, diffuse peritonitis; however in peracute disease, cell counts can be within normal limits. Cytology of peritoneal fluid should be performed routinely when peritonitis is suspected. Microscopic examination may identify bacteria, feed material contamination, or toxic neutrophils.

Serum chemistries and hematology may indicate an infectious process. Ultrasonographic examination of the peritoneal space can be extremely useful in determining the presence of effusion and/or the preferred location for the abdominocentesis. The ultrasonographic appearance of peritoneal fluid can range widely from anechoic to echogenic. In some cases of (noneffusive) peritonitis, peritoneal fluid may be difficult to identify. Therefore, the inability to visualize fluid on the ultrasound examination should *never* preclude abdominocentesis. Fibrin strands may be noted along the surfaces of abdominal organs, but these should not be confused with normal mesenteric attachments and the omentum. Gas echoes or an intra-abdominal dorsal gas cap can be seen with pneumoperitoneum. Pneumoperitoneum is often a result of a ruptured viscus. Intestines may have a thickened or "corrugated" appearance due to secondary serosal irritation in cases of peritonitis.

MANAGEMENT

Therapy consists of treatment of septic shock (see Chapter 2, Shock, Resuscitation, Fluid and Electrolyte Therapy, pp. 23–32) if indicated. The principles of treatment of any bacterial infection should be followed. Broad-spectrum antimicrobial therapy is used if an antibiotic choice cannot be made from culture and sensitivity results. Drainage of the peritoneal cavity with lavage via an exploratory celiotomy may be warranted in an attempt to find the source of infection. Drainage and lavage alone are useful and can be performed during surgery or by placing large bore drains. Peritonitis secondary to a ruptured viscus has a guarded prognosis for recovery.

HEMOPERITONEUM

KEY POINTS
- Abdominal hemorrhage is an unusual condition in the foal.
- Clinical signs of hypovolemic shock may be present.
- Abdominocentesis is diagnostic.
- Blood transfusion ± an exploratory may be necessary.

DEFINITION/OVERVIEW
Hemorrhage into the abdomen is an unusual finding in the foal.

ETIOLOGY/PATHOPHYSIOLOGY
Hemoperitoneum can be seen secondary to traumatic rupture of the spleen or, occasionally, other abdominal organs (liver, kidney), to rupture of mesenteric or umbilical vessels, and, potentially, to fractured ribs. Abdominal hemorrhage can result in hypovolemic shock.

CLINICAL PRESENTATION
Foals with hypovolemic shock show signs of pale mucous membranes, tachycardia, sweating, tachypnea, trembling, weakness, weak pulses, and distress. Abdominal distension and pain is a variable component of the presenting clinical signs.

DIFFERENTIAL DIAGNOSIS
Other conditions resulting in hypovolemic shock (see Chapter 2, Shock, Resuscitation, Fluid and Electrolyte Therapy, pp. 23–32).

DIAGNOSIS
Diagnosis is based on the presence of clinical signs suggestive of hemorrhage and by demonstration of hemoperitoneum. Ultrasonographic evaluation of the abdomen in combination with abdominocentesis can provide a definitive diagnosis. The ultrasonographic appearance of hemorrhage is that of an echogenic, homogeneous, cloudy fluid. A swirling character to the fluid is often seen. Rarely, clots (hypoechoic serum clots or echogenic fresh hemorrhagic clots) may be identified in the ventral aspect of the abdomen.

Abdominocentesis confirms the presence of blood. Examination of the blood (e.g., hematocrit) can determine whether the bleeding is a component of other conditions such as effusion rather than due to vascular rupture. The presence of platelets or erythrophagocytosis (cytologic examination) can aid in determining the duration of the presence of hemorrhage; the presence of platelets suggests a recent event, whereas erythrophagocytosis suggests that the blood has been present for a matter of hours.

MANAGEMENT
Transfusion to replace blood volume may be necessary. If a compatible donor is not available, or time does not allow for identification of a donor, an autotransfusion of blood obtained from the peritoneal cavity can be used if necessary. Exploratory surgery to search for the source of the hemorrhage may be necessary if bleeding occurs unabated.

ENTEROCOLITIS

KEY POINTS

- Enterocolitis is one of the most common conditions encountered in the foal.
- The majority of foal diarrheas are caused by infectious agents (bacteria and viruses).
- Rotavirus is the primary viral infectious agent causing diarrhea in the foal.
- *Salmonella* spp. and *Clostridium* spp. are the two most common causes of bacterial diarrhea in the foal.
- Viral or bacterial epithelial cell damage results in fluid and electrolyte loss and a loss of absorption of fluids, nutrients, and electrolytes.
- In addition to electrolyte abnormalities, leukopenia is frequently observed.
- Clinical signs are variable, but often involve fever, depression, and abdominal pain.
- Dehydration of secondary complications can be life threatening.
- A foal with enterocolitis may exhibit clinical signs before evidence of diarrhea is seen.
- If evidence of abnormal stool is not obvious, then abdominal ultrasound can be useful in diagnosis.
- The basis of treatment is fluid and electrolyte replacement, if necessary, and treatment of the underlying cause if possible.

DEFINITION/OVERVIEW

Enterocolitis (diarrhea) is the most common GI disease encountered in the foal. The terms "enteritis" and "enterocolitis" are often used interchangeably. Enteritis refers to dysfunction of the small bowel, while enterocolitis refers to dysfunction of the small and large bowel. The severity of the condition ranges from a mild self-limiting condition to a severe life-threatening disease, and it varies with the etiology, ensuing degree of dehydration, electrolyte and acid–base abnormalities, and the development of endotoxemia/exotoxemia and sepsis. Foals of all ages are affected; however, neonates are more susceptible to severe and life-threatening complications. Rapid dehydration, acid–base disturbances, and electrolyte abnormalities can occur before a significant change in fecal character is seen. This may occur as a result of massive fluid accumulation in the lumen of the GI tract (third-space loss). Infectious diseases can result in severe epidemics, with major health and economic impacts.

ETIOLOGY/PATHOPHYSIOLOGY

Foal diarrhea can be caused by infectious agents (virus, bacteria, protozoa, parasites) nutritional upsets, or changes in flora (*Table 36*). The most common cause of enteritis/enterocolitis is infectious in nature, either bacterial or viral. The major viral enteritis of foals is rotavirus, although coronavirus and adenovirus have been associated with diarrhea in foals. The pathogenicity of rotavirus in foals is well documented; however, corona and adenovirus infections have not been well established and may, in many circumstances, be secondary to other pathogens. There are two types of rotavirus infection in foals: type A results in the more typical older foal diarrhea, whereas type B results in a neonatal diarrhea affecting the foal in the first few days of life.

Table 36. Causes of diarrhea in the foal

- Rotavirus, types A and B
- *Salmonella* spp.
- *Clostridium* spp.
- Parasitism
- Foal heat
- *Escheria coli*
- *Campylobacter* spp.
- *Rhodococcus equi*
- *Actinobacillus* spp.
- *Klebsiella spp.*
- Coronavirus
- Adenovirus
- *Giardia spp.*
- *Lawsonia intracellularis*
- Cryptosporidia

Viral diarrheas can be highly contagious, with rapid development of epidemics. The major bacterial organisms resulting in foal diarrhea include *Salmonella* spp. and *Clostridium* spp. Other bacteria that may be involved in enterocolitis in the foal include *Escherichia coli*, *Rhodococcus equi*, *Campylobacter* spp., *Actinobacillus* spp., and *Klebsiella* spp. The involvement of these alternative bacterial pathogens may be secondary to septicemia or be a secondary pathogen subsequent to viral or other bacterial infections.

The critical and often life-threatening nature of the infectious diarrheas is related to their direct influence on the cells of the GI tract. Rotavirus invades the absorptive cells of the villus. These cells are destroyed, resulting in a proliferation of crypt cells (often immature) and subsequent loss of absorption of substrates and increased fluid and electrolyte loss. Decreased absorption of substrate exacerbates the diarrhea with increased fluid loss. The combination of decreased absorption and increased secretion can result in rapid dehydration, electrolyte loss, and acid–base disturbances. If uncomplicated, the diarrhea can be self-limiting; however, if complications such as secondary bacterial involvement and subsequent endotoxemia/exotoxemia result, the disease can become severe and life threatening. The pathogenesis of bacteria related to enterocolitis is through a direct adhesion to, and invasion of, intestinal epithelial cells, with cytotoxin-producing enterotoxic stimulation of hypersecretion and/or exotoxin production, which produces intestinal necrosis. Local invasion and cytotoxin production produces cellular damage and loss of absorptive surfaces. Enterotoxin stimulates fluid and electrolyte loss through the prostaglandin-mediated adenyl cyclase system. Exotoxin causes direct cell necrosis and subsequent loss of absorption surfaces, electrolytes, and fluid.

CLINICAL PRESENTATION

The clinical presentation of a foal with diarrhea will vary considerably depending on severity, age, and secondary complications (**163–165**). The etiology of the diarrhea is difficult to impossible

163–165 (163) "Pipe stream" watery diarrhea. **(164)** Perineal staining with persistent diarrhea. **(165)** Evidence of watery stool in the tail.

to interpret based on clinical signs. The initial signs of disease may well be nonspecific (e.g., fever, depression, and inappetence). Physical evidence of diarrhea may not be seen early in the course of the disease, whether it is mild or severe. Abdominal mild or severe pain may be present and can exist before clinical evidence of diarrhea. Other signs of pain, such as tachycardia and/or tachypnea, may be present. Gastric reflux may be present. Systemic evidence of shock (endotoxic, septic, and exotoxic) is variable, but it can be very severe.

DIFFERENTIAL DIAGNOSIS

Differential diagnosis includes a variety of conditions that may cause abdominal pain (*Tables 33* and *34*) or nonspecific signs of depression and inappetence plus or minus a fever.

DIAGNOSIS

Diagnosis of enterocolitis can be based on clinical signs when obvious abnormal consistency and increased frequency of stool is present (**163–165**). In the more occult case, or when passage of abnormal stool is infrequent, ultrasonographic examination of the abdomen may identify a hypermotile "fluid-filled" bowel (**166**), with or without mural thickening or edema. Diagnosis may be more obscure in cases of enteritis complicated by ileus; differentiation of functional from mechanical ileus can be difficult. Auscultation of the abdomen may identify increased GI motility. Diagnosis of the various causes of foal diarrhea requires fecal evaluation and, in some circumstances, serology. These will be discussed in more detail under individual etiologies.

Clinicopathologic information can be useful in evaluation. The acute process is usually associated with a margination of WBCs and a leukopenia. Subsequently, individuals may respond to inflammation with a leukocytosis. Serum total protein and/or albumin may be low, particularly if the condition is infiltrative or becomes chronic. Acid–base status generally reflects an acidosis, as there is an overall loss of bicarbonate with continued secretion in combination with a lack of resorption resulting in a net loss. Electrolyte status is variable, with potassium chloride and sodium

loss the most frequently seen electrolyte abnormalities. At times, potassium and/or sodium loss can be severe and life threatening. Hyponatremia can result in CNS signs.

MANAGEMENT

The basic tenet of therapy for enterocolitis is support of hydration and electrolyte loss, if necessary, and amelioration of the toxic influences of bacteria and secondary bacterial infection. Fluid loss and resultant dehydration can be life threatening. The neonate is particularly susceptible to fluid losses and may require therapy for hypovolemic as well as septic shock. Significant amounts of fluid loss can occur even before physical evidence of diarrhea. Electrolyte loss is variable and dependent on the severity of the diarrhea, the degree of secretory component of the diarrhea, and reabsorption of secreted electrolytes. A discussion of fluid/electrolyte therapy can be found in Chapter 2 (Shock, Resuscitation, Fluid and Electrolyte Therapy).

Restriction of oral intake of milk (NPO) can be very useful in the treatment of neonates or young foals with diarrhea. Diarrhea in the neonate and young foal can be exacerbated by the osmotic influences of milk intake. "Resting" of the GI tract to allow for recovery of damaged enterocytes can be a beneficial part of therapy. Neonates must be deprived of milk intake cautiously, as glucose energy stores are limited at this age. Parenteral nutrition may be necessary and this allows increased periods of time without milk intake. A strong, robust neonate may be held off milk for 24 hours without parenteral caloric support. A period of 24 hours of GI rest may greatly aid the resolution of neonatal diarrhea.

Many of the agents that produce diarrhea in the foal produce toxins that may result in systemic influences. Therapy for septic, endotoxic, or exotoxic shock may be necessary in patients with enterocolitis. A discussion of individual causes of diarrhea follows. Shock therapy is discussed in Chapter 2 (Shock, Resuscitation, Fluid and Electrolyte Therapy).

Antimicrobial therapy may be necessary, particularly in those individuals that are most susceptible to secondary bacterial infection. Bacteremia/septicemia with resultant septic arthritis is a common secondary complication of enterocolitis in the neonate. Broad-spectrum antimicrobial therapy may prevent the development of secondary infectious problems. If *Salmonella* spp. infection is suspected, antimicrobials with appropriate sensitivities should be chosen. Systemic antimicrobials do not treat the enteric infection with the exception of organisms that may invade locally (e.g., *Salmonella* spp. or *Clostridia* spp.). Oral aminoglycosides have been used with some anecdotal success when coliforms are suspected. Antimicrobial therapy for specific infections will be discussed under these specific infections.

ROTAVIRUS DIARRHEA

KEY POINTS

- Rotavirus is the most common cause of diarrhea in foals.
- Epidemics can occur.
- Cellular damage in the mucosa of the small intestine results in absorption and secretory abnormalities.
- Diagnosis is based on identification of viral particles.

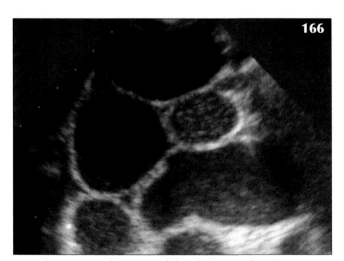

166 Ultrasonographic view of the abdomen showing fluid-filled small intestines.

DEFINITION/OVERVIEW

Rotavirus usually occurs in young foals less than 2 months of age. Rotaviral particles have been reported in up to 30% of foals with diarrhea. Most adult horses have antibodies to rotavirus. Epidemics of enterocolitis as a result of rotavirus are not uncommon. The disease can be extremely contagious and difficult to control. Group A rotavirus is the usual cause of rotavirus diarrhea in the older foal. Group B rotavirus has been associated with severe epidemics in neonates and has been frequently called neonatal or 24-hour scours.

ETIOLOGY/PATHOPHYSIOLOGY

The source of the virus is likely to be adult shedders. Subclinical infection is thought to be common in foals and may occur up to 8 months of age. The virus may persist for up to nine months in the environment. Heavy contamination of the environment occurs when population pressures and maintenance practices favor contamination.

Rotaviral infection is a small intestinal disease. The virus invades the absorptive cells of the villus. Destruction of these cells results in migration of crypt cells to the tips of the villus. This migration (hypertrophy) of secretory cells results in increased secretion and decreased absorption, and a net loss of fluid and electrolytes.

CLINICAL PRESENTATION

Variable degrees of depression, fever, and anorexia are followed by evidence of diarrhea within 12–24 hours. Abdominal pain may be present. Diarrhea may be mild to profuse-projectile watery. (See also discussion above under Enterocolitis, Clinical presentation, pp. 105–107.)

DIFFERENTIAL DIAGNOSIS

The differential diagnosis includes conditions resulting in fever, depression, anorexia, and/or abdominal pain. The differential diagnoses for a foal with diarrhea are listed in *Table 36*.

DIAGNOSIS

Diagnosis is based on fecal evaluation. Electron microscopy identifies viral particles, but is time-consuming and not practical in the clinical setting. A latex agglutination test and enzyme-linked immunosorbent assay (ELISA) test are available and do compare well with electron microscopy. Bacterial cultures may rule out other causes. The absence of positive fecal samples does not rule out the disease. Group B rotavirus is shed very early in the course of the disease and is therefore difficult to identify.

MANAGEMENT

See discussion above under Enterocolitis, Management (p. 107).

CORONAVIRUS

KEY POINTS

- Coronavirus has been definitively identified as a cause of enterocolitis in the foal.
- Enteric infections can be self-limiting; however, they may result in mortality.
- Chronically infected adults may be the source of infection.

DEFINITION/OVERVIEW

Coronavirus can cause disease in a wide variety of species. Coronavirus-like particles are not infrequently identified in foals with GI disease, however, it can be difficult to make a definitive diagnosis as other pathogens are frequently found in association. Chronically infected adults may be the source of infection for the foal. The disease may be self-limiting or result in a severe life-threatening condition.

ETIOLOGY/PATHOPHYSIOLOGY

Coronavirus can cause disease in a large variety of species including cattle, pigs, cats, poultry, mice, rats, humans, and nonhuman primates. The virus is an RNA virus that belongs to three antigenic groups. The equine coronavirus is antigenically similar to bovine coronavirus, which is a member of antigenic group II. The virus damages the intestinal villi, resulting in water, electrolyte, and protein loss. The malabsorptive diarrhea can lead to dehydration, hyponatremia, hypochloraemia, and hypoproteinaemia.

CLINICAL PRESENTATION

The clinical presentation is similar to other causes of enterocolitis in foals, particularly those that cause a malabsorptive diarrhea. (See the discussion above under Enterocolitis, Clinical presentation, pp. 105–107.)

DIFFERENTIAL DIAGNOSIS

The differential diagnosis includes other causes of fever, depression, and anorexia with or without visible signs of diarrhea. The differential diagnoses for the foal with diarrhea are listed in *Table 36*.

DIAGNOSIS

A definitive diagnosis can be problematic. Secondary infections with other pathogens can be common. However, attempts to rule out other infections can be useful. Antemortem diagnosis requires documentation of rising serum antibody titers and/or detection of coronavirus antigen in the feces (immunohistochemistry or ELISA).

MANAGEMENT

See discussion under Enterocolitis, Management (p. 107).

FOAL HEAT DIARRHEA

KEY POINTS

- Foal heat diarrhea is a mild, self-limiting diarrhea.
- Often occurs during the first estrus exhibited by the mare.
- Condition is not related to a pathogen.
- May well be a result of a nutritionally induced alteration in flora.

DEFINITION/OVERVIEW

Mild self-limiting diarrhea occurs in foals between 6 and 14 days of age. It rarely results in systemic disease unless complicated by bacterial organisms.

ETIOLOGY/PATHOPHYSIOLOGY

Suggested causes of foal heat diarrhea include hormonal changes in the mare associated with estrus resulting in flora alterations in milk composition (hence the name "foal heat diarrhea"), adaptation of the large bowel as the foal's diet begin to change, and parasitism with *Strongylus westerii*. Attempts to identify microbes such as viruses or cryptosporidia have been unsuccessful. The currently accepted and most plausible cause of foal heat diarrhea is mechanical adaptation of the GI tract, which can occur in the newborn foal at approximately 1 week of age. At this age the foal is beginning to adapt to a diet that includes roughage and other nonmilk food sources.

CLINICAL PRESENTATION
Affected foals present with mild self-limiting diarrhea with no systemic effects. If diarrhea persists or systemic complications occur, then other diseases should be considered.

DIFFERENTIAL DIAGNOSIS
See *Table 36*.

DIAGNOSIS
Diagnosis is based on signalment, history, and ruling out other causes of diarrhea.

MANAGEMENT
Therapy is not necessary if the foal shows no clinical disease other than diarrhea.

SALMONELLOSIS

KEY POINTS
- Salmonellosis is a severe, frequently life-threatening enterocolitis.
- The organism can become endemic on farms.
- Asymptomatic shedders play a role in maintenance of the organism in the environment.
- Host factors are critical in development of disease.
- *Salmonella* spp. contain numerous virulence factors, which combine to overwhelm the host's defense mechanisms.
- The intracellular survival of the *Salmonella* organism is key to its aggressive nature and severity of disease.
- Malabsorption secretory diarrhea and toxemia (endotoxin/enterotoxin) may be present.
- Secondary complications are frequent and may include septic arthritis, osteomyelitis, meningitis, or other organ system involvement.
- The hallmark of diagnosis is fecal culture.
- Appropriate antibiotic therapy is critical to successful therapy.

DEFINITION/OVERVIEW
Salmonellosis is a severe bacterial enterocolitis that can result in high morbidity and mortality. Septicemia with secondary complications such as osteomyelitis or septic arthritis is common. This bacterium can cause disease in all mammals and most vertebrates. *Salmonella* spp. organisms are widespread in nature. Epidemics of salmonellosis may be seen. The organisms can become endemic. Hospitalization has become a risk factor for development of the disease. Any age of foal may be infected.

ETIOLOGY/PATHOPHYSIOLOGY
Numerous *Salmonella* serotypes have been identified. *S. typhimurium* is the most common serotype in horses. The organism is widespread in nature. Other horses (asymptomatic shedders), other animal species, or contaminated feed/environment may provide a source of infection. Host factors play an important role in the development of clinical disease. Animals with a normal healthy intestinal flora may be resistant to transient exposure. Floral alterations (antibiotic therapy), immune suppression, stress, virulence of the bacteria, and exposure dose are factors that contribute to disease. Young foals without a developed flora may be more susceptible to virulent *Salmonella* infection.

Numerous virulent factors allow salmonellae to overwhelm the host defense mechanisms. These include endotoxins, exotoxins, flagellar motility, cytotoxins, plasmids, iron-chelating enzymes, and surface antigens. Once the bacteria gain access to the surface of the enterocyte, flagellar motility enhances contact and adhesion. Enterocyte microvilli and tight junctions undergo degeneration. Bacteria migrate from the enterocyte to the lamina propria, with a subsequent inflammatory response that includes macrophage and neutrophil phagocytosis. Salmonellae survive and remain protected within these phagocytotic cells. The organisms produces protein, which prevent fusion of the phagosome and lysosome. They multiply intracellularly and travel to lymph nodes through lymphatic circulation. From the lymph nodes the bacteria can then spread to the systemic circulation, with resultant septicemia and ensuing complications. The diarrhea that follows infection is because of malabsorption due to epithelial cell destruction and secretion (from intact epithelial cells) as a result of enterotoxin production.

Endotoxin (lipopolysaccharide) is a component of the cell wall membrane and is a major component of the severity of the disease process. Endotoxin can result in hemodynamic and vascular changes that may lead to multiorgan system failure.

CLINICAL PRESENTATION
See the discussion under Enterocolitis, Clinical presentation (pp. 105–107). Foals with salmonellosis may present with a variety of clinical syndromes. Clinical signs may be mild to severe with septic/endotoxic shock; the diarrhea can be mild to profuse and watery. The variable nature is related to host defense and the pathogenicity of the serovar of *Salmonella*. Hemorrhage in the stool can be present. Diarrhea may occasionally become chronic. Sequela of septicemia may include septic arthritis, meningitis, other organ involvement, or peritonitis.

DIFFERENTIAL DIAGNOSIS
See *Table 36*.

DIAGNOSIS
See discussion under Enterocolitis, Diagnosis (p. 107). Diagnosis is based on fecal culture. Negative culture does not rule out the disease; three–five consecutive cultures may improve the likelihood of identification. Polymerase chain reaction (PCR) testing has been used. Blood cultures may identify salmonellae in the bacteremic foal. Fecal cultures from the mare may identify the source of infection. Clinical pathology may identify leukopenia, neutropenia, and

toxic changes in neutrophils. Electrolyte changes are frequently seen (see Enterocolitis, Diagnosis, p. 107). Ultrasonography may reveal a fluid-filled colon; however, this is not specific for salmonellosis and its absence does not exclude salmonellosis.

MANAGEMENT

Treatment of shock and the fluid/electrolyte losses are described in Chapter 2 (pp. 23–32). Secondary complications (sepsis) are frequent with *Salmonella* infection, therefore antibiotics therapy is recommended. The antibiotics of choice should include those that achieve adequate intracellular levels, as the organism invades and multiplies intracellularly. Antibiotic culture and sensitivities should be performed when possible. Antibiotic resistance can be and is a frequent problem with *Salmonella* infection. Trimethoprim/sulfa combinations, chloramphenicol, and the quinilones can achieve intracellular levels.

CLOSTRIDIAL ENTEROCOLITIS

KEY POINTS

- *Clostridium perfringens* can cause severe, acute, or peracute diarrhea.
- *Clostridium difficile* is related to outbreaks of diarrhea in young foals, frequently during the neonatal age.
- *Clostridium* spp. produce a variety of toxins, which are integrally related to severity of clinical signs.
- Diagnosis is based on toxin isolation, bacterial culture, and the absence of other pathogens.

DEFINITION/OVERVIEW

Clostridium spp. can cause severe acute or peracute diarrhea with septicemia, septic/toxemic shock, and cardiovascular collapse. Acute death before evidence of diarrhea is possible. *C. perfringens* is associated with a peracute hemorrhagic enterocolitis. *C. difficile* has been associated with highly contagious or sporadic mild to severe diarrhea in neonatal foals. *C. difficile* diarrhea should be suspected when the diarrhea is a result of previous antibiotic therapy. Fecal shedding of *C. difficile* is commonly recognized in foals with diarrhea and may confuse the diagnosis.

ETIOLOGY/PATHOPHYSIOLOGY

C. perfringens types A, B, and C are associated with severe fulminating, aggressive, hemorrhagic diarrhea. Other clostridial species can also cause similar severe enterocolitis (e.g., *C. wechii*, *C. sordelli*, and *C. difficile*). *C. difficile* has recently been recognized as a more frequent cause of foal diarrhea. *C. perfringens* is more commonly associated with disease in neonatal foals. Inhibition of pancreatic trypsin by a colostral trypsin inhibitor is thought to play a role in *C. perfringens* colonization of the small intestine. Foals that overeat or are overfed (orphans) are at increased risk.

The various clostridial species produce a variety of toxins including exotoxins, endotoxins, and cytotoxins. The exotoxins cause epithelial cell necrosis and hemorrhage.

CLINICAL PRESENTATION

Clostridial diarrhea should be high on the differential list of the foal with a hemorrhagic toxic enterocolitis. Clinical signs of shock

are frequent. Abdominal pain with abdominal distension is frequently seen. Diarrhea may not be present in foals that die of peracute disease. The spectrum of disease associated with *C. difficile* is broad and includes diseases of less severity. Clostridial diarrhea does not invariably result in hemorrhage.

DIFFERENTIAL DIAGNOSIS

The differential diagnosis for clostridial diarrhea includes any other cause of diarrhea (*Table 36*). When hemorrhage is present, other bacterial causes of diarrhea or intussusception should be considered. In the neonate with diarrhea, *Rotavirus* or *Salmonella* infection would be other conditions to consider.

DIAGNOSIS

The clinicopathologic findings are nonspecific. Diagnosis must be based on a combination of clinical findings, culture of the organism, the presence of toxin, and the absence of other significant culture results. Radiographic findings include a nonspecific inflammatory process (**167**). Controversy exists as to whether culture alone is diagnostic. Shedding of *Clostridium* spp. can occur with GI upsets/diarrhea and may represent a marker of disease. Nontoxigenic strains of *C. difficile* exist, therefore identification of both the organism and the toxin provides stronger evidence of a causal relationship.

An estimate of the number of clostridial organisms can be useful in determining the significance of their presence. Culture is difficult, as fresh samples must be kept under anaerobic conditions while being delivered to the laboratory. Large numbers of *C. perfringens* ($>10^3$ colony forming units/mL) would be suggestive of the diagnosis. Direct Gram staining of stool may identify large numbers of large Gram-positive rods.

Exploratory surgery is not a standard diagnostic approach. However, unrelenting pain and a gas-filled bowel seen on ultrasound examination (**166**), in an absence of visible diarrhea, may indicate exploratory surgery as a last-ditch attempt at resolution of the pain (**168**).

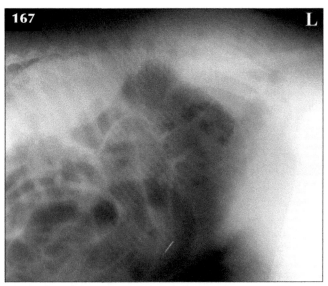

167 Radiographic appearance of clostridial enterocolitis.

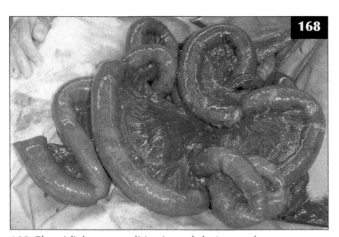

168 Clostridial enterocolitis viewed during exploratory surgery. Surgery is not a standard treatment for clostridial enterocolitis; however, there are times when a foal is so painful that exploratory surgery is performed as a "last-ditch" effort.

Regardless of the clostridial species causing the diarrhea, diagnosis can be difficult. Postmortem identification of histopathologic changes and the presence of colonization with Gram-positive rods are highly suggestive of a positive diagnosis of clostridial disease. Culture of infected intestine (refrigerated, tied-off sections) can be diagnostic. Intestinal contents can be frozen for toxin assays.

MANAGEMENT

The treatment of clostridial enterocolitis is the same as for other causes of diarrheas with respect to supportive care and treatment for shock if present (**168**) (see Enterocolitis, Management, p. 107). However, because septicemia and toxemia can be present, some specific therapies should be considered. Metronidazole orally can be used and is effective against most clostridial organisms. Oral metronidazole has been reported to be beneficial in some outbreaks of *C. difficile*. Intravenous penicillin can potentially be useful for the prevention of bacteremia/septicemia. The use of hyperimmunized plasma (hyperimmunized to the toxins of clostridial species) has met with some success. *C. perfringens* is typically an isolated problem in horses, but it can occur in outbreak situations. The practice of good hygiene may limit the spread of disease. Extensive washing of the udder, ventral limbs, and any other regions that the newborn will suckle can prevent neonatal diarrhea if the source of infection is a shedding mare. Probiotics such as *Saccharomyces boulardii* are reported to be successful in the treatment of clostridial disease in animals and humans. Vaccination of mares with toxoids prepared for ruminants has also met with reported success.

LAWSONIA INTRACELLULARIS

KEY POINTS
- *Lawsonia intracellularis* is an intracellular bacterium that results in an infiltrative enteropathy.
- Hypoproteinemia is a hallmark clinical sign.
- Diagnosis is via serology and/or PCR.

- Treatment consists of use of an antibiotic that reaches intracellular levels.
- An avirulent live vaccine has been used successfully to prevent experimental infection.
- Weanling foals are most commonly affected.

DEFINITION/OVERVIEW

L. intracellularis is an obligate intracellular bacteria. *L. intracellularis* is unique in that the infection of enterocytes results in a proliferation of the infected enterocyte and a characteristic proliferative infiltrative enteropathy. The enteropathy is typically of the small intestine. The bacterium has also been associated with an ulcerative colitis and abdominal pain. It affects a number of mammalian species, particularly swine. The condition is sporadic, but can affect multiple individuals within a farm.

ETIOLOGY/PATHOPHYSIOLOGY

L. intracellularis is an obligate intracellular bacterium. The bacteria invade the crypt (villus crypt) epithelial cells of the intestinal mucosa. This infection results in a severe hyperplasia of the distal small intestine and, potentially, a gross thickening of the bowel wall. The route of infection is fecal-oral. A variety of wild and domestic animals can shed *L. intracellularis* on farms, including dogs, cats, rabbits, opossums, skunks, mice, and coyotes. Rabbits experimentally infected with an equine isolate of *L. intracellularis* were infectious to weanling foals. In pigs it has been shown that subclinical infected individuals can act as a reservoir on infection.

CLINICAL PRESENTATION

Possible presenting clinical signs include weight loss (failure to thrive), depression, ventral edema, colic, poor hair coat/unthrifty appearance, fever, and possibly a pot-bellied appearance. Diarrhea may or not be present. Foals may also present with the primary complaint of edema only. In North America the disease is usually seen between August and January. The condition is generally seen in older foals 4–7 months of age; however, it has been seen in young adults. The most common laboratory finding is a hypoproteinemia as a result of hypoalbunemia. The hypoproteinemia may be the only consistent clinicopathologic abnormality, but there may be many nonspecific abnormalities, such as electrolyte abnormalities, serum enzyme abnormalities, and increases or decreases in white cell counts and red cell numbers. Recently, much more severe cases with poorer outcome have been presented. These patients often have severe secondary complications, and significant mortality is not uncommon.

DIFFERENTIAL DIAGNOSIS

Other diseases that result in enterocolitis (*Table 36*) should be considered. The weight loss and hypoproteinemia should lead to a suspicion of *L. intracellularis* infection. *R. equi* GI infection can produce signs very similar to *L. intracellularis* infection.

DIAGNOSIS

The initial presumptive diagnosis can be made based on farm history, typical physical exam findings, and ultrasonographic thickening of small bowel. Other diseases resulting in similar clinical signs should be ruled out. Antemortem diagnosis can be made via PCR detection of *L. intracellularis* in feces rectal swab or serum. The PCR test is specific, but has a low sensitivity. Serologic testing of infected foals is currently the most reliable premortem diagnostic test. Ultrasonography typically identifies thickening of the small intestinal wall. Postmortem examination identifies intracellular bacteria (silver stain) in the crypt epithelium. PCR analysis and immunohistochemistry can be used to confirm the presence of *L. intracellularis*. The organism cannot currently be cultured in conventional cell-free media. Cell culture techniques are available at only a few specialized laboratories.

MANAGEMENT

Antibiotic treatment can provide a successful outcome. The antibiotics that have been used are the macrolides (with or without rifampin), chloramphenicol, and the quinolones. Oxytetracycline or doxycycline have also been used. The duration of therapy may be extended, with the response to therapy used to determine the treatment end-point. Supportive care with parenteral nutrition or intravenous plasma may be necessary. An avirulent live vaccine has successfully prevented the disease in an experimental challenge model.

RHODOCOCCUS EQUI INTESTINAL DISEASE

KEY POINTS
* *Rhodococcus equi* can cause an infiltrative enteropathy.
* The bacteria colonize the GI tract, forming a granulomatous infiltrative disease.
* Clinical signs are referable to the GI tract, weight loss/failure to thrive, pot-bellied appearance, and edema.

DEFINITION/OVERVIEW

R. equi is typically a pathogen of the respiratory tract (see Chapter 8, Respiratory Disorders); however, it can cause a primary disease of the GI tract, with mesenteric lymphadenitis or ulcerative colitis. The condition is typically sporadic and can occur in association with the respiratory or other forms of the disease.

ETIOLOGY/PATHOPHYSIOLOGY

R. equi is a Gram-positive facultative intracellular bacterium. The organism is a soilborne pathogen that persists in the environment. Inoculation is via ingestion or inhalation. Ingestion of the organism results in colonization of the GI tract. Intestinal colonization may lead to several manifestations. Diffuse infiltration of the lamina propria and submucosa by infected macrophages and multinucleated giant cells can result in enterocolitis. The lesions are characterized histologically by a granulomatous inflammation of the lamina propria, which can distort villi and displace intestinal glands and crypts. Ulceration may occur. The granulomatous infiltrate involves those areas of the GI tract that contain lymphoid follicles. Grossly affected segments have thickened corrugated mucosa with foci of necrosis and ulceration (**169**). Cecal colonic and mesenteric lymph nodes may be involved (**170**). Cellular obstruction of lymph nodes and lymphatics can result in ascites.

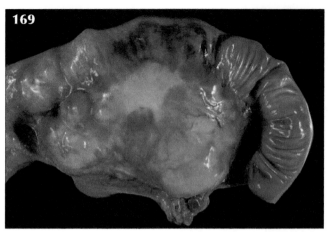

169 *Rhodococcus equi* abscess with bowel involvement.

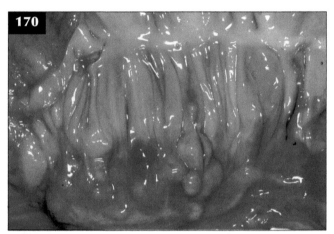

170 *Rhodococcus equi* abscessation involving the serosal surface of the large bowel.

CLINICAL PRESENTATION

Foals with enteric *R. equi* can present with variable clinical signs including fever, weight loss (unthrifty, failure to thrive), ventral edema, diarrhea, and/or a pot-bellied appearance. Diarrhea is not invariably present.

DIFFERENTIAL DIAGNOSIS

Although clinical evidence of diarrhea is not the primary clinical sign of *R. equi* infiltrative enterocolitis, other diseases resulting in diarrhea should be considered in the differential diagnosis (*Table 36*). Conditions resulting in weight loss (unthriftiness, failure to thrive) and/or hypoproteinemia, such as infiltrative *L. intracellularis* infection, should also be considered (see previous section).

DIAGNOSIS

The finding of *R. equi* in the stool can be suggestive of infection when combined with appropriate clinical signs. Serology is not diagnostic, but it can confirm exposure to *R. equi*. Clinical pathology is nonspecific; leukocytosis and hyperfibrinogenemia would be supportive of a diagnosis of *R. equi* infection.

MANAGEMENT

The treatment of *R. equi* infection is discussed in Chapter 3 (infectious Disease, pp. 53–54). Foals with the enteric form may require plasma therapy if hypoproteinemia becomes a component of the condition.

CRYPTOSPORIDIOSIS

DEFINITION/OVERVIEW

Enterocolitis as a result of infection by the protozoal parasite *Cryptosporidium parvum* can be recognized as a sporadic disease in foals or, occasionally, as a farm outbreak. The first reports of *C. parvum* infection were in immunocompromised foals. However, immunocompetent foals can develop cryptosporidial diarrhea. The condition is somewhat controversial as normal foals may shed cryptosporidia. The prevalence is higher in foals with diarrhea, and interpretation of shedding is difficult as shedding may increase with other etiologies of diarrhea. In outbreaks of disease the prevalence may reach 100%.

ETIOLOGY/PATHOPHYSIOLOGY

C. parvum is a coccidian (protozoal) organism. Infective sporulated oocysts are ingested and excyst in the small intestine. Excysted oocytes (ingested) attach to the epithelium in an intracellular yet extracytoplasmic location. Asexual and sexual multiplication occurs.

CLINICAL PRESENTATION

Clinical signs consist primarily of diarrhea. Immunocompromised foals with cryptosporidial infection may have structures other than the small intestine involved (e.g., stomach, common bile duct, pancreatic ducts, and colon). The disease usually affects younger foals, but it can cause disease in older foals and may become chronic.

DIFFERENTIAL DIAGNOSIS

Other diseases that cause diarrhea should be considered (*Table 36*).

DIAGNOSIS

Identification of oocysts in the feces is the basis of diagnosis. Oocysts can be identified by flotation, sedimentation, or staining techniques. If fresh fecal samples cannot be processed, samples can be stored in 10% formalin. During the course of disease, fecal shedding of oocysts is variable; therefore, multiple fecal samples should be evaluated.

MANAGEMENT

No antibiotic therapy has been approved or been shown to be effective in the treatment of *C. parvum* infection in foals. Paromomycin has been used effectively in calves, but no data exist for its use in foals. Sanitation practices are important considerations, as food, water, and environmental contamination can occur.

PARASITE INFESTATION

DEFINITION/OVERVIEW

Strongyloides westerii and *Strongylus vulgaris* can potentially cause diarrhea in young foals. Heavy infestation with large or small strongyles may cause chronic diarrhea in older foals. The source of infection of *S. westerii* is mares' milk. It is questionable whether this route of exposure is significant enough to result in clinical diarrhea.

ETIOLOGY/PATHOPHYSIOLOGY

S. westerii can undergo transmammary transmission or invade the skin. Unhygienic conditions including moisture and contamination with feces are situations that may lead to infection. *S. vulgaris* can penetrate the mucosa within 3 days post ingestion and migrate to the ileocecal artery by 14–21 days; therefore, foals could exhibit intestinal signs within the first two weeks of life.

CLINICAL PRESENTATION

Foals with parasitic diarrhea may present with fever, anorexia, depression, and variable manifestations of abnormal stool. Older foals may exhibit weight loss (unthrifty, failure to thrive), depression, anorexia, and abnormal stool.

DIFFERENTIAL DIAGNOSIS

Other diseases that cause diarrhea should be considered (*Table 36*).

DIAGNOSIS

Clinical signs, poor management, and parasitism in other associated individuals may lead to a suspicion of parasitic diarrhea.

MANAGEMENT

Treatment of *S. westerii* may include ivermectin, thiobendazole, cambendazole, and oxibendazole. *S. vulgaris* infection responds to ivermectin, fenbendazole, and thiobendazole. These drugs come in numerous formulations, concentrations, and combination products, so readers are advised to consult the relevant label recommendations and directions before use.

FURTHER READING

Bernard WV, Santchi EM (2002) Large and small colon disease associated with colic in the foal. In: *Manual of Equine Gastroenterology* (Mair T, Divers T, Ducharme N, Eds.). WB Saunders, Philadelphia, PA, pp. 485–488.

Davis E, Rush BR, Cox J et al. (2014) Neonatal enterocolitis associated with coronavirus infection in a foal: A case report. *Journal of Veterinary Diagnostic Investigation* 12: 153–156.

Dharma K, Pawaiya RVS, Chakraborty S et al. (2014) Coronavirus infection in equines a review. *Asian Journal of Animal and Veterinary Advances* 9: 164–176.

Fielding CL, Higgins JK, Higgins JC et al. (2015) Disease associated with equine coronavirus infection and high case fatality rate. *Journal of Veterinary Internal Medicine* 29: 307–310.

Holcombe SJ, Chaney KP (2009) Meconium impaction. In: *Current Therapy: Equine Practice*, 6th ed. (Robinson NE, Sprayberry KA, Eds.). WB Saunders, Philadelphia, PA, pp. 858–861.

Magdesian GK (2005) Neonatal foal diarrhea. *Veterinary Clinics of North America: Equine Practice* 21: 295–312.

Magdesian GK (2009) Inflammatory bowel disease in the foal. In: *Current Therapy: Equine Practice*, 6th ed. (Robinson NE, Sprayberry KA, Eds.). WB Saunders, Philadelphia, PA, pp. 870–876.

Mallicote M, House AM, Sanchez LC (2012) A review of foal diarrhoea from birth to weaning. *Equine Veterinary Education* 24: 206–214.

Murray MJ (2002) Stomach disease of the foal. In: *Manual of Equine Gastroenterology* (Mair T, Divers T, Ducharme N, Eds.). WB Saunders, Philadelphia, PA, pp. 469–476.

Orsini J (2002) Small intestinal disease associated with colic in the foal. In: *Manual of Equine Gastroenterology* (Mair T, Divers T, Ducharme N, Eds.). WB Saunders, Philadelphia, PA, pp. 477–483.

Pusterla N (2013) *Lawsonia Intracellularis* infection and proliferative enteropathy in foals. *Veterinary Microbiology* 167: 34–41.

Pusterla N, Vannicci FA, Mapes SM et al. (2012) Efficacy of a live avirulent vaccine against *Lawsonia intracellularis* in the prevention of proliferative enteropathy in experimentally infected foals. *American Journal of Veterinary Research* 73: 741–746.

Ryan CA, Sanchez CL (2005) Nondiarrheal disorders of the gastrointestinal tract in neonatal foals. *Veterinary Clinics of North America: Equine Practice* 21: 313–332.

Toribio RE, Mudge MC (2013) Diseases of the foal. In: *Equine Surgery, Medicine and Reproduction* (Mair TS, Love S, Schumacher J, Smith RK, Frazer G, Eds.). Saunders/Elsevier, Philadelphia, PA, pp. 439–444.

Wilson JH, Cudd TA (1990) Common gastrointestinal diseases. In: *Equine Clinical Neonatology* (Korterba A, Drummond W, Kosch P, Eds.). Lea & Febiger, Philadelphia, PA, pp. 412–429.

Liver Disorders

William V. Bernard

INTRODUCTION

KEY POINTS

- Hepatic disease is not common in the foal.
- Gastrointestinal (GI) disease (portal circulation) often influences the liver, resulting in increased liver enzymes.
- The excretion of bile into the biliary ductules is an energy-requiring step.
- Conjugated bilirubin is not protein bound.
- There are numerous nonhepatic causes of icterus in the foal.
- Clinical signs are nonspecific.
- Hypoglycemia is a common finding in severe, acute hepatic disease.
- A knowledge of liver enzymes, and their specificities and half-lives, is critical to the evaluation of liver disease.

DEFINITION/OVERVIEW

Hepatic disease in the foal is not as common as GI or respiratory conditions. Clinical signs are often nonspecific (*Table 37*), therefore disorders of the liver must be included in the differential diagnosis for a variety of diagnostic workups of the "sick" foal. When discussing liver abnormalities, liver disease as opposed to liver failure should be considered. As the liver is vital to the majority of metabolic processes that occur, systemic or other organ system diseases frequently affect the liver, resulting in alterations in liver enzymes or disease, but often not in liver failure. Primary liver disease can result in liver failure. The causes of liver disease can range from congenital or metabolic conditions at birth to acquired infections or toxins. The pathophysiology of foal liver disease is similar for all the conditions recognized. As the hepatocytes are progressively damaged, subsequent edema involves associated hepatocytes and adjacent structures such as biliary epithelium and vascular structures. Progressive disease further influences the anatomy and physiology of the liver, which is involved with the major metabolic pathways of the body. When liver disease is suspected, the diagnosis of liver involvement is not difficult, but biopsy may be necessary to define a definitive etiology. The management of hepatic disease subsequent to identification and treatment of the underlying disease process is based on good supportive care.

ETIOLOGY/PATHOPHYSIOLOGY

The range of causes of liver disease is wide; however, many of the conditions are seen infrequently. The neonate can be born with congenital or infectious conditions, or it can acquire disease from processes that occur shortly after birth. Neonatal asphyxia (hypoxemia/ischemia), septicemia, and isoerythrolysis can all influence hepatocytes and hepatic function. Neoplasia has been reported in a late-term aborted fetus and a stillborn term foal (see Chapter 16, Neoplasia, pp. 283–284). Inappropriate supplements can cause toxicity in the neonate. *In-utero* infections can result in evidence of hepatic disease at, or shortly after, birth. Older foals can also acquire infections and toxic conditions. Parasites, although not common, can result in liver disease, but rarely result in liver failure.

The pathophysiology of liver disease is made complex by the numerous processes with which the liver is involved. The liver functions in storage, metabolism, and secretion. Many of these processes are interrelated and function in combination with other organ systems. Disruption of hepatocytes results in hepatocellular disease and damage to associated structures. This often includes the biliary epithelium; therefore, it can be difficult to differentiate between primary hepatic and primary biliary disease.

Subclinical liver disease (anatomic or physiologic disruption that has not resulted in clinical signs of disease) is common. The liver, being such a vital structure, has an enormous capacity for reserve. Diffuse involvement of liver parenchyma (<50%), focal involvement of discrete portions of parenchyma, or hepatocyte accumulation of chemicals/toxins that do not completely disrupt metabolism may frequently result in subclinical disease. Subclinical disease may not be recognized or may be identified only when serum chemistries are evaluated. As a result of the liver's role in the majority of bodily functions, disease in other organs often results in subclinical liver disease, but not liver failure. GI disease can frequently influence hepatic function. The portal circulation is an immediate link between the GI tract and the liver.

Primary biliary disease can occur in foals, but is more frequently seen in the adult horse. As mentioned previously, chronic progressive damage to the biliary epithelium can influence hepatocyte function. Biliary obstruction secondary to a suppurative cholangitis or cholelithiasis is uncommon in the foal. Retrograde biliary disease in the foal can occasionally occur. Parasites and other obstructions can significantly obstruct flow of the common bile duct. Usually, obstructions are evident as a GI disease, with the biliary component being a secondary event. Biliary obstruction is commonly seen secondary to duodenal stricture.

Table 37. Clinical signs of liver disease

- Anorexia
- Depression
- Fever
- Weight loss
- Pain, abdominal
- Icterus
- Pigmenturia
- Encephalopathy
- Bleeding disorders
- Ascites
- Edema
- Dermatitis

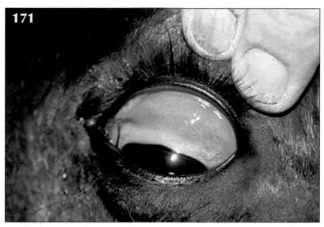

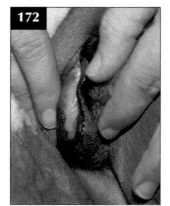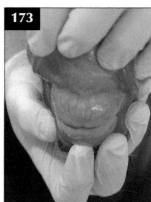

171–173 Icterus. (171) Scleral icterus. (172) Icterus of the vaginal mucosa. (173) Icteric oral mucous membranes.

Bilirubin is produced by the body's breakdown of red blood cells (RBCs). Hemoglobin is metabolized in the reticuloen-dothelial system to bilirubin; this enters the circulation (protein-bound) and attaches to a receptor site on a hepatocyte. Once reaching the hepatocyte, this unconjugated bilirubin is transferred into the hepatocyte and conjugated. The conjugated bilirubin is then transported (excreted) into the bile canaliculi. This transport step requires energy and is a rate-limiting step. Therefore, with disease of the liver, the first step of bilirubin metabolism to be affected is excretion of conjugated bilirubin. Hepatic disease results in a cellular reflux of conjugated bilirubin (from hepatocytes) into the systemic circulation. This conjugated bilirubin is not highly protein bound and "leaks" into tissues of the body to a greater degree than does the highly protein-bound unconjugated bilirubin. Therefore, the icterus of liver disease is generally greater than that of anorexia (**171–173**).

Nonhepatic causes of icterus are numerous (*Table 38*) and must be considered when faced with a jaundiced patient. Nonhepatic icterus is typically a result of elevation in unconjugated bilirubin. Anorexia is the most common cause of icterus in the adult horse and should be considered as a cause of icterus in the foal. The icterus of anorexia is thought to be caused by a competitive inhibition at the hepatic receptor site between free fatty acids, which are being mobilized from peripheral fat stores, and unconjugated bilirubin. These fatty acids are competing at the hepatic binding site for bilirubin, therefore unconjugated bilirubin remains in circulation. Hemolysis, particularly extravascular hemolysis, can result in marked levels of elevated bilirubin. The mechanism involved is an "overwhelming" of the body's ability rapidly to metabolize red cell breakdown products.

Other extrahepatic causes of icterus include sepsis, endotoxemia, and GI stasis. GI stasis can result in bile stasis. Sepsis and endotoxemia may result in a degree of bile stasis and/or

Table 38. Nonhepatic causes of icterus

- Hemolysis:
  - Neonatal isoerythrolysis
- Anorexia
- Sepsis
- Physiologic icterus
- Endotoxemia
- Plasma administration

influence the rate-limiting step of biliary excretion. In addition, the equine neonate can experience a "physiologic icterus" as a result of immature or developing biliary metabolism. A normal (or, particularly, an increased) load of red cell breakdown product can result in this physiologic icterus. Administration of plasma can provide an increased load of hemoglobin that must be metabolized.

Other clinical pathologic abnormalities that may be present with liver disease include hypoalbuminemia, hypoproteinemia, or hyperproteinemia. Clotting factors and albumin are produced in the liver. Clinical signs of coagulopathies would include hematomas or bleeding at venipuncture sites, ecchymosis, melena, epistaxis, and/or bleeding into joints or body cavities. Hypoalbuminemia can occur with liver disease. Albumin is significant in maintaining oncotic pressure; edema can be a clinical consequence of liver disease. In equine liver disease it is more common to identify a hyperproteinemia as a result of increased production of acute reacting protein and globulin.

Ascites may develop secondary to portal hypertension of liver disease. Hypoalbuminemia can contribute to ascites. The severe neurologic signs (hepatoencephalopathy) that can be seen with liver disease are multifactorial, with no definitive pathogenesis identified. Contributing factors include elevated blood ammonia, hypoglycemia, plasma amino acid alterations, altered or false neurotransmitters, and alterations in blood–brain barrier permeability.

CLINICAL PRESENTATION
Clinical signs of liver disease vary significantly with the severity. Initial signs of disease are generally nonspecific (*Table 37*). Abnormalities noted may include a combination of anorexia, depression, fever, weight loss, and abdominal pain. Icterus may be noted early in the course of the disease; however, it is not pathognomonic for hepatic disease. Icterus can also be a result of anorexia, extra- or intravascular hemolysis, or septicemia/ endotoxemia (*Table 38*). Icterus is discussed in more depth in the section on pathophysiology. Patients with fulminant, rapidly progressive hepatic disease need not routinely exhibit icterus, therefore liver disease should not be ruled out if the patient is not icteric.

As liver disease progresses, a clinical presentation including central nervous system (CNS) signs (hepatic encephalopathy, **174**), bleeding disorders, anorexia, depression, ascites, edema, and/or dermatitis may develop. Neonates with liver disease may present with nonspecific signs of sepsis, which may include fevers. Foals with liver disease can present recumbent, stuporous/ comatose, or with evidence of abdominal pain and occasionally

abdominal distension. Diarrhea may be evident, particularly in cases of bacterial hepatitis.

DIFFERENTIAL DIAGNOSIS
The differential diagnosis for liver disease is very extensive up until the illness has been attributed to primary liver disease (*Table 39*). Primary liver disease in the foal is generally infectious (viral, bacterial) in nature. Toxins that affect adult horses should be considered.

DIAGNOSIS
Subsequent to a clinical diagnosis of liver disease, confirmation is achieved through evaluation of serum enzymes, other serum chemistries, and, potentially, liver function tests. Enzymes are released into blood following damage to cellular integrity. (Enzymes of use in the evaluation of liver disease are listed in *Table 40*). These enzymes are not consistently available among laboratories. A discussion of hepatic enzymes must include their specificity. An enzyme is considered hepatospecific if it is only found within liver parenchyma and no other tissues of the body. Serum enzymes can also be classified as to whether they are located

Table 39. Differential diagnosis of liver disease in the foal
- Theiler's disease (rarely seen in the foal)
- Tyzzer's disease
- Bacterial hepatitis (other than Tyzzer's disease)
- Toxic hepatopathies (chemical, plants, drugs):
  ○ More common in the adult
- Viral hepatitis:
  ○ Equine herpesvirus I
- Birth asphyxia
- Gastroduodenal obstruction
- Abscess
- Portosystemic shunt (rare, congenital)
- Biliary atresia (rare, congenital)

Table 40. Useful serum enzymes in the evaluation of liver disease
- Sorbitol dehydrogenase
- Aspartate amino
- Gamma glutamyltransferase

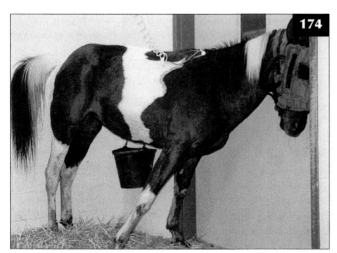
174 Head pressing with hepatic encephalopathy.

Table 41. Enzyme half-life and specificity		
Enzyme	**Specificity**	**L1/2**
Sorbitol dehydrogenase	Liver, hepatocellular	Short
Gamma glutamyltransferase	Liver, hepatobiliary	Long
Alkaline phosphatase	Nonspecific	
Lactate dehydrogenase	Nonspecific (isoenzyme-5 hepatospecific)	Short
Aspartate aminotransferase	Nonspecific	

in the cellular or biliary portion of the parenchyma. The half-life of serum enzymes may provide a time course of disease (*Table 41*). SDH is liver and hepatocellular specific. GGT is liver and biliary specific. Sequential evaluation of enzymes can be used to estimate the severity of disease or response to therapy. The degree of enzyme elevation does not always correlate with the severity of disease. Enzymes with short half-lives when compared to enzymes with long half-lives (e.g., SDH) can indicate a time course of disease and suggest whether the disease process is ongoing. In addition to being released with biliary epithelial damage, GGT is released into the serum during biliary epithelial repair, which can contribute to a prolonged elevation of GGT during the recovery phase of biliary disease.

During the evaluation of enzymes in the foal, it is a requisite to understand normal values and enzyme sources. In the foal, GGT activity is elevated for the first 45–60 days of life. AP is a nonspecific serum enzyme that is normally elevated in the foal. The isoenzyme of LDH, isoenzyme-5, is specific for liver disease; however, it is found in other areas of the body such as RBCs.

Serum bilirubin can be a measure of hepatic function, but as mentioned previously, it may be elevated from other causes. With liver failure/disease, elevations in total bilirubin are primarily of the conjugated (direct) form, contrary to the elevation with anorexia, which is primarily of the unconjugated (indirect) form. The liver conjugates and excretes conjugated bilirubin into the biliary system. Excretion of conjugated bilirubin is the rate-limiting step. The diseased liver generally maintains the ability to conjugate bilirubin; however, in the disease state the rate-limiting (energy-consuming) step may be compromised. Conjugated bilirubin then "backs up" and "leaks" into peripheral circulation.

Other function tests include measurement of clotting times, blood ammonia, bile acids, and excretion tests. Excretion tests using sulfobromophthalein (BSP; bromsulphalein) do not provide significantly more information than clinical chemistries. Blood ammonia is not reliably increased with liver disease; however, it is very useful in the diagnosis of portosystemic shunts and primary hyperammonemia. Clotting times are not invariably elevated in disease states. Bile acids, which undergo an enterohepatic circulation, can be a sensitive indication of liver disease. Bile acids may be elevated in disease states before other indicators of disruption of liver function. Anorexia can elevate serum bile acids mildly. Bile acid values are slightly higher in the foal than in the adult.

Other tests that are nonspecific but supportive of a diagnosis of liver disease include bilirubinuria, metabolic acidosis, hypoglycemia, polycythemia, and low blood urea nitrogen (BUN). Foals with acute hepatic disease may be markedly hypoglycemic and severely acidotic. The liver obviously plays a significant role in these two metabolic pathways.

Liver biopsy can be diagnostic of liver disease or at least provide guidance to appropriate therapy. The biopsy is best performed with guidance via ultrasound. Liver biopsy is generally considered safe; however, it can very occasionally result in hemorrhage from arterial puncture. The drawbacks of liver biopsy include the necessity of sedation and restraint and, most significantly, that the results of the biopsy may not be available for several days, whereas treatment usually needs to be formulated rapidly. Biopsies may be cultured and impression smears can be evaluated cytologically.

MANAGEMENT

Treatment of hepatic disease is discussed in detail under the section for each specific disorder. Knowledge of the etiology of the disease is necessary for an appropriate therapeutic plan. Anti-inflammatories and careful evaluation of acid–base status are important. Monitoring of blood glucose concentrations will indicate the potential necessity of dextrose therapy. Tranquilization may be necessary to control encephalopathy. Antibiotics are used when infection is considered.

TYZZER'S DISEASE

KEY POINTS

- Tyzzer's disease is a peracute, progressive, fulminate bacterial hepatitis caused by *Clostridium piliformis*.
- *C. piliformis* is a soil inhabitant.
- The route of infection is oral ingestion.
- Subsequent to infection, the primary lesions are hepatic and intestinal, with hepatic lesions being the typical overwhelming clinical entity.
- Hemorrhagic enterocolitis may be seen.
- In addition to septic shock, foals may present with an encephalopathy.
- Presenting patients are often acidotic and hypoglycemic, with elevation in liver-specific enzymes.

DEFINITION/OVERVIEW

Tyzzer's disease is an acute, fulminate, bacterial hepatitis that can also cause myocarditis or enterocolitis. The disease is caused by the organism *Clostridium piliformis* (previously called *Bacillus piliformis*). The organism is a mobile, spore-forming, Gram-negative, filamentous bacterium (**175, 176**). Typically, the disease is sporadic, with individual cases on a farm; however, small outbreaks

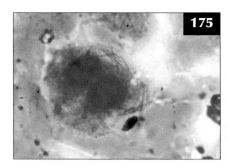

175 *Clostridium piliforme* identified in a histopathologic section of liver using Wright–Giemsa stain.

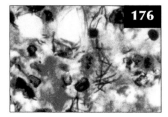

176 High-power view of *Clostridium piliforme* identified in a histopathologic section of liver using silver stain.

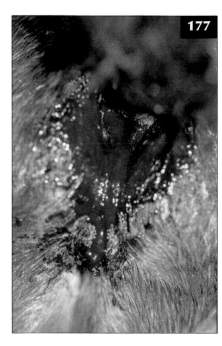

177 Blood-stained stool. Hemorrhagic enterocolitis can be seen with Tyzzer's disease.

can occur and cases can recur in a geographic location, becoming endemic in certain locations.

ETIOLOGY/PATHOPHYSIOLOGY

The route of infection is thought to be fecal/oral. Soil is contaminated by infected individuals, possibly rodents, or adult horse carriers. The disease has been identified in rabbits and rodents and rarely in dogs, cats, and calves. The causative organism has been classified as a *Bacillus* or a *Clostridium*, but taxonomically it does not fit well with either classification. It is suspected that ingestion of the organism results in GI infection and subsequent invasion of the hepatic parenchyma and myocardium via the portal circulation. The primary lesions of clinical significance are hepatic and intestinal. The lesions are peracute, with areas of coagulative necrosis surrounded by cellular debris.

CLINICAL PRESENTATION

Clinical signs can be variable. The overwhelming feature is the acute and rapidly progressive course of the disease. Tyzzer's disease should be a primary differential for a foal with no history of illness that is suddenly found dead. Clinical diagnosis of *B. piliformis* can be challenging as the signs are nonspecific and severe, often including CNS signs and septic shock with cardiovascular collapse. Foals may present in a coma/stupor or exhibit seizures. Physical examination identifies variable signs of sepsis and cardiovascular shock. Icterus of mucous membranes is variable, as the acute nature of the disease may not have resulted in a significant hyperbilirubinemia. Petechiation and high fevers may be present. Abdominal pain and/or hemorrhagic enterocolitis can be associated with the condition (**177**). The abdominal pain is likely secondary to colitis or acute swelling of the liver capsule.

DIFFERENTIAL DIAGNOSIS

Differential diagnosis should include conditions that could cause acute death, hepatitis, or overwhelming septic shock with cardiovascular collapse. Foals with Tyzzer's disease may occasionally present with primary signs of colic and/or enterocolitis.

DIAGNOSIS

Antemortem diagnosis is difficult as there is no rapid definitive diagnostic test. Signalments with appropriate age classification, acute onset, and associated clinical signs should suggest Tyzzer's as a possible diagnosis. Liver biopsy (**178**) with appropriate histopathology can be diagnostic, but biopsy is of little use in therapy unless immediate impression smears can be evaluated, due to the time frame for results. Serum or plasma liver enzymes (AST, SDH, and GGT) are moderately to markedly elevated, with increases dependent on the time course of the disease. Affected foals are often severely acidotic and hypoglycemic. Although these laboratory parameters are not specific, severe acidosis and hypoglycemia alone should suggest hepatic disease. Blood cultures are rarely diagnostic. Polymerase chain reaction (PCR) testing of fecal samples is currently being evaluated and may eventually be available on a limited basis.

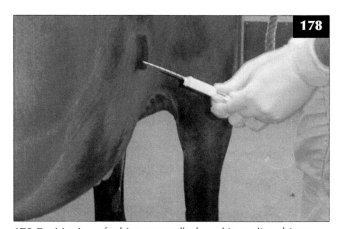

178 Positioning of a biopsy needle for taking a liver biopsy.

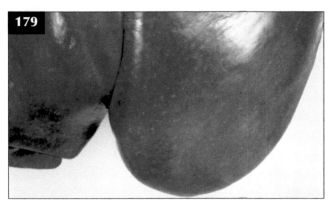

179 White spots in the hepatic parenchyma suggestive of Tyzzer's disease.

Gross necropsy identifies typical white spots in the hepatic parenchyma (**179**). Myocarditis is an occasional associated necropsy finding.

MANAGEMENT

Successful therapy of Tyzzer's disease is difficult due to the fulminate nature of the disease. There is one documented report of the successful treatment of a case of Tyzzer's disease. The lack of antibiotic sensitivity testing necessitates a choice of broad-spectrum therapy. High doses of intravenous penicillin with an aminoglycoside or other broad-spectrum intravenous therapy are appropriate choices. Emergency therapy with appropriate fluid, dextrose, and bicarbonate replacement therapy will vary dependent on the cardiovascular status and interference with intermediary metabolism. Routine therapy for shock should be provided.

BACTERIAL HEPATITIS, CHOLANGIOHEPATITIS (NON-TYZZER'S DISEASE)

KEY POINTS

- Bacteria other than *C. pilliformis* can cause hepatitis.
- Frequently, the systemic signs (septic shock) caused by these bacteria overwhelm the primary signs of hepatitis.

DEFINITION/OVERVIEW

Systemic bacterial infections are common in foals, particularly the neonate. Localization of systemic infection to bone or synovial structures and, potentially, the liver are common. However, systemic hepatic bacterial infections do not frequently manifest as primary liver disease, as is the case with the bacteremia of Tyzzer's disease. Ascending bacterial infection from the umbilical vein or portal circulation can result in hepatic disease. Invasion of bacteria (ascending) through the common bile duct to the biliary system can result in cholangiohepatitis.

ETIOLOGY/PATHOPHYSIOLOGY

A variety of bacterial organisms can cause septicemia/bacteremia in the foal. Gram-negative bacteria are the most common (see Chapter 3,

Infectious Diseases, Sepsis, pp. 39–43). *Actinobacillus equili* can cause aggressive septicemia in a foal with fulminate progression and death; hepatic involvement may contribute to the rapid demise. As mentioned previously, bacteria can invade the liver through the portal circulation, common bile duct, or umbilical vein.

CLINICAL PRESENTATION

The clinical presentation of bacterial hepatic disease is not unlike that of the bacterial hepatitis seen with Tyzzer's disease. The fulminate, rapidly progressive nature of Tyzzer's disease can clinically separate itself from the other forms of bacterial hepatitis; however, this will vary with the aggressive nature of the bacteria involved. Foals, particularly neonates, with septicemia may develop hepatitis as a secondary complication. The clinical signs may be mixed with those of septicemia.

DIFFERENTIAL DIAGNOSIS

See Tyzzer's disease, p. 119.

DIAGNOSIS

See Tyzzer's disease, p. 119.

MANAGEMENT

Broad-spectrum antimicrobials are the hallmark of therapy for the patient with suspected bacterial hepatitis. Blood cultures, biopsies, and biopsy cultures may be useful. Supportive care including fluid therapy, electrolyte supplementations, and nutritional support may increase the chances for a successful outcome.

VIRAL HEPATITIS

KEY POINTS

- Equine herpesvirus can cause primary signs of hepatitis in neonates.
- Typically, clinical signs are seen in combination with respiratory disease.
- Virus isolation confirms the diagnosis.
- The prognosis is considered guarded.

DEFINITION/OVERVIEW

EHV-1 (rhinopneumonitis virus) typically causes abortion in mares and occasional myelopathy in adult horses. However, EHV-1 infection can cause stillborn foals or diseased term or premature foals. These foals may present with signs of hepatic and respiratory disease. The condition can cause multiorgan system failure and is usually fatal.

ETIOLOGY/PATHOPHYSIOLOGY

EHV-1 infections can cause respiratory disease, abortion, neurologic disease, and fatal neonatal illnesses. Abortion may occur secondary to active infection (initially respiratory) or recrudescence of a latent form of the virus. When infection or recrudescence occurs in the near-term fetus, then stillborn or sick foals result. Foals affected usually die of an overwhelming respiratory disease, with hepatic involvement as a secondary finding.

Occasionally, a neonate with a primary viral hepatic disease may be seen. Gross necropsy identifies gray, necrotic foci in the liver.

CLINICAL PRESENTATION

The clinical presentation may be primarily of hepatic disease; however, it is usually in combination with an overwhelming respiratory disease. Foals with hepatic involvement may be icteric, show signs of clotting abnormalities, or exhibit encephalopathy.

DIFFERENTIAL DIAGNOSIS

The differential diagnosis is broad until specific hepatic involvement is identified. The foal with a herpesvirus infection may present as a typical septicemia case, with signs of toxemia, shock, and cardiovascular shock. If hepatic involvement is identified in the newborn foal, it can likely be considered as an in-utero infection (viral or bacterial).

DIAGNOSIS

Diagnosis can be suspected if pathologic evaluation of placental tissues identifies viral infection. An associated herd history of viral abortion can also lead to a presumptive diagnosis. Marked leukopenia is more typical of a viral as opposed to a bacterial infection. Confirmative diagnosis is generally based on necropsy findings and virus isolation.

MANAGEMENT

The use of antiviral drugs (acyclovir) has been attempted, but successful reports are limited. The bioavailability of acyclovir is poor and it is unlikely to reach adequate blood levels in the horse. Valacyclovir, a pro-drug of acyclovir, has greater bioavailability and is the antiherpes viral drug of choice; however, there are no reports of the use of valacyclovir in the foal. (See Chapter 17, Pharmacology, p. 307, for a more complete discussion of valacyclovir.) Aggressive supportive care is often futile; euthanasia is often warranted if herpesvirus infection is highly suspected.

PORTOSYSTEMIC SHUNTS

KEY POINTS

- Shunting of blood from the portal to systemic circulation is an uncommon finding in the foal.
- Shunts allow exposure of the brain (systemic circulation) to noxious substances normally removed by the hepatic system.
- Variable signs of encephalopathy are seen.
- Blood ammonia and/or bile acids will be elevated.

DEFINITION/OVERVIEW

Portosystemic shunts (PSSs) are an infrequent congenital abnormality that allows shunting of blood from the portal circulation to the systemic venous circulation. The onset of clinical signs may be up to 1 year of age. Clinical signs typically include a form of encephalopathy. The prognosis for survival is guarded, with or without surgical intervention.

ETIOLOGY/PATHOPHYSIOLOGY

In the normal foal the venous communications between the umbilical vein and the systemic circulation close within 2–3 days after birth. Failure of closure (intrahepatic shunt) leads to a direct communication between the umbilical vein and the caudal vena cava; however, other venous anomalies have been reported. The liver normally receives portal circulation from the GI tract, where toxic/noxious substances are removed. PSSs result in exposure of these substances to the CNS. Ammonia is one of the substances thought to be of primary significance in the development of encephalopathy. Continuous shunting of the portal circulation can result in hepatic atrophy.

CLINICAL PRESENTATION

Affected foals may be small for their age (failure to thrive) and exhibit various CNS signs (encephalopathy) from depression through seizures. The CNS signs can be intermittent and related to food consumption.

DIFFERENTIAL DIAGNOSIS

Conditions causing a failure to thrive should be considered in the list of differentials. These should include infiltrative bowel disease, parasitism, chronic pneumonia, chronic abscess/infection, peritonitis, duodenal stricture, chronic enterocolitis, renal or progressive hepatic disease, and cardiac disease. Diseases causing encephalopathy or other diffuse neurologic conditions should include other hepatic diseases, severe azotemia secondary to renal disease, or uroperitoneum.

DIAGNOSIS

Serum liver enzymes are normal. The shunting of blood does not affect the liver parenchyma directly. Blood ammonia and serum bile acids are elevated. These products are not removed from the portal circulation. The elevations in ammonia are not persistent and are related to feeding. Repeat testing may be necessary.

MANAGEMENT

Surgical ligation of the shunting vessel is required for long-term survival. Large numbers of reported surgical cases on which to base recommendations are not available. Surgical mortality is high.

OTHER HEPATIC CONDITIONS

BILIARY ATRESIA

There have been infrequent reported cases of biliary atresia in foals. Clinical signs can include depression, icterus, anorexia, and failure to thrive. Pathology may be intra- or extrahepatic, with actual atretic segments a possibility. Histopathology reveals bile stasis, biliary hyperplasia, cholestasis, fibrosis, and hepatocyte degeneration. Liver enzymes, particularly GGT, are elevated. Serum bile acids should be increased. Liver biopsy should be useful in reaching a diagnosis. Ultrasonography can identify an enlarged liver.

PARASITES

Larval stages of parasites (strongyles and ascarids) may include hepatic migration. Clinical signs are typically referable to generalized parasitism and a failure to thrive. Anthelmintic therapy towards parasite migration should be the therapy of choice. Fecal egg counts need not be positive.

LEPTOSPIROSIS

Leptospiral infection can cause abortion, stillbirths, or sick "term" foals (see Chapter 3, Infectious Diseases, Leptospirosis, pp. 54–55). Histopathology findings include a giant cell hepatopathy, which is characteristic of leptospiral infection. Typically, sick newborn foals do not have clinical evidence of hepatic disease.

HYPERAMMONEMIA

There have been rare reports of hyperammonemia in Morgan horses. Clinical signs become apparent after weaning and include encephalopathy, weight loss, and depression. Liver enzymes and blood ammonia levels were elevated. The suspected etiology is an inherited defect in ammonia metabolism.

HEPATIC ABSCESSES

Liver abscesses can occur in foals. Abscesses act as space-occupying lesions causing local parenchymal damage or, more significantly, causing obstruction of bile flow or the portal vein. A variety of organisms may be involved, with *Rhodococcus equi* or streptococci the most likely found. Ultrasound of the liver with abscess identification is diagnostic.

NEONATAL ISOERYTHROLYSIS

Foals suffering from neonatal isoerythrolysis (NI) (see Chapter 4, Immunologic and Hematologic Disorders, Increased Erythrocyte Destruction/Immune-Mediated Hemolytic Anemia, pp. 67–70) can develop marked bilirubinemia. Severe elevations in bilirubin can occur subsequent to RBC destruction or, more commonly, to RBC transfusion, usually multiple transfusions. The half-life of transfused RBCs is a matter of days. The body's ability to metabolize bilirubin can become overwhelmed. The resultant elevations in bilirubin can cause a kernicterus (with possible encephalopathy) and a disruption of metabolic pathways and/or function in other organ systems such as the hepatic or renal system.

IRON FUMARATE TOXICOSIS

Iron supplementation before or during colostrum intake can result in fatal hepatic necrosis. This can occur if the iron supplement is administered before there is closure of the ability to absorb large molecules (pinocytosis). Pinocytosis can occur up to 24 hours of age. Iron supplementation is unlikely to be necessary in the neonate.

FURTHER READING

Adolf JE (2002) Congenital disorders. In: *Manual of Equine Gastroenterology* (Mair T, Divers T, Ducharme N, Eds.). WB Saunders, Philadelphia, PA, p. 517.

Adolf JE (2002) Neoplastic conditions. In: *Manual of Equine Gastroenterology* (Mair T, Divers T, Ducharme N, Eds.). WB Saunders, Philadelphia, PA, p. 518.

Adolf JE, Divers TJ (2002) Infectious processes. In: *Manual of Equine Gastroenterology* (Mair T, Divers T, Ducharme N, Eds.). WB Saunders, Philadelphia, PA, pp. 518–521.

Bernard WV (2002) Tyzzer's disease. In: *Manual of Equine Gastroenterology* (Mair T, Divers T, Ducharme N, Eds.). WB Saunders, Philadelphia, PA, pp. 516–517.

Fortier LA (2002) Portosystemic shunts. In: *Manual of Equine Gastroenterology* (Mair T, Divers T, Ducharme N, Eds.). WB Saunders, Philadelphia, PA, pp. 513–515.

Toribio RE, Mudge MC (2013) Disease of the foal. Hepatobiliary disease. In: *Equine Surgery, Medicine and Reproduction*, 2nd ed. (Mair T, Love S, Schumaker J, Smith RK, Frazer G, Eds.). Saunders Elsevier, Philadelphia, Pennsylvania, pp. 444–445.

Cardiovascular Disorders 7

Johanna M. Reimer

INTRODUCTION

Fairly loud physiologic murmurs over the left heart base are relatively common in foals. Most such murmurs disappear by 1–2 months of age. If a murmur is grade 4/6 or louder beyond the first few days of life, echocardiography is warranted. If a coarse grade 3 to 4 murmur is present in an excited foal, tranquilization of the foal with repeat auscultation may be helpful. There are exceptions, but if the murmur diminishes in intensity or disappears with sedation, it is more likely to be physiologic or benign. Right-sided systolic murmurs and diastolic murmurs are always abnormal and require further investigation.

Arrhythmias, including atrial fibrillation (**180**), atrial tachycardia, ventricular premature complexes or tachycardia, accelerated idioventricular rhythm, and second-degree atrioventricular (AV) block, may be detected in the newborn foal within 15 minutes after birth. If arrhythmias persist, they may be secondary to hypoxemia, electrolyte and acid–base disturbances, or sepsis. Other than in the immediate postpartum period, arrhythmias are not normally detected in foals.

CONGENITAL HEART DISEASE

KEY POINTS
- Equine congenital heart disease is rare.
- Murmurs due to flow through the ductus arteriosus are not uncommon from immediately after birth up to several days of age in the foal.
- A murmur may not always be present, particularly early in the neonatal period or in cases of complex congenital heart disease.

- Hypoxemia unresponsive to oxygen in the critically ill neonatal foal may indicate reversal of flow through the ductus arteriosus or foramen ovale.

INTRODUCTION
Congenital cardiac disease occurs infrequently in the equine. The presence of congenital cardiac disease is most often manifest by a loud murmur detected during routine physical examination. However, early in the neonatal period, and in cases of complex congenital heart defects, cardiac murmurs may not be present. Other indications that congenital heart disease may exist include weakness and exercise intolerance, failure to thrive, elevated respiratory rate, and/or unresponsive or progressive cyanosis in the intensive care setting. The clinician should be particularly alert to the possibility of cyanotic congenital heart disease for neonates presenting for hypoxic ischemic encephalopathy (HIE; dummy foal syndrome) or foals with severe or progressive hypoxemia in the ICU.

PATENT DUCTUS ARTERIOSUS

DEFINITION/OVERVIEW
Although true persistent isolated patent ductus arteriosus (PDA) as a congenital defect is exceedingly rare in the horse, this discussion is important for two reasons:
- A murmur of PDA is commonly heard from birth through the first few days of life and should not be cause for alarm. Continuous machinery murmurs or very loud systolic murmurs high over the heart base are not uncommon immediately after birth and are associated with flow through the ductus arteriosus. By 3–4 days of age the murmur

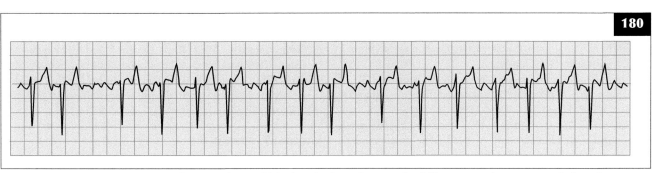

180

180 Base–apex ECG (25 mm/sec) from a 4-hour-old foal with clinical signs of mild hypoxic ischemic encephalopathy. Note the absence of "p" waves, the undulating baseline (f waves), and the irregular R–R intervals indicative of atrial fibrillation. The arrhythmia resolved by the following day.

attributable to a PDA is greatly diminished or absent in the majority of individuals.

- Reversal of flow through a PDA is not uncommon in critically ill neonatal foals with pulmonary disease or pulmonary hypertension due to sepsis and/or septicemia. The clinician needs to be on the alert for neonatal foals with a sudden deterioration in arterial oxygen values and no murmur.

PDA also occurs as a component of complex congenital heart disease, often being required for survival, and is not considered as part of this discussion.

ETIOLOGY/PATHOPHYSIOLOGY

PDA is due to a failure of the ductus arteriosus to close after birth. Left-to-right flow occurs in uncomplicated cases. If the ductus remains patent, left atrial and left ventricular dilation due to volume overload will eventually occur. In foals with pulmonary hypertension (due to viral or bacterial pneumonia, meconium aspiration, pulmonary immaturity, or septicemia) right-to-left flow through the ductus may develop, exacerbating the already existing hypoxemia.

CLINICAL PRESENTATION

A continuous machinery murmur is detected on the left side high over the heart base during a routine physical examination in cases of left-to-right PDA. In the rare instances of persistent PDA, signs of congestive heart failure may occur over months to years if there is a significant shunt.

Hospitalized neonatal foals undergoing therapy for severe respiratory disease may develop sudden worsening of hypoxemia if reversal of flow through the ductus arteriosus occurs. A murmur will not be audible in the case of reverse PDA.

DIFFERENTIAL DIAGNOSIS

The continuous machinery murmur of left-to-right PDA is fairly typical in location, on the left side over the heart base. A precordial thrill is not uncommonly present. In foals in which only the systolic component is audible, the list of differential diagnoses ranges from an innocent physiologic murmur to a severe congenital heart defect such as truncus arteriosus.

DIAGNOSIS

Echocardiography can be used to exclude other intracardiac defects as the cause of the murmur. The ductus can rarely be visualized in a left-to-right PDA due to superimposed lung. Doppler studies are required to confirm the diagnosis by demonstration of turbulent flow in the main pulmonary artery or visualization of the communication with color flow Doppler.

Reverse PDA is a far greater concern in the neonatal ICU. If severe pulmonary hypertension is present and the main pulmonary artery is quite dilated, the ductus might be visible with two-dimensional (2D) echocardiography. Otherwise, the diagnosis can be made with a bubble study. Agitated saline or saline mixed with the patient's blood is injected rapidly into the jugular vein. If bubbles are not detected in the left side of the heart, the injection is repeated while the abdominal aorta is imaged in long-axis view from either side (the left flank region just caudal to the left

kidney appears to provide the best imaging plane, since there may be less interposed intestine). The presence of bubbles in the aorta confirms a right-to-left extracardiac shunt (e.g., a PDA) if no intracardiac shunts are demonstrable.

MANAGEMENT

- *Left-to-right PDA*: If the ductus remains patent for over 1 week, NSAIDs may be of benefit as they have been shown to stimulate contraction of the ductus musculature in human infants. Surgical ligation should be contemplated if the ductus remains patent as confirmed by Doppler echocardiography. If the shunt is small, it is possible for the individual to achieve normal life expectancy. If the shunt is large, left atrial and ventricular dilation will ensue and, eventually, congestive heart failure will develop. If echocardiography reveals left ventricular and atrial dilation and no other causative defects are found, surgical ligation should be recommended. It should again be emphasized that isolated persistent PDA is extremely rare in the equine.
- *Right-to-left PDA*: In foals suffering from pulmonary hypertension, the murmur of PDA may be soft or absent due to equilibration of pressures between the aorta and the pulmonary artery. Administration of NSAIDs to stimulate closure of the ductus may reduce exacerbation of arterial hypoxemia by right-to-left shunting through a PDA in hospitalized foals with pulmonary hypertension secondary to severe pulmonary disease or sepsis. Surgical ligation should not be contemplated in these foals due to the severe pulmonary or systemic disease already present, which alone carries a guarded to grave prognosis. Regardless, once the ductus is closed in these cases, pulmonary hypertension and pressure overload of the right heart will continue until the underlying disease is corrected.

PDA may accompany complex congenital heart disease, and is generally recognized during echocardiography or at postmortem examination.

VENTRICULAR SEPTAL DEFECT

DEFINITION/OVERVIEW

Ventricular septal defect (VSD) is the most common congenital cardiac defect in the horse and is typically located in the perimembranous portion of the septum in the left ventricular outflow tract. This portion of the septum lies immediately beneath the noncoronary and right coronary cusps of the aortic valve on the left side and beneath the septal portion of the tricuspid valve annulus on the right side (**181–183**). The second most common type of VSD in the horse (in the author's practice) appears to be the subpulmonic or supracristal VSD (**184**), which is found in the right ventricular outflow tract beneath the pulmonic valve. Muscular VSDs are rare (**185**). Isolated VSDs are most common, but they are also frequently found in conjunction with, or as components of, other more severe and complex congenital cardiac defects.

ETIOLOGY/PATHOPHYSIOLOGY

Failure of closure of the affected portion of the interventricular septum results in a VSD. Breed predispositions for perimembranous VSDs have been reported in Welsh Mountain Ponies and Arabian horses.

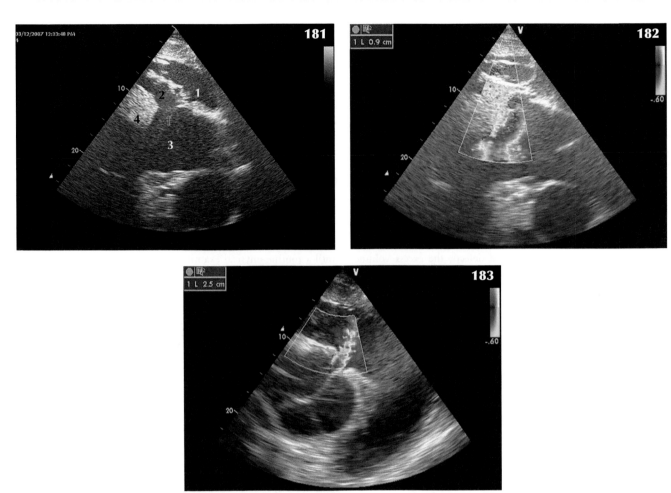

181–183 Perimembranous VSD in a horse with an enlarged left heart and exercise intolerance. Right-sided views. (**181**) Long-axis of the VSD. (**182**) Color-flow Doppler echocardiogram of same view. (**183**) Color-flow Doppler echocardiogram of short-axis view of the VSD. 1: right atrium; 2: tricuspid valve; 3: aorta; 4: septum.

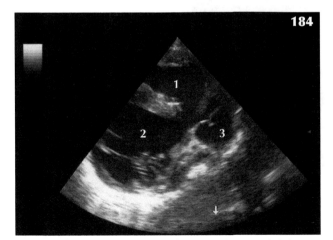

184 Subpulmonic or supracristal ventricular septal defect in a foal with loud bilateral grade 5/6 systolic murmurs over the left and right sides. Right-sided view. 1: right ventricle; 2: left ventricle; 3: pulmonary artery.

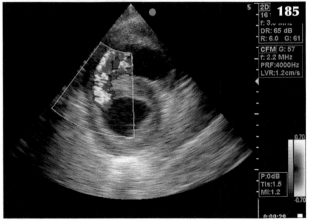

185 Short-axis color-flow Doppler image of a muscular ventricular septal defect in a foal. Right-sided view.

Due to increased pulmonary vascular resistance in the neonatal period, auscultation may fail to reveal a murmur in patients with VSD until at least several days after birth. In foals that develop pulmonary hypertension (due to lack of fetal maturation, meconium aspiration, or severe viral or bacterial pneumonia) the degree of left-to-right shunting will be reduced and, in some cases, reversed. In such cases a murmur of VSD will be absent. Exacerbation of cyanosis or lack of response to oxygen supplementation may indicate the presence of a right-to-left VSD (as well as reverse shunting of blood through a PDA or patent foramen ovale) in the neonatal intensive care setting.

In uncomplicated cases of small to medium VSDs, blood flow is left to right and with no increase in right ventricular or pulmonary artery pressures. The shunt flow is from the left outflow tract immediately into the pulmonary artery during systole, preserving the right ventricle. In medium-sized defects, the excess volume of flow through the pulmonary circulation results in dilation of the left atrium and ventricle. Very large VSDs will result in right

ventricular dilation and hypertrophy as well. Congestive heart failure ultimately develops, at which time pressure differences between the left and right ventricles will be reduced. The murmurs of the VSD may become reduced in intensity, while new murmurs of tricuspid and mitral regurgitation develop as a result of biventricular dilation (and the consequent dilation of the annulus of the AV valves). Due to the location of perimembranous VSDs beneath the aortic valve, secondary aortic valve prolapse may occur, resulting in aortic regurgitation (**186–188**).

CLINICAL PRESENTATION

Murmurs of VSD may not be detectable until several days after birth, when pulmonary vascular resistance declines and left ventricular pressures are far greater than right ventricular pressures. Therefore, in the vast majority of cases, VSDs are not suspected until a routine physical examination at a later age reveals a relatively loud murmur or murmurs. Typically, there is a loud grade 4/6 or greater holosystolic murmur far forward over the pulmonic

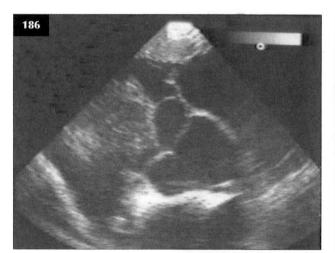

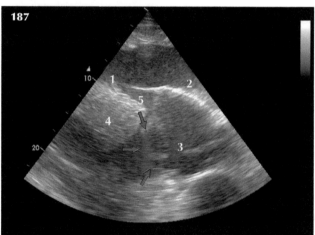

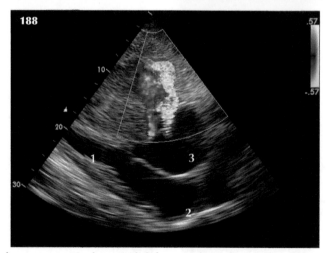

186–188 Two horses with membranous ventricular septal defects and a murmur of aortic regurgitation. (**186**) Right-sided two-dimensional echocardiogram demonstrating prolapse of an aortic valve cusp into a VSD. (Reprinted from Reimer, J.M., *Atlas of Equine Ultrasonography*, Mosby, St. Louis, MO, p. 140, Copyright 1998, with permission from Elsevier.) (**187**) Right-sided long-axis view showing prolapse of an aortic valve cusp (arrows) in a horse with a VSD. (**188**) Left-sided color-flow Doppler of the same horse as in **187**, showing a jet of aortic regurgitation directed beneath the mitral valve to the wall of the left ventricle. 1: right ventricle; 2: right atrium; 3: aorta; 4: septum; 5: ventricular septal defect.

valve region (3rd intercostal space at a point midway between the point of the shoulder and the elbow). A holo- to pansystolic murmur, often 1–2 grades louder than the murmur on the left side, is typically auscultated over the tricuspid valve region (3rd–4th intercostal spaces on the right side at approximately the same level on the chest wall as the pulmonic valve).

In foals with larger defects, failure to thrive or signs of congestive heart failure (elevated respiratory rate, jugular pulsations, and dependent edema) may be consequences of VSD.

In hospitalized neonatal foals with severe lower respiratory disease, a VSD may be suspected if there is exacerbation of hypoxemia or failure to respond to intranasal oxygen. In such cases, right-to-left shunting of blood through a VSD (but more likely the ductus arteriosus) may occur.

DIFFERENTIAL DIAGNOSIS

Small- to moderate-sized uncomplicated perimembranous VSDs often have typical auscultatory findings. Larger defects with reduced pressure differences between the left and right ventricles, those individuals in congestive heart failure, or cases in which there is concomitant aortic regurgitation due to prolapse of an aortic valve cusp into the defect may make a presumptive diagnosis based on auscultation alone more difficult. VSDs are also often found as a component of complex congenital heart disease. The author has also diagnosed three Thoroughbred horses with a single dysplastic papillary muscle of the mitral valve apparatus in conjunction with small perimembranous VSDs (see also Single Papillary Muscle, p. 128). In these three cases the murmurs characteristic of VSD were accompanied by a murmur of mitral regurgitation.

DIAGNOSIS

Echocardiography often provides direct visualization of the defect. Perimembranous VSDs are best visualized in the right parasternal long-axis, left ventricular outflow tract (LVOT) view. Such defects are also visualized at a perpendicular plane, in a short-axis view high in the LVOT (**181–183**). The aortic valve cusps should also be evaluated for any evidence of prolapse into the defect. The diameter of the VSD should be measured in at least two perpendicular planes (generally the LVOT short- and long-axis, right parasternal views). The cardiac chambers, particularly the left ventricle and atrium, should be evaluated for any evidence of dilation. It is of utmost importance to evaluate the remainder of the heart for concomitant congenital or acquired defects (see **195–198**).

Doppler studies, if available, may provide additional information. In rare instances the defect may be so small, or obscured by the tricuspid valve apparatus or by prolapse of the right or noncoronary aortic valve cusp, that the defect cannot be conclusively demonstrated. In such cases, Doppler studies may help to confirm the defect. There is often diastolic flow though the defect as well. Pulsed-wave or color-flow Doppler will reveal turbulent high-velocity systolic flow at the site of the defect (**182, 183**). Continuous-wave Doppler echocardiography can be used to estimate the pressure gradient between the right and left ventricles. If there is a pressure gradient of >60 mmHg (approximately 4 m/s peak blood flow velocity through the VSD), the defect suggests a "restrictive" VSD with a low shunt fraction and favorable long-term prognosis. In foals with pulmonary hypertension (due to

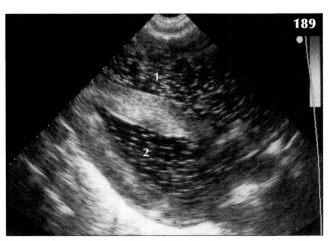

189 Bubble study in a 3-day-old foal with acute pneumonia and severe hypoxemia. Agitated saline injected through the intravenous catheter resulted in bubbles within all four heart chambers, indicating right-to-left shunting through a patent foramen ovale. 1: right ventricle; 2: left ventricle.

pulmonary immaturity, viral or bacterial pneumonia, or septicemia) a bubble study may reveal right-to-left shunting through the VSD. Agitated sterile saline (which can be mixed with the patient's blood by aspiration through an intravenous catheter to further enhance microbubbles) is rapidly injected into the foal while echocardiography is performed. A sufficient number of microbubbles will result in near opacification of the right side of the heart. The left ventricle, left atrium (for assessment of reversal of flow through a patent foramen ovale), and ascending aorta are examined for any "crossover" of microbubbles (**188**).

MANAGEMENT

Due to the tendency of this defect to appear in Welsh Mountain Ponies and Arabians, the use of affected individuals for breeding should be discouraged. Whether VSD in other breeds is a genetic disorder, a spontaneous defect, or a result of *in-utero* exposure to a fetal cardiac toxin is unknown, but discouraging the use of the animal for breeding purposes is warranted.

The prognosis for individuals with small, uncomplicated restrictive VSDs in which the defect measures under 2.5 cm appears to be favorable both for life and athletic performance. Although spontaneous closure of VSD is not uncommon in children, closure has not been observed in the horse. However, fibrosis at the edges of the defect may occur with time, resulting in a reduction in the diameter of the VSD. The defect may also be partially occluded by prolapse of either the right or noncoronary aortic valve cusp into the defect. However, aortic regurgitation, sometimes of a significant degree, may result. Rupture of an aortic valve cusp has been recognized as a complication of VSD in which prolapse of the aortic valve into the defect had been suspected to have occurred.

Individuals with large nonrestrictive defects will ultimately develop congestive heart failure. Palliative treatment for congestive heart failure (diuretics and angiotensin converting enzyme inhibitors and digoxin if secondary atrial fibrillation with tachycardia develops) may be contemplated if desired.

In foals with reversed flow through a VSD, treatment of the cause of the pulmonary hypertension is required. Bidirectional or right-to-left shunting through relatively large VSDs will also ultimately develop once congestive heart failure and pulmonary hypertension occur.

SINGLE PAPILLARY MUSCLE (PARACHUTE MITRAL VALVE)

DEFINITION/OVERVIEW

A single papillary muscle (or papillary muscle dysplasia) accompanied by a small VSD has been discovered in three asymptomatic Thoroughbred horses ranging from 7 months to 5 years of age at the time of diagnosis by the author. A recent report described a parachute mitral valve without VSD discovered in another Thoroughbred foal at 8 months of age. The abnormality results in variable degrees of mitral regurgitation.

ETIOLOGY/PATHOPHYSIOLOGY

A parachute mitral valve is a malformation of the mitral valve apparatus in which the chordae tendineae of the apparatus insert on a single dysplastic papillary muscle near the anterior location. The defect often results in mitral regurgitation of varying degree. The defect may be accompanied by other cardiac defects such as a VSD, or may be found as a sole entity.

The deformity of the mitral valve apparatus can result in mitral valve regurgitation, as well as possible mitral stenosis. Left atrial dilation will ultimately result if the degree of regurgitation is significant, and signs of congestive heart failure may eventually develop. Coexisting cardiac defects such as a VSD may also impact on the course of the disease.

CLINICAL PRESENTATION

In the three cases examined by the author, a grade 3 to 5/6 mid-to holosystolic murmur was detected over the mitral valve region, along with the murmurs typically attributable to a VSD. All three horses were asymptomatic at the time of examination and had raced or ultimately raced. In the horse diagnosed at 5 years of age, moderate left atrial and left ventricular dilation was present. The patient diagnosed as a weanling was still racing at 6 years of age.

DIFFERENTIAL DIAGNOSIS

The differential diagnosis for a murmur of mitral regurgitation detected on physical examination in horses with this defect includes mitral valve prolapse with normal papillary muscles, ruptured chordae tendineae of the mitral valve, endocarditis, and chronic valvular disease.

DIAGNOSIS

Echocardiography is diagnostic. All the chordae tendineae of the mitral valve cusps insert on a flattened, poorly defined single papillary muscle near the anterolateral location (**190, 191**).

MANAGEMENT

To date, two of the three affected horses diagnosed by the author were able to race. Therefore, it appears that in some individuals the prognosis for performance as a young horse may be better than expected, although there could be a reduction in athletic potential short term. However, as follow-up information on these horses is

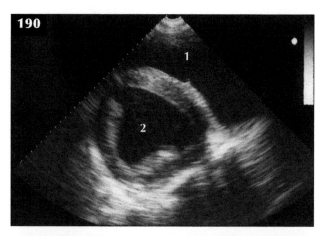

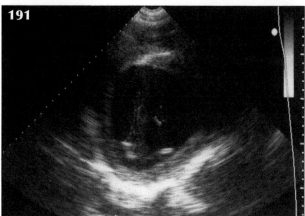

190, 191 Short-axis views of the left ventricle at the level of the chorda tendinea attachments to the papillary muscles in a normal horse (**190**) and a horse with single papillary muscle (**191**). Note the posterior positioning of the attachments in the affected horse. 1: right ventricle; 2: left ventricle. (Reprinted from Reimer, J.M., *Atlas of Equine Ultrasonography*, Mosby, St. Louis, MO, p. 141, Copyright 1998, with permission from Elsevier.)

not available, the long-term prognosis is still in question. The prognosis can be estimated in individual cases through the degree of mitral regurgitation as determined by Doppler studies. Additional important information includes the size of the VSD, if present, and aortic valve prolapse into the VSD, if present. If there is any left atrial or ventricular dilation, a poor long-term prognosis should be given.

PERSISTENT TRUNCUS ARTERIOSUS

DEFINITION/OVERVIEW

In cases of persistent truncus arteriosus a single large vessel provides outflow from the right and left ventricles through a VSD of variable size.

ETIOLOGY/PATHOPHYSIOLOGY

Persistent truncus arteriosus is a failure of the fetal truncus to partition into the pulmonary artery and the aorta. Because the truncal septum contributes to the final closure of the ventricular septum, a VSD is always present with this defect.

Flow from both ventricles courses through the VSD and out from the single great vessel. The valve may be normal, or regurgitation or stenosis may be present. Occasionally, a quadricuspid valve may be found. Pulmonary circulation is achieved via pulmonary arteries or bronchial arteries that arise from the common trunk or descending aorta, respectively.

CLINICAL PRESENTATION

Cyanosis and exercise intolerance are variably present, depending on the degree of right-to-left shunting, pulmonary vascular resistance, and the size of the obligatory VSD. A loud systolic murmur is often present over the left side; however, in some cases a murmur may be absent. Severely affected neonatal foals may present for suspected neonatal maladjustment syndrome (dummy foal or HIE).

DIAGNOSIS

Diagnosis is made by echocardiography, which demonstrates a large single vessel that straddles a variable sized VSD and provides outflow to both the left and right ventricles (**192–194**). Atresia of the pulmonary artery and pulmonic valve may be difficult to differentiate from truncus arteriosus (pseudo truncus arteriosus). Arterial blood gases reveal hypoxemia.

MANAGEMENT

The prognosis for truncus arteriosus is grave. Euthanasia is warranted, although in rare cases foals may survive to maturity.

TRICUSPID ATRESIA

DEFINITION/OVERVIEW

In cases of tricuspid atresia the tricuspid valve is absent and replaced by a dense band of tissue. There is no communication between the right atrium and right ventricle.

ETIOLOGY/PATHOPHYSIOLOGY

Tricuspid atresia is a result of a failure of the tricuspid valve to develop. Blood flow courses from the right atrium to the left atrium via an atrial septal defect (ASD) or patent foramen ovale, to the left ventricle, and through the aorta. Pulmonary circulation is achieved either through a VSD (allowing blood to flow into the right ventricle and into the pulmonary artery) and/or through a PDA or bronchial circulation. This lesion may also present with transposition of the arteries.

CLINICAL PRESENTATION

Severe cyanosis is often present. Affected foals are weak, with marked exercise intolerance, and they fail to thrive. Collapse and sudden death may occur.

DIAGNOSIS

Echocardiography reveals a dense band of tissue in the region of the tricuspid valve and a very enlarged right atrium, left atrium, and left ventricle (**195**). A VSD of variable size is often present, but not in all cases (a PDA or bronchial circulation provides circulation to the lungs). A diminutive right ventricle is often found. There may be concomitant transposition of the aorta and pulmonary artery.

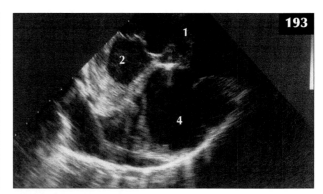

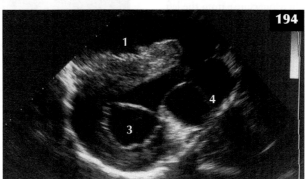

192–194 Truncus arteriosus in a 2-week-old foal with cyanosis, syncope, and a loud, coarse left-sided systolic murmur. (**192**) Long-axis left outflow tract view. (**193**) Right inflow–outflow view. (Reprinted from Reimer, J.M., *Atlas of Equine Ultrasonography*, Mosby, St. Louis, MO, p. 143, Copyright 1998, with permission from Elsevier.) (**194**) The obligatory ventricular septal defect is visible beneath the common truncus in an intermediate view. 1: right ventricle; 2: right atrium; 3: left ventricle; 4: truncus. (Reprinted from Bernard, W.V., and Reimer, J.M., *Vet. Clin. North Am. Equine Prac.*, 10, 46, 1994.)

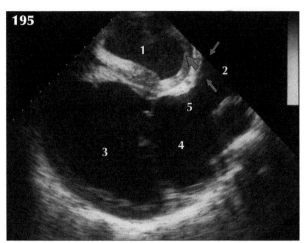

195 Tricuspid atresia in a 2-month-old Quarter Horse foal with jugular pulses and a grade 6/6 systolic murmur over the left heart base. Note the echodense band of tissue (arrows) at the normal location of the tricuspid valve. The obligatory atrial septal defect (ASD) is also present in this right-sided view. 1: right ventricle; 2: right atrium; 3: left ventricle; 4: left atrium; 5: ASD. (Reprinted from Reimer, J.M., *Atlas of Equine Ultrasonography*, Mosby, St. Louis, MO, p. 145, Copyright 1998, with permission from Elsevier.)

MANAGEMENT

The prognosis for tricuspid atresia is grave. Affected individuals rarely survive to weanling age. Euthanasia is warranted.

HYPOPLASTIC LEFT HEART

DEFINITION/OVERVIEW

The features of hypoplastic left heart include a diminutive left ventricle, with atresia of the mitral and/or aortic valves.

ETIOLOGY/PATHOPHYSIOLOGY

The defect is a result of failure of development of the mitral and/or aortic valves. There is no blood flow to the aortic valve, whether due to atresia of the mitral valve or of the aortic valve. Blood returning from the pulmonary circulation must therefore course from the left atrium in to the right atrium through the foramen ovale. From the right atrium blood flows through the right ventricle and out via the pulmonary artery. Systemic circulation is achieved through the ductus arteriosus. The very critical coronary and cerebral blood flow is then only achieved by retrograde flow to the ascending aorta from the ductus. Therefore, a PDA is essential for the patient to be alive.

CLINICAL PRESENTATION

A murmur is generally absent, but the patient is severely cyanotic and weak. Affected foals may suffer from sudden death shortly after birth when the ductus arteriosus closes.

DIFFERENTIAL DIAGNOSIS

Transposition of the great vessels or any of the other cyanotic congenital defects are included in the differentials, but they are easily differentiated with echocardiography.

DIAGNOSIS

Echocardiography reveals a diminutive left ventricle and an atretic mitral and/or aortic valve. The right atrium and ventricle are dilated (**196–198**).

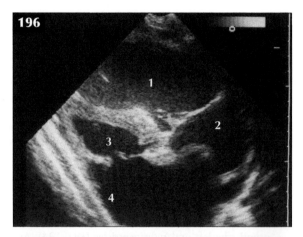

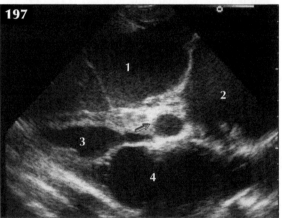

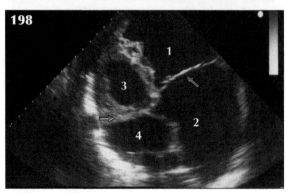

196–198 Hypoplastic left heart syndrome in two 3-day-old cyanotic foals with loud bilateral murmurs (case 1: **196**, **197**; case 2, **198**). (**196**) Right-sided four-chamber view showing the dysplastic mitral valve, diminutive left ventricle, and right-sided enlargement. (**197**) Right-sided long-axis outflow view showing the atretic aortic valve (arrow). (**198**) A second case of hypoplastic left heart syndrome with mitral atresia. Right-sided apical view. 1: right ventricle; 2: right atrium; 3: left ventricle; 4: left atrium. (Reprinted from Reimer, J.M., *Atlas of Equine Ultrasonography*, Mosby, St. Louis, MO, pp. 144–145, Copyright 1998, with permission from Elsevier.)

MANAGEMENT

The prognosis is grave; death generally occurs by 1 week of age. Sudden death is not uncommon shortly after birth when the ductus arteriosus closes.

TETRALOGY OF FALLOT

DEFINITION/OVERVIEW

The two primary and most important lesions of this defect are a perimembranous VSD and pulmonic stenosis. Pulmonary artery hypoplasia or atresia may also be seen. The aorta is classically "overriding" the VSD as the third component of this defect as a result of abnormal septation of the fetal truncus; however, the degree of right-to-left shunting is more likely dictated by the degree of right ventricular outflow tract obstruction rather than by the position of the aorta. The fourth component of right ventricular hypertrophy is secondary to right ventricular outflow obstruction (pulmonic stenosis). The right ventricular hypertrophy can be progressive as the patient matures, and this in itself leads to further right ventricular outflow tract obstruction.

ETIOLOGY/PATHOPHYSIOLOGY

The defect results from asymmetric septation of the truncus arteriosus. Tetralogy of Fallot is recognized as a heritable genetic defect in Keeshond dogs. There appears to be a tendency for this defect to occur in Arabian horses.

There is right-to-left shunting through the VSD, resulting in increased systemic blood flow and reduced pulmonary blood flow. The degree of right-to-left shunting is dictated by the degree of pulmonic stenosis.

CLINICAL PRESENTATION

Failure to thrive, exercise intolerance, dyspnea, and variable degrees of cyanosis may be present. Syncope may also be observed. Auscultation often reveals a loud systolic heart murmur over the pulmonic valve region (far forward over the left side of the chest); however, a murmur may be absent in severe cases in which there is severe pulmonic stenosis and marked right-to-left shunting through the VSD.

DIFFERENTIAL DIAGNOSIS

Severe pulmonic stenosis with a coincident VSD is a differential diagnosis with a similar pathophysiology; however, isolated pulmonic stenosis has not been recognized in the horse at the time of writing. Truncus arteriosus is also a differential and may be misdiagnosed during echocardiography if the pulmonary artery is atretic and difficult to identify (pseudotruncus arteriosus or pulmonary atresia).

DIAGNOSIS

Echocardiography reveals a fairly large VSD (typically the approximate diameter of the aorta), malalignment of the aorta over the VSD, a small dysplastic pulmonic valve and/or pulmonary artery hypoplasia, and right ventricular hypertrophy (199–201). The pulmonic valve and pulmonary artery may be completely atretic in the extreme form of this disorder. A bubble study will reveal right-to-left shunting through the VSD and arterial blood gas will demonstrate hypoxemia in tetralogy of Fallot.

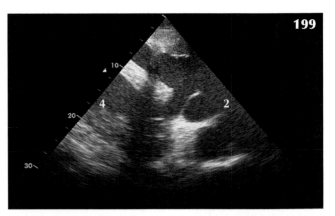

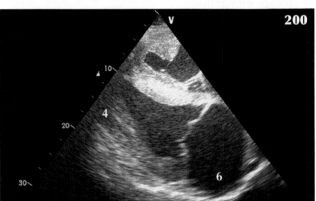

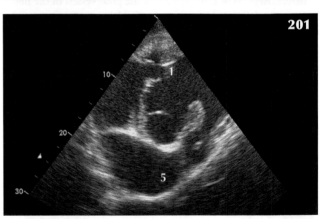

199–201 Tetralogy of Fallot in a yearling colt with a loud left-sided murmur and exercise intolerance. Right-sided views. (**199**) VSD with malalignment of the aorta over the defect. (**200**) Thickened RV (right ventricle) and flattened ventricular septum. (**201**) Short-axis view demonstrating the VSD, stenotic pulmonic valve, and poststenotic dilation of the PA. 1: ventricular defect; 2: aorta; 3: right ventricle; 4 left ventricle; 5: pulmonary artery; 6: left atrium.

MANAGEMENT

Euthanasia is warranted. Most foals fail to reach maturity, although some individuals may reach maturity if the degree of right ventricular outflow obstruction is relatively less severe (resulting in less right-to-left shunting or "pink" tetralogy).

TRANSPOSITION OF THE GREAT ARTERIES

DEFINITION/OVERVIEW

The aorta (with its coronary arteries) arises from the right ventricle, and the pulmonary artery arises from the left ventricle. Stenosis of either vessel may also be present.

ETIOLOGY/PATHOPHYSIOLOGY

Failure of normal spiral growth of the truncoconal ridges to divide the truncus into the aorta and pulmonary artery results in transposition of the great arteries. The truncus is septated in a straight, nonspiral fashion, resulting in the origination of the aorta from the morphologic right ventricle, and the pulmonary artery from the morphologic left ventricle.

Transposition of the great vessels results in two separate circuits: the pulmonary circuit (left ventricle to pulmonary artery to left atrium to left ventricle) and the systemic circuit (right ventricle to aorta to right atrium to right ventricle). In order for the patient to be alive, there must be a communication between the two circuits, either via a PDA, patent foramen ovale, or ASD, or via a VSD. Sudden death will occur in patients if a PDA closes and it is the only communication between the two circuits.

CLINICAL PRESENTATION

Cyanosis without a murmur is the typical presentation in the classic defect. Reports of transposition of the great vessels in the horse describe the defect as being accompanied by stenosis of one of the great vessels.

DIFFERENTIAL DIAGNOSIS

Other complex cyanotic congenital cardiac defects are differentials, but these can be differentiated by echocardiography.

DIAGNOSIS

Echocardiography reveals a lack of the spiral relationship of the aorta and pulmonary artery. Both vessels will be seen arising in parallel in the long-axis view of the LVOT. Careful studies will reveal coronary arteries associated with the vessel arising from the right ventricle and no coronary arteries arising from the great vessel supplying the left ventricle (**202, 203**).

MANAGEMENT

The prognosis is grave. Euthanasia is warranted.

DOUBLE OUTLET RIGHT VENTRICLE

DEFINITION/OVERVIEW

A double outlet right ventricle is where both great vessels arise from the right ventricle. A VSD and/or an ASD will be present. There may be stenosis of the pulmonic valve.

ETIOLOGY/PATHOPHYSIOLOGY

A VSD and/or an ASD must be present in order for blood from the left side of the heart to enter the circulation.

CLINICAL PRESENTATION

Cases often present with a loud systolic murmur and variable degree of cyanosis. Affected individuals fail to thrive and are exercise intolerant. Syncope may also be a clinical feature.

DIFFERENTIAL DIAGNOSIS

Other complex congenital heart defects are differentials, but they can be differentiated with echocardiography.

DIAGNOSIS

Echocardiography reveals both great vessels, generally in parallel, arising from the right ventricle. A large VSD is often present.

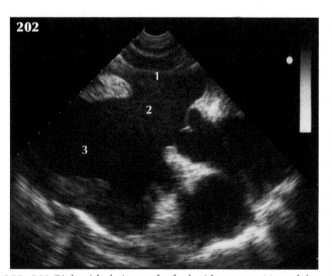 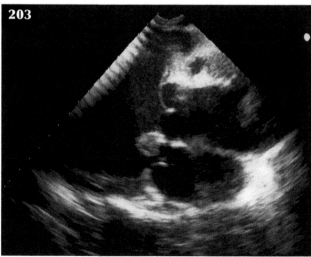

202, 203 Right-sided views of a foal with transposition of the great vessels and a large VSD and tricuspid atresia. (**202**) Coronary vessels are not present in the vessel in the middle of the image; the transposed aorta is at the bottom of the image. 1: right ventricle; 2: ventricular defect; 3: left ventricle. (**203**) Note the parallel alignment of the great vessels. (Reprinted from Reimer, J.M., *Atlas of Equine Ultrasonography*, Mosby, St. Louis, MO, p. 146, Copyright 1998, with permission from Elsevier.)

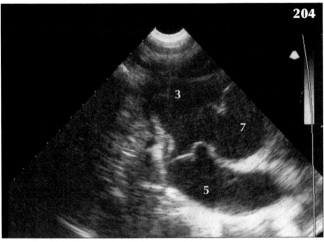

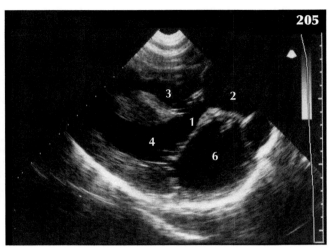

204, 205 Double outlet right ventricle in a cyanotic neonatal foal. Right-sided views. (**204**) Both great vessels arise from the RV. (**205**) An obligatory VSD is also present. 1: ventricular septal defect; 2: right atrium; 3: right ventricle; 4: left ventricle; 5: pulmonary artery; 6: left atrium; 7: aorta. (Reprinted from Reimer, J.M., *Atlas of Equine Ultrasonography*, Mosby, St. Louis, MO, pp. 146–147, Copyright 1998, with permission from Elsevier.)

There is mitral–semilunar valve discontinuity and absence of left ventricular outflow other than the VSD (**204, 205**).

MANAGEMENT
The prognosis is grave; euthanasia is warranted.

ATRIOVENTRICULAR SEPTAL DEFECT

DEFINITION/OVERVIEW
This defect has also been referred to as endocardial cushion defect or common AV canal. There is a large ASD, a VSD, and a common AV valve. All four chambers communicate; the AV valve separates the atria from the ventricles during systole.

ETIOLOGY/PATHOPHYSIOLOGY
The AV septum fails to form, so the heart functions as a two-chambered heart. Equilibration of pressures between the left and right sides is present, therefore murmurs are absent and only occur when regurgitation through the AV valve is present or they develop as a consequence of heart failure.

CLINICAL PRESENTATION
Affected individuals fail to thrive, have exercise intolerance, and develop congestive heart failure within 1 year of life. A murmur is generally absent unless the AV valve is incompetent or until secondary valvular regurgitation occurs due to the ultimate development of cardiomegaly.

DIFFERENTIAL DIAGNOSIS
The differential diagnosis includes a large VSD or other intracardiac defect with pulmonary hypertension.

DIAGNOSIS
Echocardiography reveals an echo-free space between all four cardiac chambers and a large AV valve dividing the atria and ventricles (**206**).

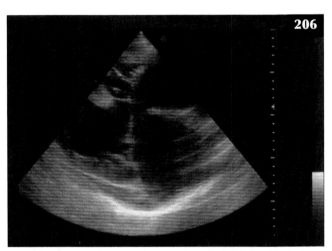

206 Atrioventricular septal defect in a foal. Right-sided view. Note the absence of the lower portion of the atrial septum and upper portion of the ventricular septum, and the common atrioventricular valve. (Courtesy of F.T. Bain.)

MANAGEMENT
The prognosis is grave; most individuals succumb to congestive heart failure within 1 year of age.

MISCELLANEOUS CONGENITAL CARDIAC DEFECTS

ASD is rare as an isolated defect. Additional cardiac defects should be ruled out, including an AV septal defect. Lone small ASDs may not have any adverse effects; large defects will eventually lead to right heart volume overload and failure.

Bicuspid pulmonic valve, aortic valve dysplasia, and interruption of the aortic arch have been observed rarely in the horse.

ACQUIRED CARDIAC DISEASE

ENDOCARDITIS

KEY POINTS

- A murmur may not be present.
- Fevers of unknown origin and unthriftiness are the most common presenting complaints.
- Prognosis depends on the valve affected, the integrity of the valve, and the degree of valvular regurgitation.
- Although the prognosis in general is poor, aggressive treatment can be successful.

DEFINITION/OVERVIEW

Bacterial endocarditis is the most common acquired cardiac disease in the pediatric equine.

ETIOLOGY/PATHOPHYSIOLOGY

The most commonly isolated organism in the author's practice in foals and weanlings is *Streptococcus zooepidemicus*. Other isolates that have been identified in cases of equine endocarditis include *Actinobacillus equuli*, *Staphylococcus aureus*, *Serratia marcenscens*, and *Candida albicans*.

Infection of one or more heart valves or the endocardium can occur. Infection of the heart valves typically develops on the atrial side of the AV valves or the ventricular side of the semilunar valves. Infection of the mitral or tricuspid chordae tendineae is not uncommon and can lead to rupture of a chorda tendineae with resultant valvular regurgitation. The most commonly affected valve in the horse is the mitral valve; however, tricuspid valve endocarditis due to Streptococcus spp infection has been noted in the pediatric patient.

Right-sided lesions may result in metastatic pneumonia, while left-sided lesions may result in hematogenous infection of synovial structures (joints, bursae, tendon sheaths). Ventricular arrhythmias may also occur either from hematogenous dissemination through the coronary circulation or via direct endocardial inflammation.

The characteristic vegetative lesions are composed of an inner layer of platelets, fibrin, and some bacteria, a middle layer of bacteria, and an outer layer of fibrin. Any leukocytes found within vegetations are often lymphocytes rather than neutrophils. Mature vegetations consist of a bed of granulation-like tissue. Older vegetations may be covered by dense fibrous tissue and endothelium and are not uncommonly mineralized.

CLINICAL PRESENTATION

Fevers of unknown origin and unthriftiness are the most common clinical signs. Pneumonia due to right-sided endocarditis or lameness due to synovitis (septic joints, bursae, or tendon sheaths) due to a left-sided lesion may be the presenting complaint. Mild tachycardia is frequently noted. Murmurs, although common, may not be detected depending on the location of the lesion(s) and whether there is any deformation of the affected valve. Infection of the chordae tendineae can result in rupture of chordae and consequent valvular regurgitation; otherwise, a murmur will not be present.

A complete blood count often reveals mild anemia, leukocytosis, hyperfibrinogenemia, and hypergammaglobulinemia in active (versus sterile) lesions.

DIFFERENTIAL DIAGNOSIS

Congenital heart defects causing a heart murmur; sterile inactive endocarditis.

DIAGNOSIS

Ideally, two criteria firmly support the diagnosis:

1. Echocardiographic demonstration of characteristic vegetative lesions on any four of the heart valves, including the chordae tendineae. Lesions appear as fleshy masses on the affected valve. Relatively active or new lesions appear relatively hypoechoic (**207**), and density increases as the vegetation becomes more mature or as a response to treatment (**208**). Mineralization with acoustic shadowing is not uncommon in older and bacteriologically cured lesions (**209**). Mural infections may be difficult to demonstrate. Pronounced valvular thickening may persist following bacterial cure (**210, 211**), therefore a diagnosis of active disease should not be made on echocardiography alone. If a lesion is fairly echodense and at least isoechoic to the surrounding unaffected portions of the valve, it may be an old "inactive" or sterile lesion.

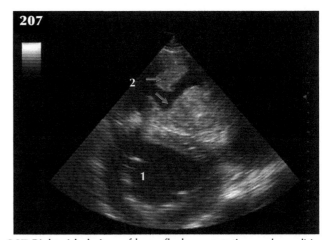

207 Right-sided view of large fleshy vegetative endocarditis lesions (arrows) of the tricuspid valve of a weanling. 1: left ventricle; 2: tricuspid valve.

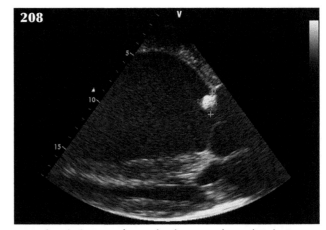

208 Left-sided view of an echodense endocarditis lesion on the aortic valve of a weanling.

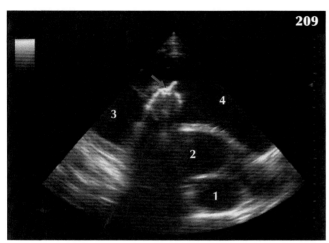

209 Right-sided view of a weanling with a mineralized vegetation of the tricuspid valve (arrow). Note the large acoustic shadow. 1: pulmonary artery; 2: aorta; 3: right ventricle; 4: right atrium.

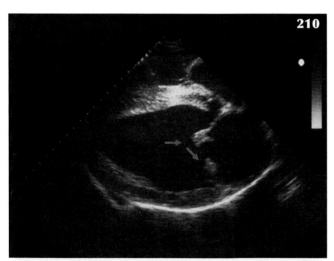

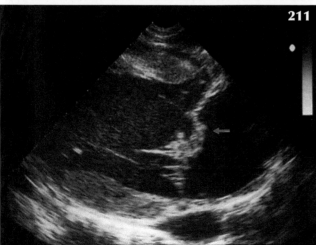

210, 211 Right-sided (**210**) and left-sided (**211**) views of thickened mitral valve leaflets (arrows) discovered in an asymptomatic murmur of mitral regurgitation found on routine physical examination.

2. Positive blood cultures: either positive cultures from two separate sites, or two positive cultures 12 hours apart, or three positive cultures over at least a 1-hour sampling period. The potential use of PCR on blood samples and/or serology in the diagnosis of infective endocarditis may eventually help identify agents in culture-negative endocarditis.

Because many patients have already received antimicrobial therapy and bacteremia may not be persistent, or the initiation of antimicrobial therapy prior to repeated blood cultures was imperative, repeated positive blood cultures may be difficult to obtain or justify. If the echocardiogram is supportive of the diagnosis, then three of the following four additional criteria should be met to firmly support the diagnosis: (1) one positive blood culture, (2) fever, (3) evidence of hematogenous dissemination or embolization, and/or (4) immune-mediated phenomenon such as polysynovitis, glomerulonephritis, or vasculitis. The author proposes that an obvious change in the echocardiographic appearance of the vegetative lesion, characterized by a reduction in size and increased echogenicity of the valve mass during the course of antimicrobial treatment, is highly suggestive of bacterial endocarditis.

MANAGEMENT

Prior to investing in therapy, a prognosis should be established as accurately as possible. If significant mitral or aortic valve regurgitation exists prior to initiation of therapy, the chances of resolution or reduction of the regurgitation are poor and treatment may prove futile. However, successful treatment of severe mitral or aortic regurgitation due to vegetative endocarditis has been achieved in two mares in the author's practice. In both cases the valvular lesions reduced markedly with intravenous antimicrobials, and in both cases the valvular insufficiencies reduced dramatically to only a mild degree. Lesions of the chordae tendineae or mitral or aortic valve in which minimal regurgitation are present may be considered for treatment. However, it should be realized that scarred chordae tendineae could theoretically rupture at any point in the future (**212, 213**) or affected valves may become scarred and incompetent during resolution of the disease. Right-sided lesions carry a more favorable prognosis due to lower pressures in the right side of the heart; however, if severe tricuspid regurgitation with noticeable right atrial and ventricular dilation is already present, a more guarded prognosis should be given.

Intravenous antimicrobial therapy is the treatment of choice for bacterial endocarditis and is most effective when administered as a 6-week course of treatment. Shorter duration of therapy can lead to recrudescence. Sensitivity patterns, if available, should be employed to determine the most appropriate antimicrobial. Otherwise, intravenous penicillin and gentamicin should be therapeutic in the majority of cases. Aspirin or other NSAIDs may reduce platelet aggregation and subsequent fibrin production of acute lesions. Response to therapy is initially ascertained by reduction and resolution of fever and improvement in hematologic parameters. During the course of treatment the endocarditis lesions typically increase in echodensity to at least that of the surrounding normal valves

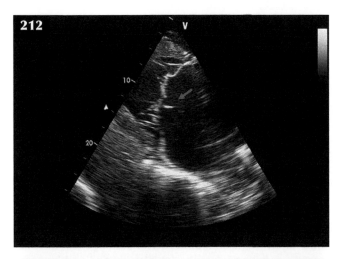

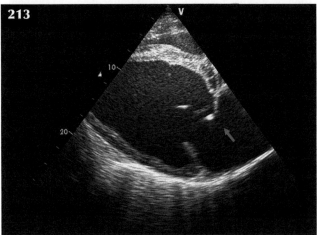

212, 213 Ruptured chordae tendineae (arrows) of the mitral valve in two weanlings with left-sided heart failure. (**212**) Left-sided view of the mitral valve showing a "flail" leaflet in the left atrium during systole. (**213**) Right-sided view of a "steplike" deformity of the mitral valve due to buckling of a leaflet from a ruptured chorda tendinea.

and progressively diminish in size. Unfortunately, contracture of valve edges can occur with scarring and more severe regurgitation can develop. Mineralization with acoustic shadowing may develop and persist in old sterile lesions.

Mitral or aortic valve endocarditis carries a grave prognosis due to the more dire consequences of AV or semilunar valve insufficiency in the higher pressures of the left heart. Tricuspid valve endocarditis is more often successfully treated, since tricuspid regurgitation is far better tolerated due to the lower pressures in the right side of the heart. Gross disruption of the tricuspid valve apparatus has resulted in early rapid development of heart failure in some cases. Pulmonary thromboembolism is a potential complication that can lead to rapid decompensation and severe right heart failure due to elevated pulmonary arterial pressures if a large fragment of the vegetation becomes dislodged.

PERICARDITIS

KEY POINTS
- Underlying bacterial infections should be suspected as a cause of either septic or sterile fibrinous effusive pericarditis in the pediatric equine.
- Pericardiocentesis is vital in cases presenting with tamponade and for diagnostic and therapeutic purposes.
- Indwelling catheters and lavage are not advocated by the author in all cases.

DEFINITION/OVERVIEW
Although sterile fibrinous effusive pericarditis is the most common type of pericarditis in the adult horse, the incidence of septic pericarditis may be greater in the foal. Constrictive pericarditis is less common, but it is an important complication of either septic or sterile pericarditis.

ETIOLOGY/PATHOPHYSIOLOGY
Exposure to eastern tent caterpillars has been correlated with fibrinous pericarditis in the horse. Bacterial agents can also result in pericarditis, whether as a primary pathogen or as an opportunistic agent in previously sterile effusions. Immune-mediated pericarditis may occur following exposure to viral or fungal agents or in conjunction with a noncardiac bacterial infection.

Subepicardial myocardial vasculitis is the underlying lesion in cases of sterile fibrinous effusive pericarditis, including that associated with exposure to eastern tent caterpillars. Occasionally, opportunistic pathogens may complicate the disease process. Hematogenous bacterial infection, often due to *Actinobacillus* spp., can also produce a primary bacterial pericarditis. Primary septic pericarditis due to *Streptococcus* spp. or *Salmonella* spp. infection has been diagnosed in foals in the author's practice.

Increased pericardial pressure from effusion results in reduced cardiac filling and signs of right heart failure due to decreased venous return. In peracute or severe chronic cases, reduced forward flow results in weakness, syncope, and decreased organ perfusion. Pericardial fibrosis may develop and constrictive pericarditis may ensue. Clinical signs of pericardial constriction may include unthriftiness, weakness, elevated respiratory rate, and jugular pulses.

CLINICAL PRESENTATION
Jugular pulses, ventral edema, and muffled heart sounds are classic signs of pericarditis. Heart sounds will not be muffled in cases with small effusions or constrictive pericarditis. Pericardial friction

rubs may be auscultable if fibrin, but little fluid, is present in the pericardial sac.

DIFFERENTIAL DIAGNOSIS

Right heart failure due to tachyarrhythmias and right heart failure due to acquired or congenital heart disease should be ruled out. Hemopericardium (which may be a result of rib fracture or trauma, or can be seen as an idiopathic condition) and hydropericardium (in which there is a noninflammatory passive transudate, often accompanied by pleural and peritoneal effusions in instances of iatrogenic fluid overload in the presence of anuria) are also differentials. Fibrin along the pericardial surfaces will not be detectable

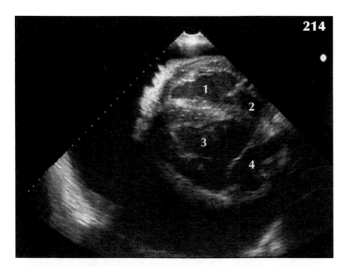

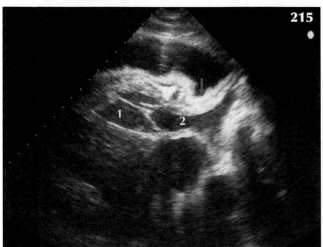

214, 215 Fibrinous pericarditis. Right-sided views. (**214**) Note the large effusion and thick shaggy layer of fibrin on the epicardial surface of the heart. (**215**) Right atrial collapse (arrow) in a case with cardiac tamponade. 1: right ventricle; 2: right atrium; 3: left ventricle; 4: left atrium.

in cases of hemopericardium or hydropericardium in the equine patient. Constrictive pericarditis is a complication of pericarditis; no effusion, or a variable degree of effusion, may be present. The prognosis for constrictive pericarditis is grave, therefore the clinician should be cognizant of this differential on initial examination.

DIAGNOSIS

Echocardiography reveals effusion within the pericardial sac. Variable amounts of fibrin may be seen along the visceral and parietal surfaces, with the thickest accumulation along the visceral pericardial surface (**214, 215**). Collapse of the right atrium and/ or right ventricle will be evident in clinically significant effusions. A "smoky" appearance to the fluid may be noted in cases of hemopericardium, but fibrin should not be evident. Pale mucous membranes and/or a decreased hematocrit with an otherwise normal CBC (complete blood count) is supportive of hemopericardium. The echocardiographic appearance of constrictive pericarditis includes small chamber diameters and abrupt cessation of septal motion at end diastole. There is a subjective "trapped" appearance to the heart during cardiac cycles. Echocardiographic findings of the pericardium in cases of constrictive pericarditis may range from a small amount of fluid and moderate accumulation of fibrin to a minimally thickened pericardium with no effusion (**216, 218**).

MANAGEMENT

Pericardiocentesis is vital in foals with effusion and tamponade. The procedure is most safely performed using ultrasound guidance and, in the author's experience, the left side is often the most easily accessible. A large-gauge over-the-needle catheter (10–14 gauge) is sufficient for initial diagnostic and therapeutic pericardiocentesis. A trocar catheter may be used for massive effusions in order to facilitate more rapid drainage, or it can be left as an indwelling catheter if a purulent effusion is suspected. In some cases, response to one-time drainage and appropriate antimicrobials and NSAIDs is surprisingly dramatic and repeat centesis may not be needed. In order to avoid contamination and further irritation of the pericardium, the author prefers to determine the need for indwelling catheters on an individual basis by follow-up ultrasound examinations. Pericardial lavage is performed by the author only if the effusion is purulent and/or septic, since any manipulation of the pericardium can lead to constrictive pericarditis. Also, systemic administration of antimicrobials can achieve high intrapericardial levels.

Systemic broad-spectrum antimicrobials should be administered even in the case of sterile effusion, since opportunistic or iatrogenic infection is possible. NSAIDs are also recommended. Most cases of pericarditis in the foal are likely associated with a concurrent bacterial infection (either primary or opportunistic septic pericarditis or presumed immune-mediated pericarditis due to a septic process involving another body system). The use of corticosteroids in cases of sterile fibrinous effusive pericarditis in the

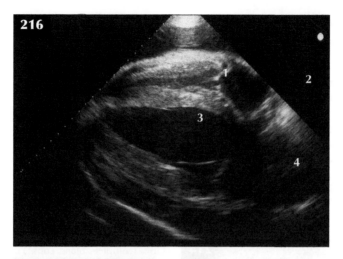

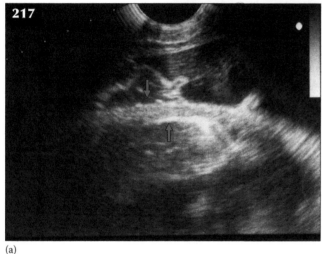

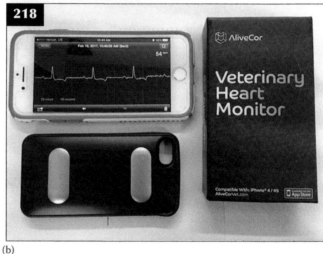

(a)   (b)

216, 217 "Thin" constrictive pericarditis. (**216**) Note the small cardiac chambers, the "trapped" appearance to the heart, and the thickened pericardium. There is no pericardial effusion, but pleural effusion is present. (**218**) Left-sided image of a minimally thickened but severely constricting pericardium (between arrows) in the same case. (**218**) Portable ECG/heart monitor designed to snap onto a cellular phone. (Courtesy of AliveCor, Inc., San Francisco, CA.)

foal should be made only after careful exclusion of the presence of an infection of any other body system.

Constrictive pericarditis is an important differential for foals presenting with small effusions and variable amounts of fibrin accumulation with clinical signs of cardiac tamponade and poor cardiac output. These foals have a grave prognosis, since constrictive pericardial disease is progressive and not reversible. Thorascopic pericardiectomy has been performed successfully at the author's hospital in adult horses that presented with suspected long-standing chronic fibrinous effusive pericarditis, and it may be considered in foals in which constrictive pericarditis appears to have developed or may be developing. Cases in which the visceral pericardium has constricted are unlikely to benefit from surgery since adequate and safe removal of the visceral pericardium is extremely difficult.

Regardless of management, including those managed with aggressive pericardial lavage, constrictive pericarditis was found to be an important and not uncommon sequela of pericarditis associated with exposure to eastern tent caterpillars. Constrictive pericarditis ultimately developed in what were initially considered to be successfully treated cases with no residual pericardial fibrin or fluid at the time of discharge. Such cases re-presented as long as 2 years later with a nonfibrinous, noneffusive constrictive pericardium. It is likely that foals with this sequela will manifest signs of constrictive pericardial disease earlier since they are growing individuals. Follow-up ultrasound examinations of patients with pericarditis should also include use of a high-frequency transducer to evaluate the pericardium for any residual thickening, since this may indicate the potential for constriction to develop.

CARDIAC ARRHYTHMIAS

KEY POINTS
- Most arrhythmias in the foal are secondary to systemic disease.
- An electrocardiogram (ECG) is necessary to characterize arrhythmias and determine appropriate treatment (**218**).

BRADYARRHYTHMIA

DEFINITION/OVERVIEW
Significant bradyarrhythmias are most often encountered in association with severe systemic disease, and they can be a precursor of cardiac arrest.

ETIOLOGY/PATHOPHYSIOLOGY
Any severe disease process (e.g., sepsis, cerebral ischemia) can potentially lead to bradycardia and, ultimately, cardiac arrest. Bradyarrhythmias, often a precursor to cardiac arrest, are a result of respiratory or cardiac failure, which leads to hypoxic acidosis and, finally, to cardiac and respiratory arrest.

CLINICAL PRESENTATION
Because most foals are obtunded due to the underlying systemic disease, bradyarrhythmias are often undetected unless there is frequent auscultation or continuous ECG monitoring in the neonatal ICU.

DIFFERENTIAL DIAGNOSIS
The differential for a slow heart rate is iatrogenic bradycardia due to recent sedation; however, it should be noted that foals with severe systemic disease may be more sensitive to sedatives. In some cases, sedation of a critically ill foal may precipitate events that will lead to cardiac arrest.

DIAGNOSIS
Diagnosis of a bradyarrhythmia is based on auscultation and further characterized by an ECG.

MANAGEMENT
Oxygen supplementation and assisted ventilation is required. Any abnormalities of arterial blood pressure (BP), serum electrolytes and acid–base status, blood glucose, and arterial blood gases should be evaluated and corrected. Dobutamine infusion should be given if necessary. In severe cases in which cardiac arrest is imminent, a low dose of epinephrine may be required.

CARDIAC ARREST

DEFINITION/OVERVIEW
Cardiac arrest is defined as an absence of effective circulation.

ETIOLOGY/PATHOPHYSIOLOGY
Cardiac arrest is often secondary to severe systemic illness, as described for bradyarrhythmia. Cardiac arrest may occur in otherwise healthy individuals in association with general anesthesia. Cardiac arrest is the end result of cardiac and/or respiratory failure resulting from severe systemic disease.

CLINICAL PRESENTATION
Clinical findings include absence of palpable or audible heartbeat, lack of palpable pulses, ashen or pale mucous membranes, agonal gasps, seizures, unconsciousness, and dilated pupils.

DIFFERENTIAL DIAGNOSIS
Causes for an inaudible heartbeat include pericardial or pleural effusion, which results in diminished heart sounds, and subcutaneous emphysema due to rib fractures resulting in inaudible heart sounds. Inadequate lead contact or faulty leads may result in an ECG artifact. The heart should be auscultated and the chest palpated for an apex beat, and an adequate lead contact should be ensured.

DIAGNOSIS
Where there are obvious clinical signs and an absent heartbeat, basic resuscitation measures should be undertaken immediately while an ECG is obtained. The ECG will reveal one of the following arrhythmias in cases of cardiac arrest:
- *Asystole*: "flat-line" ECG. This is the most common ECG finding in cases of cardiac arrest in the neonatal ICU. Atrial activity may still be present.
- *Pulseless idioventricular rhythm*: slow ventricular escape rhythm, which fails to generate mechanical contraction.
- *Pulseless electrical activity*: normal ECG tracing, but absence of myocardial contraction (a heartbeat will not be audible; the apex beat will not be palpable; no pulse pressures will be generated).
- *Ventricular flutter*: rapidly degenerates into ventricular fibrillation.
- *Ventricular fibrillation*: undulating waves on the ECG, with no organized electrical activity.

MANAGEMENT
The following steps should be taken when initiating CPR:
- Lower the head at or below the level of the heart to avoid reduction in cerebral blood flow and to avoid aspiration.
- Provide 100% oxygen and ventilate through an endotracheal tube. Hyperventilate initially at a rate of approximately 40–60 breaths per minute, followed by a rate of 15–30 breaths per minute once the patient is stabilized. If laryngospasm precludes placement of an endotracheal tube, a tracheostomy or percutaneous transtracheal insufflation with a large-gauge catheter can be employed. Arterial blood gas values should be monitored and ventilation adjusted appropriately.
- Administer chest compressions over the widest part of the chest sufficient to decrease the thoracic wall diameter by 25%–30%. Circulation is achieved by changes in intrathoracic pressures (thoracic pump mechanism) and may be more effective

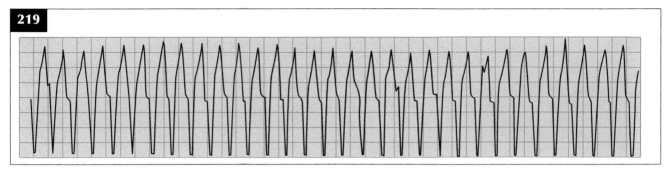

219 Ventricular tachycardia in a weanling foal. Base apex, 25 mm/s.

than pressure placed directly over the heart in animals the size of foals. The clinician should be particularly cognizant of any pre-existing rib fractures. Rib fractures, either at or 1–2 cm dorsal to the costrochondral junction, are not uncommon in the neonate as a result of birth trauma.

- Approximately 60–80 chest compressions per minute, regardless of the age or size of the equine patient, are generally recommended. Some authors recommend chest compressions of 100–120 per minute in the neonatal foal, with compressions placed directly over the heart.
- Cardiac drugs—lidocaine, epinephrine, and atropine—can be administered intravenously or endo- or transtracheally. If administered via the airway, the dose should be increased two- to threefold, given in at least 10 mL of saline at the carina, and followed by ventilation. Intracardiac administration of drugs is not recommended due to the importance of uninterrupted chest compressions and the potential for laceration of coronary vessels or lung tissue, as well as myocardial trauma and precipitation of ventricular fibrillation. Bicarbonate and calcium are not recommended as routine treatment, but may be used to correct any known pre-existing acidemia, hypocalcemia, or hyperkalemia. Epinephrine (0.01–0.02 mg/kg i/v initially, followed by 0.1–0.2 mg/kg i/v for subsequent doses) should be used to treat ventricular asystole or pulseless rhythms. If ventilation and epinephrine are ineffective, atropine may be given (0.02 mg/kg i/v).
- Defibrillation: if available, electrical defibrillation is the treatment of choice for ventricular fibrillation. However, ventricular fibrillation is an infrequent finding in cardiac arrest in the foal. In cases of ventricular flutter, lidocaine (1.5 mg/kg i/v) should be given, followed by epinephrine (or defibrillation if the rhythm degenerates to ventricular fibrillation).

CPR is rarely effective when associated with severe underlying systemic illness. Anesthesia-related cardiac arrest in otherwise healthy individuals carries a good prognosis if detected early (and is not an end result of unrecognized respiratory arrest).

TACHYARRHYTHMIAS

DEFINITION/OVERVIEW
Tachyarrhythmias are relatively uncommon in the equine pediatric patient.

ETIOLOGY/PATHOPHYSIOLOGY
Suspected causes of tachyarrhythmia include viral or bacterial myocarditis, bacterial endocarditis, immune-mediated myocarditis, and contusion. Concurrent systemic disorders, including gastrointestinal (GI) disease and sepsis, can be associated with tachyarrhythmias. Myocarditis is an infrequently recognized problem in the equine pediatric patient and cannot be confirmed without histopathology. Myocarditis is presumptively diagnosed when tachyarrhythmias of undetermined cause are discovered.

Tachyarrhythmias result in reduced ventricular filling and a reduction in cardiac output. Signs of cardiac failure ensue.

CLINICAL PRESENTATION
Foals with rapid ventricular tachycardia (**219**) present with signs of heart failure ranging from syncope and respiratory distress to more gradual signs of right-sided heart failure such as venous distension and ascites. Supraventricular tachyarrhythmias have also been observed less frequently, but rapid rates can result in similar signs. Occasionally, a moderate tachyarrhythmia is not recognized until detected on a routine physical examination.

DIFFERENTIAL DIAGNOSIS
Sinus tachycardia, a normal response to either hypoxemia, severe systemic disease, pain, or excitement, is a differential diagnosis.

DIAGNOSIS
An ECG is required to differentiate ventricular tachycardia, supraventricular tachycardia, and sinus tachycardia. An ECG is also necessary to distinguish supraventricular premature beats from ventricular premature beats. Echocardiography will invariably reveal reduced myocardial function in horses with ventricular tachycardia or rapid supraventricular tachycardia. This can easily occur secondary to the arrhythmia, and an accurate assessment of myocardial function cannot be made until the rhythm is controlled or sinus rhythm is restored. However, segmental dysfunction or myocardial fibrosis (focal areas of increased echogenicity or myocardial scarring) may indicate focal myocardial necrosis, contusion, or fibrosis. Echocardiography is also warranted to determine whether bacterial or mural endocarditis lesions are present.

A thorough search for underlying systemic disease should be made. A CBC and serum chemistry should be performed. Abdominal ultrasonography may also prove rewarding in detecting an occult disease process in some cases. Viral isolation from whole blood and nasal swabs and acute and convalescent serology can be performed if a viral etiology is suspected. Blood cultures should be performed in foals with fevers in conjunction with the arrhythmia, as mural endocarditis or early endocarditis lesions may be difficult to detect.

Cardiac troponin I levels will invariably be elevated during and shortly after resolution of tachyarrhythmias regardless of the cause. Once sinus rhythm has been restored in horses with supraventricular or ventricular tachycardia, it is the author's experience that values return to normal within one week of restoration of sinus rhythm. Should cardiac troponin I levels remain elevated, active myocardial inflammation or necrosis is likely present.

MANAGEMENT

- *Ventricular tachycardia*: Antiarrhythmic therapy is warranted if the ventricular rate is rapid (>100–120 beats per minute), multiform complexes are present, or R on T phenomenon is identified. Lidocaine is the author's preferred treatment for ventricular tachycardia and is efficacious in most cases when administered as a continuous rate infusion (CRI) (0.05 mg/ kg/min). Conversion to sinus rhythm is achieved in 2–4 hours. In more immediate life-threatening cases, the standard dose (1 mg/kg i/v) can be given as a bolus or in a small volume of fluid over 15–30 minutes, followed by a CRI if necessary. In the author's experience, horses with severe ventricular tachycardia appear to be predisposed to the toxic effects of lidocaine, and may have a seizure or develop cardiac arrest during bolus administration of lidocaine. If lidocaine is ineffective alone, oral procainamide, which can be administered orally, can be added to the treatment regimen. Other drugs that can be used to manage ventricular tachycardia include quinidine gluconate or sulfate, magnesium sulfate, propranolol or atenolol, and phenytoin. In the vast majority of foals and horses with ventricular tachycardia, long-term therapy is not needed once sinus rhythm is restored. If long-term therapy is required, oral procainamide may be the most appropriate drug to use, since it is known to be absorbed in the horse and has relatively few side-effects. Corticosteroids should also be considered if myocarditis or contusion is suspected as the cause of a recurrent arrhythmia or if cardiac troponin I levels remain elevated. If fever and/or an inflammatory leukogram are present, bacterial infection cannot be ruled out and therefore antimicrobial therapy can be justifiably added to the treatment regimen. Stall rest with hand grazing for 2 or more weeks, with frequent monitoring of heart rate and rhythm, is advisable in horses in which an underlying etiology is unknown. Horses in which an underlying disease process was the suspected cause, and has been addressed, generally do not have recurrences of the arrhythmia. Cardiac troponin I levels should be repeated after 1 week to ensure values have returned to normal and active myocardial necrosis is unlikely to be present. A 24-hour Holter monitor is also advisable to ensure that there is no increased ectopic activity prior to returning the foal to routine care.

- *Supraventricular tachycardia*: Atrial premature complexes, if frequent, can be managed by oral quinidine; however, due to hypotensive effects the animal should be confined during treatment. Beta blockers (e.g., atenolol) and calcium channel blockers (e.g., diltiazem) may be employed, although there is not much experience with these drugs in the horse and pharmacokinetic data are lacking. Corticosteroids can be given in the absence of infection if myocarditis or contusion is suspected. As described for ventricular tachyarrhythmias, the presence of fever or an inflammatory leukogram can justify the use of antimicrobials for a suspected bacterial endo- or myocarditis. Atrial fibrillation with a rapid ventricular response rate may be treated with oral digoxin. Direct current cardioversion or quinidine sulfate may restore sinus rhythm. Atrial fibrillation can occur early in the neonatal period in otherwise normal foals (**180**). Otherwise, its presence in a foal may indicate significant underlying heart disease, which should be investigated with echocardiography. It should be noted that antiarrhythmic agents are also arrhythmogenic and can result in the development of fatal arrhythmias. Such agents should not be used unless indicated.

FURTHER READING

Bonagura JD, Reef VB (2004) Disorders of the cardiovascular system. In: *Equine Internal Medicine*, 2nd ed. (Reed SM, Bayly WM, Sellon DC, Eds.). WB Saunders, St Louis, MO, pp. 355–459.

Fink BW (1985) *Congenital Heart Disease: A Deductive Approach to Its Diagnosis*. Year Book Medical Publishers, Chicago, IL.

Marr CM (Ed.) (1999) *Cardiology of the Horse*. WB Saunders, Philadelphia, PA.

Patteson MW (1997) The cardiovascular system. In: *Current Therapy in Equine Medicine*, 4th ed. (Robinson NE, Ed.). WB Saunders, Philadelphia, PA, pp. 225–272.

Reef VB (1998) Cardiovascular ultrasonography. In: *Equine Diagnostic Ultrasound* (Reef VB, Ed.). WB Saunders, Philadelphia, PA, pp. 215–272.

Reimer JM (1998) The heart. In: *Atlas of Equine Ultrasonography* (Reimer JM, Ed.). Mosby, St. Louis, MO, pp. 131–169.

Respiratory Disorders

8

Bonnie S. Barr

INTRODUCTION

Disorders of the respiratory tract are common in the equine pediatric patient. During the neonatal period respiratory disorders occur either as a primary disorder or as a sequela to other neonatal disorders such as prematurity (respiratory distress syndrome [RDS]), septicemia, or neuromuscular disorders. Congenital deformities of the respiratory tract are reported and may be diagnosed in the neonate, but they may remain unidentified until the foal is older. Lower respiratory tract (LRT) disorders are common in weanling and suckling foals, with pneumonia being the most common cause of morbidity in these individuals. This chapter will begin with an overview of the diagnosis of respiratory disorders followed by a description of specific disorders of the upper respiratory tract (URT) and LRT.

HISTORY

In the neonatal foal, gestational age and maturity of the foal are important, along with the history of an abnormal delivery. Periparturient problems (e.g., systemic illness of the mare, placental abnormalities, and exposure to infectious diseases) can affect the foal *in utero* and result in the conditions that compromise the foal. In the older foal, history of exposure to infectious diseases or a history of respiratory problems on the farm may aid in the identification of respiratory disorders.

PHYSICAL EXAMINATION

A thorough and complete physical examination should be carried out on all equine pediatric patients. Note that diagnosis of a respiratory disorder by physical examination could be either straightforward or vague. The head should be observed and palpated for any asymmetry. Airflow through both nostrils should be assessed along with evidence of ocular or nasal discharge. The character and location of the nasal discharge should be taken into consideration. Mucous membrane color, moistness, and capillary refill time (CRT) should all be assessed, although mucous membrane color can often be misleading in the neonate. The diagnosis of a lower respiratory problem in the newborn foal can sometimes be challenging because of the insidious nature of the onset of pulmonary disease in these individuals. When assessing a neonate it is important to differentiate normal from abnormal and have in mind the normal finding of a physical examination of a neonate.

Careful attention should be paid to the respiratory rate (*Table 42*) and respiratory pattern. Nonrespiratory disorders of the neonate can mimic respiratory disease by causing tachypnea.

The respiratory pattern, the degree of effort, and any abnormal noises associated with respiration should be noted. Inspiratory noises are most commonly associated with upper airway disorders. Expiratory grunting may be noted in neonates with atelectasis, pneumonia, or pulmonary edema. Normal neonates show a slight abdominal component to their breathing (compliance of the ribs makes respiratory efforts differ from that of adults). Marked abdominal component is abnormal, with paradoxical movement of the ribs and abdomen suggesting a respiratory disorder. The respiratory pattern is regular in a normal standing foal, but is often erratic in a normal sleeping foal. Increased nostril flare or periods of apnea also suggest a respiratory disorder. Thoracic auscultation is often not reliable as an indicator of lower respiratory disease in the neonate because often only subtle abnormalities are appreciable on auscultation, even in the presence of very severe pulmonary disease. Immediately postpartum the lung sounds are very moist. Significant differences between the sounds of the upper and lower lung in lateral recumbency have been appreciated in normal neonatal foals. A change from lateral to sternal recumbency may cause crackles to be auscultated in the previously down lung. Lung sounds in the neonate are much easier to hear than in adults and they can be harsh, especially with tachypnea. Physical examination findings in the older foal are usually more straightforward than in the neonate. In the older individual with pulmonary compromise there is usually evidence of cough, nasal discharge, depression, and fever. Changes in respiratory rate, respiratory pattern, and abnormal noises associated with respiration can often lead to similar

Table 42. Respiratory rates in the foal		
Newborn (1 day old)	**7 days old**	**30 days old**
60–80 bpm	40–50 bpm	<40 bpm
bpm = breaths per minute.		

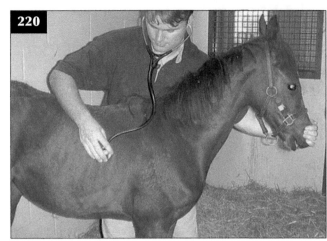

220 Auscultation of the thorax. Occluding the nares provides a faster and deeper respiration pattern, making it easier to detect abnormalities.

conclusions in older foals, as in the neonate. Auscultation of the thorax should be performed at rest and if needed, and if the foal can tolerate it, with a soft plastic bag or occlusion of the nares to allow a faster and deeper respiratory pattern, making it easier to detect abnormalities (**220**). Adventitial sounds can be classified as crackles or wheezes and identified as diffuse or focal. Quiet or absent lung sounds may indicate consolidation or fluid accumulation in the thorax. The trachea should be auscultated and abnormal tracheal sounds should not be confused with abnormal lower airway sounds.

RADIOGRAPHY

Good-quality thoracic radiographs with all the lung fields well aerated should clearly define the heart, posterior vena cava, aorta, and thymus (**221**). The ribs should be assessed for fractures, especially in the neonate. Radiographs can help to evaluate the type, severity, and location of pulmonary disease. The infiltrates can be characterized as interstitial, alveolar, or bronchiolar patterns and as focal or diffuse (*Table 43*; **222–224**).

Table 43. Radiographic lesions in the pediatric thorax

- Diffuse infiltrates:
  - Atelectasis
  - Interstitial pneumonia
  - Bacterial pneumonia
  - Viral pneumonia
  - Fungal pneumonia
  - Pulmonary edema
  - Hyaline membrane disease
- Cranioventral infiltrates:
  - Aspiration pneumonia
- Caudodorsal infiltrates:
  - *In-utero* acquired pneumonia
  - Hemorrhage
- Focal areas of opacity:
  - Abscessation

In the neonate, lateral and dorsoventral views are sometimes obtained, although standing radiographs are most often performed in older foals. Interpretation of thoracic radiographs of the neonate can often be challenging because immature lungs can appear radiographically similar to diseased lungs. Serial thoracic radiographs are

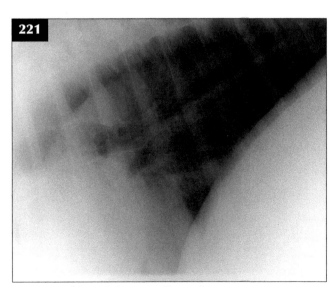

221 Normal lateral thorax radiograph.

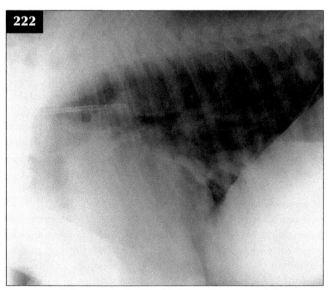

222 Lateral thoracic radiograph demonstrating a diffuse interstitial pattern. Note the generalized increased lung opacity and inability to visualize fine vascular margins.

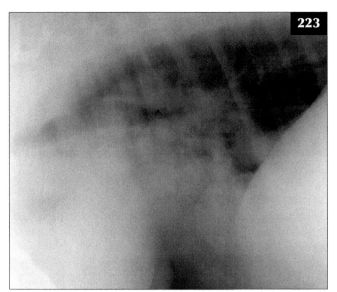

223 Lateral thoracic radiograph demonstrating aspiration pneumonia. Note that the majority of the pathology is localized in the cranioventral lung field.

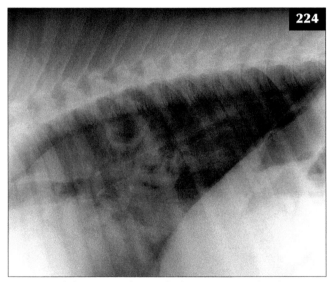

224 Lateral thoracic radiograph demonstrating focal areas of opacity (abscessation). Note the two large, rounded, cavitated abscesses.

useful in monitoring the progression of the disease and response to therapy; however, radiographic changes may either follow or precede changes in the clinical condition. Skull radiographs image the URT allowing for assessment of the sinuses, pharynx, and larynx (**242**).

ULTRASONOGRAPHY
Ultrasound of the thorax of the neonate with pulmonary disease, regardless of the etiology, often reveals the nonspecific finding of a loss of the normal reverberation artifact pattern. Rib fractures, hemothorax, and diaphragmatic hernias can be identified by ultrasound. Other abnormalities that can be identified include pulmonary abscess or pneumothorax. The examination

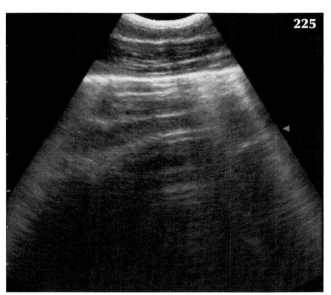

225 Ultrasound view of normal lung.

must be performed with the foal standing or in sternal recumbency. A 5.0 or 7.5 MHz straight or curved linear array transducer provides a good image and fits between the foal's ribs (**225**). Ultrasound can also be performed on the structures of the laryngeal region.

ENDOSCOPY
Endoscopy is useful for evaluation of the URT and diagnosis of congenital abnormalities. This procedure can allow careful evaluation of the nasal passages, the integrity of the palate, and the function of the pharyngeal structures. Indications for endoscopy include a pattern of breathing or respiratory noises suggestive of obstruction, milk observed at one or both nostrils, other nasal discharge, or external swellings.

HEMATOLOGY
The most common hematologic abnormality in the pediatric patient with pulmonary disease is usually a leukocytosis and hyperfibrinogenemia. Those with a more chronic process may also have an anemia and hyperproteinemia. Acutely compromised neonates may demonstrate a leukopenia due to an overwhelming systemic inflammatory response. Serial monitoring of the hemogram can help to assess the response to therapy.

ARTERIAL BLOOD GAS ANALYSIS
Arterial blood gas analysis is most often performed in the neonatal foal to define the severity of the disease and to assess response to therapy. In neonatal foals, arterial blood can be obtained from the great metatarsal artery (**226**) or the brachial artery. In older foals the sample can also be obtained from the facial artery. Several factors can influence the interpretation of the arterial blood gas analysis including the position of the foal (lateral versus sternal), room air contaminating the sample, accidentally obtaining venous blood, struggling, machine error, and gestational and postnatal age of the individual. The two most common derangements of respiratory origin noted on arterial blood gas analysis, especially in the neonate, are hypoxemia (low or normal $PaCO_2$) and hypoxemia with hypercapnia. Right-to-left

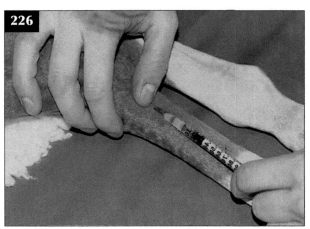

226

226 Obtaining an arterial blood gas sample from the great metatarsal artery.

vascular shunting and ventilation–perfusion mismatch most often causes hypoxemia in the neonate. Hypoventilation due to neurologic dysfunction or an inability of the neonate's respiratory muscles to work hard enough to ventilate abnormal lungs adequately would result in hypoxemia with a hypercapnia.

BLOOD CULTURES

Blood cultures are often obtained in the neonatal patient and may help to identify a causative agent. These samples should be taken prior to the administration of antimicrobials and should be obtained using careful aseptic technique.

TRANSTRACHEAL ASPIRATE

The technique for transtracheal aspirate is similar to that performed in adult horses. A sample obtained percutaneously has less of a chance of URT contamination (*Table 44*; **227, 228**). If this is not

---

Table 44. How to perform a percutaneous transtracheal aspirate

- **Equipment needed:**
  - Sedation (if needed, 0.2–0.5 mg/kg xylazine i/v with 0.01 mg/kg butorphanol i/v; caution: do not sedate a foal in respiratory distress)
  - Clippers
  - Sterile scrub
  - Sterile gloves
  - Transtracheal wash kit (such as BD Intracath made by Becton Dickson or a 14 gauge 2 inch needle and 16 gauge 24 inch catheter tubing)
  - Sterile saline (two syringes each with 6 mL of saline)
  - Lidocaine for block

- **Procedure:**
  - Clip and prep (sterile) a site on the upper two-thirds of the ventral aspect of the neck, over the trachea
  - Lidocaine block
  - Wearing sterile gloves, palpate the trachea and stabilize it with one hand (**227**)
  - With the bevel of the needle downward, place the needle through the skin and between the tracheal rings into the tracheal lumen
  - Feed the catheter one-half to two-thirds down the trachea and remove the stylet (if one is present)
  - Inject one syringe of 6 mL of sterile saline
  - Aspirate fluid back into the syringe (**228**); reposition the catheter by pulling it in or out to help obtain a sample
  - Withdraw the catheter first and finally the needle

- **Complications:**
  - Subcutaneous abscess, cellulitis, or emphysema at site of needle placement
  - Catheter laceration—usually coughed out
  - Coughing, which can retroflex the catheter cranially, resulting in a pharyngeal sample
  - Accidental puncturing of the carotid artery
  - Excessive trauma to the trachea

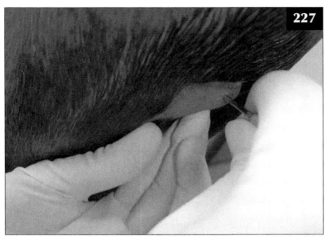

227 When performing a percutaneous transtracheal aspirate, stabilize the trachea with one hand and place the needle between tracheal rings.

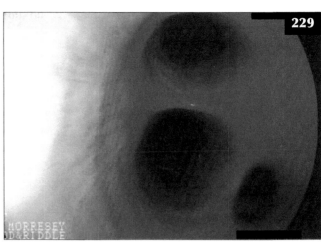

229 Endoscopic view of the bronchial airways prior to performing a bronchioalveolar lavage. (Courtesy of P. Morresey.)

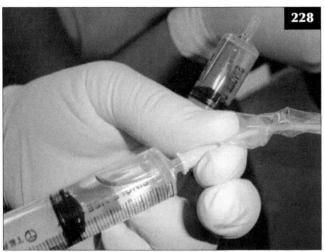

228 When performing a percutaneous transtracheal aspirate, aspirate fluid back into the syringe.

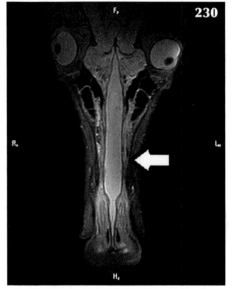

230 MRI of a foal skull—STIR dorsal image displaying a large nasal septal cyst. The hyperintense signal (arrow) is consistent with a fluid-filled cyst. (Courtesy of K. Garrett.)

practical various specialized catheters are available to reduce the risk of contamination when the sample is collected via biopsy channel of an endoscope. A positive culture is useful in identifying a septic process, and the sensitivity can help to fine-tune the antimicrobial therapy. Cytologic evaluation of the aspirate may help to identify a septic process and give an early indication of the type of organism involved. A transtracheal aspirate should not be performed if the individual is critical or in respiratory distress.

Bronchioalveolar lavage
This procedure is not often performed in the pediatric patient. Bronchial alveolar lavage (BAL) is used primarily for cytologic examination of nonseptic conditions. Because only a localized region of the lung is sampled, BAL is most commonly used for the diagnosis of diffuse processes involving the lower airway. The procedure can be performed blindly using a double-lumen catheter or under visual guidance with a flexible endoscope (229).

Other imaging modalities
Computed tomography (CT) and magnetic resonance imaging (MRI) are two additional imaging modalities available to aid in the characterization of certain upper respiratory disorders such as sinonasal disease or laryngeal dysplasia (230).

DISORDERS OF THE UPPER RESPIRATORY TRACT

This section of the chapter will discuss specific disorders of the URT and will include both congenital and acquired disorders of the nares, nasal passages, sinus, palate, guttural pouch, and trachea.

WRY NOSE

KEY POINTS
- Wry nose is a deviation of the maxilla (± mandible) to one side.
- In severe cases, respiratory stridor may be noted.
- Surgical intervention may be indicated.

DEFINITION/OVERVIEW
Wry nose is a deviation of the premaxilla to one side due to a deformity of the maxilla, nasal, incisive, and vomer bones (**231, 232**). There may be a corresponding milder deviation of the mandible.

ETIOLOGY/PATHOPHYSIOLOGY
This deformity is thought to be genetically transmitted, but it may be due to abnormal fetal positioning *in utero*. The clinical signs observed are secondary due to the distortion and compromise of the nasal airway.

CLINICAL PRESENTATION
If the deviation is mild, clinical signs may not be present. In more severe cases, respiratory stridor and difficulties in nursing may be noted.

DIFFERENTIAL DIAGNOSIS
Tables 45 and *46.*

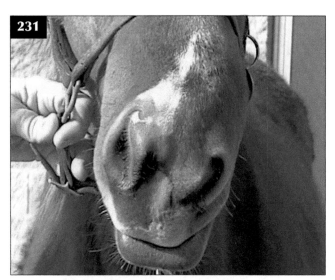

231 A 1-month-old foal with a wry nose. (Courtesy of R. Embertson.)

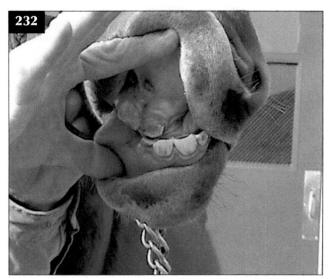

232 A 1-month-old foal with wry nose. Note the deviation of the maxilla. (Courtesy of R. Emberston.)

Table 45. Causes of respiratory distress in the pediatric patient

- **Respiratory causes:**
  - Choanal atresia
  - Guttural pouch empyema
  - Guttural pouch tympany
  - Nasopharyngeal dysfunction (pharyngeal collapse)
  - Laryngeal web
  - Laryngeal paresis
  - Tracheal stenosis/collapse/perforation
  - Bacterial pneumonia
  - Viral pneumonia
  - Retropharyngeal mass/abscess
  - Pleuritis/pleuropneumonia
  - Cleft palate
  - Pharyngeal/subepiglottic cysts
  - Foreign body (nasal, laryngeal)
  - Bronchointerstitial pneumonia (acute respiratory distress syndrome)
  - Neonatal respiratory distress syndrome
  - Meconium aspiration syndrome
  - Aspiration pneumonia
  - Pneumothorax
  - Hemothorax
  - Idiopathic or transient tachypnea
  - Atelectasis
  - Pulmonary edema
- **Nonrespiratory causes:**
  - Hyperkalemic periodic paralysis
  - Cardiac disease/anomalies

(Continued)

Table 45. (*Continued*) Causes of respiratory distress in the pediatric patient

- ◦ Shock/sepsis
- ◦ Neonatal isoerythrolysis
- ◦ Anemia
- ◦ Hyperthermia
- ◦ Blood or plasma transfusion reaction
- ◦ Intracarotid injection
- ◦ Gastrointestinal lesion
- ◦ Electrolyte/metabolic derangements
- ◦ Toxins
- ◦ Anaphylaxis
- ◦ Excitement
- ◦ Diaphragmatic hernia
- ◦ Persistent pulmonary hypertension
- ◦ Pain (musculoskeletal)
- ◦ Rib fractures

Table 46. Causes of respiratory stridor in the pediatric patient

- • **Respiratory causes:**
  - ◦ Dorsal displacement of the soft palate
  - ◦ Epidermal inclusion cysts (atheroma)
  - ◦ Sinus cysts
  - ◦ Progressive ethmoidal hematomas
  - ◦ Unilateral choanal atresia
  - ◦ Pharyngeal cysts
  - ◦ Rostral displacement of the palatopharyngeal arch
  - ◦ Pharyngeal collapse
  - ◦ Guttural pouch tympany/empyema
  - ◦ Nasopharyngeal dysfunction
  - ◦ Laryngeal web
  - ◦ Laryngeal paresis
  - ◦ Tracheal stenosis/collapse/perforation
  - ◦ Retropharyngeal mass/abscess
  - ◦ Foreign body (nasal, pharyngeal, laryngeal, tracheal, bronchial)
  - ◦ Abnormalities of nasal septum
- • **Nonrespiratory causes:**
  - ◦ Anaphylaxis
  - ◦ Hyperkalemic periodic paralysis
  - ◦ Dystrophic myodegeneration (white muscle disease)

DIAGNOSIS

Diagnosis is based on physical examination. Radiography may need to be performed to assess the severity.

MANAGEMENT

In those foals with very mild deviation, spontaneous improvement may be noted with time. Most often, surgical intervention is indicated.

DEVIATION OR THICKENING OF NASAL SEPTUM

KEY POINTS

- • Can be acquired or congenital.
- • Acquired may be the result of trauma, infection, or a space-occupying mass.
- • May result in a restriction of air flow.
- • Endoscopy or a dorsal ventral radiograph may be useful.
- • Surgical resection may be required.

DEFINITION/OVERVIEW

Deviation or thickening of the nasal septum can be an acquired or congenital anomaly. Invariably, this deformity is present in cases of a wry nose, but it can occur as an independent entity.

ETIOLOGY/PATHOPHYSIOLOGY

Acquired deviation or thickening of the nasal septum may result from an infection, a space-occupying mass, or following a traumatic incident. A congenital deviation may occur alone or in conjunction with deviation of the premaxilla. Deformation of the nasal septum, if severe enough, may result in restriction of airflow due to the narrowing of the nasal passages.

CLINICAL PRESENTATION

Clinical presentation varies depending on the degree of narrowing. Clinical signs may be subtle and evident only during strenuous exercise. If the deformation is severe, restricted airflow through one or both nostrils may result in respiratory distress. A respiratory stridor and nasal discharge may also be observed.

DIFFERENTIAL DIAGNOSIS

Tables 45 through *47*.

DIAGNOSIS

Diagnosis can be made by palpating the rostral septum or by endoscopically observing the deformity or the narrowing of the ventral meatus caused by the deformity. A dorsoventral radiograph of the nasal septum can help to establish the extent of the deformity. A good-quality radiograph is obtained by centering on the midline just caudal to the rostral extremity of the facial crest.

Table 47. Causes of nasal discharge in the pediatric patient

- Bacterial pneumonia
- Viral pneumonia
- Pharyngitis
- Sinus/paranasal cysts
- Progressive ethmoidal hematomas (serosanguineous)
- Cleft palate
- Pharyngeal cysts
- Guttural pouch tympany
- Dorsal displacement of the soft palate
- Nasopharyngeal dysfunction/pharyngeal collapse
- Laryngeal web
- Persistent frenulum of the epiglottis
- Laryngeal paresis
- Tracheal stenosis/collapse/perforation
- Foreign body (nasal, pharyngeal, laryngeal, tracheal, bronchial)
- Trauma to the upper airway
- Pulmonary edema
- Pleuritis
- Esophageal obstruction/choke
- Gastric distension due to GI dysfunction
- Neurologic deficits affecting swallowing and resulting in dysphagia (e.g., botulism)
- Hyperkalemic periodic paralysis
- White muscle disease/nutritional myodegeneration
- Electrolyte or metabolic derangements
- Cardiac disease

MANAGEMENT

In cases in which the deformity is restricting performance, surgical resection of the nasal septum can be performed.

EPIDERMAL INCLUSION CYSTS (OR ATHEROMA)

KEY POINTS

- Epidermal inclusion cysts are fluid-filled cysts.
- They are located at the caudal aspect of the false nostril.
- Usually they do not cause functional impairment.

DEFINITION/OVERVIEW

Epidermal inclusion cysts (or atheroma) are fluid-filled, cyst-like structures located at the caudal aspect of the false nostril (**233**).

ETIOLOGY/PATHOPHYSIOLOGY

The exact etiology is unknown, but most likely represents a congenital ectopic sequestration of epithelium. Epidermal inclusion cysts do not usually cause any functional impairment.

CLINICAL PRESENTATION

The epidermal inclusion cysts are most often single, spherical nodules that vary in size from 3 to 5 cm in diameter located on the caudal dorsal aspect of the false nostril. These cysts are nonpainful on palpation. If large enough, a respiratory stridor may result during exercise.

DIFFERENTIAL DIAGNOSIS

Table 46.

DIAGNOSIS

The epidermal inclusion cysts are easily identified by visual appearance, location, and palpation of the caudal extent of the nasal diverticulum. Diagnosis can be confirmed by cytologic examination of a fine needle aspirate, which reveals a whitish-gray, thick odorless fluid (**234, 235**).

MANAGEMENT

Specific treatment is not needed because these lesions are seldom associated with problems in the foal. Epidermal inclusion cysts may be removed for cosmetic appearance by drainage or surgical removal (surgical extirpation).

SINUS CYST (PARANASAL SINUS CYST)

KEY POINTS

- Sinus cysts are fluid-filled cavities that originate in the maxillary sinuses.
- If large enough, they can cause deformity of the nasal septum and alteration of airflow.
- Clinical presentation may include facial deformity, airway obstruction, or nasal discharge.
- Surgical removal is generally required.

DEFINITION/OVERVIEW

Sinus cysts (paranasal sinus cysts) are fluid-filled cavities that originate in the maxillary sinuses and ventral conchae and occasionally extend into the frontal sinus and nasal cavity (**236**). The cysts are single or loculated with epithelial lining and contain a yellow acellular fluid. Sinus cysts are usually unilateral, but bilateral cysts have been reported in foals. If large enough, the cyst can result in deformity of the nasal septum.

ETIOLOGY/PATHOPHYSIOLOGY

Sinus cysts occur infrequently in the foal and are considered congenital anomalies of unknown etiology. In some instances the cysts have been hypothesized to be due to abnormal placement of

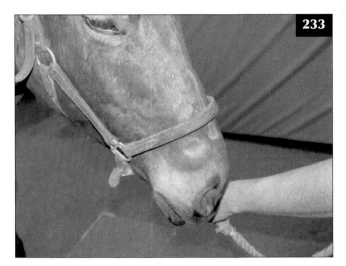

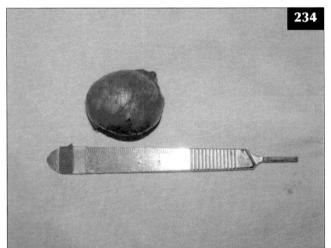

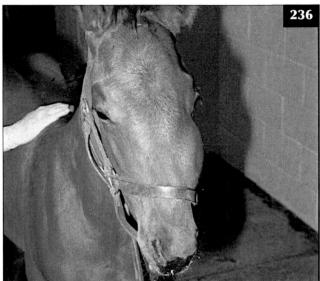

236 A 1-month-old foal with a maxillary sinus cyst. (Courtesy of R. Emberston.)

CLINICAL PRESENTATION

The most common clinical signs of sinus cysts are facial deformity (often unilateral), nasal discharge, dullness on percussion of the sinus, and partial airway obstruction. The nasal discharge is characterized as serous to mucopurulent, and rarely malodorous unless a secondary infection is present.

DIFFERENTIAL DIAGNOSIS

Tables 46 and *47* or skull trauma.

DIAGNOSIS

Nonspecific physical examination abnormalities would include facial deformity, nasal discharge, and decreased air movement from the nostrils. Endoscopic examination of the upper airway would identify a narrowed nasal passage due to a soft tissue mass or deviation of the nasal septum. Radiographs of the skull may demonstrate fluid lines in the sinus and delineate the cyst as a soft tissue density. The radiographs will also help to assess the degree of nasal septal deviation or facial bone deformity. Often the definitive diagnosis and degree of involvement is not made until surgery.

MANAGEMENT

The best treatment is surgical removal of the cyst and the involved conchal lining. Early diagnosis and complete surgical removal can result in a functionally sound and cosmetically acceptable individual. The above-mentioned therapy carries a good prognosis and low recurrence rate.

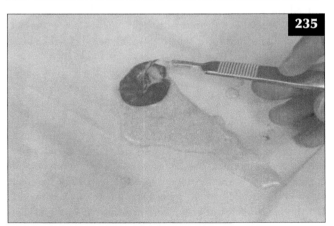

233–235 (233) Epidermal inclusion cyst in a 4-month-old foal. **(234)** Excised cyst from the foal in **233**. **(235)** Fluid contained within the cyst. (Courtesy of B. Woodie.)

dentigerous tissue. Sinus cysts can result in dynamic change in the airflow through the nasal passage due to facial deformity or physical obstruction by the soft tissue mass. Congenital cyst may be slowly expanding and may not produce any clinical signs until the cyst is large and the foal is older.

PROGRESSIVE ETHMOIDAL HEMATOMA

KEY POINTS
- Rare in foals.
- Clinical signs include facial deformity, respiratory stridor, and/ or serosanguineous nasal discharge.
- Endoscopy and/or radiography are useful in diagnosis.

DEFINITION/OVERVIEW

Progressive ethmoidal hematoma is a slowly enlarging, encapsulated, hemorrhagic mass originating from the mucosal lining of the ethmoidal conchae. This condition rarely develops in foals.

ETIOLOGY/PATHOPHYSIOLOGY

The etiology is unknown. The hematoma enlarges by fibrotic reaction in zones of repeated hemorrhage. Local pressure by the mass causes erosion and resorption of bone. In the foal, facial deformity is often noted due to the relatively softer bones. Respiratory stridor results from the mass changing the dynamics of airflow in the nasal passage.

CLINICAL PRESENTATION

The clinical presentation of a progressive ethmoidal hematoma would include facial deformity and respiratory stridor. Varying degrees of serosanguineous nasal discharge may also be present.

DIFFERENTIAL DIAGNOSIS

Tables 46 and *47.*

DIAGNOSIS

Endoscopic evaluation of the nasal passages and nasopharynx may identify a portion of the hematoma protruding into these regions from the ethmoid area, which is suggestive of an ethmoid hematoma (**237**). Radiographs of the head may reveal the appearance of a soft tissue opacity that involves the area of the ethmoturbinate, paranasal sinus, and nasal passage. CT can help to differentiate between the different structures of the nasal passages. Definitive diagnosis is from biopsy of the mass.

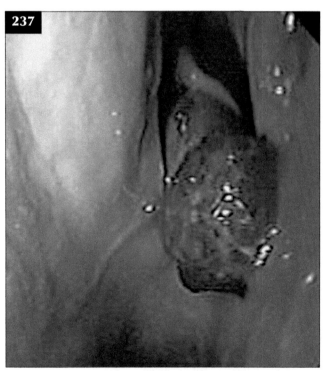

237 Endoscopic view of an ethmoid hematoma. (Courtesy of B. Woodie.)

MANAGEMENT

The rate of progression of the lesion is unknown. Complete surgical removal or laser ablation of the mass is the best therapy. The recurrence rate is unknown in the foal, but in the adult it is reported to be 50%.

CHOANAL ATRESIA

KEY POINTS

- Choanal atresia is a rare congenital abnormality of embryonic development.
- Unilateral or bilateral failure of communication between the nasal cavity and the nasopharynx.
- Clinical signs include complete to partial airway obstruction from birth.
- Complete obstruction requires emergency tracheotomy or oral–tracheal intubation.

DEFINITION/OVERVIEW

Choanal atresia is a rare congenital abnormality reported in the neonate.

ETIOLOGY/PATHOPHYSIOLOGY

Choanal atresia results from a failure of the bucconasal membrane located at the caudal extent of the nasal cavity to rupture during embryonic development. The lesion can either be unilateral or bilateral. The failure of the rupture of this membrane results in an absence of communication between the nasal cavity and the nasopharynx. When both nasal passages are affected, the result is complete airway obstruction.

CLINICAL PRESENTATION

Complete airway obstruction will result if the foal is born with bilateral complete choanal atresia. If only one side is affected, the neonate will not be in distress, although it will only have normal airflow through one nostril. This individual may also make a loud respiratory noise and have evidence of exercise intolerance.

DIFFERENTIAL DIAGNOSIS

Tables 45 and *46.*

DIAGNOSIS

Nasal endoscopy reveals an inability to pass the endoscope into the nasopharynx and a failure to visualize the pharyngeal anatomy caudal to the membrane on the affected side or sides. Positive contrast radiography with instillation of contrast media into the nares (of the affected side) delineates only the caudal limits of the nares.

MANAGEMENT

An emergency tracheostomy should be performed in those cases that present in respiratory distress. Surgical correction can be performed by resection of the occluding membrane. Appropriate postoperative nursing care includes broad-spectrum antimicrobials, anti-inflammatories, and fluid and nutritional support. The prognosis is unclear because there are no reports of long-term follow-up.

CLEFT PALATE (OR PALATOSCHISIS)

KEY POINTS
- Cleft palate is an uncommon congenital deformity.
- The cleft results in a communication between the oral and nasal cavities.
- The cleft may include the soft palate or the soft and hard palate.
- Bilateral milk discharge is typically noted.
- Palpation or endoscopic evaluation aid diagnosis.
- Surgical repair can be attempted.
- The prognosis is dependent on the size of the cleft.

DEFINITION/OVERVIEW
A cleft palate is an uncommon congenital deformity that has been reported in approximately 0.1%–0.2% of equine births. Occasionally, other congenital deformities (i.e., wry nose, cyclops) are observed with the cleft palate. The heritability in horses is unknown.

ETIOLOGY/PATHOPHYSIOLOGY
The exact etiology is unknown, although possible causes include genetic anomalies or factors, nutritional disorders, or teratogens. The cleft is caused by an interruption in the embryologic closure of the lateral palatine process. The cleft results in a direct communication between the oral and nasal cavities and may involve the soft palate only or the hard and soft palate. In the horse the most common defect reported involves the caudal half to three-quarters of the soft palate.

CLINICAL PRESENTATION
In the newborn foal, bilateral nasal discharge (usually milk) is observed after the foal has been nursing (238); however, if the defect in the palate is small, clinical signs may not be observed until the foal is older.

DIFFERENTIAL DIAGNOSIS
Immature pharynx, nasopharyngeal dysfunction, laryngeal paresis, hypoxic ischemic encephalopathy/disease, dorsal displacement of the soft palate, laryngeal web, persistent frenulum of the epiglottis, nutritional myodegeneration, hyperkalemic periodic paralysis

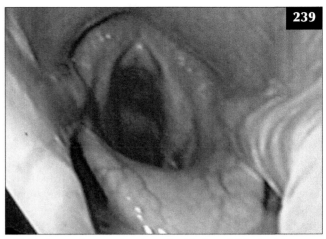

239 Endoscopic examination of a 14-day-old foal with a cleft palate. (Courtesy of R. Embertson.)

(HYPP), botulism, electrolyte/metabolic derangements, esophageal obstruction/choke, gastric distention.

DIAGNOSIS
Observation of the foal after nursing will reveal evidence of milk in both nostrils. An incomplete palate can be palpated on an oral examination. Endoscopic examination of the URT allows for a definitive diagnosis and assessment of the extent of the defect. The margins of the soft palate will be visible and the epiglottis will be positioned in the oropharynx (**239**).

MANAGEMENT
Treatment involves surgical correction of the palatal defect and intensive management of any secondary medical problems such as aspiration pneumonia. Postsurgical complications reported include mandibular osteitis or nonunion and dehiscence failure of the palatal repair. Compromised pharyngeal function, despite successful palate repair, has been reported. The prognosis depends on the size of the defect and involvement of the hard palate.

PHARYNGEAL CYSTS

KEY POINTS
- Pharyngeal cysts are congenital cystic abnormalities of the pharynx.
- Clinical signs may include airway noise, nasal discharge, exercise intolerance, and/or cough.
- Treatment is by surgical excision.

DEFINITION/OVERVIEW
Pharyngeal cysts have been reported to occur in three locations: the dorsal pharyngeal wall, the subepiglottic region, and the soft palate. They are usually evident at a young age, can occur in any breed, and have been commonly reported in male horses.

ETIOLOGY/PATHOPHYSIOLOGY
Pharyngeal cysts are believed to be congenital anomalies. Cysts located on the dorsal pharyngeal wall result from a persistent remnant of the craniopharyngeal duct or Rathke's pouch.

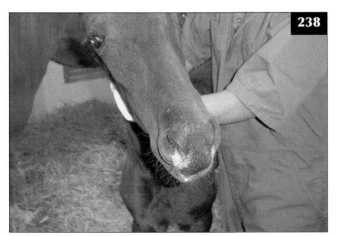

238 Foal with milk coming out of its nostrils.

Subepiglottic cysts have been associated with a congenital remnant of the embryologic thyroglossal duct or trauma. Cysts located on the soft palate are histologically similar to a mucocele.

The presence of a cyst in the pharyngeal region may change the dynamics of airflow through the upper airway, resulting in a respiratory noise on inspiration and expiration. In addition, the cyst could cause a mechanical obstruction, resulting in pharyngeal dysfunction and an inability to protect the airway.

CLINICAL PRESENTATION

Clinical signs associated with pharyngeal cysts include abnormal upper airway noise, cough, exercise intolerance, and nasal discharge. Dysphagia has also been documented. In foals, chronic pneumonia and persistent nasal discharge have been a common clinical presentation reported.

DIFFERENTIAL DIAGNOSIS

Tables 46 through 48.

Table 48. Causes of cough in the pediatric patient

- **Respiratory:**
  - ○ Viral infection
  - ○ Bacterial pneumonia
  - ○ Pleuritis
  - ○ Pharyngitis
  - ○ Strangles
  - ○ Retropharyngeal mass/abscess
  - ○ Pharyngeal paresis
  - ○ Guttural pouch empyema/tympany
  - ○ Subepiglottic cyst
  - ○ Tracheal collapse/stenosis/perforation
  - ○ Aspiration pneumonia (feed material, meconium)
  - ○ Rostral displacement of the palatopharyngeal arch
  - ○ Ethmoidal hematomas
  - ○ Foreign body (nasal, pharyngeal, laryngeal, tracheal, bronchial)
  - ○ Pneumothorax
- **Nonrespiratory:**
  - ○ Esopharyngeal obstruction
  - ○ Neonatal septicemia
  - ○ Left heart failure
  - ○ Congestive heart failure
  - ○ Tetralogy of Fallot
  - ○ Endocarditis

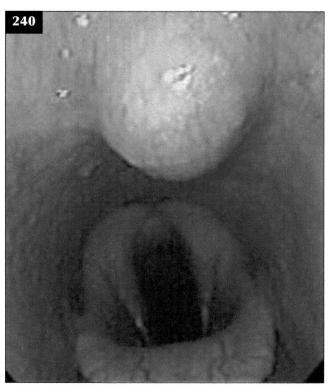

240 Endoscopic examination of pharyngeal cysts. (Courtesy of B. Woodie.)

DIAGNOSIS

Endoscopic evaluation of the pharyngeal region is the best procedure to identify a pharyngeal cyst (**240**). A soft tissue mass is visualized directly under the epiglottis in the aryepiglottic fold, in various dorsal locations close to the pharynx, or within the soft palate. Dorsal displacement of the soft palate may be observed in those individuals with a cyst involving the soft palate. Radiographs of the skull and pharyngeal region may be used to evaluate the extensiveness of the cyst below the epiglottis and those involving the soft palate. Contrast radiography after oral administration of barium sulfate can be helpful in isolating cysts located on the soft palate.

MANAGEMENT

Surgical excision is the best treatment for pharyngeal cysts. The surgery can be accomplished through a laryngotomy, pharyngotomy, transnasal, or transoral approach. Noncontact laser ablation is another successful treatment option and obviates the need for a surgical incision. To prevent recurrence, the cyst and its lining must be completely removed. The prognosis is considered favorable if recognized early.

ROSTRAL DISPLACEMENT OF THE PALATOPHARYNGEAL ARCH

KEY POINTS

- Rostral displacement of the palatopharyngeal arch is due to a malformation of the supporting structures of this region.
- Results in dysfunction of the pharynx and abnormal airflow.

- Clinical signs include dysphagia, cough, stridor, exercise intolerance, and possibly chronic aspiration pneumonia.
- Prognosis for athletic performance is poor.

DEFINITION/OVERVIEW

Rostral displacement of the palatopharyngeal arch is a congenital anomaly that causes pharyngeal dysfunction. This anomaly may be seen in conjunction with other anomalies such as absence of the cricopharyngeal muscle, deformed thyroid cartilage, absence of the cricothyroid articulation, and degeneration of the recurrent laryngeal nerve.

ETIOLOGY/PATHOPHYSIOLOGY

Rostral displacement of the palatopharyngeal arch is believed to be secondary to malformation or agenesis of laryngeal cartilages (primarily the thyroid cartilage) and associated laryngeal muscles. The palatopharyngeal arch forms the caudal border of the intrapharyngeal ostium and normally the larynx protrudes through this ostium. Due to the malformation of the supporting structures of this area, the palatopharyngeal arch is displaced rostrally, resulting in dysfunction of the pharynx and an abnormal airflow pattern in the upper airway.

CLINICAL PRESENTATION

Clinical signs include dysphagia, persistent cough, respiratory stridor, and exercise intolerance. Secondary aspiration pneumonia may also be present.

DIFFERENTIAL DIAGNOSIS

Tables 46 and *48*.

DIAGNOSIS

Endoscopic evaluation of the larynx reveals that the corniculate process of one or both arytenoids cartilages is partially or completely obstructed from view by the displaced palatopharyngeal arch (**241, 242**).

MANAGEMENT

Surgical laser ablation of the displaced palate has been performed successfully, although the prognosis for an equine athlete is poor. Concurrent anomalies may also limit the effectiveness of surgical treatment.

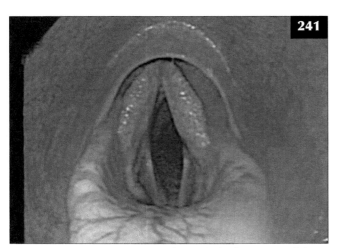

241 Endoscopic examination of rostral displacement of the palatopharyngeal arch. (Courtesy of B. Woodie.)

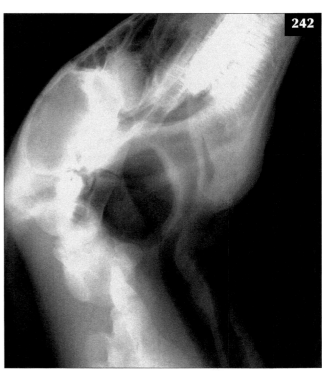

242 Lateral radiographs of the pharyngeal region of a 2-month-old foal with rostral displacement of the palatopharyngeal arch.

RETROPHARYNGEAL ABSCESS

See Chapter 3, Infectious Diseases, *Streptococcus equi*, pp. 48–50.

PERILARYNGEAL ACCESSORY BRONCHIAL CYSTS AND BRANCHIAL CYSTS

KEY POINTS

- These are rare cysts that form around the structures of the larynx.
- Usually they do not cause clinical signs without exercise.
- Transcutaneous ultrasound may identify the cysts.

DEFINITION/OVERVIEW

Perilaryngeal accessory bronchial cysts and branchial cysts are congenital and developmental anomalies that are very rarely reported because they generally do not cause clinical signs in the foal.

ETIOLOGY/PATHOPHYSIOLOGY

Perilaryngeal accessory bronchial cysts and branchial cysts result from an alteration in normal embryologic development in the laryngeal region. The glottis and trachea are derived from the tracheal bud of the foregut and the supraglottic region of the larynx is branchial in origin. It is possible for cysts to develop as these structures join around the larynx. The cysts can cause a change in the dynamics of airflow in the laryngeal region, which may become more evident at exercise.

CLINICAL PRESENTATION

The most common clinical presentation is a respiratory noise at exercise, which may not be evident until the foal is older.

8

DIFFERENTIAL DIAGNOSIS
Table 46.

DIAGNOSIS
Deep palpation of the laryngeal region may identify the presence of a fluctuant swelling. Endoscopic evaluation of the upper airway may reveal laryngeal hemiplegia, most likely due to possible damage to the recurrent laryngeal nerve or malformation of the cricoid and thyroid cartilages. A cyst-like structure may be noted on transcutaneous ultrasound of the laryngeal region. Aseptic aspiration may help provide a tentative diagnosis. Definitive diagnosis is ultimately made by histopathology of the cystic tissue.

MANAGEMENT
The treatment of choice is complete resection of the cystic tissue. The prognosis is good if complete resection of the cyst is accomplished and if irreparable damage to adjacent structures has not occurred.

PHARYNGEAL COLLAPSE

KEY POINTS
- Dorsal and lateral collapse of the pharyngeal walls.
- May be congenital or a result of space-occupying lesions, muscular weakness, neuropathies, or inflammation.
- HYPP should be considered in the Quarter Horse.
- Tachypnea or respiratory distress is present.

DEFINITION/OVERVIEW
Pharyngeal collapse is defined as dorsal and lateral collapse of the pharyngeal walls due to mechanical or functional disorder.

ETIOLOGY/PATHOPHYSIOLOGY
Collapse of the pharyngeal area may result from a space-occupying mass (abscess), guttural pouch empyema/tympany, inflammation, deformity, muscular weakness (HYPP), or neuropathies causing weakness of the musculature. Rostral obstruction to the pharynx results in increased negative pressures in the pharyngeal cavity. Neuropathies cause dysfunction of the supporting musculature of the pharynx that result in collapse due to increased negative pressures within the pharyngeal region.

CLINICAL PRESENTATION
The foal may present tachypneic or in respiratory distress. Most affected foals have a history of a respiratory noise (primarily expiratory).

DIFFERENTIAL DIAGNOSIS
Tables 45 and 46.

DIAGNOSIS
Endoscopic examination of the upper airway reveals collapsing of the pharyngeal region (**243**). To further assess the primary

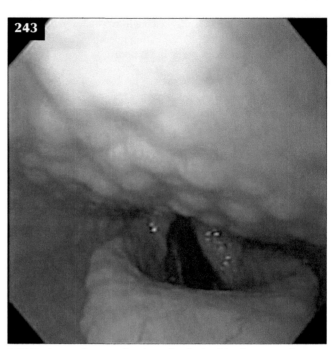

243 Endoscopic examination of a foal with pharyngeal collapse.

cause, radiographs or ultrasonograms of the pharyngeal region may be needed.

MANAGEMENT
The best treatment depends on the inciting cause. Medical management may be adequate if the cause is an abscess or a metabolic disorder (HYPP or neuropathy). A surgical approach may be needed if the cause is a deformity or a space-occupying mass.

GUTTURAL POUCH TYMPANY

KEY POINTS
- Unilateral/bilateral distension of the guttural pouch with air.
- Can be congenital or acquired.
- Congenital guttural pouch tympany is a result of an abnormality of the guttural pouch opening (redundant mucosa).
- Acquired guttural pouch tympany is a result of infection or inflammation.
- Results in formation of a one-way valve, which allows air in but not out.
- Unilateral/bilateral retropharyngeal swelling may be noted.
- With severe distension, stridor or dysphagia may be noted.
- Radiographs or catheterization with deflation of the pouch can be diagnostic.
- Surgical intervention is often required.

DEFINITION/OVERVIEW
Guttural pouch tympany is characterized by unilateral or bilateral distension of the guttural pouch with air due to a malfunctioning of the pharyngeal orifice. This condition affects foals

from birth to 1 year of age. For unknown reasons, more cases have been documented in fillies.

ETIOLOGY/PATHOPHYSIOLOGY

This condition can be either congenital or acquired. The congenital form is due to a redundancy of the mucosa on the ventral aspect of the guttural pouch opening (plica salpingopharyngea). It has also been postulated that upper airway infection and inflammation may result in edema of the tissue on the ventral aspect of the guttural pouch opening. The dysfunction results in the opening of the guttural pouch acting as a one-way valve, only allowing air to enter the pouch.

CLINICAL PRESENTATION

A nonpainful, unilateral soft fluctuant swelling may be noted in the retropharyngeal space. Bilateral swelling may indicate a bilateral condition, although unilateral involvement can give the appearance of bilateral involvement. Variable respiratory distress has been reported. Early in the disease an inspiratory stridor may be noted to worsen with excitement. In cases with severe distension, respiratory distress can result due to collapse of the dorsal pharyngeal wall obstructing the larynx. Dysphagia and milk coming from the nostril may also be observed in cases of severe distension.

DIFFERENTIAL DIAGNOSIS

Tables 45 and *46.*

DIAGNOSIS

Swelling in the retropharyngeal region will be noted on physical examination (**244, 245**). Radiography of the retropharyngeal region will reveal gas distension of one or both guttural pouches (**246**). Endoscopy of the upper airway may reveal pharyngeal collapse. Catheterization of the guttural pouches through the pharyngeal opening deflates the pouch, confirms the diagnosis, and identifies unilateral or bilateral involvement. Percutaneous centesis can also confirm the diagnosis. Ultrasound of the area may identify gas distension and may help differentiate between unilateral and bilateral involvement.

MANAGEMENT

Conservative medical management includes antimicrobials, antiinflammatories, and decompression by insertion of an indwelling catheter into the guttural pouch if the tympany is not severe (**54**). If the foal is in respiratory distress, a tracheotomy may be required to provide a patent airway. More commonly, surgical intervention is required. Several procedures have been described and include fenestration of the septum between the guttural pouches by excision and electrosurgery, or photoablation, or surgical excision or photoablation of the redundant plica salpingopharyngea tissue. An alternative procedure involves creation of a fistula with the pharynx to achieve drainage. Prognosis is good with surgical treatment provided that care is taken to avoid iatrogenic neurologic damage and that secondary complications (aspiration pneumonia) have not arisen.

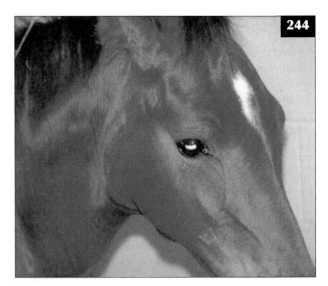

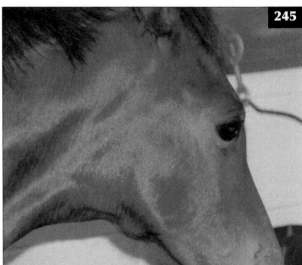

244, 245 A 2-month-old foal with guttural pouch tympany.

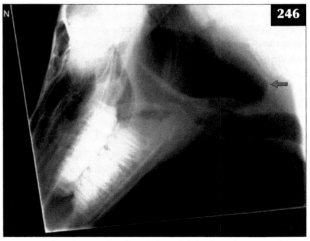

246 Lateral radiograph of a 3-day-old foal with guttural pouch tympany. Note that the guttural pouch extends to the cranial aspect of C3 (arrow).

GUTTURAL POUCH EMPYEMA

KEY POINTS

- Guttural pouch empyema is an accumulation of purulent exudate.
- Results from extension of upper airway infection or abscess rupture into the guttural pouch.
- *Streptococcus equi* is the most common pathogen involved.
- Mucopurulent nasal discharge is often noted.
- Endoscopy identifies purulent discharge from the guttural pouch opening.
- Medical therapy and local lavage are required.

DEFINITION/OVERVIEW

Guttural pouch empyema is an accumulation of purulent exudates within one or both of the guttural pouches.

ETIOLOGY/PATHOPHYSIOLOGY

Empyema results from extension of an upper airway infection or rupture of a retropharyngeal abscess into the guttural pouch. Infection can become established because drainage from the guttural pouch is poor. More chronic infection can result from scarring of the pharyngeal opening and failure of drainage from the pouch. The most common bacteria isolated are beta-hemolytic streptococci, especially *Streptococcus equi* (see Chapter 3, Infectious Diseases, *Streptococcus equi*, p. 48).

CLINICAL PRESENTATION

Mucopurulent nasal discharge and lymphadenopathy are the most common clinical signs. Occasionally, fever, respiratory stridor, and dysphagia may be observed on clinical presentation.

DIFFERENTIAL DIAGNOSIS

Tables 19, 46, and *47.*

DIAGNOSIS

Endoscopy of the upper airway identifies purulent exudates at the guttural pouch opening. Exudates or chondroid can be seen within the affected pouch (**247**). Lateral radiographs of the skull can help to identify material within the pouches or retropharyngeal abscesses (**248**). An aspirate of the purulent material through the pharyngeal opening enables the causative organism to be identified by culture.

MANAGEMENT

Medical management includes local and, often, systemic therapy, as well as addressing secondary complications (aspiration pneumonia or dysphagia). Local lavage of the pouch with balanced electrolyte solution is accomplished by catheterization blindly (**54**) or through the biopsy port on the endoscope. If inspissated material or chondroids are present, surgical drainage may need to be pursued.

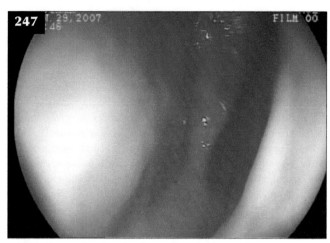

247 Endoscopic examination of guttural pouch empyema. Note the purulent material on the floor of the pouch.

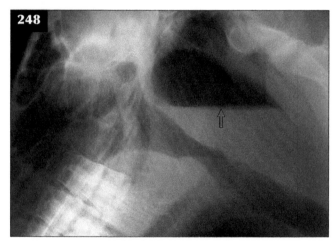

248 Lateral radiograph of a 2-month-old foal with guttural pouch empyema due to *Streptococcus equi* infection. Note the enlarged retropharyngeal lymph nodes and the fluid line in the guttural pouch (arrow).

DORSAL DISPLACEMENT OF THE SOFT PALATE

KEY POINTS

- Caudal free edge of the soft palate displaces dorsally over the epiglottis.
- Condition is uncommon in foals.
- Results in partial obstruction of the upper airway, with potential tachypnea and dysphagia.

DEFINITION/OVERVIEW

Dorsal displacement of the soft palate is described as the intermittent or persistent malpositioning of the caudal free edge of the soft palate dorsal to the epiglottis. The displacement results in obstruction of the upper airway by the soft palate and disruption of the airtight seal of the intrapharyngeal ostium around the laryngeal cartilages. The condition is uncommon in foals.

ETIOLOGY/PATHOPHYSIOLOGY

The exact etiology is unknown. It may be due to primary pharyngeal and palatal muscular laxity or inflammation in the pharyngeal region. Muscular laxity may prevent proper coordination of the muscles of the soft palate or result in flaccid pharyngeal musculature and dynamic collapse of the pharynx, thus narrowing the nasopharyngeal lumen. Because of the flaccidity and redundancy of the pharyngeal structures, when the foal nurses or inspires the flaccid soft palate is sucked upward and into the larynx, resulting in respiratory strider, dysphagia, and food regurgitation. If the soft palate has sufficient muscle tone, but there is evidence of redundant or inflamed surrounding soft tissue, strider only may be present without regurgitation.

CLINICAL PRESENTATION

Common presenting signs include respiratory stridor, tachypnea, dysphagia, and the presence of milk in the nostril. Secondary aspiration pneumonia can develop as a result of the dysphagia.

DIFFERENTIAL DIAGNOSIS

Table 46 and neurologic deficits affecting swallowing, esophageal obstruction/choke, and electrolyte/metabolic derangements.

DIAGNOSIS

Endoscopic evaluation of the upper airway provides the best diagnosis and may reveal redundancy of the soft tissues of the soft palate or dorsal displacement of the soft palate (**249**). Radiographs of the upper airway may reveal edematous pharyngeal structures.

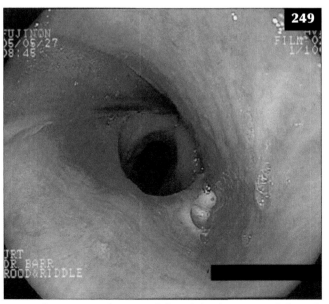

249 Endoscopic evaluation of dorsal displacement of the soft palate. (Courtesy of B. Woodie.)

MANAGEMENT

Medical management includes anti-inflammatories, antimicrobials, and nutritional support. Resolution has been reported within 4 days. Surgical excision of the caudal margin of the soft palate (staphylectomy) may be needed if medical management is not effective. The prognosis for these foals is difficult to determine because there are only a few reports in the literature.

NASOPHARYNGEAL DYSFUNCTION

KEY POINTS

- The condition is rare in foals.
- Immature neural circuit of nasopharynx and larynx.
- Supportive medical therapy.
- Long-term prognosis unknown.

DEFINITION/OVERVIEW

Nasopharyngeal dysfunction rarely occurs in the foal, but when it does it occurs during the first month of life.

ETIOLOGY/PATHOPHYSIOLOGY

The etiology is unknown, although as described in the human literature this dysfunction may be due to an immaturity of the neuromuscular reflexes and defense mechanisms that support the nasopharynx and larynx. It is suspected that these neonates have an immature neural circuit that results in muscular dysfunction and incoordination in the nasopharynx. The result is dysphagia and nasopharyngeal collapse.

CLINICAL PRESENTATION

Clinical signs include respiratory stridor, dysphagia, milk noted in the nostrils, and occasionally respiratory distress.

DIFFERENTIAL DIAGNOSIS

Tables 45 and *46*.

DIAGNOSIS

A definitive diagnosis can be difficult and only made after ruling out other differentials. Endoscopic examination of the upper airway may reveal flaccidity of the nasopharyngeal region, nasopharyngeal edema, pooling of milk in the nasopharynx, and persistent dorsal displacement of the soft palate (**250, 251**).

MANAGEMENT

Most cases respond to supportive medical therapy including broad-spectrum antimicrobials and anti-inflammatories. If the foal is dysphagic, enteral feeding can be performed through a nasogastric tube or parental feeding can be initiated. A tracheotomy may need to be performed if the foal is in severe respiratory distress. Recovery in most foals is usually within 10–14 days. One report documents that prognosis for life is favorable but for athleticism is only fair.

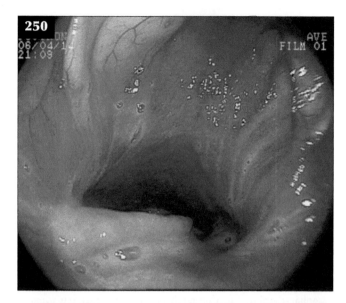

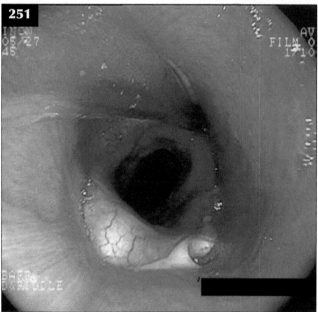

250, 251 Endoscopic evaluation of a 1-day-old foal with nasopharyngeal dysfunction. (Courtesy B. Woodie.)

LARYNGEAL WEB

KEY POINTS
- Often reported with other congenital abnormalities.
- Web of tissue on the central aspect of the rima glottis.
- Treatment is surgical resection of the tissue.

DEFINITION/OVERVIEW
Laryngeal web is a congenital problem infrequently reported in foals. This disease has been reported with other congenital abnormalities such as cleft palate, epiglottic hypoplasia, and abnormal movement of the arytenoid cartilage.

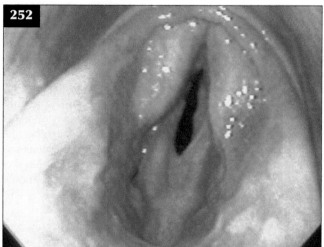

252 Endoscopic view of a laryngeal web. (Courtesy of B. Woodie.)

ETIOLOGY/PATHOPHYSIOLOGY
During development the larynx fails to completely recanalize and a piece of tissue remains on the rima glottides. The laryngeal web results in fusion of the vocal folds due to a web of tissue on the ventral aspect of the rima glottides.

CLINICAL PRESENTATION
Foals present with respiratory stridor, respiratory distress, and dysphagia. Milk may be noted coming from the nostrils after nursing.

DIFFERENTIAL DIAGNOSIS
Tables 45 and *46*, botulism, and esophageal obstruction/choke.

DIAGNOSIS
Definitive diagnosis is based on endoscopic examination of the larynx in which a web of tissue is noted on the ventral aspect of the rima glottis (**252**). Lateral radiographs of the laryngeal region may reveal abnormalities of the laryngeal cartilages.

MANAGEMENT
If the foal appears in respiratory distress, a patent airway may need to be established with a tracheotomy. Surgical resection of the tissue (with the foal under general anesthesia) by laser excision or through a laryngotomy is the most logical treatment. The prognosis is unknown, although one possible complication of surgical correction would be stricture of the larynx during healing.

PERSISTENT FRENULUM OF THE EPIGLOTTIS

KEY POINTS
- Congenital anomaly.
- Dorsal displacement of soft palate due to frenulum.
- Treatment is surgical resection of the frenulum.

DEFINITION/OVERVIEW
Persistent frenulum of the ventral aspect of the epiglottis is a congenital anomaly that results in consistently dorsal displacement of the soft palate. It is a rare condition.

ETIOLOGY/PATHOPHYSIOLOGY

Several possible developmental scenarios exist for the presence of the frenulum including inappropriate divergence of the epiglottis and the base of the tongue, altered closure of the thyroglossal duct, or fibrosis of the normal glossoepiglottic fold and hypoepiglottis muscle. A membranous band of tissue (frenulum), located between the ventral aspect of the epiglottis and the base of the tongue, causes persistent dorsal displacement of the soft palate. This ridge of tissue may be thin and membranous or rounded and thickened.

CLINICAL PRESENTATION

Clinical signs are usually present at birth and include dysphagia and oronasal reflux of milk. If the condition goes undiagnosed for several days, the risk of aspiration pneumonia is great.

DIFFERENTIAL DIAGNOSIS

Cleft palate, nasopharyngeal dysfunction, laryngeal web, dorsal displacement of the soft palate, pharyngeal cysts, esophageal obstruction/choke, gastric distension due to gastrointestinal (GI) dysfunction, botulism, HYPP, nutritional myodegeneration, and electrolyte/metabolic derangements.

DIAGNOSIS

Endoscopy of the upper airway reveals persistent dorsal displacement of the soft palate. Definitive diagnosis is made under general anesthesia by oral endoscopy. This procedure identifies the tip of the epiglottis directed ventrally under the soft palate and a ridge of tissue on the ventral aspect of the epiglottis.

MANAGEMENT

Surgical resection of the frenulum is the best treatment. If the condition is recognized and treated early before the establishment of severe aspiration pneumonia, the prognosis is excellent.

TRACHEAL STENOSIS AND TRACHEAL COLLAPSE

KEY POINTS

• An uncommon condition; may be congenital or acquired.
• Clinical signs are dependent on the severity of the condition and may be as severe as respiratory distress.

DEFINITION/OVERVIEW

Tracheal stenosis is a narrowing or stricture of the tracheal lumen. Trachea collapse is a widespread or segmental dorsoventral flattening of tracheal cartilage. Both disorders are uncommon in the equine pediatric patient.

ETIOLOGY/PATHOPHYSIOLOGY

Tracheal stenosis can be divided into two categories depending on whether the defect is intrinsic to the cartilaginous supporting structure (primary) or the result of external structures impinging on the trachea (secondary). Primary tracheal stenosis can result from trauma to the tracheal rings by external foreign body penetration, iatrogenic trauma to the tracheal rings secondary to tracheotomy, or damage to the tracheal mucosa and cartilage after endotracheal intubation. Possible causes of secondary tracheal stenosis include abscessation of regional lymph nodes and peritracheal hematomas. The exact etiology of tracheal collapse has not been determined, although it may be a sequela to trauma to the trachea or secondary to a congenital abnormality in cartilage development or degeneration of cartilage.

Tracheal stenosis occurs due to excessive fibrosis associated with mucosal inflammation in foals where there is a primary cause for the stenosis. Peritracheal abscesses and hematomas cause external compression on the trachea. Tracheal collapse results from changes in pressure gradients across the abnormal area of the tracheal cartilage.

CLINICAL PRESENTATION

Regardless of the cause of the tracheal stenosis or collapse, the severity of clinical signs depends on the severity and location of the narrowing. In mild cases, clinical signs may only be evident at exercise and may include increased inspiratory stridor and increased respiratory rate. These signs may not be evident until the foal is older. In those cases with severe tracheal narrowing, nostril flaring, respiratory stridor, tachypnea, respiratory distress, and cyanosis may be present while the animal is at rest. Additional clinical signs include laryngeal hemiplegia and fever secondary to peritracheal abscesses or bronchopneumonia.

DIFFERENTIAL DIAGNOSIS

Tables 45 and *46*.

DIAGNOSIS

Historical information such as endemic *Streptococcus equi* infection or recent trauma may help in establishing a diagnosis. A complete physical examination may identify the presence of external wounds, deformities, or swelling in the cervical trachea. Palpation of the cervical trachea may reveal the lateral edges of the flattened trachea in the jugular groove. Radiographs can localize the area of stenosis to the cervical or thoracic trachea and differentiate an intraluminal from an extraluminal lesion. Ultrasound of the cervical trachea may assist in identifying an abscess or hematoma. Endoscopic examination of the trachea is invaluable in confirming the location of the stenosis and eliminating the URT as a source of noise, exercise intolerance, and dyspnea (**253**). This modality also provides visualization of anatomic abnormalities associated with stenotic lesions such as tracheal ring and mucosal abnormalities.

MANAGEMENT

If the individual is in severe respiratory distress, a temporary tracheotomy may be needed. An extraluminal lesion such as an abscess or hematoma can be drained with or without ultrasound guidance and the fluid submitted for bacterial culture and antimicrobial sensitivity. Broad-spectrum antimicrobials such as penicillin and an aminoglycoside or a third-generation cephalosporin should be administered until culture results are available. In addition, anti-inflammatory therapy with flunixin meglumine may help to reduce inflammation. In cases of both tracheal stenosis and tracheal collapse, surgical intervention may be necessary to restore the luminal shape. This includes procedures such as tracheal resection and anastomosis, and extraluminal or intraluminal prosthesis.

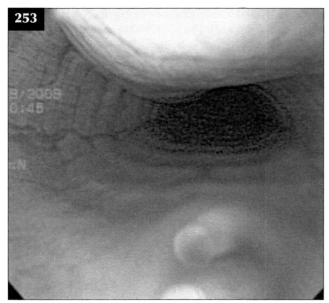

253 Tracheal stenosis or collapse. (Courtesy of B. Woodie.)

However, the approach depends on etiologic factors, the length of trachea involved, and accessibility.

TRACHEAL PERFORATION

KEY POINTS
- Blunt trauma to the trachea.
- A subcutaneous, crepitant swelling may be noted.
- Continued leakage of air may result in air in the mediastinum and possibly pneumothorax.
- Small tears may respond to conservative therapy.

DEFINITION/OVERVIEW
Tracheal perforation rarely occurs in the equine pediatric patient and is the result of blunt trauma.

ETIOLOGY/PATHOPHYSIOLOGY
Tracheal perforation results from a traumatic condition. Trauma in the cervical region from a kick is the most likely cause. Perforations of the trachea tend to occur dorsally or dorsolaterally in the tracheal soft tissue. Blunt trauma can exacerbate the normal dorsoventral flattening of the trachea, resulting in an increased shear stress at the junction of the cartilaginous rings (dorsolaterally) and tracheal muscle (dorsally). The trauma can also cause increased tension of the dorsal structures with resultant ventral compression. Tracheal perforation allows air to dissect into the peritracheal tissue, resulting in subcutaneous emphysema.

CLINICAL PRESENTATION
The only noticeable clinical sign may be a subcutaneous swelling along the cervical region of the neck that is nonpainful, soft, easily indented, mobile, and crepitant. Obvious skin damage may be observed along with the subcutaneous emphysema. Continued leakage of air into the mediastinum may predispose to pneumothorax and result in respiratory distress.

DIFFERENTIAL DIAGNOSIS
Esophageal rupture, skin wounds in the axillary region, cellulitis, fasciitis and myositis from gas-forming bacteria (*Clostridium* spp.), and iatrogenic procedures such as percutaneous transtracheal aspirate. See also *Table 45*.

DIAGNOSIS
Physical examination may reveal an area of skin damage along the cervical trachea region and the presence of subcutaneous emphysema. Sometimes, in more severe cases, subcutaneous emphysema may involve the head, ventral abdomen, and proximal extremities (**254**). Radiographs often do not identify defects in the trachea, but dissecting planes of air may be observed in the soft tissue of the neck (**255**). Thoracic radiographs are helpful for identifying a pneumomediastinum, marked air contrast around both the esophagus and trachea, and a pneumothorax. Tracheoscopy is the ideal modality to diagnosis a tracheal perforation.

MANAGEMENT
Treatment of perforations of the trachea in the cervical region depends on the extent of the injury. Small tears can be managed

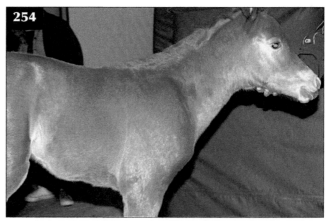

254 A 2-month-old foal with subcutaneous emphysema due to trauma resulting in a small perforation of the trachea.

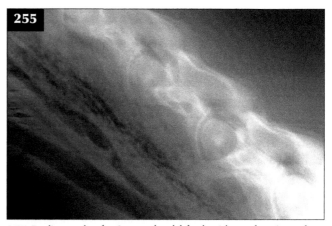

255 Radiograph of a 2-month-old foal with perforation of the trachea. Note the dissecting planes of air in the soft tissue.

conservatively with broad-spectrum antimicrobial therapy, anti-inflammatories, and careful monitoring for complications. In most cases a fibrin seal forms within 48 hours. Generally, both subcutaneous emphysema and pneumomediastinum resolve without specific therapy. If a large mucosal defect is present, it may need to be sutured once the foal is stabilized. A tube thoracotomy with a suction drain may need to be placed if a severe pneumothorax is present.

DISORDERS OF THE LOWER RESPIRATORY TRACT

BACTERIAL PNEUMONIA

KEY POINTS
- Common in neonatal and older foals.
- Due to immature immune system.
- May be secondary to viral infection.
- Clinical signs vary from depression, fever, nasal discharge, cough, and respiratory distress.
- Abnormalities diagnosed on radiographs or ultrasound.
- Transtracheal aspiration needed to identify bacterium.
- Antimicrobial therapy should be for several weeks.

DEFINITION/OVERVIEW
Bacterial pneumonia is a concern in the neonatal and older foal. Both age groups are susceptible due to a compromise in their immunologic protection. In the neonate, bacterial pneumonia is often secondary to sepsis and failure of passive transfer (FPT), whereas in the older foal, bacterial pneumonia is a primary disease and susceptibility may be due to waxing of the maternal antibodies and a delay in the production of their own antibodies.

ETIOLOGY/PATHOPHYSIOLOGY
The organisms that most commonly cause bacterial pneumonia in neonates include *Escherichia coli*, *Klebsiella* spp., *Actinobacillus equuli*, and *Streptococcus* spp., whereas in the older foal, *Streptococcus zooepidemicus* and *Rhodococcus equi* are the most common organisms isolated (*Table 49*).

The respiratory system can serve as a primary portal of entry of bacteria into the body or the individual may be infected secondarily as a result of septicemia and hematogenous spread of bacteria. In the neonate, bacteria can gain entry by inhalation, ingestion, or through the umbilicus and spread hematogenously to the lungs. Infection most commonly occurs shortly after birth, but it also can occur *in utero* or during parturition. In the older foal, bacterial pneumonia often follows viral infections or other stressful events that affect the pulmonary defense mechanism. In addition, pneumonia may result secondary to any condition that causes dysfunction of the larynx or pharynx.

CLINICAL PRESENTATION
Early in the course of the disease the foal may only be weak or depressed. As the disease progresses, nostril flare, tachypnea, or an increased abdominal component may be present. The older foal may have a fever, nasal discharge, and a cough, whereas the neonate may have clinical signs of septicemia. Both age groups can present in severe respiratory distress.

Table 49. Bacteria that cause pneumonia in the pediatric patient
- *Streptococcus zooepidemicus*
- *Streptococcus pneumonia*
- *Streptococcus equi*
- *Actinobacillus* spp.
- *Pasteurella* spp.
- *Klebsiella* spp.
- *Bordetella bronchiseptica*
- *Escherichia coli*
- *Enterobacter* spp.
- *Staphylococcus* spp.
- *Salmonella* spp.
- *Bacteroides* spp.
- *Pseudomonas* spp.
- *Rhodococcus equi*
- *Clostridium* spp.
- *Peptostreptococcus* spp.
- *Fusobacterium* spp.

DIFFERENTIAL DIAGNOSIS
Tables 19, 45 through *48*.

DIAGNOSIS
History/physical examination
History of endemic problems on the farm and, in the case of the neonate, gestational length is important. Auscultation of the thorax may reveal decreased or adventitial bronchovesicular sounds, which is typically more evident in the older foal. The number and type of abnormal lung sounds may not correlate well with the degree of pulmonary dysfunction, especially in the neonate.

Hematology
The hematological changes may vary from a leukocytosis to leukopenia. Often, a hyperfibrinogenemia is noted.

Radiography
The presence of radiographic infiltrates can confirm the diagnosis of pneumonia, although radiographic changes may lag behind clinical signs (*Table 43*; **254–256**). Thoracic radiographs can also help in following the progression of the disease in response to treatment. In the neonate, radiographic interpretation may be difficult because of the similarities between the abnormalities associated with pneumonia and other respiratory conditions such as atelectasis or immature lungs.

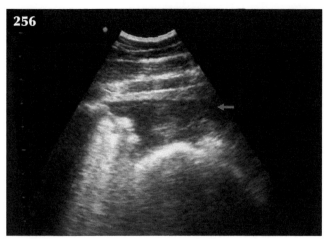

256 Ultrasonogram of consolidated lung (arrow).

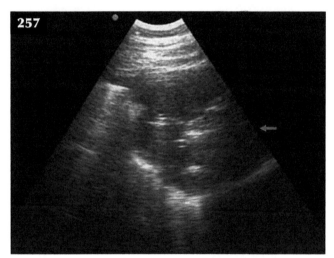

257 Ultrasonogram of a pulmonary abscess (arrow).

Ultrasound

Ultrasound may be useful in identifying consolidated lung (**256**) and pulmonary abscesses (**257**).

Arterial blood gas

Arterial blood gas analysis is most often performed on the newborn foal. This procedure can be useful to define the severity of the disease and the type of therapy needed.

Blood culture

A blood culture is most often performed in the septic neonate to help identify the causative agent.

Transtracheal aspiration

This procedure can be very important for confirming the diagnosis and identifying a causative organism (*Table 44*; **227, 228**). Gram stains of material obtained from a transtracheal aspirate may help to establish a tentative identification of the organism, which is then confirmed by culture and sensitivity (**258**). A compromised septic neonate or a severely distressed foal may not be a good candidate for a transtracheal aspirate.

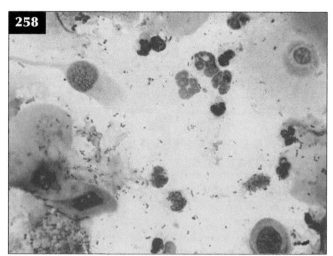

258 Cytology of a percutaneous transtracheal aspirate from a foal with pneumonia. Note the inflammatory cells and mixed bacteria (rods and cocci).

Culture of endotracheal tube

This procedure is only performed on intubated neonatal foals receiving mechanical ventilation; often the results are not very rewarding.

MANAGEMENT

Antimicrobial therapy is an essential part of medical treatment of bacterial pneumonia. Prior to the results of bacterial cultures (transtracheal aspirate/blood culture), broad-spectrum antimicrobial therapy should be instituted. A combination of penicillin and an aminoglycoside or third-generation cephalosporin will provide the best initial intravenous coverage. Oral options include trimethoprim–sulfonamide, doxycycline, or chloroamphenicol, but if *R equi* is suspected a macrolide agent alone or with rifampin is better. Once the culture results are available, the antimicrobial therapy can be changed accordingly. The length of antimicrobial therapy normally ranges from 2 to 5 weeks. The foal should be closely monitored for response to therapy and the possibility of resistant pneumonia. When administering an aminoglycoside to a compromised foal, aminoglycoside peaks/troughs and careful evaluation of renal function should be performed. A positive response to treatment will be noted by resolution of the abnormal clinical signs (lack of fever, return to normal respiratory rate/effort), improvement in the hemogram, and improvement in thoracic radiographs. In severe cases, intranasal oxygen, bronchodilators, and anti-inflammatories may also be important as part of the treatment. Septic neonates may require additional supportive treatment including parental nutrition, appropriate positioning and turning if recumbent, respiratory stimulants, cardiovascular/hemodynamic support, or mechanical ventilation.

An adjunct to systemic treatment is aerosol administration of therapeutic agents. (**259a and b**). This means of delivery allows the rapid achievement of high concentrations of therapeutic agents in the pulmonary epithelial lining and bronchiolar fluid. Antimicrobials that have been aerosolized are gentamicin (50 mg/mL) and ceftiofur (25 mg/mL). Bronchodilators, steroids, and mucolytic agents have also been administered by this method.

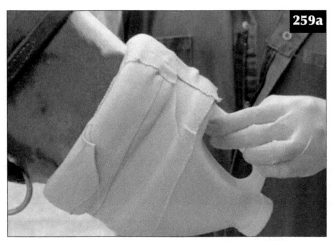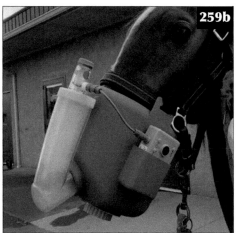

259 (a) Nebulization of a foal with a homemade mask in which the nebulization chamber is inserted at the bottom. (b) Nebulization with Flexineb™. (Courtesy of Nortev, Galway, Ireland.)

The prognosis for bacterial pneumonia is variable depending on the severity of the disease and the age of the individual.

VIRAL PNEUMONIA

KEY POINTS
- In the newborn foal, viral pneumonia can be fatal.
- Viral infections may predispose to bacterial pneumonia or other respiratory abnormalities.
- Most common viruses identified are EHV-1/4 (equine herpesvirus), influenza virus, and equine viral arteritis (EVA) virus.
- The neonate may present in respiratory distress and cardiovascular collapse.
- The older foal presents with a variable combination of fever, cough, nasal discharge, and malaise.
- Definitive diagnosis is dependent on virus isolation.

DEFINITION/OVERVIEW
Viral pneumonia in the newborn foal is often fatal. In the older foal, viruses can induce changes in the respiratory tract defenses that make the foal more susceptible to secondary bacterial infections. Some of the viruses can also cause rhinitis, pharyngitis, and tracheitis and have been implemented in the acute RDS of 1- to 8-month-old foals.

ETIOLOGY/PATHOPHYSIOLOGY
The most commonly identified causes of viral pneumonia are EHV-1/4, influenza virus, and EVA virus. Adenovirus has been reported in immune-compromised Arabian foals. There has been speculation of an association between EHV-2 and LRT disease, but the exact role has not been established. Details for each virus infection can be found in Chapter 3 (Infectious Diseases).

Transmission is primarily through the respiratory tract from contact with a subclinically infected individual. The neonate can be infected *in utero*.

CLINICAL PRESENTATION
In the neonate, clinical signs are similar to those of severe sepsis (see Chapter 3, Infectious Diseases, pp. 39–43), and the disease is often fatal. The older foal may present with a dry cough, fever, and serous nasal discharge or be in acute respiratory distress.

DIFFERENTIAL DIAGNOSIS
Tables 19, 45 through *47.*

DIAGNOSIS
A presumptive diagnosis can be made from the history, clinical signs, and the rapidity of spread of infection through a group of animals. Hematology may initially reveal a leukopenia characterized by a moderate to marked lymphopenia and, later, a monocytosis. Virus isolation can be attempted, but is most successful within the first 24–48 hours of infection. Polymerase chain reaction (PCR) testing is a quick and sensitive way to identify viral agents. The best method for virus isolation or PCR is from a nasal swab, although fluid from a transtracheal aspirate can sometimes be submitted. A polyester-tipped sterile swab is inserted into the nasal passage (**227**). The swab is placed in a special virus transport medium or sterile saline and delivered to the appropriate laboratory. Acute and convalescent serum antibody titers may be helpful in the diagnosis in an older foal, but consideration must be given to age, vaccination status, and presence of maternal antibodies when interpreting the results.

MANAGEMENT
Treatment depends on the severity of the disease and the age of the foal. Broad-spectrum antimicrobials are often administered to the neonate, whereas the older foal is simply monitored closely for any signs of secondary bacterial infections. Anti-inflammatories can be administered as needed and the foal should be isolated.

PLEURITIS

KEY POINTS

- Rare in foals.
- Usually secondary to pneumonia.
- Clinical signs of pneumonia.
- Diagnosis is based on auscultation and confirmed with ultrasound.

DEFINITION/OVERVIEW

Pleuritis is defined as inflammation of the pleural membrane. When this condition is associated with pneumonia, it is referred to as pleuropneumonia. Pleural effusion is associated with pleuritis, but may not always be present. Pleuritis is rare in foals.

ETIOLOGY/PATHOPHYSIOLOGY

Pleuritis is usually secondary to pneumonia or lung abscessation. Causative agents include the bacterial organisms and viral organisms that typically cause pneumonia. Inflammation of the pleura results in the accumulation of fluid within the pleural space due an increase in production of pleural fluid and to changes in vascular capillary permeability of the visceral pleura.

CLINICAL PRESENTATION

The clinical presentation depends on the severity and duration of disease. Fever, depression, and changes in respiratory rate or effort are most commonly observed. In severe cases, respiratory distress may be present.

DIFFERENTIAL DIAGNOSIS

Tables 19 and *45.*

DIAGNOSIS

Physical examination may reveal quiet lung sounds ventrally, pain when palpated over the thoracic wall, and restricted thoracic movements. Hematology reveals an abnormal leukogram and increased fibrinogen. Ultrasound is most useful for detecting pleural effusion (**260, 261**) and allows for characterization of the fluid and evaluation of the severity of the disease. Radiographs of the thorax reveal diffuse opacity ventrally (**262**). Thoracocentesis is often attempted if there is a significant amount of fluid and the foal is in respiratory distress. A 16–20 French gauge trocar catheter (**263, 264**) or an 18 gauge 1.2 cm (3 in) catheter can be used. The fluid sample should be submitted for cytology and culture. More often a causative agent (bacteria) is isolated from the culture of a fluid sample obtained from a transtracheal aspirate rather than from a culture of pleural fluid.

MANAGEMENT

Initially, intravenous broad-spectrum antimicrobial therapy is administered. A combination of penicillin and an aminoglycoside or third-generation cephalosporin will provide the best initial coverage. Once culture results are available, the therapy may need to be modified. Anti-inflammatories may help with pain and inflammation. Additional therapies that may be administered depending on the severity of the disease include intranasal oxygen and intravenous fluids. Thoracocentesis may need to be repeated if the fluid level rises and causes respiratory compromise. Response to therapy

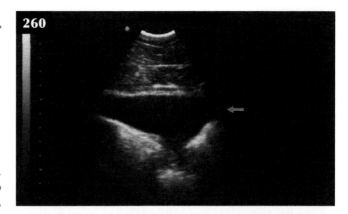

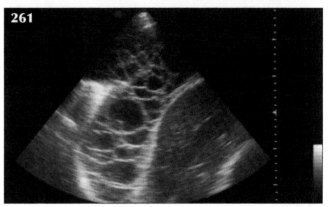

260, 261 (**260**) Ultrasonogram showing pleural effusion and consolidation. (arrow) (**261**) Ultrasonogram showing pleural effusion and strands of fibrin between the lung and thoracic wall giving a "honeycomb" appearance.

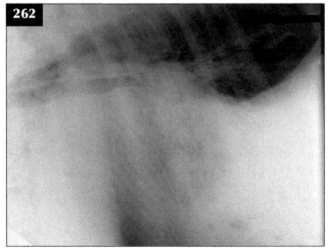

262 Lateral radiograph of a 2-month-old foal with pleural effusion caused by *Streptococcus zooepidemicus*. Note the fluid line.

is noted by improvement in vital parameters, hematology/serum chemistry, and no reaccumulation of pleural fluid. Possible complications include adhesions between the lung and parietal pleura or abscess formation. The prognosis depends on the severity and duration of the disease.

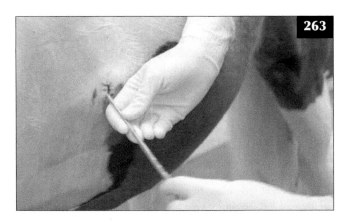

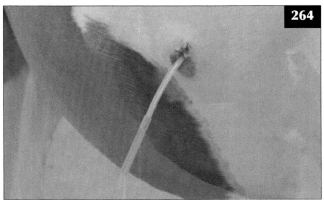

263, 264 Thoracocentesis. (**263**) Insertion of a 16 French gauge trocar chest tube through the intercostal muscle in a 6-month-old foal. (**264**) Freely flowing fluid from the pleural space after placement of a 16 French gauge trocar chest tube.

ACUTE RESPIRATORY DISTRESS SYNDROME (BRONCHOINTERSTITIAL PNEUMONIA)

KEY POINTS
- Etiology is unknown.
- Involves diffuse pulmonary fibrosis.
- Clinical presentation includes a sudden onset of tachypnea, increased respiratory effort, nostril flare, and dyspnea.
- Fever may be present.
- Diagnosis is supported with an increased radiographic opacity as a result of bronchointerstitial pulmonary pattern.
- Treatment includes steroidal/nonsteroidal anti-inflammatories, broad-spectrum antimicrobials, and supportive care.
- Prognosis for recovery is guarded to poor.

DEFINITION/OVERVIEW
An acute RDS has been reported in foals between the ages of 1 and 8 months. It manifests as interstitial or bronchointerstitial pneumonia. Foals are either found dead or present with an acute onset of respiratory distress.

ETIOLOGY/PATHOPHYSIOLOGY
Several etiologies have been suspected including viruses, bacteria, *Pneumocystis carinii*, toxins, allergic response, and heat stroke.

No definitive agent has been identified. The inciting agent initiates damage to the cells of the alveoli and terminal airways. This results in pulmonary congestion and interstitial edema. The alveoli and terminal airways are flooded with inflammatory cells, fibrin, and cellular debris. Damaged type I pneumocytes are replaced by type II pneumocytes. All this results in diffuse pulmonary fibrosis and scarring of the interlobular septa and pleura.

CLINICAL PRESENTATION
Clinical signs include a sudden onset of respiratory distress with marked tachypnea, dyspnea, nostril flare, and increased inspiratory and expiratory effort. Also, the foal may be febrile.

DIFFERENTIAL DIAGNOSIS
Tables 19 and *45*.

DIAGNOSIS
Thoracic auscultation reveals loud bronchial sounds over the large airways, with quieter sounds over the periphery. Adventitial sounds can range from crackles to wheezes in all lung fields. The most common radiographic abnormality is a bronchointerstitial pulmonary pattern of increased opacity, which varies in severity from an interstitial opacity with variable bronchial thickening to a more serve coalescing nodular pattern of increased interstitial opacity (**265**). Ultrasound will reveal diffuse coalescing comet tails radiating from the lung surface. If the foal is stable, a transtracheal aspirate can be performed for cytology and culture. Virus isolation from a nasopharyngeal swab is another method of attempting to identify a causative agent.

MANAGEMENT
Treatment is broad based and includes administration of oxygen, NSAIDs, antimicrobial therapy, nebulization, intravenous fluids,

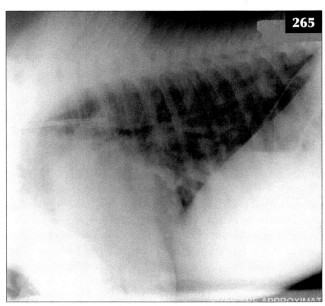

265 Lateral thorax radiographs of a 2-day-old foal with acute respiratory distress syndrome. Note the diffuse interstitial pattern.

and nutritional support. Corticosteroid administration has been reported to help some foals. The prognosis is very guarded.

NEONATAL RESPIRATORY DISTRESS SYNDROME

KEY POINTS
- Progressive respiratory distress as a result of inadequate surfactant function.
- Often associated with prematurity.
- Inadequate surfactant results in alveolar collapse.
- History and progressive clinical signs are suggestive, an alveolar pulmonary radiographic pattern is supportive.
- Exogenous surfactant can be administered.
- Prognosis is guarded.

DEFINITION/OVERVIEW
Neonatal RDS is defined as progressive respiratory failure caused by inadequate surfactant function superimposed on a structurally immature lung. It is primarily seen in premature foals. This syndrome has been reported in other species, although it has not been well documented in foals.

ETIOLOGY/PATHOPHYSIOLOGY
The exact etiology is unknown. Surfactant dysfunction may result from either low surfactant levels or conditions known to interfere with the activity of surfactant such as asphyxia, acidosis, hypercapnia, pulmonary edema, sepsis, and shock.

The pathophysiology of neonatal RDS possibly involves an interaction of an immature chest wall, incomplete surfactant lining, and asphyxial damage. Without adequate surfactant the alveolar walls collapse and, as the process continues, there is an increase in capillary permeability. This increase in permeability predisposes to wet lung and worsening of pulmonary function. Asphyxia may interfere with alveolar stability and pulmonary perfusion by causing a decrease in surfactant production and vasoconstriction of the pulmonary arterioles.

CLINICAL PRESENTATION
Neonatal RDS presents as a premature neonate with tachypnea, increased respiratory effort, and respiratory distress.

DIFFERENTIAL DIAGNOSIS
Congestive heart failure secondary to congenital heart defect, severe meconium aspiration, and *in-utero* bacterial or viral pneumonia. See also *Table 45*.

DIAGNOSIS
Diagnosis is often made on history and clinical impression (i.e., a neonate born at a gestational age of younger than 320 days that displays immature physical characteristics such as low birth weight, general weakness, short silky hair coat, and soft pliant ears). The neonate may progress to respiratory distress over 24 hours. The breathing pattern may have more of an abdominal effort and auscultation of the thorax may identify quiet areas. Thoracic radiographs demonstrate a diffuse, alveolar pattern. Ultrasound may demonstrate consolidation with coalescing comet tails. An arterial blood gas analysis would identify characteristics of respiratory failure such as hypoxemia, hypercapnia, and respiratory acidosis.

MANAGEMENT
The primary objective of therapy is to provide an increased percentage of inspired oxygen and decrease carbon dioxide in the blood. This is most often accomplished by mechanical ventilation, although intranasal oxygen may be sufficient. Synthetic surfactant has been administered. Appropriate antimicrobials, nutrition, and nursing care are also important. The prognosis is grave.

MECONIUM ASPIRATION SYNDROME

KEY POINTS
- Aspiration of meconium by the fetus *in utero* subsequent to release of meconium into the amniotic fluid.
- Premature meconium release may be a result of fetal distress.
- Meconium in the lower airways causes obstruction of gas exchange and chemical pneumonia.
- Clinically, foals are stained with meconium.
- Duration of meconium in amniotic fluid (with aspiration) dictates whether respiratory signs will develop.
- With moderate to severe aspiration, prognosis is guarded.

DEFINITION/OVERVIEW
Meconium aspiration syndrome occurs only in neonatal foals.

ETIOLOGY/PATHOPHYSIOLOGY
Meconium aspiration syndrome is caused by aspiration of meconium by the fetus while *in utero* or during the birthing process. *In-utero* asphyxia, stress, or umbilical cord compression can result in fetal distress and expulsion of meconium into the amniotic fluid. Fetal gasping while *in utero* or during parturition results in meconium in the airway. The meconium may obstruct the airways and interfere with gas exchange, causing respiratory distress or providing a medium for growth of bacteria.

CLINICAL PRESENTATION
The newborn foal may be meconium stained or have a brown-tinged nasal discharge (**266**). A mild increase in respiratory rate and effort may be noted or the neonate may be in respiratory distress.

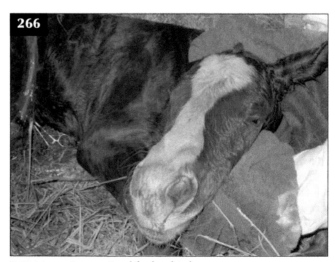

266 Meconium-stained foal at birth.

DIFFERENTIAL DIAGNOSIS
Table 45.

DIAGNOSIS
Diagnosis relies on the observation of meconium-contaminated amniotic fluid or a meconium-stained newborn. Auscultation of the thorax may reveal an increased harshness to the lungs, although changes are not always evident. The changes on thoracic radiographs may be a cranioventral distribution of pulmonary infiltrates characteristic of aspiration. Ultrasound may demonstrate consolidation with coalescing comet tails.

MANAGEMENT
If there is evidence of meconium contamination of amniotic fluid at parturition and the veterinarian is present, gentle suction of the mouth, nose, and trachea can be performed. Postparturient therapy includes broad-spectrum antimicrobials, respiratory support, nutritional support, anti-inflammatory agents, and appropriate nursing care. The foal should be closely monitored for any secondary complications.

ASPIRATION PNEUMONIA

KEY POINTS
- Most common cause in neonates is aspiration of milk; older foals may aspirate feed material.
- Occurs as a result of a defect in the upper airway.
- Signs of lower airway disease may ensue.
- Coughing, nasal discharge, or regurgitation of milk may be noted.

DEFINITION/OVERVIEW
Pneumonia results most often from aspiration of milk in the newborn. Older foals might aspirate food material or saliva secondary to other systemic diseases.

ETIOLOGY/PATHOPHYSIOLOGY
The bacteria most often involved are a mixed population of Gram-negative and Gram-positive organisms, with anaerobes occasionally being documented. Aspiration pneumonia occurs as a result of a physical defect in the upper airway (cleft palate, dorsal displacement of the soft palate) or of a functional abnormality of the larynx that affects swallowing (neuromuscular disorders, guttural pouch disease, myopathies, hypoxic ischemic encephalopathy, weakness secondary to sepsis, and esophageal obstruction). Poor nursing behavior or improper bottle feeding may also result in aspiration pneumonia.

CLINICAL PRESENTATION
After nursing, the foal may have nasal regurgitation of milk, sneezing, coughing, or a gurgling sound in the trachea. Other abnormalities include fever, depression, tachypnea, and respiratory distress.

DIFFERENTIAL DIAGNOSIS
Tables 19 and *45.*

DIAGNOSIS
Diagnosis is supported by historical information such as the nasal regurgitation of milk, having to be bottle fed, or having been treated for a systemic illness. Adventitial lung sounds may or may not be auscultated, although abnormal tracheal noises can be auscultated, especially while the foal is nursing. Additional diagnostics that can be performed to help establish the degree of pulmonary involvement include thoracic radiographs, thoracic ultrasound, arterial blood gas analysis, and transtracheal aspirate. With both thoracic radiographs and ultrasound the presence of consolidation is typically localized cranioventrally (**266**), although other patterns and locations may exist. Endoscopy may identify a deformity of the upper airway.

MANAGEMENT
Initial therapy includes the administration of broad-spectrum antimicrobials such as penicillin and an aminoglycoside, which eventually may be changed based on culture results. If the foal shows evidence of respiratory distress, oxygen insufflation may be beneficial. An indwelling feeding tube may need to be placed if a neuromuscular problem such as botulism is suspected or the foal may need intravenous fluids. The underlying cause should be pursued and treated. Antimicrobial therapy is often long term. Prognosis depends on the cause of the aspiration pneumonia and the severity of the pulmonary involvement.

PERSISTENT PULMONARY HYPERTENSION OF THE NEWBORN

KEY POINTS
- Reversion to, or persistent, fetal circulation.
- Right-to-left shunting of blood through patent fetal conduits.
- Cyanosis and respiratory distress.
- Arterial blood gas analysis reveals persistent hypercapnic hypoxemia.

DEFINITION/OVERVIEW
Persistent pulmonary hypertension (PPHN) is also referred to as reversion to fetal circulation or persistent fetal circulation. It is due to either the failure of the neonate to make a successful respiratory and cardiac transition to extrauterine life or the reversion of the neonate to fetal circulatory patterns in response to hypoxia or acidosis.

ETIOLOGY/PATHOPHYSIOLOGY
PPHN occurs when the pulmonary vascular resistance fails to decrease below systemic vascular resistance (SVR). This results in shunting of blood from right to left through the foramen ovale and ductus arteriosus, resulting in hypoperfusion of the lungs and severe hypoxemia. The exact mechanisms involved are unknown, but may include an imbalance of vasoconstrictor and vasodilator substances such as endothelin-1 and nitric oxide. Numerous factors can contribute to this disorder, including chronic *in-utero* hypoxia, birth asphyxia, prematurity, dysmaturity, and meconium aspiration.

CLINICAL PRESENTATION
The neonate may present recumbent and tachypneic with evidence of cyanosis. A heart murmur may be auscultated or the neonate may be in respiratory distress.

DIFFERENTIAL DIAGNOSIS
Tables 6 and 45.

DIAGNOSIS
PPHN should be suspected when serial blood gas analyses indicate a persistent, worsening hypercapnic hypoxemia. Echocardiographic evidence suggestive of increased pulmonary arterial pressure includes dilation of the main pulmonary artery, demonstrable shunts across the ductus arteriosus or foramen ovale, and the absence of other cyanosis-causing heart defects.

MANAGEMENT
Many neonates will respond to treatment with intranasal oxygen. Correction of acidosis and any underlying condition will help to optimize oxygen delivery to tissues. Appropriate systemic BPs should be maintained to minimize right-to-left shunting. Some cases require mechanical ventilation with 100% oxygen and a few require the addition of nitric oxide or other pulmonary vasodilators. The prognosis is poor, with possible secondary complications including lung and brain damage.

PNEUMOTHORAX

KEY POINTS
- Trapping of air within the pleural space.
- Usually secondary to trauma (rib fractures).
- Can be secondary to necrotizing pneumonia.
- Clinical signs include respiratory difficulties or distress.
- Diagnostic auscultation of the thorax is supported by radiographs or ultrasound.

DEFINITION/OVERVIEW
Pneumothorax is the trapping of air within the pleural space. It occurs infrequently in the equine pediatric patient and is usually secondary to trauma.

ETIOLOGY/PATHOPHYSIOLOGY
Pneumothorax may occur spontaneously or result from birth trauma (secondary to rib fractures). A pneumothorax may also be a consequence of excessive positive pressure ventilation of diseased lungs or, rarely, can occur secondary to necrotizing bronchopneumonia. In the older foal, trauma is most often the cause.

During mechanical ventilation, uneven alveolar ventilation leads to alveolar rupture and dissection of air into the interstitium. The air moves along bronchioles and other lung structures to pleural surfaces, forming blebs. This air may rupture into the pleural space. Pneumothorax can be closed, where air is trapped in the pleural space, or open, where there is free communication between the pleural space and the external environment.

CLINICAL PRESENTATION
The clinical signs of pneumothorax are nonspecific and include respiratory distress and possible decreased air movement in a lung field. The mechanically ventilated foal's condition will suddenly worsen through developing respiratory distress, hypoxemia, and hypotension.

DIFFERENTIAL DIAGNOSIS
Table 45.

DIAGNOSIS
Auscultation of the thorax
Auscultation may reveal decreased breath sounds on one or both sides of the thorax or absence of lung sounds dorsally. The foal's breathing pattern may be irregular, with it taking several shallow breaths followed by a prolonged pause.

Radiography
Thoracic radiographs may show retraction of the lungs away from the diaphragm and spinal column and an increased lucency along the cranial border of the diaphragm. If radiography is not available, and the foal is in respiratory distress, a direct needle aspirate can be diagnostic and therapeutic.

Ultrasound
Pneumothorax is noted by a break in the normal reverberation air artifact (**267**). Occasionally, pleural fluid will also be evident and this will make it easier to identify the pneumothorax.

MANAGEMENT
If the neonate is showing mild signs, no distress, and the condition appears stable, conservative management is best. This includes minimizing stress, possible antimicrobial therapy, and placing the foal on high inspired intranasal oxygen if warranted. In foals with a large pneumothorax, or where the pneumothorax is causing circulating insufficiency, a thoracocentesis may be needed to decrease the amount of free air in the thoracic cavity. A small leak should seal within a few days. The prognosis is good for foals with a small pneumothorax, but guarded for foals with a large pneumothorax.

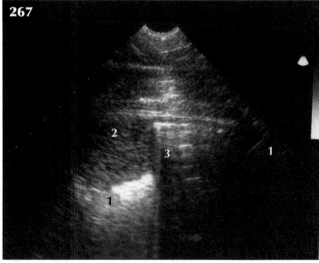

267 Ultrasound of a foal with a pneumothorax. 1: lung; 2: pus; 3: gas cap.

HEMOTHORAX

KEY POINTS
- Due to rib fractures in neonate or trauma in the older foal.
- Clinical signs depend on amount of blood loss.
- Ultrasound examination confirms diagnosis.

DEFINITION/OVERVIEW
Hemothorax, the accumulation of blood in the pleural space, occasionally occurs in the foal.

ETIOLOGY/PATHOPHYSIOLOGY
In neonatal foals, hemothorax can be a sequela to unstable rib fractures. In older foals, hemothorax can be secondary to trauma. Most commonly an unstable rib fracture punctures the highly vascular lung parenchyma or a thoracic vessel, resulting in blood accumulation in the pleural space. A traumatic episode may result in contusion to the lung surface and accumulation of fluid.

CLINICAL PRESENTATION
The clinical presentation depends on the amount of blood accumulating in the pleural space. With a large amount of blood, recumbency, hypovolemic shock, and pale mucous membranes may be present. If only a small amount of blood is present, the foal may be weak with minimal signs of respiratory and cardiovascular compromise.

DIFFERENTIAL DIAGNOSIS
Sepsis, trauma, neonatal isoerythrolysis (NI). See also *Table 45*.

DIAGNOSIS
Historical information can be supportive of the diagnosis including dystocia (neonate) or a traumatic incident. Crepitance or clicking may be noted when palpating over the ribs, or chest wall asymmetry may be visualized. With a large amount of blood, auscultation of the thorax reveals decreased lung sounds bilaterally. A complete loss of detail ventrally with a fluid line is noted on thoracic radiographs, although a definitive diagnosis is made with ultrasound.

Ultrasound reveals homogeneous echogenic fluid, which may be swirling (268). Thoracocentesis can be both diagnostic and therapeutic (263, 264).

MANAGEMENT
In foals that present in hypovolemic shock, cardiovascular stabilization with fluid resuscitation and blood products should be performed immediately (269; see also Chapter 2, Shock, Resuscitation, Fluid and Electrolyte Therapy, p. 17). Once the foal is stabilized, conservative management should include antimicrobial therapy and minimizing of stress. If there is a significant amount of fluid that is causing respiratory compromise, thoracocentesis, with ultrasound guidance, may need to be performed once the foal is stabilized and it is evident that it is not actively bleeding. The prognosis depends on the severity of the lesion and the degree of hypovolemic shock.

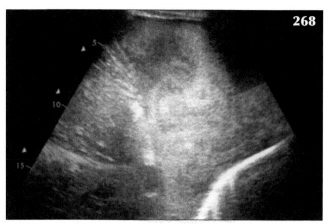

268 Ultrasonogram of a foal with hemothorax secondary to fractured ribs. Note the homogeneous echogenic fluid and the heterogeneous mass in the ventral thorax, which is most likely a blood clot.

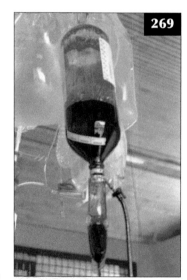

269 Whole blood being administered to a 1-day-old foal with blood loss secondary to rib fractures.

RIB FRACTURES

KEY POINTS
- Significant in newborn foal.
- Usually identified during physical examination.
- Treatment depends on location of the fractured ribs.

DEFINITION/OVERVIEW
Rib fractures are a significant cause of morbidity and mortality in the neonatal foal. Newborn foals should be examined for this injury, especially those born in complicated or difficult deliveries.

ETIOLOGY/PATHOPHYSIOLOGY
Rib fractures occur secondary to trauma, especially dystocia. They occur during parturition due to mechanical pressure exerted on the foal's thoracic cavity as it travels through the pelvic canal.

CLINICAL PRESENTATION

Neonatal foals with rib fractures often present with tachypnea, tachycardia, or respiratory distress. Other signs include plaques of subcutaneous edema overlying the ribs or along the ventrum of the thorax, and flinching when the rib area is palpated.

DIFFERENTIAL DIAGNOSIS

Table 45.

DIAGNOSIS

Rib fractures are frequently found during physical examination by palpation of the ribs or by auscultation over the fracture sites. Audible or palpable crepitation or a clicking sensation is noted when the hand is gently pressed over an affected area (**270**). Ultrasound or radiography is useful to confirm the diagnosis (**271**). Often, multiple ribs are affected on one side. The fracture usually occurs at or within several centimeters of the

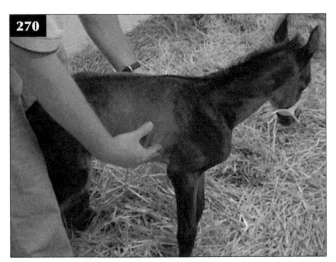

270 Palpation for rib fractures in a newborn foal.

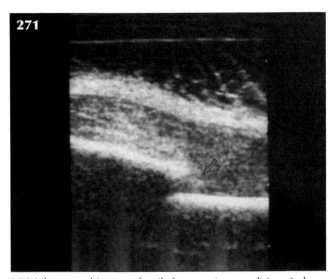

271 Ultrasound image of a rib fracture (arrowed) in a 1-day-old foal. (Courtesy of J. Reimer.)

costochondral junction. The distal rib fracture tends to displace axially, which can result in secondary injury to the pleural cavity or the myocardium. Flail chest occurs when several consecutive ribs are fractured, leading to an incompetent segment of chest wall.

MANAGEMENT

If there is no evidence of complications, stall confinement for 2–4 weeks is recommended. Neonatal foals with fractures overlying the heart may be considered for surgical stabilization. Surgical techniques include a dynamic compression plate placement or stabilization using the Securos Cranial Cruciate Ligament Repair System (SCCLRS; Securos Veterinary Orthopedics, Charleston, MA). Potential complications of rib fractures include pneumothorax, hemothorax, or fatal myocardial puncture.

NEONATAL APNEA AND IRREGULAR BREATHING PATTERNS

KEY POINTS

- Associated with nonrespiratory problem.
- Due to central nervous system (CNS) or metabolic disorders.
- Treat the primary condition.

OVERVIEW/DEFINITION

Abnormal breathing patterns have been documented in the neonatal foal and are commonly associated with nonrespiratory factors.

ETIOLOGY/PATHOPHYSIOLOGY

The exact etiology is unknown, but it is usually associated with an infection (nonrespiratory), a CNS disorder, hypothermia, or metabolic causes.

There are two mechanisms of apnea: central apnea, which results from cessation of diaphragmatic activity, and obstructive apnea, which results from obstruction of the airway, usually at the pharyngeal level.

CLINICAL PRESENTATION

The foal may present weak with an abnormal breathing pattern, which is often characterized by frequent pauses in breathing activity.

DIFFERENTIAL DIAGNOSIS

Sepsis, bacterial and viral pneumonia, electrolyte/metabolic derangements. See also *Table 45.*

DIAGNOSIS

Diagnosis involves identifying a nonrespiratory problem. Neurologic problems or metabolic disorders (hypoglycemia) are most often identified.

MANAGEMENT

Management involves appropriate therapy for the diagnosed primary condition. Additional therapy includes external stimulation, intranasal oxygen, antimicrobials, and respiratory stimulants (caffeine or doxapram). Occasionally, positive pressure ventilation is needed.

IDIOPATHIC OR TRANSIENT TACHYPNEA

KEY POINTS
- May be due to dysfunction of the thermoregulatory system.
- Rule out other causes of pulmonary disease or metabolic disease.
- Good prognosis.

OVERVIEW/DEFINITION
This disease syndrome has been reported in a number of Clydesdale, Thoroughbred, and Arabian neonatal foals. The clinical signs usually develop a few days after a normal birth and may persist for several weeks.

ETIOLOGY/PATHOPHYSIOLOGY
The exact cause of idiopathic or transient tachypnea is unknown. It is generally seen when environmental conditions are warm and humid and is thought to result from immature or dysfunctional thermoregulatory mechanisms.

CLINICAL PRESENTATION
The typical presentation has been a combination of fever (38.8°C–42.2°C [102°F–108°F]) and tachypnea. The foal is often noted to be "panting" (respiratory rate >80 breaths per minute).

DIFFERENTIAL DIAGNOSIS
Bacterial pneumonia, viral pneumonia, aspiration pneumonia, meconium aspiration, PPHN of the newborn, metabolic acidosis. See also *Tables 19* and *45*.

DIAGNOSIS
Before this condition can be diagnosed, other causes of tachypnea such as pulmonary disease, infection, and metabolic acidosis must be ruled out.

MANAGEMENT
Therapy for idiopathic or transient tachypnea generally involves moving the foal to a cooler environment, body clipping, and cool water or alcohol baths. Generally, there is a poor response to antipyretics. Until an infectious process can be ruled out, antimicrobial therapy should be included. Recovery is good.

FURTHER READING

Altmaier K, Morris EA (1993) Dorsal displacement of the soft palate in neonatal foals. *Equine Veterinary Journal* 25: 329–332.

Colbourne CM, Rosenstein DS, Steficek BA, Yovick JV, Stick JA (1997) Surgical treatment of progressive ethmoidal hematoma aided by computed tomography in a foal. *Journal of the American Veterinary Medical Association* 221: 335–338.

Couetil LL, Hawkins JF (2013) Congenital abnormalities. In: *Respiratory Diseases of the Horse: A Problem-Oriented Approach to Diagnosis and Management.* Manson Publishing, London, UK, pp. 201–212.

Dunkel B, Dolente B, Boston RC (2005) Acute lung injury/acute respiratory distress syndrome in 15 foals. *Equine Veterinary Journal* 37: 435–440.

Freeman KP, Cline JM, Simmons R, Wilkins PA, Cudd TA, Perry BJ (1989) Recognition of bronchopulmonary dysplasia in a newborn foal. *Equine Veterinary Journal* 21: 292–296.

Fultz L, Giguere S, Berghaus LJ, Grover GS, Merritt DA (2015) Pulmonary pharmacokinetics of desfuroylceftiofur acetamide after nebulisation or intramuscular administration of ceftiofur sodium to weanling foals. *Equine Veterinary Journal* 47: 473–477.

Garrett KS, Woodie JB, Cook JL, Williams NM (2010) Imaging diagnosis—Nasal septal and laryngeal cyst-like malformations in a thoroughbred weanling colt diagnosed using ultrasonography and magnetic resonance imaging. *Veterinary Radiology & Ultrasound* 51: 504–507.

Holcombe SJ, Hurcombe SD, Barr BS, Schott HC 2nd (2012) Dysphagia associated with presumed pharyngeal dysfunction in 16 neonatal foals. *Equine Veterinary Journal* Suppl 41: 105–108.

Lascola KM, Joslyn S (2015) Diagnostic imaging of the lower respiratory tract in neonatal foals: Radiography and computed tomography. *Veterinary Clinics of North America: Equine Practice* 31: 497–514.

Mair TS, Lane JG (2005) Diseases of the equine trachea. *Equine Veterinary Education* 17: 146–149.

Manso-Diaz G, Dyson SJ, Dennis R, Garcia-Lopez JM, Bigg M, Garcia-Real MI, San Roman F, Taeymans O (2015) Magnetic resonance imaging characteristics of equine head disorders: 84 cases (2000–2013). *Veterinary Radiology & Ultrasound* 56: 176–187.

McKenzie HC (2003) Characterization of antimicrobial aerosols for administration to horses. *Veterinary Therapeutics* 4: 110–119.

Prange T (2015) Management of tracheal perforations: Potential complications and pitfalls. *Equine Veterinary Journal* 27: 566–568.

Reuss SM, Cohen ND (2015) Update on bacterial pneumonia in the foal and weanling. *Veterinary Clinics of North America: Equine Practice* 31: 121–135.

Sanders-Shamis M, Robertson JT (1987) Congenital sinus cyst in a foal. *Journal of the American Veterinary Medical Association* 190: 1011–1012.

Shappell KK, Caron JP, Stick JA, Parks AJ (1989) Staphylectomy for treatment of dorsal displacement of the soft palate in two foals. *Journal of the American Veterinary Medical Association* 195: 1395–1398.

Siger L, Hawkins JF, Andrews FM, Henry RW (1998) Tracheal stenosis and collapse in horses. *Compendium on Continuing Education for the Practicing Veterinarian* 20: 628–636.

Sprayberry KA (2015) Ultrasonographic examination of the equine neonate: Thorax and abdomen. *Veterinary Clinics of North America: Equine Practice* 31: 515–600.

Stick JA, Boles C (1980) Subepiglottic cyst in three foals. *Journal of the American Veterinary Medical Association* 177: 62–64.

Trostle SS, Semrad SD, Hendrickson DA (1995) Tracheal perforation in horses. *Compendium on Continuing Education for the Practicing Veterinarian* 17: 952–959.

Yarbrough TB, Voss E, Herrgesell EJ, Shaw M (1999) Persistent frenulum of the epiglottis in four foals. *Veterinary Surgery* 28: 287–291.

Urinary and Umbilical Disorders

9

Johanna M. Reimer and William V. Bernard

INTRODUCTION

Diseases of the urinary system of the equine pediatric patient encompass congenital, traumatic, infectious, toxic, and iatrogenic causes that affect the upper and/or lower segments of the urinary tract. Foals with urogenital disease can present with abdominal distension, colic, fever, abnormal hematology/serum chemistry, stranguria/dysuria (*Table 50*), hematuria (*Table 51*), or central nervous system (CNS) signs. Serum electrolytes and creatinine values, urinalysis, ultrasonography, contrast radiography, cystoscopy, and biopsy are utilized in the investigation of these diseases.

The results of urinalysis in foals differ from that of adult horses in part due to their milk diet. Foal urine is often dilute and acidic, and may contain protein for the first 1–2 days of life. Serum creatinine is slightly higher in the normal neonatal foal. Some clinically normal neonatal foals may have a marked elevation in serum creatinine, which declines to normal values by 3–5 days of age. Similar transient elevations in serum creatinine, sometimes >531 µmol/L (6 mg/dL), may be observed in foals that become hypoxemic due to dystocia. These elevations are not necessarily due to renal disease and are thought by some to be a result of placental malfunction.

Table 50. Causes of dysuria/stranguria
- Urachal diverticulum
- Ureterocele (**272, 273**)
- Mural bladder trauma/mural hematoma
- Cystitis
- Bladder or urachal rupture
- Ectopic ureter

Table 51. Causes of hematuria
- Trauma to structures of the urinary tract
- Infection
- Leptospirosis
- Cystic hematomas
- Hydronephrosis
- Renal abscessation
- Ectopic ureter

272, 273 Ultrasound images of the bladder of a 1-month-old foal with stranguria due to a large right ureterocele. Note the "bladder within a bladder" appearance and dilation of the right ureter. The ureterocele was surgically transected and the foal made a full recovery. 1: Foley catheter; 2: bladder; 3: ureterocele; 4: right ureter.

UROPERITONEUM

KEY POINTS
- Uroperitoneum in the foal is not uncommon.
- Uroperitoneum can result from bladder or urachal defects or, less commonly, ureteral abnormalities.
- Bladder distension with rupture during parturition is presumed to be the most common cause.
- Electrolyte disturbances are significant sequelae to uroperitoneum.
- Clinical signs may be varied and nonspecific.
- Abdominal distension is the most common presenting clinical sign.
- Serum chemistries and ultrasonography form the basis of diagnosis.
- Surgical repair is generally successful.
- Prognosis with surgical repair is good.

DEFINITION/OVERVIEW
Uroperitoneum resulting from disruption of the urinary bladder or urachus is not uncommon and can affect as many as 2.5% of hospitalized equine neonates. Ureteral defects are much less frequently recognized causes of uroperitoneum in the neonatal foal. Males and females are at equal risk for bladder and/or urachal rupture. The prognosis with surgical repair is very good; however, sepsis may be a complicating factor in nearly half of all hospitalized cases and adversely affects outcome.

ETIOLOGY/PATHOPHYSIOLOGY
Fetal bladder distension with traumatic rupture during parturition is presumed to be the most common cause of disruption of the urinary tract in the neonate. Ischemia and necrosis, with associated infection at the site of bladder or urachal disruption (**274**), can be found in septic neonates with uroperitoneum, although it is unclear whether infection in such cases is a primary or an opportunistic process.

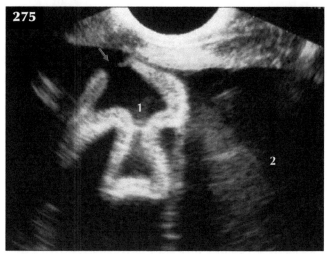

275 Transverse image of a ruptured bladder in a neonatal foal. Note the collapsed appearance to the bladder (1) and the large amount of peritoneal fluid (uroperitoneum) (2). The tear (arrow) is along the ventral aspect of the bladder. In most cases the site of rupture is not as readily apparent as in this case. 6 MHz microconvex linear array transducer.

The dorsal bladder wall is the most common site of tearing, followed by the urachus, ventral bladder wall, or bladder apex (**275**). Two sites of disruption are present in as many as one-quarter of cases, necessitating a thorough examination at the time of surgery. Bladder or urachal rupture is not an unusual complication in hospitalized foals that are recumbent (e.g., in cases of botulism or sepsis) or in foals that are heavily sedated with barbiturates for control of seizures. The authors have encountered two instances of marked fetal urinary bladder distension discovered during ultrasound studies in late gestation; in both cases the bladder ruptured on parturition (**276**). It was not determined whether the inciting cause was defective bladder development or *in-utero* obstruction.

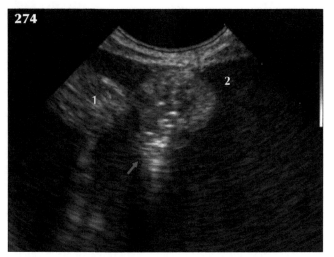

274 Transverse image of a necrotic urachus in a foal with uroperitoneum. Note the gas echoes (arrow) in the urachus. 1: small intestine; 2: uroperitoneum. 6 MHz microconvex linear array transducer.

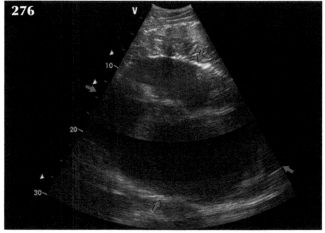

276 Long-axis view of the abdomen of a late gestation fetus. Note the marked fetal bladder distension (arrows). Centimeter markings are to the left of the image. The bladder was ruptured on parturition. 3 MHz convex linear array transducer.

Uroperitoneum results in hyponatremia, hypochloremia, and hyperkalemia due to equilibration of electrolytes between the peritoneum and extracellular fluid space. Azotemia ultimately develops; however, creatinine does not cross the peritoneal barrier. This means that the peritoneal fluid:serum creatinine ratio is a valuable diagnostic tool. Depression and inappetence may develop as a result of azotemia and electrolyte disturbances or possible sepsis. Serum electrolytes are often normal in foals that rupture their bladder while receiving intravenous fluid therapy.

CLINICAL PRESENTATION

Clinical signs of uroperitoneum may be nonspecific and vary widely (*Table 52*). Abdominal distension is the most common presenting clinical sign (**277**). In addition, severe ventral, preputial, and/or umbilical edema may be seen (**278**). Stranguria (**279**) is not usually observed; rather absence of urination is more often reported. Uroperitoneum may become severe enough to lead to tachypnea due to either abdominal distension or the secondary accumulation of pleural effusion. Abdominal pain (colic) may be evident as abdominal distension progresses. In long-standing uroperitoneum, foals may present on rare occasions with CNS signs

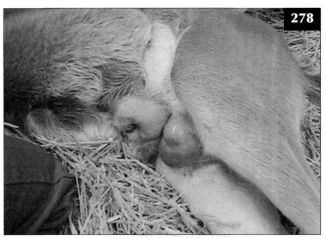

278 Uroperitoneum can result in preputial and/or ventral edema.

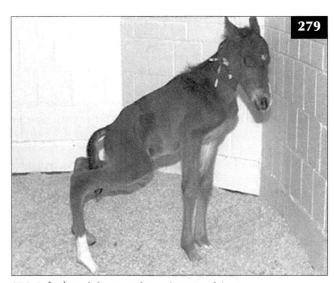

279 A foal straining to urinate (stranguria).

Table 52. Clinical signs of uroperitoneum

- Inappetence
- Depression
- Abdominal distension
- Straining to urinate
- Absence of visible urine production
- Tachypnea
- Abdominal pain
- CNS signs due to uremic encephalopathy

---

secondary to a uremic encephalopathy. CNS signs include head pressing, circling, or aimless wandering. Veterinary attention is often not sought until 3 or more days of age, when abdominal distension becomes apparent. In the hospital setting, abdominal distension is the most common clinical finding followed, in intensively monitored foals, by reduced or absent urine production.

DIFFERENTIAL DIAGNOSIS

Abdominal distension can also be caused by peritoneal effusion due to a ruptured viscus or gas or fluid accumulation within the intestinal tract. Dysuria and stranguria, uncommonly seen with uroperitoneum, is observed in foals with urachal diverticulum. Foals with meconium impaction may present with abdominal distension due to a gas-filled colon, but they are often under 3 days of age and exhibit tenesmus. Benign azotemia of newborn foals (a differential for elevation in serum creatinine) is not associated with any clinical signs; there is no accumulation of peritoneal fluid, serum electrolyte values remains normal, and there is progressive reduction in serum creatinine over a period of a few days.

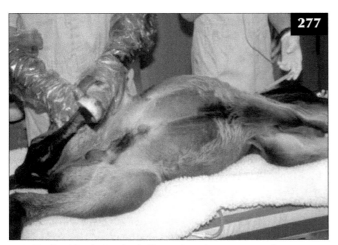

277 Foal with abdominal distension due to uroperitoneum.

DIAGNOSIS

Ultrasonography is an invaluable tool in the diagnosis of uroperitoneum, as it can be used to determine whether abdominal distension is due to excessive fluid accumulation within the peritoneal cavity (**274, 275, 280**) or intestinal distension. A collapsed or folded appearance to the urinary bladder may be noted in cases of bladder rupture (**275, 281**) in addition to peritoneal fluid accumulation. A normal appearance to the bladder may be found in cases with small bladder perforations, urachal disruption, or ureteral defects. Ureteral defects will result in retroperitoneal accumulation of fluid, prior to the development of uroperitoneum. It is generally wise to evaluate the kidneys ultrasonographically for gross defects or retroperitoneal fluid accumulation as part of a complete examination of the urinary tract in cases with suspected uroperitoneum. Small perforations in the urachus or bladder may be investigated through a "bubble study" in which agitated saline is injected into the bladder via a urinary catheter and the peritoneal fluid is examined ultrasonographically for escaped bubbles (**282**). This study can be of particular value in cases in which postoperative dehiscence of the repair site is suspected. Ureteral defects often require the use of contrast radiography with percutaneous injection of contrast medium into the renal pelvis.

An elevated peritoneal fluid:serum creatinine ratio is invaluable in the diagnosis of uroperitoneum and is not confounded by fluid therapy. A ratio of 2:1 is highly suggestive of uroperitoneum. Hyperkalemia, hyponatremia, and hypochloremia are typically present; however, these electrolyte derangements may also be found in foals with gastric rupture or severe acute enteritis. Conversely, electrolyte values are often normal in foals that have received intravenous fluid therapy.

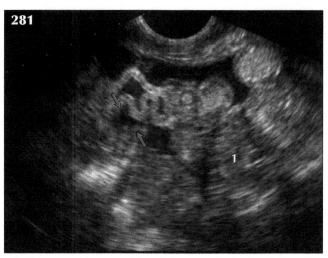

281 Transverse image of the abdomen of a foal with a ruptured bladder. Note the folded appearance to the bladder (between arrows). 1: small intestine.

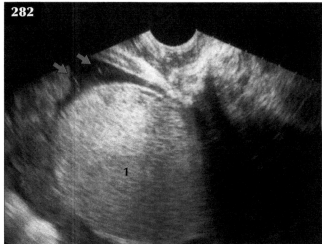

282 "Bubble study" of the bladder of a foal that had undergone surgical repair of a ruptured bladder 2 days earlier and had developed slight abdominal distension. The bladder lumen is opacified with bubbles. Note the slight anechoic peritoneal effusion and the two "escaped" bubbles within the fluid (arrows). The postoperative leak was presumed to be small, and a second surgery was not required. Cranial is to the left. 6 MHz microconvex linear array transducer. 1: bladder.

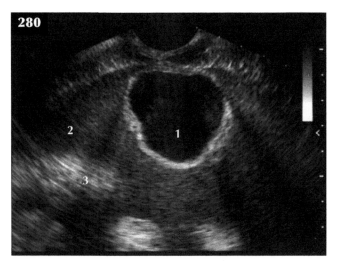

280 Transverse image of the abdomen of a foal with a ruptured bladder. Note the large accumulation of echogenic peritoneal fluid and the slightly flaccid appearance to the bladder wall. The peritoneal effusion is more echogenic than the urine within the bladder in this particular case due to a high WBC count within the peritoneal fluid from secondary peritonitis. 1: bladder; 2: peritoneal fluid; 3: small intestine. 6 MHz microconvex linear array transducer.

MANAGEMENT

Surgical exploration (**283**) and repair of the site of the defect is recommended in almost all cases. Rare instances of a small bladder or urachal perforation have been managed by indwelling urinary catheters (**284**) and close monitoring; however, ascending infection with spread to the peritoneal cavity is a potential serious complication.

If hyperkalemia is present (>55 mmol/L [5.5 mEq/dL]), the foal may be predisposed to fatal bradyarrhythmias precipitated by xylazine administration or general anesthesia. Intravenous bicarbonate

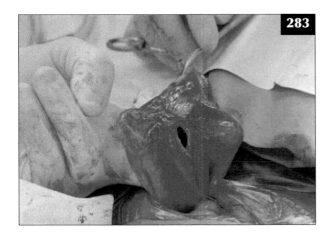

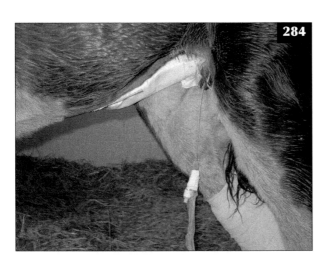

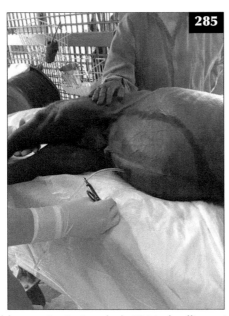

283 Bladder tear *in situ* in a foal. 284 Indwelling urinary catheter in a neonatal foal. 285 Percutaneous catheter to allow for drainage of peritoneal fluid in a neonatal foal with a suspected rupture bladder.

containing fluids (1–2 mEq/kg over 5–15 minutes) or normal saline should be administered in an attempt to lower serum potassium. Percutaneous catheter drainage (285) of potassium-laden peritoneal fluid may also be necessary to reduce serum potassium to a concentration that is safe for induction and anesthesia. Preoperative drainage may also be required in some cases to facilitate adequate ventilation during anesthesia.

The entire bladder and urachus should be examined carefully during surgery, since more than one site of disruption may be present. The prognosis for foals following surgical repair of defects is excellent if the foal is otherwise healthy. A small number of foals develop leakage at the repair site and require a second surgery. Repair of ureteral defects is more difficult, but the outcome in the few cases described in the literature was favorable.

PATENT URACHUS

KEY POINTS
- The urachus usually closes shortly after birth.
- The condition may be congenital or acquired.
- Excessive human manipulation/intervention of the umbilical cord can be problematic.
- The umbilical stump may appear wet, or urine may drip/stream from the umbilical remnants.
- Surgical resection is rarely necessary.

DEFINITION/OVERVIEW
The urachus normally closes soon after birth and regresses by 1–3 months of age. In cases of patent urachus, failure of initial closure may be a result of a congenitally widened lumen or trauma to the cord during birth. Patent urachus may also develop at days to weeks of age, possibly as a result of urachal infection or large volume of fluid administration. The severity ranges from a large stream of urine passing from the umbilical region during micturition to slight moisture noted on examination of the umbilical stump.

ETIOLOGY/PATHOPHYSIOLOGY
Patent urachus is not uncommon in foals up to 1 month of age and it may be congenital or acquired. Acquired patent urachus is often secondary to infection or precipitated by large-volume fluid administration and/or recumbency. Clamping, cutting, or tying of the umbilical cord before allowing the natural breaking of the umbilicus may predispose the foal to patent urachus.

Congenital patent urachus is due to failure of the urachus to contract after birth due to either congenital widening or trauma to the cord during birth. In acquired cases the urachus regains patency secondary to infection. High volumes of intravenous fluids, leading to a persistently full bladder, can result in pressure on the urachal remnant causing a patent urachus.

CLINICAL PRESENTATION
Foals may be present at any age, from birth to (rarely) more than 1 month of age. Urine is voided from the umbilical stump either as a few drops to a full stream (286). A wet and inflamed umbilical stump is the most common clinical finding (287). Most foals with acquired patent urachus due to infection have normal hematology/serum chemistry findings and are afebrile; if abnormalities in these

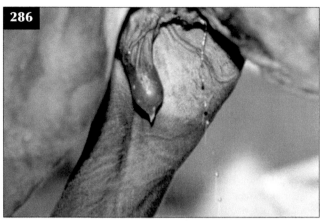

286 Patent urachus in a neonatal foal.

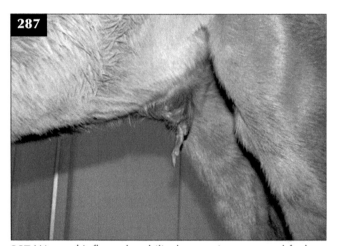

287 Wet and inflamed umbilical stump in a neonatal foal.

parameters are noted, a coincident source of infection should be suspected. Swelling in the umbilical region due to dissection of urine into the surrounding tissues has been observed in a few foals with severe umbilical cord trauma during parturition. Some swelling may also be seen in cases with concurrent internal umbilical remnant infection.

DIFFERENTIAL DIAGNOSIS
Patent urachus resulting from failure of the urachal tissue to contract, versus patency due to infection, is in part determined by age at onset and ultrasonographic and clinical findings.

DIAGNOSIS
Patent urachus is a diagnosis based on clinical signs; the cause is determined by history and ultrasonographic findings. Umbilical infections subsequently resulting in patent urachus are relatively common. A normal ultrasound study is not uncommon once the infected material is extruded via the patent urachus; it is also difficult to visualize the urachal lumen once this has occurred. Abnormal findings that may be discovered include thickening of the urachal wall or fluid within the lumen, as found with infection, or seromas or generalized soft tissue thickening involving

the urachal sheath and/or lumen as in cases of cord trauma. The umbilical arteries and vein should also be examined for evidence of infection, since abnormal findings could further influence therapy.

MANAGEMENT
Surgical resection is rarely necessary unless urine is leaking into layers of the abdominal wall. Most cases are probably a consequence of mild infection and can be managed with oral antibiotics and gentle cleansing of the umbilical stump until drainage ceases. Infected material and urine is allowed to continue to exit through the urachus while keeping the umbilical stump clean and dry. Systemic antibiotics such as trimethoprim/sulfa combinations are not always necessary, but they may speed healing and prevent a compounding infection. Topical medications can trap dirt and debris. Iodine-based solutions and silver nitrate sticks are irritating and should be avoided in most cases. Cautery with a silver nitrate applicator, gently swabbed on the urachal opening at the umbilical stump, is appropriate for congenital patent urachus; the irritation produced by the cautery promotes closure of the urachus and prevents ascending infection.

UMBILICAL REMNANT INFECTIONS

KEY POINTS
- Most likely cause of umbilical remnant infection is contamination shortly after birth.
- Beta-streptococcal organisms and coliforms are the most common pathogens.
- Swelling and/or purulent discharge are common, but not always present.
- Fevers and/or an inflammatory leukogram are not always present, but are more likely in foals with "closed" infections.
- Ultrasonography is excellent for diagnosis.
- Medical management (antibiotic therapy) is usually successful.
- Hygiene is significant in prevention.

DEFINITION/OVERVIEW
The internal umbilical remnants consist of the urachal sheath, which is comprised of the urachal lumen and the umbilical arteries from the bladder apex to the umbilical stump, the umbilical arteries as they extend caudally along both the left and right sides of the bladder, and the umbilical vein, which courses from the umbilical stump to the liver. Infections can occur in one or more of these structures, as well as in the external stump.

ETIOLOGY/PATHOPHYSIOLOGY
Infection of the umbilical remnants is generally presumed to be due to contamination of the umbilical stump at birth resulting in ascending infection. Beta-streptococcal organisms are invariably involved, with coliforms a common second pathogen. *Staphylococcus aureus*, *Klebsiela* spp., and anaerobes are also recognized pathogens and may occur alone or in conjunction with other bacteria.

CLINICAL PRESENTATION
Discharge of purulent material from the umbilical stump (**288**), umbilical swelling, or patent urachus (**286**) are the most common

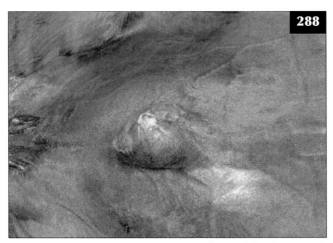

288 Purulent discharge material from the umbilical stump of a neonatal foal with an umbilical infection.

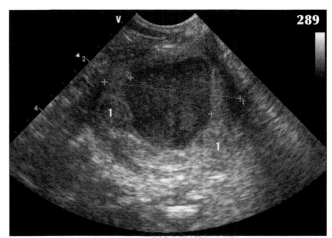

289 Short-axis image of a urachal abscess in a foal. Note the thick capsule surrounding echogenic fluid. "1" denotes each umbilical artery. Medical treatment was successful. 6 MHz microconvex linear array transducer.

clinical signs. Closed umbilical infections may not result in any clinical signs, and are instead discovered on investigation of fevers, elevations in the white blood cell (WBC) count and/or fibrinogen, or investigation of the source of septic arthritis.

DIFFERENTIAL DIAGNOSIS
Enlarged umbilical structures may be a result of fibrous tissue or seromas, and not infection. Pyrexia and an abnormal leukogram may also be caused by other diseases such as occult septic physitis and pneumonia, therefore a diagnosis of internal umbilical remnant infection in foals with fevers and/or abnormalities on hematology/serum chemistry should be made after a thorough physical examination to exclude other diseases. Peritoneal tears in older foals at the umbilical stump or umbilical hernias are differentials for swelling in the umbilical region.

DIAGNOSIS
Ultrasonographic evaluation (**289**) can be used to support or exclude the diagnosis. Enlargement of and/or fluid within lumen of the urachus, umbilical vein, and/or an umbilical artery are consistent with infection. An inflammatory leukogram may or may not be present.

MANAGEMENT
The vast majority of umbilical remnant infections resolve with medical therapy. Oral or intravenous broad-spectrum antimicrobial therapy directed against streptococci and coliforms is successful in most cases. Adjunct treatment with metronidazole should be considered if a foul odor is noted to any umbilical discharge or high fevers are present. Gas may be noted within the remnants on ultrasound examination in foals with anaerobic infections; however, gas is not uncommonly found within the urachal lumen of foals with patent urachus, presumably due to ascending migration of air. Surgical resection is a consideration for management if a large accumulation of purulent material is present. Extensive umbilical vein infections may be most safely managed medically, since transection of the vein may result in

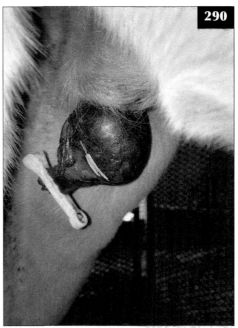

290 Umbilical stump swelling caused by bleeding resulting in a hematoma.

contamination of the peritoneum and the portion remaining within the liver will still require medical treatment. A 2–3-day course of antimicrobial treatment followed by surgical excision may decrease contamination of the surgical site and incision, while also providing an opportunity to assess the potential success of medical treatment through a repeat ultrasound examination prior to surgery.

If there is purulent material at the umbilical stump in close proximity to the skin surface, a simple stab incision to allow drainage is a reasonable management option. If drainage is already present, the stump should be kept clean to allow continued drainage.

In foals being treated for concurrent septic arthritis, it may be best to monitor affected internal remnants with repeat ultrasound examinations instead of immediate excision. Continued antimicrobial administration is required anyway for the septic arthritis, and, with the possible exception of very young (neonatal) foals, continued dissemination of infection from internal umbilical infection is unlikely by the time septic arthritis has been recognized.

Prevention of umbilical remnant infection is best achieved through good hygiene. Clean foaling facilities with clean/fresh bedding reduce the frequency of infection. Minimal handling of the umbilical structure reduces the chances for infection. Clean hands/hand washing reduces exposure to potential pathogens. If personnel cannot be relied on to wash their hands, wearing of disposable latex gloves should be a requirement. Dipping/cleansing the umbilical stump is generally recommended. The product used for the dipping/cleansing is not as significant as the care/cleanliness employed in the procedure. Repeat dipping of the umbilicus is not necessary unless the structures remain moist or patent. Overzealous dipping can cause irritation and inflammation and result in discomfort and tissue that can become susceptible to infection.

The prognosis for resolution of umbilical remnant infections is excellent in cases that show an initial ultrasonographic response. Complications in cases managed surgically are infrequent and are usually a result of contamination at the time of excision. Such complications include intestinal adhesions, incisional infections, and dehiscence.

UMBILICAL SWELLING

KEY POINTS

- Common causes include hernias, infections, and peritoneal rents.
- Ultrasonography is the diagnostic method of choice.

DEFINITION/OVERVIEW

The umbilical stump may become swollen due to a variety of causes from the time of birth to several months of age. The nature of the swelling (firm, fluctuant, pitting, warm, and cool) may help the clinician determine the underlying cause of the problem.

ETIOLOGY/PATHOPHYSIOLOGY

Umbilical cord trauma with edema and/or seroma formation, or leakage of urine, can result in umbilical swelling early in the neonatal period (**290**). Infection of the umbilical remnants, including the umbilical stump, may result in abscessation or fibrous tissue formation in the stump region, which may not become manifest until 1 or more months of age. Herniation of intestines or omentum can develop if the umbilical defect is large. Foals from one to several months of age may develop a rent in the peritoneum at the umbilical site. This results in leakage of peritoneal fluid into the subcutaneous tissues.

CLINICAL PRESENTATION

Parturient traumatic injuries to the cord may result in seroma formation or edema of the umbilical stump, usually within the first 1–2 days of life. Swellings resulting from such incidents may be firm to fluctuant, cool, and nonpainful. If the urachal remnant is traumatized, and the urachus does not contract, urine may leak into the subcutaneous tissues from the umbilical stump region, resulting in progressive warm, firm, or pitting edema originating from the stump. Umbilical herniation of intestines or omentum may result in swellings that are often reducible, although incarceration of the herniated material can occur and the contents may not be reducible. Rents in the peritoneum at the umbilical stump generally develop at 2 to several months of age, resulting in progressive warm pitting edema originating from the umbilical region.

DIFFERENTIAL DIAGNOSIS

The differential diagnosis for umbilical swelling includes umbilical hernias, umbilical remnant infections, fibrous tissue swelling, peritoneal rents, and parturient traumatic injuries to the umbilical stump that may involve the urachus. Since the treatment for specific disorders includes medical, surgical, and no treatment options, the diagnosis of the cause of an umbilical swelling is very important.

DIAGNOSIS

Ultrasonography is the diagnostic method of choice for determining the etiology of an umbilical swelling.

MANAGEMENT

The management of an umbilical swelling depends on the cause, which is most appropriately determined by ultrasonography. Traumatic swelling in the neonate can be carefully monitored without treatment. Umbilical stump infections often respond to medical therapy, particularly if drainage is present or created with a stab incision. Peritoneal rents, seen in older foals, generally need no treatment and resolve in about one week. Umbilical hernias generally require surgical repair (see Chapter 5, Alimentary Tract Disorders, Umbilical hernias, p. 90).

RENAL FAILURE/RENAL DISEASE

KEY POINTS

- Causes of renal failure may be congenital or acquired.
- Iatrogenic causes (drug toxicities) are a common etiology.
- Clinically, foals with renal failure are often depressed and inappetent.
- Chronic renal failure often results in weight loss/failure to thrive.
- Diagnosis is supported by an elevated serum creatinine, low urine specific gravity (SG), and abnormal serum electrolytes.
- Diuresis and supportive care are the basis of management.

DEFINITION/OVERVIEW

Renal failure in the foal may result from congenital or acquired conditions, including iatrogenic causes.

ETIOLOGY/PATHOPHYSIOLOGY

Congenital causes of renal failure include renal agenesis, dysplasia (**291, 292**), hypoplasia, and polycystic kidneys (**293**). A syndrome of renal failure associated with hydroureter and hydronephrosis in neonatal foals has also been recognized. Fatal anuric renal failure in neonatal foals, associated with echogenic renal cortices on ultrasound examination, with otherwise structurally normal kidneys (**294**), has been observed and was suspected to be a result of antibiotic administration to the mare during gestation.

Congenital mild to moderate hydronephrosis in the neonatal foal, not associated with ectopic ureters, has also been seen. Affected foals are azotemic with electrolyte abnormalities; some cases resolve with supportive care. Unilateral ureteroceles have been diagnosed on ultrasonography by the authors on two foals that presented with stranguria and azotemia (**272, 273**).

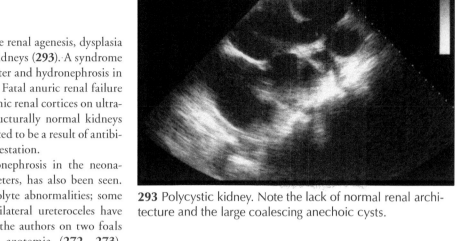

293 Polycystic kidney. Note the lack of normal renal architecture and the large coalescing anechoic cysts.

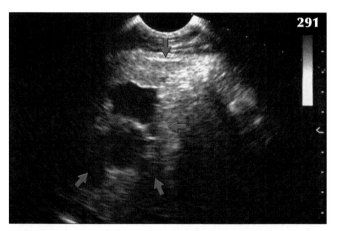

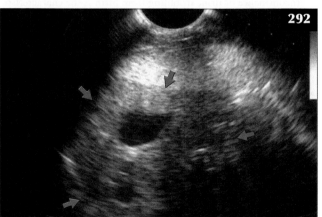

291, 292 Right (**291**) and left (**292**) kidneys (delineated by arrows) of a foal with anuric renal failure due to renal dysplasia. Note the large anechoic cyst-like regions, the absence of corticomedullary demarcation, and the atypical shape to both kidneys. 5 MHz sector transducer.

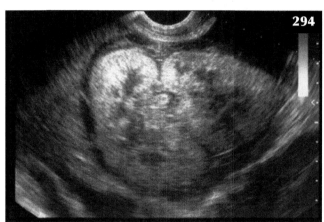

294 Ultrasound image of the right kidney in a foal with congenital anuric renal failure. Note the echogenic renal cortex and perirenal edema. 6 MHz microconvex linear array transducer.

The ureteroceles were so large that they obstructed the opposite ureteral orifice.

The pathogenesis of the disorders mentioned earlier is not known, but possibilities include fetal viral infection, drug administration to the mare during pregnancy, or *in-utero* urinary tract obstruction. Familial renal dysplasia has been recognized in other species, but a breed predilection has not been recognized in the horse. The suspected cases of antibiotic-induced congenital renal disease were in mares being treated for protozoal myelitis. These mares were being treated with trimethoprim/sulfa combinations, pyrimethamine, and supplementation with folic acid. It is presumed that the oral supplementation with folic acid blocked, or competed with, the absorption of the activated form of folic acid from the gastrointestinal (GI) tract.

Acquired causes of renal failure include pigment nephrosis (often a result of neonatal isoerythrolysis [NI]), nephrotoxic drugs such as aminoglycosides and oxytetracycline, overdose of NSAIDs, leptospirosis, hemodynamic collapse, endotoxemia, ischemia, hypoxemia (as seen in some cases of severe periparturient hypoxia), and immune-mediated glomerulonephritis.

Although both kidneys are affected in most cases of renal diseases, unilateral cases may be asymptomatic, with a normal life expectancy provided the opposite kidney remains functional. Bilateral cases will become symptomatic anytime from birth up to a few years of age depending on the extent of the pathology.

CLINICAL PRESENTATION

Foals with renal failure due to any cause become dull and inappetent. A marked reduction in urine output may be seen in acute renal failure and may be accompanied by subcutaneous edema in foals receiving intravenous fluids. Polyuria may be seen in other cases. Ataxia, abnormal mentation, or seizures may be observed in cases of renal failure complicated by severe hyponatremia. Chronic renal failure results in weight loss and failure to thrive.

DIFFERENTIAL DIAGNOSIS

Failure to thrive from disease of other organ systems or infection can often be excluded by physical examination and results of laboratory testing. CNS disorders or liver failure can cause seizures, but it should be remembered that seizures may also result from severe hyponatremia in foals with renal failure. Prerenal azotemia and benign idiopathic transient azotemia in neonatal foals are disorders that may result in elevations in serum creatinine that are not due to renal disease.

DIAGNOSIS

Laboratory findings of an elevated serum creatinine and low urine SG support a diagnosis of renal failure. Benign transient azotemia in the neonatal foal is an exception, since foals often have dilute urine normally. Differentiation of chronic from acute failure is made by history, body condition, and ultrasonography. Ultrasonography is also of value in ruling out congenital renal disorders. In cases of renal dysplasia (**291, 292**), ultrasonograms typically reveal small misshapen echodense kidneys with decreased corticomedullary demarcation and abnormal internal architecture. Renal cysts or dilation of the ureters may also be seen. In some cases the kidneys may appear grossly normal in spite of the microscopic changes. One or both kidneys may be affected. Ultrasonography may reveal normal to increased renal size with normal echogenicity, while chronic renal disease typically reveals smaller than normal kidneys with increased echogenicity of the cortex and/or medullary region; perirenal edema may be seen (**294**). Renal biopsy may be considered in some cases; however, there is a high risk for hemorrhage and the etiology often remains unclear.

MANAGEMENT

Any underlying or complicating factors such as administration of nephrotoxic drugs, hemoglobinuria, dehydration, or sepsis should be addressed. Diuresis with correction of any underlying electrolyte or acid–base abnormalities is the primary method of treatment in cases of acute renal failure. Measurement of central venous pressure (CVP) is advisable to avoid volume overload and is of particular importance in patients with oliguric renal failure. If elevations in CVP occur, a dopamine infusion (3–5 µg/kg/min) and furosemide (1 mg/kg q2h) may be necessary.

Antimicrobial therapy is required for the treatment of leptospirosis. Effective antimicrobial therapy includes doxytetracycline (provided severe azotemia is not present and serum creatinine is monitored closely). Penicillins are otherwise very effective against leptospirosis.

Immune-mediated glomerulonephritis is uncommon in younger horses, but if suspected or confirmed with biopsy, corticosteroid therapy would be indicated.

Hemo- and peritoneal dialysis have been used in the horse to manage acute renal failure refractory to conventional therapy. Dialysis enables correction of acid–base and electrolyte abnormalities and removal of toxins, allowing the patient to improve clinically while giving the kidneys time to repair.

Chronic renal disease is managed by ensuring adequate nutritional support, fluid intake, and removal of any potential conditions that may acutely exacerbate the disease.

ECTOPIC URETER

KEY POINTS

- Ectopic ureters are a rare condition in the foal; however, they are the most commonly identified anomaly of the urinary tract.
- The majority of the reported case are fillies, but this number may be biased as ectopic ureters entering the pelvic urethra of the colt may pass retrograde into the bladder.
- Ectopic ureters are a developmental abnormality in which one or both ureters exit in an aberrant location (do not enter the bladder).
- Incontinence or urine dribbling from birth is the characteristic clinical presentation.
- Diagnosis is based on endoscopic or speculum examination of the urethra, vagina, and/or bladder, most recently computed tomographic imaging has been used to diagnose this condition.
- Surgical repair is the only option for correction.

DEFINITION/OVERVIEW

Ectopic ureters are extremely uncommon in foals. They are a developmental anomaly. In the normal foal the ureters enter the bladder in the region of the trigone. Ectopic ureters open in the urethra, vagina, or other area of the reproductive tract. Fillies appear to be more commonly affected than colts. Ectopic ureters may be unilateral or bilateral.

ETIOLOGY/PATHOPHYSIOLOGY

Ectopic ureters are a result of failure of the metanephric duct to migrate to the trigone or be incorporated in the urogenital sinus.

In fillies, a mesonephric duct may fail to regress and the ureter opens into the uterus or vagina. There is no known breed predilection.

CLINICAL PRESENTATION

Foals typically present with a history of urine dribbling since birth (incontinence). Fillies may present with perineal dermatitis due to urine scalding. Colts may present with chronic urinary tract infections and may or may not have urine scalding.

DIFFERENTIAL DIAGNOSIS

Neurologic conditions may cause a similar clinical scenario.

DIAGNOSIS

Diagnosis of ectopic ureters is made via speculum or endoscopic examination of the urethra, bladder, and vagina. Cystoscopic examination should reveal urine emptying into the bladder periodically from the ureteral openings. Pigmentation of the urine to facilitate identification of the ectopic ureter may be achieved with intravenous administration of phenolsulfonphthalein, neopontosil, or indigo carmine.

Percutaneous pyelography can be used to delineate the ureters. Retrograde ureterography can also be used in such cases, but usually does not outline the kidney. Ultrasound examination of some cases may reveal hydroureter (**295**) and hydronephrosis of the affected side. The condition may also be bilateral.

MANAGEMENT

Unilateral disease can be addressed surgically, providing the other kidney is functioning normally. A normally functioning contralateral kidney and ureter can be determined by evaluation of blood urea nitrogen (BUN) and creatinine, the ultrasonographic appearance of the other kidney and ureter, and the endoscopic appearance of the ureteral opening into the bladder. Surgical reimplantation of the ureter into the bladder wall may be accomplished by submucosal tunneling or side-to-side anastomosis of the ureter and dorsolateral bladder wall. The patient will be at risk for ascending

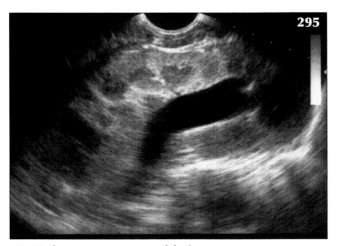

295 Hydroureter in a neonatal foal.

pyelonephritis, therefore removal of the affected kidney and ureter is justifiable. Ureteral ectopia has been associated with renal dysplasia of the affected side; therefore, nephrectomy may be further justified.

NEUROGENIC BLADDER

KEY POINTS

- Neurogenic bladder is not a common finding in the equine pediatric patient.
- Bladder atony may be seen in the neonatal patient as a result of recumbency, drug therapy, congenital weakness, or trauma.
- Spinal cord trauma or spinal cord disease is a frequent cause.
- Typical clinical presentation is urinary incontinence.
- Ultrasonographic identification of persistent bladder distension can support the diagnosis.
- Pharmacologic intervention is often unrewarding.

DEFINITION/OVERVIEW

Neurogenic bladder is an infrequently encountered problem in the equine pediatric patient. Bladder atony may be observed in some recumbent foals during hospitalization for birth asphyxia and it could be a complication of phenobarbital administration. Bladder atony may also be due to bladder trauma during delivery without bladder rupture (*Table 50*) or to a congenital weakness of bladder tone.

ETIOLOGY/PATHOPHYSIOLOGY

Neurogenic bladder in the foal can be caused by damage to the spinal cord as a result of traumatic or hypoxic injury. Inflammatory lesions resulting in compression of the spinal cord can also result in a neurogenic bladder. Damage to the spinal cord cranial to the sacral segments results in an "upper motor neuron" (UMN) bladder. Damage to the actual sacral segments results in a "lower motor neuron" (LMN) bladder. The UMN bladder (intact sacral segments) results in loss of conscious voiding of the bladder. The detrusor muscle can contract and empty the bladder when it is full. The LMN bladder loses detrusor muscle function and it is continuously distended and atonic.

CLINICAL PRESENTATION

Urinary incontinence, urine dribbling, and urine scalding are typical clinical signs. Neurologic signs referable to the spinal cord may be associated with a history or evidence of trauma.

DIFFERENTIAL DIAGNOSIS

Differential diagnosis includes ectopic ureters and possibly obstruction of the urethral outflow of urine.

DIAGNOSIS

Ectopic ureters must be ruled out. The presence of continuous bladder distension suggests an atonic bladder, as ectopic ureters are continually evacuating the bladder. Identification of spinal cord injury or an injury damaging sacral segments innervating the bladder may be observed.

MANAGEMENT

Treatment of the underlying cause, when possible, may resolve a neurogenic bladder. Pharmacologic intervention with alpha-adrenergic antagonists or parasympathomimetics is usually unrewarding. Indwelling catheters can provide relief of distension and may aid in the return of bladder function.

The prognosis for pharmacologically induced paralysis is good once the agent is discontinued. A recumbent foal can improve with time and physical improvement. The neonate with a suspected hypoxic insult resulting in bladder dysfunction may also improve as long as secondary complications are avoided. The prognosis for a traumatic neurogenic bladder is dependent on resolution of the underlying cause.

FURTHER READING

Adams R (1990) The urogenital system. In: *Equine Clinical Neonatology* (Korterba A, Drummond W, Kosch P, Eds.). Lea & Febiger, Philadelphia, PA, pp. 443–531.

Bayly WM, Schott HC II (2004) Disorders of the urinary system. In: *Equine Internal Medicine*, 2nd ed. (Reed SM, Bayly WM, Sellon DC, Eds.). WB Saunders, St Louis, MO, pp. 1169–1295.

Chaney K, Schott HC (2007) *Veterinary Clinics of North America: Equine Practice* 23: 691–696.

Richardson DW (1985) Urogenital problems in the neonatal foal. *Veterinary Clinics of North America: Equine Practice* 1: 179–189.

Neurologic Disorders

10

William V. Bernard

EXAMINATION OF THE NERVOUS SYSTEM

The neurologic examination begins with the signalment and a thorough history, including information regarding age, sex, breed, previous medical history, age at onset of neurologic signs, and any treatments administered. The neurologic examination should include a complete physical examination, as systemic diseases that involve the central nervous system (CNS) are common in the foal.

A systematic approach to the neurologic examination should begin with an assessment of the mental state and progress to an evaluation of the head position and the cranial nerves (CNs). A lesion of either the cerebrum or, occasionally, the brainstem results in some degree of depression. If the foal is bright and alert, then it is unlikely that a central lesion exists; however, critically ill neonates are often weak, depressed, or recumbent. These foals must be differentiated from those with primary neurologic disease.

The vestibular system aids in the maintenance of balance and the orientation of the head with the body. When evaluating the vestibular system, the clinician must take into account that the neonate often holds its head in a flexed position and responds to stimuli with quick, jerky movements. The vestibular system includes the inner ear and its efferents, the brainstem nuclei, and the cerebellar tracts. A lesion of the vestibular system results in a head tilt with the poll deviated laterally and the muzzle and caudal neck on a median plane. Severe lesions can produce a deviation of the entire neck to one side and a tendency to lean or circle in one direction. Asymmetric cerebral lesions can also result in a head tilt and circling in one direction. Foals with cerebral lesions are often severely depressed, and their circling is continuous and progressive.

Evaluation of the CNs is performed as in the adult horse; however, a few normal variations should be noted. The palpebral reflex is present shortly after birth. The menace response (blinking subsequent to a menacing gesture) does not develop until several weeks of age, but the foal should withdraw its head from a menacing gesture. The pupillary light reflex can be slow in an excited foal. The ability to swallow can be evaluated by observing the foal's ability to nurse. Lip and tongue tone and recognition of the udder are necessary for adequate nursing. If large amounts of milk are seen coming from the mouth or nostrils, then a swallowing deficit should be considered.

Examination of the eye should be a routine part of the basic physical and neurologic examination (see Chapter 13, "Ophthalmologic Disorders"). Vision can be evaluated by observation of the foal's behavior, navigation through obstacles, and response to a menacing gesture. Direct and consensual light reflexes should be present. The normal cornea is clear and oval. Foals commonly have persistent papillary membrane tags that may extend freely into the aqueous humor or span the circumference of the iris collarette. Persistent hyaloid structures are common in the foal up to 4 months of age. The foal's fundus is similar to that of the adult.

Spinal cord reflexes can easily be evaluated in the neonate and are useful when trying to localize a spinal cord lesion. Neonates and young foals are often hyperreflexic until they are several weeks of age. In the hindlimb, the patellar, flexor, gastrocnemius, and cranial tibial reflexes can be tested. The patellar reflex is tested with the foal in lateral recumbency and the limb to be tested supported in a relaxed flexion. A brisk extension of the limb (stifle) is expected when the patellar ligaments are struck with the side of the hand. This reflex involves spinal segments L4 and L5 and is mediated through the femoral nerve. The hindlimb flexor or withdrawal reflex involves spinal segments L3 to S3 and is mediated through the sciatic nerve. Pinching the skin of the distal limb, the coronary band, or the bulbs of the heel should elicit a withdrawal of the limb and/or central recognition of pain. The gastrocnemius reflex is performed by bluntly striking the gastrocnemius tendon and observing for extension of the hock. This reflex involves spinal cord segments L5 to S3 and is mediated through the tibial branch of the sciatic nerve. The cranial tibial reflex is performed by holding the limb in relaxed extension and balloting the cranial tibial muscle. The expected response is hock flexion.

Reflex testing in the forelimbs includes evaluation of the flexor and triceps reflexes. The triceps reflex is tested by holding the limb in relaxed flexion and tapping the biceps tendon above its insertion at the olecranon. This reflex is mediated by the radial nerve through the cervical intumescence (C6–T1). The flexor or withdrawal reflex of the forelimb is mediated through the last three cervical and first two thoracic spinal cord segments. The expected response is flexion of the digit, carpus, elbow, and shoulder. A central response to pain should be observed.

Thoracolumbar lesions can be localized by evaluating the cutaneous reflex along the lateral body wall. Gentle pinching or poking of the skin along the lateral thorax elicits a twitching of the cutaneous trunci muscle. The sensory input is carried to the spinal cord at the level of the stimulation. It then travels cranially in spinal cord white matter to the last cervical and first thoracic nerves. The lateral thoracic nerve innervates the cutaneous trunci muscle. Damage to any portion of this pathway results in an absence of the cutaneous trunci reflex. The perineal reflex evaluates the last sacral segments and the caudal spinal cord segments. Stimulation of the perineal area results in flexion of the tail and closure of the anus.

The gait of the foal should be examined for weakness or ataxia. The newborn foal often has a choppy, springy, dysmetric gait. Signs of weakness include stumbling, knuckling, dragging a toe, or trembling. Further evaluation of weakness is performed by pushing or pulling from side to side and/or backing. Ataxia or incoordination suggests the presence of proprioceptive deficits (lack of recognition of limb position) and these are most easily identified at slower gaits. Circling, turning, backing, and traveling up and down slopes in a straight line and with the head held elevated should be used to detect ataxia. In a straight line, the patient may weave or sway. Circling may elicit limb circumduction, delayed protraction, and crossing over and/or stepping on the opposite foot. Holding the head in an elevated position while walking may elicit or worsen a dysmetric forelimb gait.

DISEASES OF THE FOREBRAIN (CEREBRAL HEMISPHERES)

KEY POINTS

- The most common cause of forebrain disease in the neonate is hypoxia/ischemia. In the older foal, trauma is the more common cause. Clinical signs of forebrain dysfunction include changes in behavior, altered consciousness, seizures, and/or central blindness.
- Seizures are a result of sudden abnormal electrical activity.
- Diagnosis is based on history, signalment, clinical signs, cerebrospinal fluid (CSF) analysis, radiographs, and advanced imaging when available.
- Control of clinical signs (self-inflicting trauma) is the first step in case management.

DEFINITION/OVERVIEW

Disease of the forebrain is characterized by changes in behavior, altered consciousness, seizures and/or central blindness. A wide variety of insults to the integrity of the CNS can lead to neuronal dysfunction that results in the clinical signs mentioned. The most common forebrain disease in the neonate is hypoxic/ischemic insult at birth, with congenital, infectious, and metabolic disorders less commonly seen. With the nature and activity level of the older foal, head trauma is the most common cause of forebrain disease in the non-neonate or older foal.

ETIOLOGY/PATHOPHYSIOLOGY

Disease of the CNS can result from a wide variety of causes: trauma, infection, compression, toxicity, vascular (blood flow) disorders, hypoxia/ischemia, or metabolic disorders. Any of these conditions can influence the CNS through acute disruption of neural tissue or disruption of neural pathways or metabolism. Seizures are a result of sudden abnormal electrical activity, which may occur in one area of the brain or spread to the entire brain. Changes in behavior or paroxysmal movements are a result of the sudden abnormal neural discharge.

CLINICAL PRESENTATION

Disease of one or both of the cerebral hemispheres can result in a variety of clinical signs referable to the CNS (*Table 53*). Disease processes disrupt normal neuronal function, which can lead to abnormalities of consciousness, behavior, seizures (**296**), or central blindness. Mild central lesions may be exhibited by drifting to one side, partial seizures (facial twitching), intermittent depression, or continual yawning (*Table 54*). Signs of more severe involvement include severe depression, circling, a dramatic uncontrollable lean to one side, seizures, blindness, maniacal behavior, or head pressing (*Table 55*). Diffuse cerebral involvement (both cerebral hemispheres) results in clinically symmetric signs. Lesions on one side of the forebrain result in asymmetry of neurologic signs. Seizures can be classified as partial, general, or partial with generalization. Diffuse cerebral involvement results in generalized seizures. Generalized seizures may be preceded by abnormal behavior, tachycardia, tachypnea, teeth grinding, abnormal facial expressions, restlessness, or disorientation. Generalized

---

Table 53. Classifications of clinical signs of central nervous system disease

- Abnormalities of consciousness
- Abnormalities of behavior
- Seizures
- Central blindness

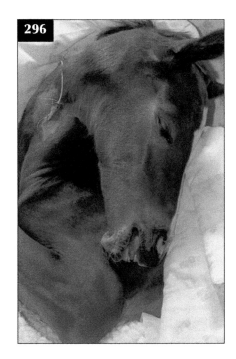

296 A foal with forebrain disease seizing.

Table 54. Mild signs of central nervous system disease

- Intermittent depression
- Drifting to one side
- Partial seizures (facial twitch/grimace)
- Continual yawning

Table 55. Severe signs of central nervous system disease

- Severe depression
- Circling (intermittent or continuous)
- Uncontrollable lean to one side
- Seizures (continuous or intermittent)
- Blindness
- Maniacal behavior
- Head pressing

Table 56. Differential diagnosis of central nervous system disease

- Meningitis
- Hypoxic ischemic encephalopathy
- Hydrocephalus
- Epilepsy
- Hyponatremia, hypocalcemia
- Hypoglycemia
- Cerebral trauma
- Viral encephalitis
- Leukoencephalomalacia
- Hepatic encephalopathy

seizures are manifested by a diffuse muscle rigidity, recumbency, and unconsciousness, with variable association of paddling movements and abnormal activity such as urination, defecation, or salivation. Abnormal discharge in a focus (seizure focus) of the brain results in a partial seizure. If this activity is in the motor cortex, a range of paroxysmal–clonic motor activity can occur. Seizure foci in other parts of the brain may result in other signs such as blindness, abnormal behavior, depression, or unconsciousness.

DIFFERENTIAL DIAGNOSIS
See *Table 56*.

DIAGNOSIS
Diagnosis of CNS disease is based on history, signalment, and localization of the lesion to the CNS. Radiographs of the skull may be useful in identifying trauma (fracture of the skull). CSF analysis can identify inflammatory lesions and possibly trauma. Pleocytosis (increased CSF cell count) indicates viral or bacterial diseases. Increased protein content is also compatible with inflammatory conditions. Xanthochromia (yellow tinge) indicates a possible injury. Red blood cells (RBCs) can indicate traumatic injury to the CNS. Increases in RBCs must be differentiated from a traumatic centesis. Magnetic resonance imaging

(MRI) and computed tomography (CT) scans provide an image of the brain within the calvarium.

MANAGEMENT
The initial approach to the foal with forebrain disease should be to control clinical signs that could result in self-inflicted trauma and, when possible, to provide a safe environment. Seizure control can include a variety of medications; these are discussed in more detail in Chapter 17 (Pharmacology). Diazepam and phenobarbital are the more commonly used anticonvulsants (*Table 57*). Diazepam is a safe but short-acting anticonvulsant. Phenobarbital can influence temperature regulation and gastrointestinal (GI) motility. Diazepam is often the first choice in seizure control as it is safe and relatively fast acting; however, diazepam is also short acting and may not have the potency to control severe seizure activity. When diazepam is not effective, phenobarbital becomes the most common drug of choice. Phenobarbital must be administered slowly over 15–30 minutes; an initial dose may require titration, with additional doses to control severe seizures. Supportive/nursing care becomes an important factor in management of the seizuring foal. Temperature regulation, urination, defecation, musculoskeletal factors, and nutrition need to be addressed.

Table 57. Anticonvulsant therapy

- Diazepam
- Alpha-2 antagonists
- Chloral hydrate
- Glycol guaiacolate
- Phenobarbital

MENINGITIS

KEY POINTS

- Meningitis is an inflammatory lesion of the meninges as a result of bacterial, viral, or protozoal disease.
- Bacterial meningitis is most common.
- Gram-negative organisms are most commonly involved.
- A wide variety of CNS signs may be seen.
- The presence of a high fever in association with CNS signs is suggestive.
- A CSF analysis can be diagnostic.
- Broad-spectrum antibiotic therapy (with an aggressive Gram-negative spectrum) must include drugs with the ability to cross the blood–brain barrier.

DEFINITION/OVERVIEW

Meningitis is a bacterial, viral, or protozoal disease of the meningeal structures, with bacterial meningitis being the most commonly diagnosed. The condition occurs more commonly in young foals than in neonates or older foals. Bacterial meningitis can be seen in compromised hospitalized neonates that develop nosocomial infections, or it can develop secondary to bacterial infections in other body systems. Viral infections of foals are the same as those that affect adult horses. As in adult horses, protozoal meningitis is rare. The prognosis for survival of foals with bacterial meningitis is poor.

ETIOLOGY/PATHOPHYSIOLOGY

Bacterial infection is the most common cause of meningitis in the foal. Bacteria may reach the brain via bacteremia or, possibly, with the migration of infected monocytes through normal pathways to the meninges. The bacteremia may result from infection involving any mucous membrane surface (respiratory or GI) abscess or internal infection with subsequent migration to the CNS. The damage that results directly from bacterial infection, or from secondary inflammatory response, disrupts the local structures adjacent to the meninges. Gram-negative organisms (often coliforms) are the more common causes of bacterial meningitis. Gram-positive organisms such as *Staphylococci* spp. or *Streptococci* spp. can be seen. The viral agents that cause CNS disease in adult horses generally cause clinical signs more typical of encephalitis.

CLINICAL PRESENTATION

Foals with meningitis may present with multiple signs of CNS disease (e.g., hyperesthesia, hyperhidrosis, tonic–clonic seizures [**297**], or more focal evidence of CNS abnormality) (*Table 58*). High fevers are often present. Foals may be depressed (**298**) and show signs of neck stiffness and blindness. Other CNS signs may include abnormal facial expressions (**299, 300**) (lip chomping, grimace), wandering, circling, or stargazing.

DIFFERENTIAL DIAGNOSIS

See *Table 56*.

DIAGNOSIS

The condition may be initially differentiated from other causes of forebrain disease based on signalment and the presence of fever. Neurologic signs may differ from those caused by hypoxic ischemic

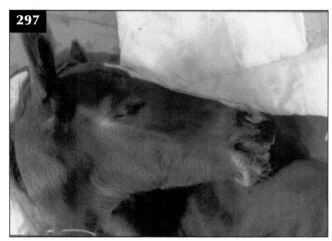

297 Tonic–clonic seizure activity in a foal with CNS disease.

Table 58. Clinical signs of meningitis

- Fever
- Hyperesthesia
- Hyperhidrosis
- Tonic–clonic seizures
- Neck stiffness
- Blindness
- Wandering
- Circling
- Stargazing
- Abnormal facial expressions
- Lip chomping
- Grimace

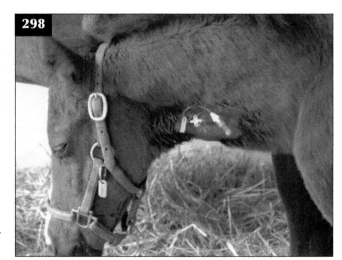

298 Central depression in a foal with CNS disease.

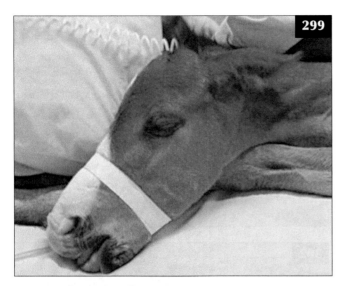

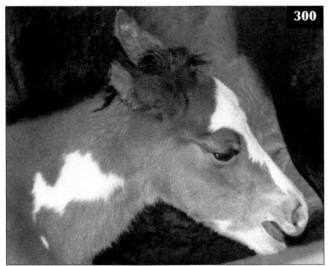

299, 300 Abnormal facial expression associated with CNS disease showing (**299**) twitching of the lip and (**300**) open mouth with lip chomping.

encephalopathy (HIE) in that HIE usually causes more diffuse symmetric cerebral involvement. Meningitis typically results in more focal CNS signs. The other neurologic signs such as hyperhidrosis, hyperesthesia, teeth grinding, lip chomping, and neck pain are typical of meningitis. The definitive diagnosis of meningitis is based on collection of CSF. Pleocytosis with neutrophils or occasionally mononuclear cells is expected. Bacteria may be observed in the CSF; cultures of fluid should be performed. Blood cultures may be positive. A complete blood count (CBC) is not specific and may be normal to low, or elevated. When viral or protozoal disease is suspected, serology or virus isolation should be attempted.

MANAGEMENT
Control of CNS signs with anticonvulsants (*Table 57*) and supportive care in addition to antibiotic therapy are the principles of therapy. Antibiotic therapy needs to be aggressive and rapid and should be based on culture and sensitivity results. When culture results are negative or not available, broad-spectrum antibiotics

with good CSF penetration should be chosen, although this aspect of antibiotic choice may be less important with inflammation of the meningeal vasculature. The Gram-negative spectrum of the antibiotic therapy is most significant as the majority of organisms causing sepsis in the foal are Gram negative. Third-generation cephalosporins with excellent Gram-negative spectrum and CSF penetration (see Chapter 17, Pharmacology) should be considered. Anti-inflammatories are of benefit and can include steroidal or non-steroidal drugs. Steroids can be immunosuppressive and should be used only when clinical signs are progressive or life threatening. When steroids are used, the duration of therapy should be limited.

HYPOXIC ISCHEMIC ENCEPHALOPATHY

KEY POINTS
* HIE describes a deficiency of oxygen reaching the brain resulting from either hypoxemia or ischemia, which ends in an encephalopathy, HIE is also known as neonatal maladjustment syndrome (NMS) or perinatal asphyxia syndrome.
* Events before, during, or after birth may lead to HIE.
* Clinical signs vary from mild nonspecific to tonic–clonic seizures.
* The onset of clinical signs is typically within 24 hours, but it can be up to several days of age.
* Diagnosis is based on signalment/history and ruling out other possible causes of CNS signs in the neonate.
* Factors frequently associated with the condition include placental insufficiency, emergency cesarean section, and dystocia.
* Hematology/serum chemistries are nonspecific, but an elevated creatinine level is suggestive of placental insufficiency.
* Therapy for HIE is primarily supportive in nature.

DEFINITION/OVERVIEW
The term "neonatal maladjustment syndrome" has been used to describe newborn foals that are exhibiting behavioral or neurologic abnormalities that are not related to infectious or toxic conditions, congenital or developmental abnormalities, or metabolic disorders. These foals have previously been classified as barkers, wanderers, dummies, or convulsants. The incidence of the syndrome is estimated to be 1%–2% of all foal births. Numerous theories are given as to the cause of the syndrome. These include CNS trauma and hemorrhage and CNS anoxia. In some instances increased proinflammatory cytokines associated with placental infection and fetal inflammation may play a role. It appears that the majority of neonates exhibiting CNS signs within the first few days of life have suffered a lack of cerebral oxygen delivery resulting from either a lack of blood flow (ischemia) or decreased arterial oxygen tension (hypoxemia). Therefore, the descriptive term "HIE," which has been adapted from human medicine, will be used in the remainder of this discussion.

The history of a foal with HIE may include a report of gestational problems in the mare. Examples include vaginal discharge suggesting uterine or placental infection, colic or other medical problems during gestation, premature lactation, and prolonged or shortened gestational length. Some mares have a history of repeatedly delivering foals that develop CNS signs. It is possible that these mares may have repeated problems during parturition or an inability to form an adequate

Table 59. Risk factors for the development of hypoxic ischemic encephalopathy

• Gestational abnormalities

• Placental insufficiency

• Premature placental separation

• Dystocia

• Nonelective cesarean section

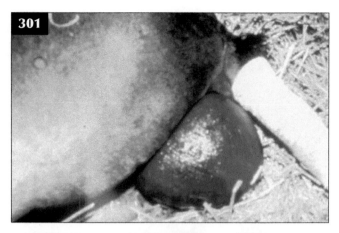

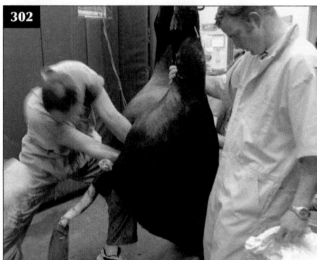

301, 302 Premature placental separation (**301**) and dystocia requiring manipulation under general anesthesia (**302**) are very common circumstances in the mare that result in a lack of oxygen delivery to the foal and subsequent hypoxic ischemic encephalopathy in the foal.

placental unit. Premature placental separation is also commonly reported in the history of neonates with HIE. Previous reports suggest that delivery of affected neonates may be fast and uncomplicated; however, more recent reports suggest that dystocia is not uncommon in neonates with HIE. Delivery via emergency cesarean section is another risk factor for the development of hypoxic insults before or shortly after delivery (*Table 59*). A very important point to consider is that these neonates may be normal at birth and show no evidence of CNS disease for hours to days after delivery. Alternatively, these foals may exhibit evidence of violent CNS activity immediately or shortly after birth. This variation in onset of clinical signs is likely to be related to the degree of cell damage occurring as a result of the hypoxia–ischemia and possibly to the degree of edema that occurs as a result of cell death.

ETIOLOGY/PATHOPHYSIOLOGY

Intracranial hemorrhage as a result of increased CNS pressure during birth or subsequent to trauma has been proposed as a cause of CNS disease in the neonate. Many newborn foals with CNS disturbances have a history suggestive of decreased oxygen delivery during the perinatal period. This, coupled with histopathologic findings similar to those described in other species with experimentally induced asphyxia, suggests that hypoxia and ischemia are important components of this syndrome in foals.

Interference with blood flow and oxygen delivery before birth can result from placental insufficiency or interference with uterine blood flow. A wide variety of conditions can result in interference with blood flow and oxygen delivery during parturition (e.g., obstruction of umbilical blood flow, premature placental separation [**301**], decreased uterine blood flow, and prolonged parturition (dystocia) [**302**]). During normal foaling the fetus experiences a transient period of anoxia. The normal healthy foal is not affected by this period of oxygen deprivation; however, the compromised foal may not be able to compensate and a cycle of events leading to exacerbation of the anoxia may result.

Events subsequent to birth can also lead to hypoxia and ischemia. Inadequate cardiac output can result in insufficient pulmonary or cerebral blood flow. The transition from fetal to adult circulation is critical to adequate oxygen delivery and can result in periods of inadequate delivery if delayed or if there is a reversion to fetal circulation.

The primary event in the initiation of brain injury is a hypoxic event as a result of reduction in cerebral blood flow. This event occurs during the antepartum, peripartum, or postpartum period. The hypoxia initiates a cascade of events that in combination result in the ensuing neuronal damage. Hypoxia results in a transition to anaerobic metabolism and an inability to maintain normal

cellular homeostasis. Transcellular ion pumps are disrupted leading to an intracellular increase in calcium and water. In addition, the excitatory neurotransmitter glutamate increases in the extracellular space. Glutamate results in cell swelling/lysis by stimulating sodium entry, followed by a passive influx of chloride and water. The process of reperfusion also includes the generation of free radicals that can exacerbate cellular injury. The high content of polyunsaturated fatty acids and the relative low level of antioxidants make the brain highly susceptible to oxidative damage.

CLINICAL PRESENTATION

Clinical signs of HIE in neonatal foals are highly variable. The original descriptions of these foals as "barkers," "wanderers," or "convulsants" indicate the variation in clinical signs. Signs can be mild (*Table 60*) (e.g., a loss of affinity for the mare, an inappropriate suckle reflex, wandering, intermittent depression [**298**], and stargazing). Facial spasms, lip curling and chomping (**299, 300**), or abnormal respiratory patterns may occur. The abnormal vocalizations (barking) are rarely identified. These foals may sleep deeply and may be difficult to arouse.

Table 60. Mild signs of hypoxic ischemic encephalopathy

- Loss of affinity for the mare
- Inappropriate suckle reflex
- Intermittent depression
- Stargazing
- Abnormal facial expressions (spasms, lip curling/ chomping, grimace)
- Abnormal respiratory patterns
- Abnormal vocalizations

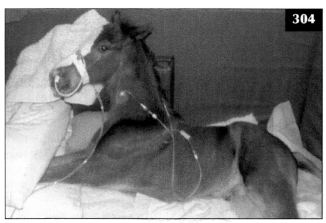

304 A foal with hypoxic ischemic encephalopathy showing generalized seizure with extensor rigidity.

These "mild" signs may be all that is seen and the patient may recover without complication. On the other hand, signs may progress to more prominent and severe indications of CNS disease (*Table 61*). Foals may become totally unaware of the environment (**303**) and appear to have blindness of central origin. Seizures may follow and are usually very sudden in onset, but they are often preceded by one or more of the earlier mentioned signs. One of the more frequent premonitory signs of seizure is a "stretching" activity that may in fact be a mild seizure. While lying down, the foal extends its forelimbs outward and lifts its head before relaxing

Table 61. Severe signs of hypoxic ischemic encephalopathy

- Total unawareness of the environment
- Central blindness
- Grand mal seizures with oposthonus, extensor rigidity, paddling
- Stupor/coma

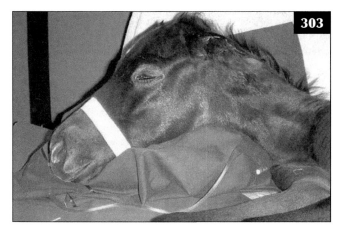

303 Stuporous foal with hypoxic ischemic encephalopathy showing signs of being nonresponsive to the environment.

again into a sternal sleeping position. Seizures can be of short duration and with no subsequent evidence of obvious CNS disease. In more severe cases, seizures are severe and generalized with tonic–clonic convulsions, opisthotonus, and extensor rigidity (**304**). Some patients may paddle violently. If the seizures are repetitive or continuous, affected foals are generally stuporous or comatose in the interictal period. Not all HIE patients develop seizures before progressing into a state of stupor.

The onset of clinical signs is extremely variable, and many foals may appear completely normal for hours to days. The onset of seizures has been reported to be as late as 4–5 days of age. Neonates can also be seen with CNS signs immediately after birth. The duration of clinical signs can also vary. These signs can be very brief, with single or no seizures to persistent stupor or coma for several days. Usually, foals recover in the reverse order in which the CNS signs developed (i.e., stupor to awareness of the environment, standing, walking, and suckling). Typically, when foals recover from prolonged CNS derangement, relapses do not occur; however, recurrence of seizures subsequent to prolonged stupor has been seen.

DIFFERENTIAL DIAGNOSIS
See *Table 56*.

DIAGNOSIS
The diagnosis of HIE is based on typical clinical signs, historical information (potential hypoxic event), and elimination of other possible causes of CNS disease in the newborn foal. As mentioned, the history often includes such factors as prepartum problems in the mare, problems during delivery, and placental separation or delivery via emergency cesarean section (*Table 59*). When parturition includes any of these factors, close observation should ensue with special attention to evidence of CNS disease. The signs of CNS disease are not pathognomonic for HIE. Conditions that may also result in seizures include hyponatremia, hypocalcemia, hypoglycemia, hypomagnesemia, metabolic acidosis, generalized sepsis, parasite migration, Tyzzer's disease, viral encephalitis, drug-induced toxicities, hydrocephaly, liver failure, idiopathic epilepsy, and heat stroke. These conditions must be considered in the differential diagnosis, but they rarely cause seizures in the

newborn foal. Conditions, other than HIE, that more frequently cause CNS derangement in the neonate or newborn foal are hydrocephalus and bacterial meningitis.

The differentiation of the foal with hydrocephalus from one with HIE can be difficult. CNS abnormalities are not always present at birth in either case. The seizures in foals with hydrocephalus can be very severe, violent, and difficult to control. Foals with meningitis may have fever. The CNS signs may first appear as periods of agitation accompanied by pawing, grinding of teeth, or sweating. The CNS signs in foals with meningitis may appear more like those in the adult horse with encephalopathy and may include continuous and persistent wandering and circling, maniacal behavior, and head pressing.

Results of laboratory data of the equine neonate with HIE are neither specific nor diagnostic; however, an elevated creatinine level and, less commonly, elevated muscle enzyme levels are occasionally present in foals with HIE. The elevation in creatinine that is seen at birth is related to placental insufficiency, which may be related to a lack of adequate oxygen delivery *in utero*. The elevation in the muscle enzymes CK and AST may correlate with muscle hypoxia/ischemia or trauma at birth. Severe muscle trauma during a dystocia can result in marked elevations in muscle enzymes. The leukogram in a foal with meningitis may suggest infection; however, it is not diagnostic. Serum chemistry levels can be useful in excluding some of the less likely causes of CNS disease such as metabolic or hepatic disease. CSF analysis is not diagnostic in the foal with HIE or hydrocephalus; however, increased CSF cell counts can be diagnostic of meningitis.

Radiographs of the skull may be useful in cases of severe trauma. CT (axial) or MRI can be used to diagnose hydrocephalus. In human medicine, brain imaging or electroencephalography has been used to identify hypoxic encephalopathy. These modalities have not been evaluated extensively in the horse.

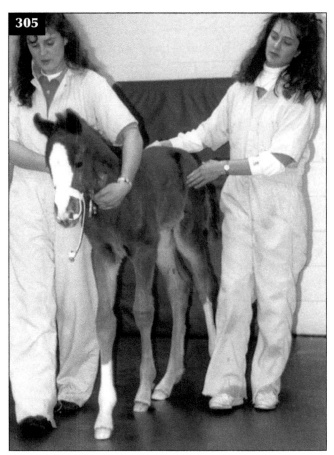

305 Nursing care is critical to the recovery of the patient with CNS disease.

MANAGEMENT

Primary treatment of HIE is symptomatic. Supportive and nursing care is critical to the outcome of the case (**305**). The treatment of seizures varies depending on their severity. A seizure that is mild and brief may not need to be controlled; however, if seizures are recurrent or severe, treatment becomes necessary. The control of seizure activity can prevent trauma, reduce the energy consumption of seizures, and allow for better nursing care. A variety of anticonvulsants can be used. Diazepam (0.1 mg/kg i/v) is the drug of choice for the immediate short-term suppression of seizures. If this is not effective, repeated doses can be given. Diazepam is safe and fast acting, but its duration of action is short. If seizures persist, alternative choices of drugs include phenobarbital, phenytoin, or sodium pentobarbital used to effect. Phenobarbital can provide prolonged seizure control and is safe if given slowly and used to effect. The dosage is 10–20 mg/kg as a loading dose (10 mg/kg is often sufficient), diluted in isotonic saline and given over a period of 20–30 minutes. Administration should stop if the desired effects are achieved before the full dose is administered. Phenobarbital can be repeated as needed. Once the seizures are controlled, oral administration (10–20 mg/kg q12h) can be used for maintenance. Phenytoin (5–10 mg/kg i/v initially followed by 1–5 mg/kg i/v,

i/m, or p/o q6–12h) may also be used. The disadvantages are the frequency of administration and cost. Intravenous sodium pentobarbital to effect (approximately 2–4 mg/kg) may be used in foals with uncontrollable seizures. Marked sedation or anesthesia may occur at higher or more frequent doses.

Broad-spectrum antimicrobial therapy should be considered for the prevention of secondary infection in the compromised patient. Nutritional therapy is of the utmost importance and varies with the severity of the condition. If the foal can stand but not suckle, an indwelling nasogastric tube may be used to provide adequate caloric support. The foal requires a minimum of 10% of its body weight in milk over a 24-hour period. Feeding every 1–2 hours is preferred. If the patient is recumbent but is able to maintain sternal recumbency, cautious enteral feeding is still possible, but care must be taken not to overfeed a recumbent foal. Enteral feeding must be provided sparingly in the stuporous foal. In these cases, caloric supplementation should be provided with continuous intravenous dextrose administration or more complete parenteral nutrition.

Intravenous fluids should be used judiciously in foals with HIE as overhydration may worsen cerebral edema. It is wise to restrict fluid administration unless a secondary complication requires additional fluid therapy. When determining maintenance fluid requirements (2 mL/kg/hour), oral fluid intake must be taken into account.

A foal that is receiving 10% of its body weight in milk may not need additional intravenous fluids.

Medications to reduce cerebral edema may be helpful, however, none of these therapies can be well supported due to the lack of adequate clinical trials. Intravenous dimethyl sulfoxide (DMSO) (0.5–1.0 g/kg as a 10% solution i/v) or mannitol can be useful in the acute stages of cerebral edema. Other unsubstantiated therapies include opioid antagonists, magnesium, thiamine, allopurinol, ascorbic acid, and theophylline. Hypertonic solutions such as mannitol should be used only if it can be definitively shown that cerebral hemorrhage is not present. In the presence of cerebral hemorrhage, hypertonic solutions can exacerbate edema. The use of corticosteroids is controversial as they can increase cerebral blood flow, which may contribute to cerebral edema. Additionally, corticosteroids can result in immune suppression and potentially exacerbate secondary infection. In human medicine, therapeutic hypothermia is the only treatment that has withstood clinical trials. Therapeutic cooling can decrease brain injury by slowing metabolism and the pathways that lead to cell death and edema.

The prognosis for survival is dependent on the severity of the initial insult and the progression of the edema and cellular damage. Overwhelming hypoxia can result in a rapid onset of respiratory arrest. If cerebral damage results in fixed, dilated, nonresponsive pupils, the prognosis is grave. The CNS signs in many affected foals may not progress beyond a minimal loss of recognition of the environment, with gradual recovery over a 1- to 2-day period. The prognosis for foals that have seizures is worse than for those that do not; however, if seizures can be controlled, adequate nursing care provided, and secondary complications avoided, the prognosis for these foals is good. Persistence of residual neurologic signs is unusual. When recovery does occur, there does not appear to be a long-term effect on growth or development.

HYDROCEPHALUS

KEY POINTS
- Hydrocephalus is a collection of CSF in the ventricles or subarachnoid space.
- Hydrocephalus is typically a congenital condition.
- Internal hydrocephalus (ventricular) is a result of obstructed CSF outflow.
- External hydrocephalus (subarachnoid) is a failure of development of brain parenchyma (hydranencephaly).
- A physical appearance of a domed skull may be seen at birth.
- Clinical signs with congenital disease are of CNS origin and are present at birth or within days.
- Ruling out other conditions and lack of response to therapy forms a presumptive diagnosis.
- Advanced imaging techniques are diagnostic.

DEFINITION/OVERVIEW
Hydrocephalus is defined as increased CSF in either the ventricles (internal) or subarachnoid space (external) and is most frequently recognized as a congenital disorder. Internal hydrocephalus is more common than external hydrocephalus. Clinical signs are related to forebrain involvement and are frequently present at, or shortly

after, birth. In acquired hydrocephalus, CNS signs appear as CSF outflow is obstructed over time. Survival of foals with hydrocephalus is limited and the prognosis for survival is guarded.

ETIOLOGY/PATHOPHYSIOLOGY
External hydrocephalus is typically a congenital disorder. Internal hydrocephalus can be congenital or acquired. Acquired disease may be seen secondary to space-occupying lesions, inflammatory lesions, or aplasia of the conducting pathways. Congenital internal hydrocephalus is secondary to hypoplasia of the conducting pathways.

External hydrocephalus results from a failure of development (hypoplasia) of normal brain parenchyma. This failure of development is known as hydranencephaly. CSF passively fills the space normally occupied by brain tissue. External hydrocephalus is normotensive, therefore it is usually a result of, and not the cause of, the CNS disease.

Internal hydrocephalus results from obstruction of CSF flow between the sites of production and sites of absorption. CSF is produced in the choroid plexus of the lateral third and fourth ventricles and then circulates to the subarachnoid space, where it is absorbed by the arachnoid villi. Abnormalities of this pathway result in a "buildup" of CSF with increased intracranial pressure. Hypertensive hydrocephalus progressively results in clinical signs as a result of pressure-induced damage to structures surrounding the ventricles.

CLINICAL PRESENTATION
Physical clinical signs of hydrocephalus may be seen at birth. Newborn foals with hydranencephaly may have a misshaped calvarium or other congenital abnormalities (306). Signs of hypertensive hydrocephalus can occasionally be manifested by an enlarged calvarium with open sutures; however, the absence of these external features does not rule out the presence of hydrocephalus. Foals born with hydrocephalus may show dramatic CNS signs at birth or develop CNS signs within days of birth. Seizures manifested can be violent and difficult to control. Alternatively, the CNS signs can be manifested as mental disorders (loss of cerebral white matter).

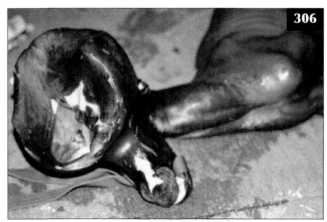

306 Hydranencephaly in a foal. Note the abnormally shaped calvarium.

These disorders may include a loss of affinity for the dam, blindness, an inability to suckle, or a disoriented wandering. Foals with acquired hydrocephalus may progressively develop intermittent depression and unthriftiness.

DIFFERENTIAL DIAGNOSIS
See *Table 56*.

DIAGNOSIS
Diagnosis is based on ruling out other disease processes with similar clinical signs. Normal CSF cell counts can be useful in ruling out meningitis. Patients with persistence of neurologic signs should be considered as candidates for advanced diagnostics. Advanced imaging techniques (CT or MRI) are the definitive premortem tests of choice.

MANAGEMENT
Treatment options are limited and generally unsuccessful.

EPILEPSY

KEY POINTS
- Epilepsy can be defined as disturbed electrical rhythms of the CNS.
- Clinical manifestation of epilepsy is seizures/convulsions.
- Epilepsy in horses can be defined as juvenile or acquired.
- The etiology of epilepsy is a focus of intermittent abnormal electrical activity.
- Diagnosis is based on ruling out other causes of seizures/convulsions.
- Pharmacologic control of seizures may allow for long-term resolution.

DEFINITION/OVERVIEW
Epilepsy is defined as a disorder marked by disturbed electrical rhythms of the CNS. The condition is manifested by seizures/convulsions. Juvenile epilepsy has been described in foals, with an onset at weeks to months of age. The condition is most common in Arabian foals and may have a familial tendency. Acquired epilepsy may also be seen in foals. Successful therapy can be achieved with long-term anticonvulsants.

ETIOLOGY/PATHOPHYSIOLOGY
The etiology of juvenile epilepsy is unknown. An abnormal focus of paroxysmal electrical activity with a possible lowered seizure threshold results in uncontrollable motor activity. Seizures may be mild (manifestations of lip chomping, grimace, and chewing), with progression to generalized seizures and variations of nystagmus, opisthotonus, tonic–clonic convulsions, and loss of consciousness. The seizures are usually symmetric. Asymmetric localizing signs may suggest an acquired form of epilepsy. The acquired form of epilepsy is considered to be secondary to an epileptic focus. The epileptic focus may be secondary to a previous disease process (inflammation, physical injury, or hypoxia/ischemia).

Seizure activity results from rapidly spreading paroxysmal discharges of electrical activity.

CLINICAL PRESENTATION
Foals may present in an active form of either a partial seizure or generalized seizures. Foals presenting in the interictal period may have physical evidence of trauma. When trauma is noted, the gums, lips, eyes, and/or head are often involved, as the seizing foal moves forward at the start of a seizure. Foals may present with varying degrees of depression or blindness in the interictal period. The interictal abnormalities may last for minutes to days.

DIFFERENTIAL DIAGNOSIS
Any condition resulting in partial or generalized seizures should be considered. Nonepileptic causes of seizure are generally continuous and progressive, whereas the epileptic foal may act completely normal in the interictal period. See also *Table 56*.

DIAGNOSIS
Diagnosis is based on history, clinical signs, and ruling out other causes of seizures. CSF is normal, as are serum chemistry and leukogram findings. Advanced imaging techniques should be considered. Epilepsy should be considered in a foal that responds well to anticonvulsants with subsequent regression when therapy is abruptly discontinued.

MANAGEMENT
Control of seizures is advisable if they are repeatable and generalized. Trauma secondary to generalized seizures can be life threatening. The basis of treatment is to raise the seizure threshold with anticonvulsants (*Table 57*). One to three months of anticonvulsant therapy is the usual course of therapy, followed by a gradual reduction in therapy over weeks. Phenobarbital is the most frequently used drug for long-term control of seizures. This drug is long acting and relatively inexpensive. Dosages are adjusted based on seizure control and the degree of sedation produced. Juvenile or familial epilepsy patients generally recover subsequent to weeks/months of seizure control.

HYPONATREMIA

KEY POINTS
- Hyponatremia can result in CNS signs.
- Hyponatremia is generally seen as a result of an underlying disease process.
- Management is based on resolution of the underlying disease process and gradual correction of the sodium imbalance.

DEFINITION/OVERVIEW
Neurologic dysfunction in foals secondary to electrolyte abnormality is occasionally seen. Blood sodium concentrations of 110 mmol/L (mEq/L) or less, depending on the status of other electrolytes and osmolality, may result in clinical signs of CNS disease. Neonatal or older foals may be affected. An underlying disease process is typically the cause of the electrolyte abnormality.

ETIOLOGY/PATHOPHYSIOLOGY

Hyponatremia may be seen secondary to severe sodium loss with enterocolitis, uroperitoneum (the accumulation of sodium-containing fluid in the abdomen), acute renal failure, or inappropriate renal excretion of sodium. Sodium loss in severe secretory enteritis/enterocolitis, particularly with a secretory component, can result in significant losses of total body sodium. If this fluid is replaced with nonsodium-containing (water) fluids, then a hyponatremia can ensue. Uroperitoneum can result in hyponatremia as total body sodium equilibrates between blood and peritoneal fluid. The blood sodium concentration decreases as sodium diffuses from the blood (higher sodium concentration) to the peritoneal fluid (lower sodium concentration). Hyponatremia is a common abnormality associated with acute renal disease. Inappropriate secretion of sodium can occur secondary to renal disease and it has been seen in neonates (in the absence of renal disease) shortly after birth.

CLINICAL PRESENTATION

Foals with hyponatremia present with generalized seizures, which may be preceded by partial seizures.

DIFFERENTIAL DIAGNOSIS

Other conditions resulting in foal seizures (see *Table 56*).

DIAGNOSIS

The presence of hyponatremia, with or without azotemia and other electrolyte abnormalities, or other concurrent electrolyte abnormalities may include hypochloremia and/or hyperkalemia. This electrolyte pattern can be seen with uroperitoneum, ruptured bladder, or enterocolitis. Foals with an idiopathic inappropriate secretion of sodium will have hyponatremia with an increased fractional excretion of sodium.

MANAGEMENT

Treatment of hyponatremia includes sodium replacement therapy in an attempt to control clinical signs. If CNS signs are persistent and progressive, then a hypertonic saline solution can be used, with frequent monitoring of blood sodium concentrations. Hypertonic saline should be followed by or concurrently administered with isotonic solutions. A more judicious replacement of sodium is via the use of an isotonic fluid; this produces a more gradual correction of sodium levels.

HYPOGLYCEMIA

KEY POINTS
- Hypoglycemia is a common metabolic disorder of the equine neonate.
- The limited glycogen stores of the neonate prevent a rapid response to glucose requirements.
- The liver plays a key role in glucose metabolism. Foals with hepatic disease may be severely hypoglycemic.
- Clinical signs of hypoglycemia vary from CNS depression to CNS seizures.
- Hypoglycemia is most easily corrected with cautious intravenous administration of glucose.

DEFINITION/OVERVIEW

Hypoglycemia is one of the more common metabolic abnormalities of the neonate, although older foals can also develop hypoglycemia. Hypoglycemia in older foals is generally secondary to hepatic disease.

ETIOLOGY/PATHOPHYSIOLOGY

Causes of hypoglycemia are numerous and are exacerbated by the lack of glycogen stores and the immaturity of gluconeogenic pathways in the newborn, and in particular the premature, foal. In these individuals the lack of glycogen stores and the immature gluconeogenic pathways, in combination with the increased consumption of glucose during disease processes (e.g., sepsis, asphyxia, shock, and hypothermia), can lead to hypoglycemia. A delay in the normal progression of a foal to suckle after birth, or inappropriate milk production in the mare, may also contribute to hypoglycemia. The older foal with adequate glycogen stores is much less susceptible to low blood glucose levels. The liver plays a major role in the gluconeogenic pathways; foals with acute hepatitis can be severely hypoglycemic.

CLINICAL PRESENTATION

Clinical signs of hypoglycemia are not specific for the condition, are vague, and may contribute to the signs of the primary disease process. Common signs noted include weakness, lethargy, collapse, poor suckle, inappetence, and, in the neonate, occasional seizures. Older foals with hypoglycemia are more prone to seizure than the hypoglycemic neonate.

DIFFERENTIAL DIAGNOSIS

As the clinical signs of hypoglycemia are very nonspecific, the differential is broad and can include any condition resulting in the weak, depressed, lethargic foal. The seizuring foal differential is listed in *Table 56*.

DIAGNOSIS

Blood glucose determinations are made via laboratory analysis, reagent strips, or glucometers. Blood tests for determination of blood glucose should be run shortly after collection, as RBCs can continue to consume glucose after collection and result in falsely low values. Collection of blood in a sodium fluoride/potassium oxalate blood tube (which inhibits the gluconeogenic process) provides more accurate results if samples cannot be evaluated rapidly.

MANAGEMENT

When hypoglycemia is severe and potentially life threatening, glucose (dextrose) solutions can be given rapidly over minutes; however, the preferable method of administration is by constant rate infusion (CRI). Boluses of hypertonic glucose can be irritating to veins, exacerbate CNS signs, and result in diuresis or rebound hypoglycemia. Rapid infusions of 200 mg/kg/min over several minutes of a 5%–10% solution can be given intravenously to treat severe hypoglycemia. Preferably, a CRI of a 50% solution at a rate of 10 g/kg/day should be used, with continuous monitoring of blood glucose levels. In a 50 kg foal this calculates to 20 g/hour and 40 mL/hour of a 50% dextrose solution. When starting this infusion rate, it is advisable to start at 50%–75% of the calculated dose; this avoids a period of hyperglycemia. Continuous glucose can be administered with microdrip sets or fluid pumps. Monitoring the blood glucose concentration frequently is advisable.

CEREBRAL TRAUMA

KEY POINTS
* Trauma should be considered as a differential for any foal with CNS signs.
* Radiographs of the skull may identify fractures.
* Treatment is aimed at reducing the inflammation that is causing an increase in intracranial pressure.

DEFINITION/OVERVIEW
Because of the active nature of horses, trauma to the CNS is common. Trauma should be considered in the differential of any foal with CNS signs. Blunt trauma is common due to running into objects, kicks, or, particularly, rearing over backward. A foal that rears over backward creates blunt force trauma to the parietal or occipital bones. This can directly damage neural tissues or indirectly displace the basisphenoid and basioccipital bones beneath the brainstem.

ETIOLOGY/PATHOPHYSIOLOGY
The pathophysiology of head trauma is complex and has been categorized as being the result of concussion, contusion, compression, laceration, or hemorrhage. Tissue damage results from one of the above events. Acute physical trauma can result in disruption of neural tissue. Physical trauma is generally associated with fractures; however, acceleration/deceleration injuries can be as damaging as direct trauma secondary to fractures. Delayed changes that result from secondary vascular damage occur gradually and insidiously. Vascular changes result in ischemic injury and subsequent edema and progressive loss of vascular perfusion.

CLINICAL PRESENTATION
Foals with cerebral trauma can present with signs varying from depression to violent seizures and coma. These clinical manifestations vary with the region of the brain or brainstem traumatized. Signs of mentational changes such as depression, stupor, or coma may be present. CN deficits, miosis, mydriasis, anisocoria, nystagmus, strabismus, dysphagia, head tilt, facial nerve deficits, and blindness may be seen. Midbrain lesions resulting in nonresponsive, dilated pupils (mydriasis) suggest a poor prognosis. Ataxia may be present and is often difficult to interpret in the disoriented patient.

DIFFERENTIAL DIAGNOSIS
See *Table 56*.

DIAGNOSIS
A diagnosis can be made when physical evidence (**307, 308**) or a history of trauma is present; however, significant trauma can occur

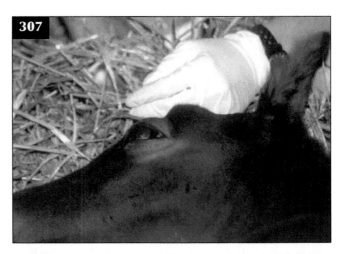

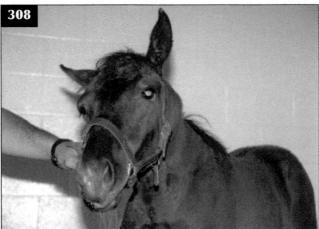

307, 308 Physical evidence of head trauma in a foal.

without obvious physical evidence. Additionally, patients with other forms of CNS disease (*Table 56*) may have physical evidence of trauma as a result of the primary disease process. Radiographs of the skull can identify fractures of the skull, calvarium, orbit, and sinus, and the petrous temporal, occipital, basisphenoid, and basioccipital bones. CSF collection may identify hemorrhage. Hemorrhage may be noted from a nostril (**309, 310**) or ear canal (**311**). Radiography or endoscopy may identify hemorrhage into a guttural pouch (**312**).

MANAGEMENT
Treatment of cranial trauma is directed at reducing inflammation and slowing the progression of increasing intracranial pressure. Anti-inflammatories may include steroids and NSAIDs (*Table 62*). Broad-spectrum antimicrobials should be considered in order to prevent secondary bacterial infections (see Chapter 17, Pharmacology). Surgical reduction of fractures should be considered when feasible. A head trauma case that is recumbent or maniacal/incoherent provides a treatment challenge. Head padding (helmets) or stall padding can be useful (**313**). Recumbent patients must be turned frequently and supported nutritionally.

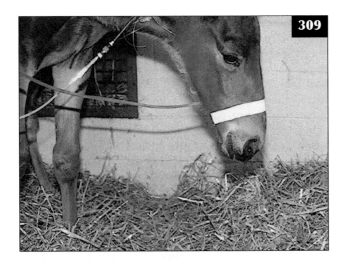

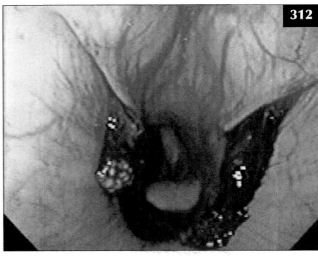

312 Endoscopic view of hemorrhage from the guttural pouch.

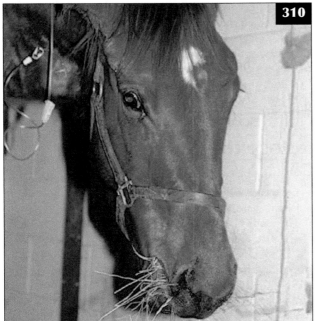

Table 62. Anti-inflammatories for use in central nervous system disease

- Flunixin meglumine (1.1 mg/kg i/v q12h)
- Dexamethasone (0.05–0.2 mg/kg i/v q12–24h)
- Prednisolone sodium succinate (1.0–2.5 mg/kg i/v)
- Prednisolone (oral) (0.25–1.0 mg/kg p/o q24h)

309, 310 Epistaxis. Hemorrhage from the nostrils.

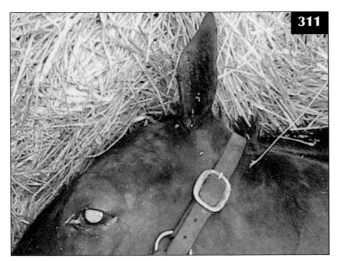

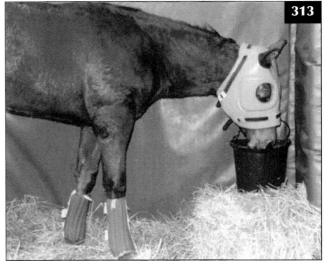

311 Hemorrhage from the inner ear.

313 Head gear and padding protecting a foal with cerebral trauma and CNS signs from further injury.

VIRAL ENCEPHALITIS

Key points
- Viral encephalitis is more common in adult horses.
- Clinical signs are typically referable to the CNS.
- Early signs of rabies virus infection does not always immediately suggest neurologic disease.
- Serologic response can be useful when interpreted in the light of vaccination history.
- CSF response can be variable.

Definition/overview
Viral encephalitis is generally more commonly identified in the adult horse; however, viral diseases should be considered when evaluating the foal with CNS signs. Encephalitic viruses are distributed throughout the world. The epizoology of these viral infections often involves maintenance of the viruses in feral reservoirs, with insect vectors involved in transmission. Equine encephalitis viruses are also often of concern because of their zoonotic potential.

Etiology/pathophysiology
Equine viral encephalitis can be caused by viruses of the families *Rhabdovirus* (rabies), *Flavivirus* (West Nile virus [WNV], St. Louis encephalitis virus, Kunju virus and Murray Valley encephalitis virus), *Alphavirus* (Eastern, Western, Venezuelan, Japanese, Highlands J.), and *Borna* virus (Borna disease).

The histologic lesions associated with neurotrophic viruses are similar: a nonsuppurative encephalomyelitis and vasculitis with perivascular cuffing and monocytic cell infiltration.

Clinical presentation
Foals with viral encephalomyelitis typically present with signs referable to the CNS (*Table 53*). However, both WNV and rabies do not classically fit this characteristic. As the term "encephalomyelitis" indicates, spinal cord involvement can be present and is quite typical with WNV. Rabies infection eventually progresses to encephalitis; however, the presenting clinical signs can be quite variable and do not always immediately suggest neural disease. These early clinical signs of rabies include recumbency, lameness, hyperesthesia, colic, ataxia, and muscle tremors. Early nonspecific signs of viral encephalomyelitis may include fever, depression, and anorexia.

Differential diagnosis
See *Table 56* for other disease conditions resulting in clinical signs similar to those produced by viral encephalitis. A fever may be useful in differentiation.

Diagnosis
Diagnosis is based on identification of compatible neurologic signs and epidemiologic features that suggest the possibility of infection. Epidemiologic factors include the appropriate time of year when insect vectors would be active, the presence of an endemic disease, and seasonality of feral hosts (rabies). Serologic diagnostics can be confused/influenced by vaccination or maternal transfer of antibodies. A fourfold rise in convalescent titer has been suggested to be diagnostic. Immunoglobulin subclass (IgM) titers, when available, are useful to identify recurrent/active infection and are considered to be diagnostic of WNV.

CSF analysis can be useful; however, normal CSF does not rule out viral encephalitis. Cellular changes in CSF are related to the time course of the disease, therefore CSF may be normal early in the course of the disease. Elevations in protein and/or a mononuclear pleocytosis are the typical CSF changes expected. A neutrophilic pleocytosis should not be considered to rule out viral encephalitis. Serum chemistry and leukogram findings may suggest infection/inflammation, but are nonspecific. Definitive diagnosis is usually dependent on postmortem histopathologic changes, viral isolation, immunohistochemical staining, and/or PCR testing.

Management
Initial therapy should include control of CNS signs if present (*Table 57*). The use of anti-inflammatories should be considered (*Table 62*). The use of steroids is controversial (potential immune suppression), but should be considered in the patient that is severe or rapidly progressive. Supportive and nursing care becomes crucial in the patient that is recumbent or anorectic. The pharmokinetics of the antiviral drug valacyclovir have recently been determined. This drug, contrary to the parent drug acyclovir, is well absorbed by the horse. Valacyclovir should be considered in viral disease of the foal.

LEUKOENCEPHALOMALACIA

Key points
- Leukoencephalomalacia (moldy corn poisoning) can affect foals that are of an age to eat solid foods.
- The condition results from corn contaminated with a fungus.
- The fungus produces a neuro/hepatic toxin (fumonisin).
- Clinical signs are referable to the CNS and/or liver.

Definition/overview
Leukoencephalomalacia, also known as "moldy corn poisoning" or "blind staggers," is a CNS disease that results from the ingestion of moldy corn containing neuronal toxins. Leukoencephalomalacia can affect foals that are of an age to consume solid food, but the toxicity is more common in adult horses. The disease should be considered whenever an outbreak of CNS disease is being investigated.

Etiology/pathophysiology
The condition has been associated with the ingestion of moldy corn that is contaminated with *Fusarium* spp. fungi. The most commonly associated fungi is *F. moniliform*. Other commercially prepared feedstuffs can be contaminated with *F. moniliform*. The toxins produced are fumonisin toxins, which can result in neuro- or hepatotoxicity. The disease is usually associated with a dry growing season followed by heavy moisture (a wet harvest) and the feeding of cracked corn.

Clinical presentation
Clinical signs are referable to the CNS and/or the liver and may vary from depression to acute death. Fever is not usually present.

Neurologic signs consist of depression, anorexia, lethargy, ataxia, blindness, head pressing, excitability, and delirium.

DIFFERENTIAL DIAGNOSIS
Other conditions causing CNS signs (*Table 56*). The concurrent presence of hepatic disease or the occurrence of outbreaks may be useful in establishing a presumptive diagnosis; however, hepatic encephalopathy may produce similar clinical signs. The absence of a fever may suggest that the condition is not infectious.

DIAGNOSIS
Diagnosis is based on clinical signs, history, and epidemiologic factors compatible with the disease. The majority of corn samples will have *Fusarium* spp. fungi present; a finding of large numbers of fungi is suggestive of contaminated feed. Identification of fumonisin toxins can be diagnostic. CSF analysis may identify a neutrophilic pleocytosis. Necropsy findings are a hepatic necrosis and focal areas of hemorrhagic necrosis in the white matter of the cerebrum.

MANAGEMENT
Treatment of leukoencephalomalacia is supportive. Treatment of the CNS signs (*Table 57*) is usually necessary. Survival is related to the amount of toxin ingestion. Severe cases have a guarded prognosis.

HEPATIC ENCEPHALOPATHY

KEY POINTS
- Hepatic encephalopathy is characterized by diffuse cerebral involvement.
- The neuronal dysfunction resulting in clinical signs is multifactorial.
- Serum chemistries (elevated liver specific enzymes) can be diagnostic.

DEFINITION/OVERVIEW
Hepatic encephalopathy is a CNS dysfunction secondary to liver disease or portasystemic shunts. Liver disease in the foal is primarily infectious in nature. Bacterial infections are the primary causes, with viral infection an occasional factor. The neurologic signs are diffuse and cerebral. Portasystemic shunts are rare.

ETIOLOGY/PATHOPHYSIOLOGY
Liver disease in the foal is discussed in Chapter 6 (Liver Disorders). The pathogenesis of hepatic encephalopathy is multifactorial. The influence of toxins such as ammonia and long-chain fatty acids on the CNS may alter cerebral energy metabolism, damage neuronal membranes, or influence synaptic transmission. An imbalance of chemicals in the brain, particularly excitatory and inhibitory neurotransmitters, may contribute to the encephalopathy that is seen.

CLINICAL PRESENTATION
The signs of hepatic encephalopathy are usually symmetric, indicating diffuse cerebral involvement. A variety of signs such as depression, yawning, wandering, head pressing, dementia, ataxia, blindness, seizure, and coma may be seen. Physical signs of liver disease (icterus) may be observed, but should not be used to rule out liver disease. Acute hepatitis may not result in clinical icterus. Patients with liver disease may present with abdominal pain, as swelling of the liver capsule is painful.

DIFFERENTIAL DIAGNOSIS
Disease conditions resulting in CNS signs (*Table 56*).

DIAGNOSIS
Symmetry of CNS signs or the presence of icterus may help the initial differentiation of hepatic encephalopathy from other CNS conditions. CSF analysis is normal. Serum chemistries can be diagnostic of hepatitis (see Chapter 6, Liver Disorders). Ultrasonography of the foal's abdomen can identify hepatic changes and, particularly, an enlarged liver (see Chapter 6, Liver Disorders).

MANAGEMENT
Treatment of hepatic encephalopathy consists of controlling the CNS signs and supportive care. Correction of metabolic disturbances (i.e., hypoglycemia [see Hypoglycemia, pp. 197–198] and metabolic acidosis, if present) may provide a significant improvement in CNS signs. The underlying disease process must be determined and treated.

VESTIBULAR DISEASE

KEY POINTS
- The vestibular system maintains the body's orientation in space.
- The most common lesion of the vestibular system is trauma to the receptor organs (inner ear).
- The hallmark clinical sign of vestibular disease is a loss of balance.

DEFINITION/OVERVIEW
The vestibular system maintains the orientation of the body with respect to gravity and influences the eyes, trunk, and limbs in relationship to the position of the head and to movement of the head and limbs. It also maintains balance and orientation to the environment. The vestibular system consists of the receptor organ, vestibular nerves, and vestibular nuclei. The receptor organs are located in the inner ear and consist of the semicircular canals, utricle, and saccule. The fluid, which is contained in the semicircular canal (endolymph), senses changes in the position of the head and sends impulses to the vestibular nuclei via the vestibular nerve. Vestibular efferents travel to the cerebellum, eye, brainstem, reticular formation, and spinal cord. The facial nerve travels in close proximity through the middle ear.

ETIOLOGY/PATHOPHYSIOLOGY
Trauma and otitis are the most common causes of vestibular disease, with trauma being much more common in the foal. Temporohyoid osteoarthropathy, as seen in adults, is unlikely to be seen in foals. Other causes of vestibular disease are equine

protozoal myeloencephalitis (EPM), parasite migration, space-occupying lesions, and lightening strike. Ototoxicity from aminoglycosides has also been reported. Trauma can be a result of kicks, falls, blows, or collisions involving the skull. Hemorrhage from the ear or nares suggests fracture of the ethmoid or petrosal bones.

Lesions of the vestibular system result in alterations in efferent output to CNs III, IV, and VI (which control eye movement), the cerebellum, cortex, reticular formation, and vestibulospinal tracts. An absence of vestibular input to these CNs results in an abnormal eye position and movement. The vestibulospinal tract facilitates and inhibits ipsilateral and contralateral extensors and flexors. An asymmetric vestibular lesion results in an asymmetric ataxia, resulting in a circle or tendency to lean or move to one side. The direction is toward the side of the lesion. This directional ataxia is a result of loss of inhibitory neural influence in the contralateral extensors and a loss of facilitatory neuronal influence in the ipsilateral extensors.

CLINICAL PRESENTATION

General signs of vestibular disease are staggering/loss of balance, leaning/rolling or circling to one side, a head tilt to the affected side, a base wide stance (the horse stands with its limbs spread wide instead of squarely under the body in a normal support position; 314), strabismus, and nystagmus. Acute vestibular lesions can result in severe and sometimes violent disorientation. It can be anthropomorphized that this would be similar to the vertigo (dizziness) that is described in humans with vestibular lesions.

Clinical presentations of central versus peripheral vestibular disease are very similar and can be difficult to differentiate. Peripheral vestibular disease results in nystagmus, with the fast phase away from the side of the lesion. In central vestibular lesions, the nystagmus can be horizontal (head elevation exaggerates eye movements). Central lesions should result in more evidence of limb weakness (descending motor tract involvement), depression (reticular formation), and signs of involvement of other CNs. Facial nerve involvement (muzzle deviation, ptosis, ear droop) can frequently be seen in association with peripheral lesions due to the proximity of CN VII to the inner ear.

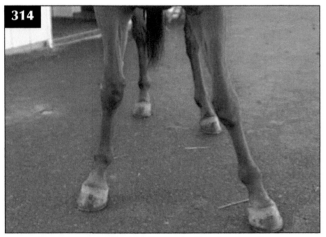

314 A late weanling foal with cerebellar disease demonstrating a base wide stance.

DIFFERENTIAL DIAGNOSIS

Other conditions that can cause similar clinical signs include asymmetric cerebral disease and cerebellar disease. Due to the variation in severity of vestibular lesions, the typical clinical signs exhibited can be partial and not all inclusive, therefore cerebellar and unilateral forebrain disease can be difficult to differentiate from vestibular disease.

DIAGNOSIS

Diagnosis is based on clinical signs. Blindfolding the foal during the neurologic examination can dramatically exacerbate signs of vestibular disease. Identification of fractures and evidence of hemorrhage from the nares or ear canal can support the diagnosis. Examination of the external and inner ear may identify inflammation or hemorrhage. CSF analysis may identify trauma or be used to rule out EPM. Lightening strike can be suspected if the foal is found after a severe storm or if singed hair is observed.

MANAGEMENT

Treatment of the inflammation (*Table 62*) can provide a degree of improvement. Supportive care to avoid further injury and nutritional/fluid support may need to be considered. Antibiotic therapy is necessary if otitis or infection is suspected.

CEREBELLAR DISEASE

KEY POINTS
- The cerebellum regulates motor activity.
- Cerebellar disease is usually either a congenital hypoplasia or a degenerative abiotrophy.
- Abiotrophy is most commonly seen in the Arabian breed.
- Intention tremors with a base wide stance are common clinical signs.

DEFINITION/OVERVIEW

Cerebellar disorders are manifested by abnormalities in rate, range, and force of movement. The cerebellum receives efferents from the entire body including the brainstem and the vestibular system. The cerebellum processes this information and, through its efferent pathways, regulates motor activity. Clinical signs most typically seen are intension tremors, hypermetria, and spasticity.

ETIOLOGY/PATHOPHYSIOLOGY

Cerebellar disease is generally either a congenital hypoplasia or a degenerative abiotrophy. Viral or toxic etiologies have not been identified as in other domestic species. Congenital hypoplasia (cerebellar hypoplasia at birth) is seen most commonly in the Arabian breed and has been reported in the Thoroughbred, Paso Fino, and Morgan breeds. Breeding studies of the congenital hypoplasia have shown a recessive mode of inheritance for this condition. More typical is the abiotrophy that develops as a progressive cerebellar disease. This abiotrophy has been seen in Gothand Ponies, Arabians, Arabian crosses, and Thoroughbreds. In degenerative cerebellar disease, degeneration of cerebellar neurons (Purkinje and granular cells) is thought to be secondary to a deficiency of a cerebellar trophic substance.

Table 63. Clinical signs of spinal cord disease in the foal

- Paresis/paralysis
- Ataxia
- Proprioceptive deficits
- Spasticity
- Dysmetria
- Muscle atrophy
- Weakness
- Abnormal spinal cord reflexes
- Abnormal sense of joint position

CLINICAL PRESENTATION

Clinical signs of cerebellar disease can be present shortly after birth, but typically clinical signs are progressive over subsequent weeks to months. In Thoroughbreds, cerebellar disease has been seen as late as 1 year of age. Clinical signs include a head bob or sway, base wide stance (**314**), intention tremors, absent menace response, and hypo- or hypermetria with spasticity or dysmetria. The gait can be described as "goose stepping." Signs may be exacerbated by activity or excitement. There is no weakness and vision is unaffected.

DIFFERENTIAL DIAGNOSIS

The clinical signs of cerebellar disease are characteristic; however, spinal cord disease may present with similar clinical signs and should be considered (*Table 63*). Typically, spinal cord diseases do not exhibit intention tremors, head bob or sway, or a dramatic base wide stance. Patients with spinal cord disease may definitely be dysmetric or spastic.

DIAGNOSIS

Typical clinical signs with appropriate epidemiologic correlates can be highly suggestive of cerebellar disease. There have been reports of elevated CSF protein concentrations in some foals with abiotrophy.

MANAGEMENT

There is no effective treatment. There are reports of degrees of improvement; however, the prognosis should be considered poor to guarded.

BRAINSTEM DISEASE

KEY POINTS

- The cranial nerve nuclei are located in the brainstem, with upper motor neuron (UMN) input from the cerebral cortex.
- Trauma to the head is the most common cause of injury.
- Other causes include space-occupying or inflammatory lesions.
- The presence of multifocal cranial nerve signs suggests localization of the lesion.

DEFINITION/OVERVIEW

The 12 CNs are involved with specialized senses such as smell, sight, balance, hearing, and innervation of the eyes, facial muscles, larynx, pharynx, and tongue. The CN nuclei are contained in the brainstem, with UMN input from the cerebral cortex. Injury to the CNs may involve the nuclei centrally or the nerves peripherally. Injury to the peripheral nerves can be multiple. Injuries to the nuclei often occur in combination with other adjacent portions of the brainstem.

ETIOLOGY/PATHOPHYSIOLOGY

Trauma

Trauma is the most common cause of brainstem injury in the foal. Rearing or falling over backward and striking the poll can lead to brainstem and/or other associated neurologic deficits. Trauma to the back of the head can result in skull fractures and/or hemorrhage in the inner ear (**311**). Trauma to the head without skull fractures (closed head injury) can result in midbrain hemorrhage and cerebral edema. Optic nerve trauma can occur with blows to the head that are not severe enough to cause other CNS signs. The facial nerve (CN VII) is commonly involved with head trauma. CN VII travels in close association with CN VIII through the internal acoustic meatus and then crosses the dorsal aspect of the guttural pouch, where branches travel to the ear. From the guttural pouch the nerve passes across the vertical ramus of the mandible and branches into dorsal and ventral branches. Injury to the nerve proximal to the ramus of the mandible produces complete facial paralysis/paresis. Damage near or within the inner ear results in associated vestibular signs (**315**). Distal (peripheral) facial nerve injury is usually a result of direct trauma or pressure. Facial nerve

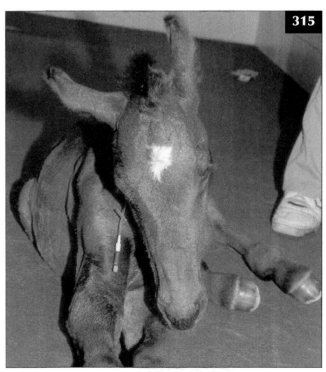

315 Damage to the inner ear has resulted in a head tilt to the side of the lesion in this foal.

paralysis centrally at the CN nuclei results in complete facial paralysis/paresis and possibly other CN signs.

Lesions other than trauma

Miscellaneous causes of CN abnormalities include space-occupying lesions such as abscesses or tumors, infectious conditions such as EPM, and otitis media.

CLINICAL PRESENTATION

The clinical presentation of CN abnormalities is dependent on the nerve or nerves involved; frequently, other CNS signs will be seen or will overshadow the presence of CN signs. The presence of multifocal CN signs may provide clues to the location of the lesion. Combinations of CN VII and VIII signs are frequent and can be produced by a peripheral or central lesion. Optic nerve injury is characterized by blindness. Severe injury to the midbrain can result in profound depression, coma, or a "decerebrate" of extensor rigidity. Trauma to the inner ear results in both CN VII and VIII signs. CN VII signs include deviation of the nose to the normal side, reduced response of the ipsilateral nostril during inspiration, and drooping of the lip, eyelid, and ear on the ipsilateral side. Exposure keratitis can occur as a sequela to inability to close the lid.

DIFFERENTIAL DIAGNOSIS

The differential diagnosis for brainstem lesions includes trauma, space-occupying lesions such as abscesses or tumors, and infectious conditions such as EPM or otitis media.

DIAGNOSIS

Diagnosis is based on clinical examination. Findings such as palpable swelling or hemorrhage are suggestive of trauma. Localization of the lesion can often be determined by interpretation of the clinical signs (see Clinical presentation, above). Hematology and serum chemistries may indicate inflammation/infection. Radiographic evaluation will identify fractures, osteomyelitis, or soft tissue densities. The nasal passages can be evaluated by endoscopic examination. Pharyngeal and guttural pouches and hemorrhage may be noted in or involving these structures. The evaluation of EPM is discussed later (Equine protozoal myeloencephalitis, see pp. 211–212).

MANAGEMENT

Management of cerebral trauma is dependent on the diagnosis. The treatment of CNS trauma is discussed in a previous section (see pp. 198–199). If the trauma patient can be safely maintained and nutritional support provided, then the clinician is allowed time to pursue therapy. Infections are treated with an appropriate antimicrobial based on the diagnosis or knowledge of the most likely organism involved.

SPINAL CORD DISEASES

KEY POINTS

- The patient with spinal cord disease does not have CNS signs (i.e., he/she is bright and alert).
- The commonality of spinal cord diseases are compression inflammation and/or contusions of the spinal cord.
- Radiographs and CSF analysis are useful diagnostic tools.

DEFINITION/OVERVIEW

Spinal cord disease in the foal results in varying degrees of ataxia, weakness, and/or spasticity. Muscle atrophy may also be seen. Cerebellar disease must be ruled out as a cause of ataxia. Patients with CNS disease can show other clinical signs referable to forebrain disease.

ETIOLOGY/PATHOPHYSIOLOGY

There are numerous causes of pediatric spinal cord disease. Many adult spinal cord diseases may also occasionally affect foals. Individual etiologies will be discussed later. The commonality of these conditions is that the spinal cord is compromised through inflammation, compression, or contusion resulting in axonal damage and leading to clinical signs of spinal cord disease.

CLINICAL PRESENTATION

The clinical signs of spinal cord disease (*Table 63*) consist of varying degrees of paresis/paralysis, ataxia, proprioceptive deficits, and spasticity. With lower motor neuron (LMN) lesions, muscle atrophy may ensue. Abnormal reflexes may be present. Spinal cord disease should be considered in the foal that is found recumbent. Localization of a spinal cord lesion can be aided by knowledge of spinal cord segments and UMN and LMN clinical signs (*Table 64*). LMN signs include paralysis, hyporeflexia/areflexia, early or severe muscle atrophy, and anesthesia of the innervated area. UMN signs include paresis/paralysis, normal to hyperreflexia, and late and diffuse muscle atrophy.

DIFFERENTIAL DIAGNOSIS

The differential diagnosis of spinal cord disease is listed in *Table 65*. A wide variety of conditions can result in spinal cord abnormality. Trauma is the most common cause of spinal cord disease. Numerous other conditions such as infections and space-occupying lesions can compromise spinal cord function.

Table 64. Upper motor and lower motor neuron signs of spinal cord disease

UMN

- Paresis/paralysis
- Normal to hyperreflexia
- Late and diffuse muscle atrophy

LMN

- Paralysis
- Hyporeflexia/areflexia
- Early or severe muscle atrophy
- Anesthesia of innervated area

> **Table 65. Differential diagnosis of spinal cord disease in the foal**
> - Cervical compressive myelopathy
> - Trauma
> - Equine degenerative myelopathy
> - Vertebral body abscess cerebellar disease
> - West Nile virus
> - Malformations of the cervical vertebrae
> - Myelodysplasia
> - Hypoxic injury at birth
> - Equine herpesvirus infection
> - Equine protozoal myelitis

DIAGNOSIS

In addition to the neurologic examination and localization of neurologic deficits to the spinal cord, other diagnostics may include hematology/serum chemistry, radiography, CSF analysis, advanced imagining (CT/MRI), and electrodiagnostics. The neurologic examination should include evaluation of spinal reflexes. Spinal reflexes can localize a lesion, thus improving evaluation via radiography. Deep palpation of the vertebral column may elicit pain in cases of trauma or space-occupying lesions. Swelling associated with the vertebral column may or may not be identified in cases of trauma.

Hematology/serum chemistry is generally nonspecific, but an inflammatory leukogram suggests infection. Abnormal concentrations of serum enzymes and electrolytes help identify hepatic, muscle, or metabolic diseases. When indicated, radiographs of the skull and cervical spine can be performed. In the neonate or young foal, radiographs of the entire spine are possible.

A CSF tap can be performed in either the atlanto-occipital or lumbosacral space. Minimal CSF analysis should include determination of total protein content, WBC and RBC count, and WBC differential.

Lumbosacral tap

A lumbosacral tap can be performed in a quiet or sedated, standing or recumbent, foal. The lumbosacral space is identified as a depression on the midline caudal to the spinous process of the last lumbar vertebrae and cranial to the spine of the sacrum. This depression is bordered laterally by the cranial edge of tuber sacrale. A 3.5 inch needle with a stylet is adequate for foals as large as 180 kg (400 lb). The area is clipped and surgically prepared. Following a local block, the needle is advanced perpendicular to the spinal cord. Frequent, gentle aspiration with a small syringe will determine when the subarachnoid space has been entered. A sudden flicking of the tail or kicking with the hindlimbs also marks entry into the space.

Atlanto-occipital tap

An atlanto-occipital tap is performed with the foal anesthetized or heavily sedated in lateral recumbency. A 1.5–3.5 inch 20 gauge needle is used. The site is aseptically prepared. The tap is performed on the midline, on a line connecting the cranial edges of the wings of the atlas. While the head is held in a flexed position, the needle is directed toward the lower lip. A slight "pop" or decrease in resistance is felt when the subarachnoid space has been entered; however, it is prudent to remove the stylet from the needle frequently to determine if the subarachnoid space has been entered.

MANAGEMENT

The management of individual spinal cord diseases is discussed under the specific disease.

MALFORMATIONS

KEY POINTS
- The majority of malformations are of the atlas, axis, and occipital condyles.
- Clinical signs are usually apparent within the first few months of life and are referable to compression of the spinal cord.
- An abnormal carriage of the head and neck or enlargement of the cranial cervical region may be noted.
- Radiography is diagnostic.

DEFINITION/OVERVIEW

Congenital malformations of the CNS, skull, and spinal cord are not commonly observed abnormalities in the horse. Hydrocephalus has been discussed previously (pp. 195–196). There is a breed predilection for other congenital malformations. Occipito-atlanto-axial malformation is most common in the Arabian breed and is thought to be inherited. The condition is a malformation of the occipital condyles, atlas, and axis. These may include malformations of the dens and an ankylosed or absent atlanto-occipital articulation.

ETIOLOGY/PATHOPHYSIOLOGY

The condition is considered to be inherited in some breeds (Arabians), but it can be seen in a variety of light breed horses. Malformations of the occipital condyles, atlas, and axis frequently result in stenosis of the spinal canal.

CLINICAL PRESENTATION

Clinical signs of a spinal cord lesion may be seen at birth or within the first few months of life. The signs are referable to the cervical spine and can include varying degrees of ataxia/weakness involving the hindlimbs and forelimbs. Severely affected foals may be dead at birth as a result of parturient compression of the spine. Foals may be born with tetraparesis or tetraplegia. Mild cases may not become apparent until adulthood. Affected foals may walk with a head and neck extension.

DIFFERENTIAL DIAGNOSIS

Breed predilection and the rapidity of onset of clinical signs are highly suggestive of occipito-atlanto-axial malformation. Other differentials should be considered (*Table 65*).

DIAGNOSIS

Diagnosis is confined by radiography and demonstration of various malformations. Observation of head/neck extension and/or an abnormal appearance to the cranial cervical region with ataxia can result in a high degree of suspicion.

MANAGEMENT

Medical management is generally unrewarding. Dorsal decompression (decompressive laminectomy) has been performed with some success. The prognosis for future athletic performance is very poor.

MYELODYSPLASIA

KEY POINTS

- Congenital abnormal development of the spinal cord (myelo-dysplasia) is rare.
- Paraparesis, ataxia, and paraplegia are common and often present at birth.

DEFINITION/OVERVIEW

The term "myelodysplasia" describes developmental abnormalities of the spinal cord. The condition is uncommon. Congenital abnormalities of the axial skeleton may be seen in association with myelodysplasia. Clinical signs are present at birth or within days.

ETIOLOGY/PATHOPHYSIOLOGY

The cause of these developmental abnormalities is not known. The skeleton surrounding the spinal cord develops in conjunction with the neural tube; foals with myelodysplasia may often also have skeletal abnormalities. These abnormalities may include failure of fusion of the vertebral dorsal arches, block or hemivertebrae, contractures of the axial skeleton (contracted foal syndrome), scoliosis, lordosis, kyphosis, and torticollis. Myelodysplasia may include spina bifida, cystic dilations, tubular cavitations, and dilations of the central canal or spinal cord duplication.

CLINICAL PRESENTATION

Clinical signs are present at birth or develop shortly thereafter. Signs include paraparesis, ataxia, and paraplegia. Affected foals may have a bunny-hopping gait. Reflexes may be bilaterally active at the level of the deficit. Vertebral and/or skeletal abnormalities may be evident (see Malformations, p. 205).

DIFFERENTIAL DIAGNOSIS

Associated skeletal abnormalities and age of onset may lead to a high degree of suspicion. Other differentials considered should include other spinal cord diseases (*Table 65*) or, more specifically, neonatal paresis/paralysis as a result of a hypoxic lesion, birth trauma, or congenital malformation.

DIAGNOSIS

Clinical signs of paresis/paralysis at, or shortly after, birth suggest the possibility of myelodysplasia. Radiographic evidence of vertebral abnormalities with clinical signs is highly suggestive. A myelogram may provide further evidence of cysts or compression of the spinal cord. If the diagnosis cannot be confirmed,

then a persistence of clinical signs or failure to respond to therapy suggests a congenital abnormality.

MANAGEMENT

These conditions are generally severe and progressive. Treatment is unsuccessful.

TRAUMA (SPINAL CORD)

KEY POINTS

- Trauma of the spinal cord is relatively common.
- Lesions can be located to specific regions of the cord using reflexes and motor neuron signs.
- Treatment is geared towards a reduction in inflammation and compression.

DEFINITION/OVERVIEW

As in the case of CNS disease, trauma to the spinal cord is fairly common in foals and compatible with their active lifestyle. Trauma can occur to any segment of the spinal cord. The regions of the spinal cord most commonly affected are those referring to weight bearing (T18–L6), the site of most dorsal ventral motion (T9–T16), the occipital–atlanto-axial region, and the site corresponding to the anchor points of the vertebral column (T1–T3).

ETIOLOGY/PATHOPHYSIOLOGY

The pathophysiology of neuronal injury in spinal cord trauma is similar to injury of the CNS. When edema develops within a confined space, further damage to the spinal cord can occur. Spinal cord injuries can lead to vascular tears, with resultant hemorrhage and hematomas. Heavily myelinated tracts are more susceptible to deterioration following compression injury. Proprioceptive deficits may be seen before loss of motor function or deep pain.

CLINICAL PRESENTATION

The clinical presentation of spinal cord trauma is referable to a spinal ataxia, which may be as severe as quadraparesis/paralysis. Lesions of the different regions of the spinal cord can be localized by a physical examination and knowledge of the UMN versus LMN signs (*Table 64*). Evaluation of the cutaneous trunci reflex and the level of cervical hypalgesia can indicate the cranial extent of a lesion. Patches of sweating may be seen if nerve roots are damaged. Sweating in the neck or Horner's syndrome can be seen with lesions cranial to the cervical intumescence. Whole body sweating may be present with severe pain or disruption of spinal sympathetic pathways.

DIFFERENTIAL DIAGNOSIS

Includes other conditions that result in spinal cord disease (*Table 65*).

DIAGNOSIS

Thorough examination, looking for evidence of trauma of the vertebral column, and/or evidence of trauma of the axial skeleton can suggest trauma. Swellings or palpable pain over the cervical, thoracic, or lumbar spine may be observed. Hemorrhage from the ears or nostrils, swellings, and lacerations may be noted.

However, trauma should not be ruled out if external evidence is not observed. Conversely, a foal that is recumbent for other reasons can rapidly develop traumatic injuries.

Radiography can confirm the presence of vertebral fractures. The entire vertebral column can be evaluated in the foal; however, nondisplaced fractures can be difficult to locate. Dorsal ventral views provide an additional plane of observation. CSF evaluation can identify hemorrhage. Past hemorrhage can be distinguished cytologically.

MANAGEMENT

Treatment of spinal cord trauma is initially directed at stabilization of the vertebral column and control of pain and inflammation. The use of a stretcher, heavy bandages, and splints may be helpful in stabilization. Medical therapy (anti-inflammatories) is similar to that for cranial trauma (*Table 62*). Nursing care becomes critical to the recumbent patient. Surgical intervention (when possible) provides stabilization and/or decompression. The prognosis for the recumbent patient is generally limited by its ability to perform and willingness to accept the long-term therapy of recumbency. The patient suffering from spinal cord injury that does not become recumbent and/or can stand following recumbency has a good prognosis for recovery. Complete recovery to expected athletic performance is directly related to the severity of the initial injury.

VERTEBRAL BODY ABSCESS

KEY POINTS

- Vertebral body abscesses typically result in posterior paresis/paralysis, although any region of the spinal cord can be affected.
- The source of bacteria is hematogenous spread from a mucous membrane or foci of infection to the vertebrae.
- *R. equi* and *Streptococcus* spp. are the most common offending organisms.
- Radiographs, CSF analysis, and hematology/serum chemistries are not routinely diagnostic.

DEFINITION/OVERVIEW

Vertebral infections can cause cord compression and result in paraparesis or quadraparesis/paralysis. Vertebral body abscess (VBA) is typically a condition seen in young foals; however, adults have been diagnosed with this condition. Affected foals often have a history of previous systemic infection. Clinical signs are referable to the spinal cord. Paraparesis/paralysis of the hindlimbs (the "dog-sitting" foal) is the more common presentation; however, any region of the spinal cord can be affected.

ETIOLOGY/PATHOPHYSIOLOGY

The condition occurs secondary to septicemic/bacteremic spread of bacteria from a septic focus or mucous membrane, with localization to a vertebral body or vertebral arch and process. Secondary osteomyelitis results in swelling and potential cord compression (**316**). If the infection invades through cortical bone, it can involve intervertebral disks or expand to involve abscessation of paravertebral structures. A variety of organisms may be cultured from

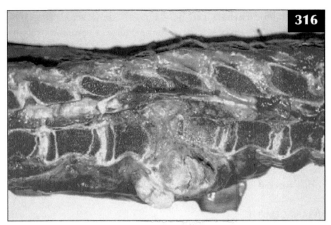

316 Vertebral body abscess with osteomyelitis and cord compression.

vertebral infections. *R. equi* and *Streptococcus* spp. are among the more common organisms cultured.

CLINICAL PRESENTATION

Clinical signs are referable to a focal spinal cord lesion (*Table 63*). Posterior paresis/paralysis is often noted (**317**). The neurologic signs may be gradual and progressive. Palpable pain or swellings may be identified on physical examination. A history of fever or other infectious processes such as enteritis, pneumonia, umbilical infection, or osteomyelitis of the axial skeleton may be present. A farm history of *R. equi* or *S. equi* infection should be noted. The leukogram may identify a leukocytosis. Hyperfibrinogenemia may be present. The absence of abnormalities of the leukogram does not rule out a VBA.

DIFFERENTIAL DIAGNOSIS

Other causes of spinal ataxia (*Table 65*) should be considered.

DIAGNOSIS

The suspicion of vertebral infection is based on clinical signs of a spinal cord lesion. Identification of palpable pain (rarely present), the presence of inflammatory changes in the leukogram (inconsistently present), along with a history of a current or previous infectious process, can suggest the presence of a VBA as a possible cause of spinal ataxia. The absence of hematology/serum chemistry changes should not be used to rule out the condition.

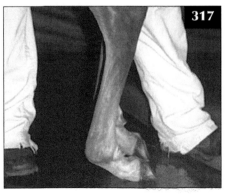

317 Posterior paresis/paralysis in a foal with a vertebral body abscess.

Radiographic changes can be diagnostic; however, radiographic changes are not often seen early in the course of vertebral osteomyelitis. Additionally, radiographs of the thoracic and lumbar spine can be difficult to interpret because of the size of the patient and overlying shadows created by the lungs or GI tract. A myelogram can confirm cord compression. Nuclear scintigraphy may be useful. CSF analysis is generally normal as it is unusual for these infections to penetrate the dura. If the dura is penetrated, an elevated CSF white cell count is expected. Attempts to culture affected areas are difficult; however, if a primary source of infection can be found (umbilical infection, abscess, diarrhea, pneumonia, and other osteomyelitis), bacterial cultures should be performed.

MANAGEMENT
Antibiotic therapy should be based on culture results when available or on the most likely expectations of the offending organism. Historical information regarding previous infections or history of farm diseases may aid the choice of antibiotic. Surgical drainage should be considered, but access to the vertebra can be limited. Anti-inflammatories and supportive care should be provided.

EQUINE DEGENERATIVE MYELOPATHY

KEY POINTS
- Equine degenerative myelopathy (EDM) is a neuroaxonal dystrophy that is causally related to vitamin E deficiency.
- A genetic predisposition exists in some breeds.
- Spasticity is a prominent component of clinical signs.
- Determination of vitamin E levels can aid the diagnosis.
- Individuals may respond to supplementation with vitamin E.

DEFINITION/OVERVIEW
EDM is a degenerative disease of the spinal cord and/or brainstem. The disease has been recognized in the United States and in Europe. Most breeds, including captive Equidae, can be affected. The disease can occur in an individual or in groups on a farm.

ETIOLOGY/PATHOPHYSIOLOGY
EDM is characterized histopathologically by neuroaxonal dystrophy (NAD) for which a precise etiology has not been determined. EDM is likely caused by an interaction of many factors (e.g., dietary deficiencies or excesses, nutrient absorption or interaction, and heredity). Vitamin E is very likely involved through its link as an antioxidant. Oxidative stress is a result of an imbalance between available antioxidants and the presence of pro-oxidants. Excessive oxidation can result in cell damage. The CNS, with its high rate of oxygen consumption, is particularly susceptible to oxidative stress; therefore, it is possible that young foals with a genetic predisposition and an imbalance of antioxidants (vitamin E or other nutrients) may develop EDM.

Vitamin E deficiency has been shown to be cause related. Affected individuals have low vitamin E levels and often respond to vitamin E therapy. One study on a farm where there was a high incidence of EDM demonstrated low vitamin E levels. Supplementation with vitamin E reduced the incidence of EDM dramatically. In another study, foals housed on a dry lot showed dramatic clinical signs of EDM. Histopathologic confirmation of NAD was determined at necropsy. The surviving foals improved

dramatically following access to grass pasture. Low vitamin E concentrations have been found in rats, monkeys, humans, and captured Prewalski's horses that were affected with NAD. Oral vitamin E absorption tests have not showed a difference in affected versus unaffected individuals. This suggests that abnormal vitamin E absorption from the GI tract is not related to the development of EDM. Pathologic changes in experimentally induced vitamin E deficiency and naturally occurring cases are similar. A genetic predisposition for the condition appears to exist. Eight of nine foals sired by the same stallion had clinical signs of EDM and low serum vitamin E levels. Age-matched controls had normal vitamin E levels.

CLINICAL PRESENTATION
The onset of clinical signs can be acute or insidious and they are referable to the spinal cord. Clinical signs are often more severe in the hindlimbs and they can be similar to the signs of cervical stenotic myelopathy; however, other diseases causing spinal ataxia should be considered (*Table 65*). Affected individuals may have prominent spasticity (lack of joint flexion). The gait can be described as "stiff-legged" or "tin-soldier" like. Muscle atrophy is not seen.

DIFFERENTIAL DIAGNOSIS
Clinical signs of ataxia, with a prominent component of spasticity (lack of joint flexion) (**318**), in a patient with the appropriate

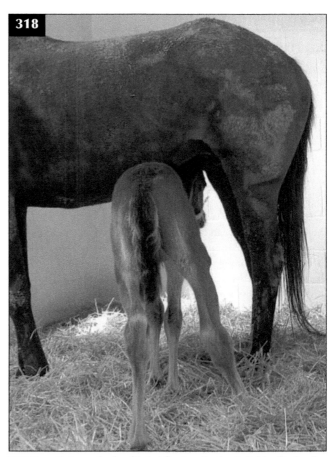

318 Spasticity or lack of joint flexion in the left hindlimb of a foal.

signalment suggests the need to rule out EDM. Other conditions resulting in spinal cord disease (*Table 65*) should be considered.

DIAGNOSIS

A diagnosis of EDM can be made by ruling out other spinal cord diseases (particularly cervical compressive myelopathy) and determining serum vitamin E levels. The levels should be compared with laboratory normals and with normal individuals on the same premises. Serum vitamin E levels can vary with the stage of the disease and are considered to reflect accurately the total body vitamin E status. Vitamin E levels of <1 mcg/mL have been associated with EDM.

MANAGEMENT

Supplementation with vitamin E is the treatment of choice. Response to therapy is dependent on the severity and duration of the disease. Affected individuals can be supplemented with 5,000–10,000 IU vitamin E p/o q24h. Intramuscular vitamin E in oil can be given at 1,000–3,000 IU q24h.

CERVICAL COMPRESSIVE MYELOPATHY

KEY POINTS

- Cervical compressive myelopathy (CCM) is a compression of the spinal cord as a result of a narrowed spinal canal or vertebral abnormalities.
- A genetic predisposition may exist with a narrowed spinal cord as a component.
- Typical clinical signs are a symmetric ataxia, spasticity, and/or weakness.
- Hindlimbs are often more severely affected than the forelimbs.
- Survey radiography is not diagnostic, but can lead to an increased suspicion of the disease.
- Myelography is diagnostic.

DEFINITION/OVERVIEW

CCM is a spinal cord disease with variable components of vertebral malformation, narrowing of the vertebral canal, and spinal cord compression. The typical age of onset is considered to be 1–3 years of age, but weanling foals can frequently be affected. CCM continues to be one of the more frequently diagnosed causes of neurologic disease in the horse. The condition is reported in most horse breeds, with some breeds (e.g., Thoroughbreds) being more frequently affected. The disease predominates in males.

ETIOLOGY/PATHOPHYSIOLOGY

The etiology of the disease is not precisely determined; however, a genetic predisposition may be involved with development of the disease in some breeds. The pathophysiology of the disease includes components of spinal cord narrowing (possibly genetic related), vertebral malformation or malalignment, and osteoarthrosis of the articular facets. The correlation of CCM to developmental or orthopedic disease, and the histopathologic observation of osteochondrosis of articular facets in affected horses, has lead to a speculative relationship to developmental orthopedic disease (DOD). Dietary factors (rapid growth, elemental deficiencies) may play a role. More recent evidence that horses with narrowed canals are more likely to suffer from CCM implicates a narrowed spinal canal as a factor in the disease.

CLINICAL PRESENTATION

The onset of disease can be acute or insidious and at onset may be mild to severe (recumbency). CCM has occasionally been reported as the cause of acute death. The history of a patient with CCM often includes reports of a traumatic episode; however, the traumatic episode is usually the result of and not the cause of the compressive lesion. Clinical signs of disease are generally characteristic and referable to a focal cervical spinal cord lesion. The typical clinical signs are of symmetric weakness, ataxia, and spasticity. The hindlimbs are generally more severely affected than the forelimbs. If the spinal cord involvement is in the caudal cervical region (involving the cranial intumescence), forelimb signs can be more severe than hindlimb signs.

DIFFERENTIAL DIAGNOSIS

CCM should be considered as one of the top differentials in a foal with spinal cord disease. Typical clinical signs of symmetric ataxia are highly suggestive of a compressive myelopathy. Other diseases to consider are listed in *Table 65*.

DIAGNOSIS

CSF analysis is not of use in the diagnosis of CCM, but it can rule out other differentials. Survey radiographs can be evaluated objectively and subjectively. Radiographs of the cervical spine are not diagnostic, but they can suggest the necessity of confirmation via myelography. Standing cervical films are evaluated for canal diameter and for vertebral malformation. In horses with CCM, malformations that may characteristically be identified include flare of the caudal epiphysis of the vertebral body (vertebral endplate remodeling), caudal extension of the dorsal laminae, malalignment between vertebrae, and degenerative joint disease/abnormal ossification of the articular facet. Degenerative joint disease of the articular process of the caudal cervical vertebrae is the most common malformation identified in horses with CCM; however, degenerative disease of the articular process is also the most frequent cervical radiographic abnormality observed in horses that are not affected with CCM. Subjective evaluation of articular facet abnormalities often results in a false-positive diagnosis of CCM. Identification of characteristic vertebral malformations supports, but does not confirm, the diagnosis of CCM. Subjective evaluation of radiographic malformation does not reliably differentiate between CCM-affected horses and unaffected horses. Determination of the sagittal ratio (ratio of two intervertebral measurements) is a useful method of determining canal diameter. The minimum sagittal diameter (a) is divided by the corresponding body width (b) at its widest point (**319**). The use of the ratio adjusts for magnification and difference focal-film distance.

When the canal is determined to be narrowed at more than one location from C3–C6, there is a statistically significant increased likelihood that the affected individual will have CCM.

Myelography is considered the premortem diagnostic test of choice for CCM. However, subjectivity exists in interpretation of the cord compression and in positioning of the cervical vertebrae

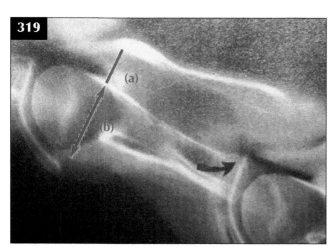

319 The minimum sagittal diameter (MSD) (a) is divided by (b) the body width.

for the dynamic radiographic views that are performed. A 50% loss of the dorsal contrast column with associated loss ventrally is considered diagnostic of CCM. CT and MRI are likely to be of considerable use in the diagnosis of cervical vertebral abnormalities. However, difficulties arise while the aperture openings are not large enough to evaluate the entire cervical spine, dynamic positioning is difficult, and equipment costs are high.

MANAGEMENT

Treatment of CCM is typically unrewarding. Dietary management has been suggested. Alterations in rate of growth via caloric restriction have met with variable success. Supplementation with vitamin E and concurrent anti-inflammatory therapy has benefited milder affected individuals. Surgical intervention can be beneficial if cases are selected cautiously. The goals of surgery are stabilization of the cervical vertebrae, with subsequent remodeling at the affected site. Many patients improve subsequent to stabilization, but the degree of improvement may be slight. Possibly the most important factor influencing postoperative prognosis is duration of clinical signs prior to surgical intervention.

EQUINE HERPESVIRUS MYELOENCEPHALITIS

KEY POINTS

- Equine herpesvirus (EHV) infection can occasionally cause a myeloencephalitis in foals.
- Outbreaks of the disease can be seen.
- Fever and respiratory signs may precede neurologic signs.
- Characteristic clinical signs are a posterior paresis/paralysis.
- CSF xanthochromia and elevated protein levels can lead to a presumptive diagnosis.
- Anti-inflammatories are the hallmark of therapy.

DEFINITION/OVERVIEW

EHV-1 myeloencephalitis is generally a sporadic disease, but outbreaks can occur. The disease is frequently seen following a respiratory infection and it can affect any equine population (e.g., racetrack and farm). Morbidity and mortality can be high in outbreaks of the disease. The disease can be seen at any age. Foals are occasionally affected, but young adults and aged individuals appear to be most commonly affected. The disease has been reported in most countries with a large equine population. EHV-1 infection resulting in neurologic disease also causes abortion in the mare.

ETIOLOGY/PATHOPHYSIOLOGY

The disease is caused by EHV-1, which is also known as equine rhinopneumonitis virus or equine abortion virus. The virus appears to have a tropism for endothelial cells and particularly CNS blood vessels. This results in a vasculitis of arterioles and ischemic necrosis in the gray and white matter of the brain and spinal cord. White matter of the spinal cord seems to be more preferentially affected. The pathogenesis of the disease is considered to be a secondary immune-mediated reaction or direct viral damage resulting in inflammation and involvement of contiguous nervous tissue. Demonstration of EHV-1 antigen in endothelial cells of vessels in the CNS suggests that the most likely pathogenesis of the disease is direct viral involvement with subsequent induced inflammatory response.

CLINICAL PRESENTATION

The predominant presentation is an acute symmetric ataxia and weakness. The hindlimbs are most commonly affected; these animals present as the "dog sitting" horse with paralysis/paresis of the limbs. Paralysis/paresis can progress to, or present, in all four limbs, resulting in recumbency. Cauda equina syndrome (bladder distension, overflow incontinence, rectal impaction, perineal analgesia, and penile prolapse) is an additional common clinical sign. Less frequently, involvement of CNs may be seen. A fever and respiratory disease may precede the neurologic signs. Fever may be absent at the onset of neurologic signs.

DIFFERENTIAL DIAGNOSIS

Other spinal cord diseases should be considered. The presence of fever, respiratory disease, or other affected individuals in a group of horses should lead to a strong suspicion of EHV-1 infection.

DIAGNOSIS

Diagnosis of EHV-1 infection is based on clinical signs and evaluation of CSF. The vasculitis of viral infection results in a characteristic xanthochromia and protein elevation of the CSF. There should be no increase in the nucleated cell count of the CSF. Virus isolation from CSF is usually unsuccessful, but it may be more rewarding from nasal swabs or blood. A fourfold change in virus titer is consistent with a diagnosis of EHV-1.

MANAGEMENT

Antiviral drugs such as valacyclovir are likely to be useful (see Chapter 17, Pharmacology, p. 307). As a result of the inflammatory component of vasculitis, steroid, and/or aggressive anti-inflammatory therapy should be considered (*Table 62*). In addition, other anti-inflammatories (e.g., flunixin meglumine and dimethyl sulfoxide [DMSO]) are suggested. Nursing care with particular attention to bladder dysfunction is critical to a successful outcome. The recumbent patient requires particular attention to nutrition, hydration, defecation, urination, and decubital ulceration.

EQUINE PROTOZOAL MYELOENCEPHALITIS

KEY POINTS

- Equine protozoal myeloencephalitis infection is unusual in foals.
- Spinal cord dysfunction is a prominent clinical sign; however, any area of the nervous system can be affected.
- EPM must be considered on the differential for a wide variety of neurologic disease.
- A premortem definitive diagnostic test is not available.
- Several antiprotozoal therapies are available.

DEFINITION/OVERVIEW

EPM is a neurologic condition that can affect any area of the nervous system. It is a disease found in North, Central, and South America and in horses that have been shipped from these countries. Any age horse can be affected; however, the infection is unusual in foals.

ETIOLOGY/PATHOPHYSIOLOGY

The protozoal organism responsible for EPM is *Sarcocystis neurona*. The American opossum is the definitive host. A variety of birds and the skunk (intermediate host) are likely involved in the life cycle. The horse is an aberrant, dead-end host. The organism is ingested by the horse (through a pathway that is yet unknown), then migrates to the CNS. Multiplication of the organism within neurons results in local inflammation and damage to affected and associated neurons.

CLINICAL PRESENTATION

Ataxia and/or paresis of suspected spinal cord dysfunction are the predominant clinical signs observed with EPM. Any portion of the spinal cord can be affected (C1–C6, C6–T2, T3–L3, or L4–S5), as well as either the gray or white matter. The location of the lesion can result in a wide variety of clinical signs. Gray matter involvement results in focal muscle atrophy (**320**). Cerebral,

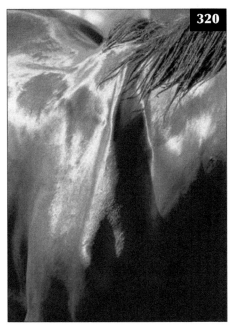

320 Muscle atrophy over the scapula in a foal with equine protozoal myeloencephalitis.

cerebella, or brainstem involvement is less frequent. Brainstem infection results in CN signs, which are frequently asymmetric. Cerebral involvement (rare) may cause seizures. The onset of clinical signs may be insidious or acute and the progression may be gradual or rapid. The onset of CN signs appears to be acute, while gait abnormalities may be acute or insidious. A very difficult (controversial) clinical challenge is identifying the EPM case that has a mild gait abnormality or a progressing failure of performance. Subtle asymmetric gait abnormalities, weakness, toe dragging, upward fixation of the patella, or focal muscle atrophy are considerations.

DIFFERENTIAL DIAGNOSIS

As EPM can infect any region of the CNS, the disease must be considered in the differential for a wide variety of equine neurologic disorders. Diseases to consider must include conditions involving all areas of the nervous system, including the forebrain (rare), brainstem, and spinal cord.

DIAGNOSIS

As a result of the lack of definitive premortem diagnostic tests, it is essential to rule out other causes of the presenting clinical signs. Establishing a list of rule outs with a systematic approach to diagnostics is essential for a presumptive diagnosis. EPM should be considered in the foal; however, other conditions are often more likely.

There is a high prevalence of exposure to EPM in most parts of the United States; therefore, serum antibody testing is of little use. However, it is rare for a horse with clinical signs of EPM to have a negative serum antibody test; therefore, serum antibody testing can be used as a screening test.

A serum negative horse is unlikely to have clinical disease. The Western blot test assay for *S. neurona* antibody in CSF is very sensitive, but not specific for clinical disease. The reasons for the lack of specificity are numerous:

- Blood/plasma contaminated tap
- Previous infection
- Movement of peripheral immune-primed lymphocytes into the CNS
- Movement of antibody across an intact blood–brain barrier
- Movement of antibody across a damaged blood–brain barrier
- Cross reactivity
- Persistence of organisms in the absence of clinical disease

Therefore, a positive CSF antibody test does not diagnose the disease, but a negative test suggests that the organism is not present in the CNS. A diagnosis of EPM is made by the degree of suspicion, ruling out other neurologic conditions, and the presence of antibodies to *S. neurona* in CSF.

MANAGEMENT

A variety of antiprotozoal agents are available, one of which (ponazuril) is currently approved for use in horses.

Pyrimethamine/sulfonamide combinations (the pyrimethamine dose should be at least 1 mg/kg p/o q24h) have been the standard therapy for EPM for many years. This combination of folate synthesis inhibitors produces a response to therapy in approximately

60% of patients. However, the combination can influence folate production in mammalian cells and it has been reported to cause a macrocytic anemia or leukopenia. Teratogenic influences in pregnant mares have been reported. Supplementation with folic acid has been associated with this toxicity; therefore, folic acid supplementation should not be given at the same time as pyrimethamine/sulfonamide therapy. Because these drugs reach marginal concentrations in CSF, which may not be adequate to kill *S. neurona*, the duration of therapy should be extended to 1–6 months. Relapses may occur. Using CSF-negative results as an end-point of therapy is dubious.

Diclazuril (2.5 g/455 kg [1,000 lb]) has been evaluated at the University of Kentucky, Lexington, Kentucky for its efficiency against EPM. Diclazuril is an antiprotozoal (benzeneacetonitrile derivative) used in poultry, calves, and humans. In humans it has been used to treat *Toxoplasma* encephalitis. In one study, 60% of the horses treated improved by at least one neurologic grade (the horses were graded from 1 to 5). Ponazuril, which is chemically similar to diclazuril, is also being used for therapy of EPM. Ponazuril has been approved for use in the United States and is marketed in a paste formulation (see data sheet for information regarding dosage and route of administration).

Anti-inflammatory therapy can be beneficial in the acute stage. DMSO may reduce oxidative damage to the CNS. The drug can be administered via a nasogastric tube or intravenously (10% solution) at 1 mg/kg q12–24h. NSAIDs are frequently used to decrease the inflammatory response. Flunixin meglumine is the NSAID most commonly used. Even though experimental evidence contradicts the use of corticosteroids, they are useful in situations where the patient's condition warrants rapid anti-inflammatory benefit.

Management considerations may be useful in prevention of the disease. Limiting opossum contact with feed sources and, potentially, the direct environment is advisable. Feeding grain products on the ground should be avoided. If the intermediate host returns nightly to a ground feed source, the possibility of contamination is increased dramatically. Intermittent dosing of horses with antiprotozoal drugs is difficult to recommend as the life cycle of the organism in the horse is not known. If, however, merozoite development from sporocysts can be prevented with timely, intermittent use of drug therapy, this form of preventative medicine may prove to be effective.

PERIPHERAL NEUROPATHIES

KEY POINTS
- The most common cause of monoplegia is trauma.

DEFINITION/OVERVIEW
Paresis or paralysis (monoplegia) of one limb is an occasional neurologic lesion identified in the foal. Traumatic injuries are the first consideration when monoplegia is identified.

ETIOLOGY/PATHOPHYSIOLOGY
Lesions resulting in paresis or paralysis of one limb are found in the ventral gray matter, nerve roots, or brachial and lumbosacral plexus, and the peripheral nerves or muscles that they innervate.

Trauma is the most frequent case of damage to the plexi, nerve roots, or peripheral nerves.

CLINICAL PRESENTATION
- *Suprascapular nerve*: This nerve is injured frequently with blows to the shoulder region. Atrophy of the supraspinatus and infraspinatus muscle occurs (swelling). Lateral subluxation of the shoulder may be seen with weight bearing.
- *Radial nerve*: Affected animals cannot bear weight on the limb as a result of an inability to extend the elbow or flex the shoulder. They cannot extend the knee, fetlock, or interphalangeal joints. Affected foals stand with their elbow dropped and the dorsum of the foot on the ground. Severely affected foals may have trouble rising or may collapse on the limb when attempting to bear weight. Mildly affected foals may advance the limb by flipping or flinging it forward from the shoulder. Atrophy of the triceps muscle develops 2–3 weeks subsequent to injury. Trauma is a common cause of this injury.
- *Brachial plexus*: Injuries to the brachial plexus are frequently seen with shoulder injuries. The suprascapular and radial nerves are often involved.
- *Femoral nerve*: Damage to the femoral nerve results in an inability to extend the stifle. The limb is advanced with difficulty and buckles with weight bearing. Injury to the femoral nerve can be a result of femoral fractures occurring at the time of foaling or with spinal cord gray matter lesions.
- *Sciatic nerve*: This nerve can be damaged with spinal cord gray matter lesions (L5–S3), fractures of the pelvis, or deep injections. Affected individuals have weak flexion of the limb. Weight can be supported if the foot is placed flat on the ground. Individuals have difficulty advancing the limb and stand with the hock and stifle extended and the dorsum of the hoof on the ground.
- *Tibial nerve*: Damage to this nerve can result in a hypermetria or a stringhalt-like gait with flexion of the hock at rest.
- *Peroneal nerve*: Paralysis due to perineal nerve damage causes an inability to flex the hock and extend the digits. Hyperextension of the hock and flexor of the digit results in a dragging of the foot.

DIAGNOSIS
Diagnosis is based on clinical signs and identification of any associated injuries.

MANAGEMENT
Treatment consists of anti-inflammatories and nursing care. Short-term glucocorticoid therapy, DMSO intravenously or locally, cold/hot hydrotherapy, and NSAID therapy may be useful.

FURTHER READING

Bernard WV (1997) Hypoxic ischemic encephalopathy. In: *Current Therapy in Equine Medicine*, 4th ed. (Robinson NE, Ed.). WB Saunders, Philadelphia, PA, pp. 589–591.

Ferriero DM (2004) Neonatal brain injury. *The New England Journal of Medicine* 351(19): 1985–1995.

Green SL, Mayhew IG (1990) Neurologic disorders. In: *Equine Clinical Neonatology* (Korterba A, Drummond W, Kosch P, Eds.). Lea & Febiger, Philadelphia, PA, pp. 496–530.

Johnson AL (2011) Equine cerebellar abiotrophy: Searching the genome for an explanations. *Equine Veterinary Education* 23: 135–136.

Mackay RJ (2005) Neurologic disorders of neonatal foals. *Veterinary Clinics of North America: Equine Practice* 21: 387–406.

Shalak LF, Laptook AR, Jafri AS et al. (2002) Clinical chorioamnionitis, elevated cytokines and brain injury in term infants. *Pediatrics* 100(4): 673–680.

Torbio R, Mudge MC (2013) Diseases of the foal. Diseases of the nervous system. In: *Equine Medicine Surgery and Reproduction*, 2nd ed. (Mair TS, Love S, Schumacher J, Smith RK, Frazer G, Eds.). WB Saunders, Philadelphia, PA, pp. 433–438.

Vaala W (1994) Peripartum asphyxia. *Veterinary Clinics of North America: Equine Practice* 10(1): 187–218.

Volpe JJ (2001) Hypoxic-ischemic encephalopathy: biochemical and physiological aspects. In: *Neurology of the Newborn*, 4th ed. (Volpe JJ, Ed.). WB Saunders, Philadelphia, PA.

Wong DM, Wilkins PA, Bain FT et al. (2011) Neonatal encephalopathy in foals. *Compendium Continuing Education for Veterinarians* 33: E1–E10.

Muscle and Neuromuscular Junction Disorders

William V. Bernard

INTRODUCTION

Muscle disorders are not commonly identified in the foal. They need to be recognized alone and as differentials for neurologic, musculoskeletal, or metabolic disorders. The stiff gait or rigid paralysis seen with muscle diseases must be differentiated from the neuromuscular paralysis of disorders such as tetanus, botulism (flaccid paralysis), or calcium disorders (*Table 66*). Hyperkalemic periodic paralysis (HYPP) and myotonia are a result of electrolyte conduction disturbances, while the other muscle diseases of foals (e.g., nutritional myodegeneration [NM]) are nutritionally based.

DIAGNOSIS OF MUSCLE DISEASE

HISTORY AND SIGNALMENT

Breed characteristics are important data in the evaluation of muscle disorders; HYPP has been confirmed to have a genetic basis, while myotonia is suspected to be genetically based. Quarter Horses affected with HYPP are most commonly the heavily muscled types used for conformation or performance. Males appear to have a higher prevalence of HYPP. NM is geographically distributed based on soil type and nutrient content. It can be present from birth to adulthood. Necropsies of aborted fetuses have noted histologic evidence of NM (white muscle disease). Myotonia is usually present in the first year of life, while HYPP has been reported in foals as young as 2 months of age. Foals with HYPP may present with recurrent episodes of weakness, muscle tremors, collapse, or respiratory distress. Foals with NM may present with a complaint

---

Table 66. Diseases causing paralysis/muscle stiffness

- Tetanus
- Botulism (flaccid paralysis)
- Hyperkalemic periodic paralysis
- Hypocalcemia
- Nutritional myodegeneration
- Myotonia
- Tick paralysis

---

of weakness, recumbency, stiff gait, or colic (misinterpreted due to struggling to stand).

PHYSICAL EXAMINATION

Frequently, the patient with muscle disease presents with a complaint that suggests abnormalities of some system other than the muscular system. In addition, patients with suspected muscle disease may have other conditions that result in stiffness, abnormal gaits, or an inability to rise.

A complete physical examination should be followed by observation of the patient at rest, a gait analysis, and observation and palpation of muscles and muscle groups. Palpation should include comparison of muscle groups bilaterally and with other muscle groups. Pain, firmness, or asymmetry can be observed. If proprioceptive deficits are identified, neurologic disorders should be suspected. Weakness can be difficult to differentiate from a primary muscle disorder, neurologic disease, or muscle loss resulting from weight loss.

DIAGNOSTICS

Diagnostics that can be used to evaluate muscle disorders include biopsy, electromyography, and clinical pathology. Alterations in muscle enzymes are frequently present with muscle disorders. Determination of muscle enzymes are the simplest and least invasive test to perform when evaluating the muscle system. The serum enzymes that are of primary use are creatine phosphokinase (CPK) and aspartate aminotransferase (AST). Lactate dehydrogenase (LDH) is also indicative of muscle disorders; however, LDH contains isoenzymes, which must be fractionated to specify muscle disease. CPK is very specific for muscle injury (skeletal and cardiac); values increase shortly after the muscle insult occurs. Exercise (training) may result in mild elevations in serum CPK. Muscle fatigue can result in moderate CPK elevations (>1,000 μL), which rapidly return to normal values. CPK values subsequent to muscle injury can be variable and may not always relate to the severity of the injury. This variability is linked to the relatively short half-life of serum CPK and also to the time at which the blood sample was drawn in relation to the injury. Severe muscle injury can result in CPK values ranging from thousands of units per liter to hundreds of thousands of units per liter. The values may remain elevated with progression of muscle damage or begin to decrease as muscle damage reduces.

Serum AST can also be used to evaluate muscle damage. This enzyme is not specific for muscle damage; it can be found in other

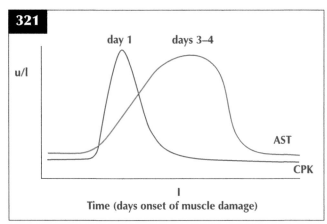

321 Half-life of AST compared with half-life of CPK. Muscle enzymes increase following muscle damage. CPK has a shorter $t_{1/2}$ than AST and rapidly returns to normal if muscle damage/inflammation does not continue. AST = aspartate aminotransferase; CPK = creatine phosphokinase.

tissues of the body, with the liver being the most significant. Serum AST values increase more slowly than CPK and AST has a much longer half-life (~7 days) compared with the rapidly rising short half-life of CPK (~1–2 days) (**321**). These differences in enzyme characteristics can be used to evaluate the severity and time course of muscle damage.

Electromyography is of more use for evaluating neuromuscular than muscular disorders. Muscle biopsy can be a very useful diagnostic technique. High-quality samples are produced with open dissection techniques using local or general anesthesia. Routine microscopy, electron microscopy, specialized staining, and *in-vitro* responses to stimuli can be performed.

NUTRITIONAL MYODEGENERATION (WHITE MUSCLE DISEASE)

KEY POINTS
- White muscle disease is a nutritional deficiency.
- The disease occurs primarily in areas of selenium-deficient soils.
- Inadequate dietary intake of vitamin E may contribute to the condition.
- Selenium/vitamin E combat oxidative stress (peroxide), therefore stabilizing muscle cell membranes.
- Clinical signs can include weakness, stiff gait, dysphagia, and inability to stand or difficulty standing.
- Muscle groups may be palpably firm.
- Botulism is a primary differential.
- Muscle enzymes are typically elevated.

DEFINITION/OVERVIEW
NM, commonly known as white muscle disease, is a nutritional deficiency observed in horses from birth to adulthood, with clinical signs generally presenting in the first year of life. The disease occurs primarily in geographic areas that have selenium-deficient soils. These areas will in turn produce selenium-deficient grains and forage. There is no breed or sex predilection. Clinical signs vary from weakness to rigid paralysis.

ETIOLOGY/PATHOPHYSIOLOGY
NM occurs as a result of inadequate dietary intake of vitamin E and/or selenium. Vitamin E and selenium act synergistically in their roles as antioxidants. The exact role of vitamin E and selenium jointly or independently in the development of NM remains controversial. Selenium supplementation alone is successful in both the treatment and prevention of NM. This suggests that inadequate intake of selenium may be more important than inadequate intake of vitamin E in the development of the disease.

Selenium and vitamin E function together to protect cell membranes (including muscle cell membranes) against oxidative stress. Selenium and vitamin E "protect" and "stabilize" muscle cell membranes by decreasing the formation of, or destroying, peroxides. Vitamin E is a first-line antioxidant decreasing the formation of peroxides. Selenium, as a component of the tissue enzyme glutathione peroxidase, destroys excessive tissue peroxides. Inadequate tissue antiperoxide activity allows for the formation of elevated tissue peroxide activity, disruption of cell metabolism, and cellular destruction.

CLINICAL PRESENTATION
Foals with NM present from areas where there is selenium-deficient soil. The mare and the foal are generally fed foodstuffs that are locally grown. The age of onset can be from birth through the pediatric period. Physical examination is referable to abnormalities of muscular function. Affected foals may be found recumbent and unable to stand or have difficulty when attempting to stand, or stand only with assistance. Affected foals may have a stilted, stiff gait. Dysphagia may be exhibited by difficulty nursing or masticating. Affected foals often drop milk from the mouth (**322**) or nares when nursing. Occasionally, respiratory stridor secondary to pharyngeal paresis may be noted. Depending

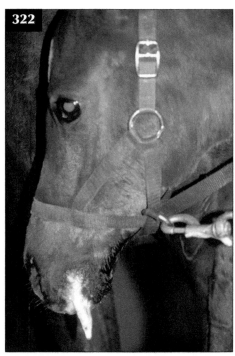

322 Foal with nutritional myodegeneration with milk dripping from its mouth.

on the muscle group affected, pain can be exhibited at a walk, when attempting to stand or when suckling the mare. Tachycardia and tachypnea are typically present. Cyanotic oral mucous membranes may be noted if the respiratory tract is involved. A pigmenturia may be present. Palpably firm muscle groups may be identified.

DIFFERENTIAL DIAGNOSIS

Other conditions causing a paralysis should be considered (*Table 66*). Although these conditions are not numerous, they can be difficult to differentiate based on physical examination alone. Botulism is a primary differential. Although not typically seen in the neonate, botulism can be seen in the young foal. The foal with clinical signs of botulism has a flaccid neuromuscular paralysis, whereas the foal with NM has more of a rigid paralysis with palpable firm musculature. Geography and knowledge of soil conditions can be integral in diagnosis of the disease.

DIAGNOSIS

Diagnosis of NM is based on physical examination findings suggestive of neuromuscular disease, soil or nutritional predisposition for the disease, and clinicopathologic evidence of muscle inflammation, decreased blood selenium/glutathione peroxide activity, and/or response to vitamin E/selenium treatment. Muscle enzymes (CK or AST) are elevated. The serum half-life of these enzymes must be considered when they are used diagnostically (**321**). If the insult resulting in muscle enzyme elevation is of short duration and not excessive, then the elevation of CK is of short duration. Electrolyte abnormalities may also be noted in some affected foals (i.e., hyperkalemia with moderate hyponatremia and hypochloremia). The hyperkalemia is considered to be a result of cellular release from damaged muscle cells. Pigmenturia, if present, is a result of a myoglobinemia. Blood glutathione peroxidase or selenium levels are low in foals with myodegeneration; however, these values alone should not be considered diagnostic, as values from unaffected foals (in deficient areas) are typically low.

MANAGEMENT

Treatment of the deficiency with parenteral vitamin E/selenium, in addition to correction of electrolyte imbalances and anti-inflammatories, helps to minimize pain. Nursing care, including restriction of activity, is critical, in addition to enteral feeding if necessary. The outcome is dependent on the severity of the condition. Long-term supplementation with vitamin E/selenium may be required.

MYOTONIA

KEY POINTS

- A breed predilection likely exists.
- The disease is characterized by repeated muscle contractions after stimulation.
- Etiology is likely to involve abnormalities in muscle membrane transport; however, the exact etiology is unknown.
- Clinically, a stiff hindlimb gait is frequently noted.
- Muscle groups may appear overdeveloped or bulging (particularly the gluteals).
- Definitive diagnosis is based on histopathology and/or electromyography.

DEFINITION/OVERVIEW

Myotonia is a disease of muscle that is generally manifested before one year of age. The condition is characterized by repeated muscle contractions after stimulation. There appears to be a breed predilection; however no heritable trait has been proven. Myotonia is also recognized in humans, goats, and dogs.

ETIOLOGY/PATHOPHYSIOLOGY

The precise etiology of myotonia in horses is not known. A genetic basis is suspected, particularly in some families of Quarter Horses, but not proven. Abnormalities in membrane transport mechanisms are likely to be involved; sarcolemmal chloride transport mechanisms are involved with some forms of myotonia in goats and humans.

CLINICAL PRESENTATION

Gait abnormalities (stiffness, typically of the hindlimbs) are usually the first signs noticed. Hindlimb stiffness (gait abnormality) is most obvious at the start of exercise and often improves with exercise. Muscle groups (particularly the gluteals) may appear overdeveloped or bulging. Percussion leads to muscle contraction or dimpling, which may be prolonged.

DIFFERENTIAL DIAGNOSIS

Differential diagnosis includes other conditions causing gait abnormalities and, in particular, a bilateral stiff-gaited appearance. Abnormal appearance of muscle groups and response to percussion can differentiate myotonia from other musculoskeletal diseases.

DIAGNOSIS

A presumptive diagnosis can be made from the characteristic clinical signs. Definitive diagnosis is based on histopathology and/or electromyography. Histopathology identifies abnormal (enlarged) muscle fiber size. Muscle fibers may be mixed, with normal to double-sized fibers present; increased perimysial and endomysial connective tissues, with rounded yet irregular muscle fibers, are also present. Electromyography of abnormal muscle reveals high-frequency repetitive crescendo–decrescendo bursts that are produced by repetitive firing of muscle fibers subsequent to stimulation. These characteristic bursts have been described as a "dive bomber" sound.

MANAGEMENT

Currently, therapies for treating myotonia in foals have been adopted from human medicine; however, they have not been routinely successful. Useful therapy is unlikely to be available until the exact etiology of the condition in adult horses and foals is elucidated. The prognosis is dictated by the severity of the disease. Severely affected individuals may progress to levels of severe pain and have difficulty ambulating. Mildly affected individuals have been reported to heal spontaneously over a period of months.

HYPERKALEMIC PERIODIC PARALYSIS

KEY POINTS

- HYPP is a familial disease of the Quarter Horse breed.
- The gene responsible for the condition is inherited as an autosomal dominant.

- The pathogenesis involves an altered permeability of muscle membrane to sodium and potassium.
- Clinical presentation may include stiffness, sweating, weakness, muscle fasciculations, and recumbency.
- Foals may present with upper respiratory stridor.
- A hyperkalemia may be noted during an episode.
- DNA (hair) testing is definitive.
- Severe episodes can be managed with intravenous calcium, bicarbonate, or dextrose.
- Long-term management can be achieved with acetazolamide.

DEFINITION/OVERVIEW

HYPP is a familial disorder that affects pure and crossbred Quarter Horses and foals. Affected animals experience intermittent episodes of muscle tremors and weakness, which may result in collapse. The gene responsible has been identified in descendants of the Quarter Horse stallion named Impressive.

ETIOLOGY/PATHOPHYSIOLOGY

HYPP is inherited as an autosomal dominant trait. The condition is due to a point mutation, which results in a resting membrane potential that is closer to activation than in the normal individual. The pathogenesis involves an altered permeability of muscle membranes to sodium and potassium by affecting the sodium ion channel. The altered permeability to potassium results in an uncontrollable influx of sodium, causing depolarization of muscle fibers and resulting in uncontrollable muscle twitching and weakness. The cellular influx of sodium results in an outward flux of potassium, resulting in persistent depolarization of muscle cells, which results in weakness.

CLINICAL PRESENTATION

The clinical signs often include episodes of muscle weakness, tremors, and collapse, which may be recurrent. Episodes begin with stiffness, sweating, and muscle fasciculations. Patients can "dog sit," have difficulty rising, and become recumbent. Mental status is normal; horses remain bright and alert during an "attack," respond to noxious stimuli, and are normal between episodes. Upper respiratory stridor may be noted and is a frequent representation of HYPP in the foal. The stridor is a result of pharyngeal/laryngeal paralysis. The severity of paralysis necessitates a permanent tracheostomy in some cases.

DIFFERENTIAL DIAGNOSIS

Differential diagnosis includes other causes of weakness, tremors, stiffness, upper respiratory stridor, and collapse. Central nervous system (CNS) diseases can be ruled out as individuals remain bright and alert. Musculoskeletal diseases should be considered as causes of stiffness or collapse, but generally not of persistent tremors or stridor. Other conditions resulting in pharyngeal/laryngeal paralysis are listed in *Table 67*. Muscular and neuromuscular disorders that should be considered in the differential are listed in *Table 66*.

DIAGNOSIS

The disease can be tentatively diagnosed on the basis of clinical signs and signalment. Hyperkalemia, hemoconcentration, and hyponatremia are typically observed during an episode; however,

> **Table 67. Conditions causing pharyngeal paresis/ paralysis**
> - Laryngeal hemiplegia
> - Laryngitis/pharyngitis
> - Retropharyngeal abscess or lymphadenopathy
> - Lead poisoning
> - Hypocalcemia
> - Hyperkalemic periodic paralysis
> - Botulism
> - Nutritional myodegeneration
> - Central nervous system lesions; encephalopathy
> - Brainstem lesions
> - Tick paralysis

this is not invariable. Potassium concentrations may reach values of 6–9 mmol/L (6–9 mEq/L) during episodes of weakness. A potassium chloride challenge test (90–50 mg/kg potassium chloride given in water via a nasogastric tube following an overnight fast) can produce signs of HYPP within 2–4 hours. A low dose of potassium chloride to start with is suggested and patients should be monitored continuously. The definitive diagnosis is through DNA testing of hair samples.

MANAGEMENT

Mild cases (muscle fasciculations) can be managed by hand walking, which encourages an influx of intracellular potassium, or oral acetazolamide (carbonic anhydrase inhibitor). Acetazolamide increases potassium secretion by the kidneys. Severe "attacks" can be treated with calcium gluconate, bicarbonate, and/or intravenous dextrose. Management of HYPP includes nutritional and exercise recommendations. High potassium-containing feedstuffs (alfalfa hay) should be eliminated from the diet. Turnout is preferable to stall rest. When management is not effective, oral acetazolamide (q8–12 h) can be used. Dilantin has also been used with some success.

POLYSACCHARIDE STORAGE MYOPATHY

KEY POINTS

- This is a common condition of Quarter Horses and related breeds.
- The disorder is an inherited trait.
- It is characterized by an accumulation of glycogen and an abnormal polysaccharide in skeletal muscle.

ETIOLOGY/PATHOPHYSIOLOGY

Polysaccharide storage myopathy (PSSM) is an inherited trait in Quarter Horses, Paints, Appaloosa, Draft Horse Breeds, Warmbloods, and more recently numerous other breeds including the Thoroughbred and Standardbred. The inherited trait is a defect in an enzyme involved in glycogenolysis, glycolysis, or energy metabolism. Glycogen accumulates as a result of the abnormality of muscle energy metabolism.

CLINICAL PRESENTATION

In the adult horse, clinical signs are usually seen at the onset of exercise. These signs include muscle stiffness, muscle fasciculations, reluctance to exercise, and pain. Foals of PSSM lineage may have subclinical elevations in muscle enzymes which can be exacerbated by unrelated conditions such as bacterial pneumonia. These foals may develop clinical signs of rhabdomyolysis.

DIFFERENTIAL DIAGNOSIS

Differential diagnosis includes other causes of weakness, tremors, stiffness, fasciculation's, and difficulty rising. Muscular and neuromuscular disorders that should be considered in the differential are listed in *Table 66*.

DIAGNOSIS

A presumptive diagnosis is based on clinical signs and elevation in muscle enzymes. Confirmation requires muscle biopsy or genetic testing on whole blood or hair roots.

MANAGEMENT

Management includes minimal stall confinement, access to as much turnout as possible, and a diet that is low in starch and high in fat.

GYLCOGEN BRANCHING ENZYME DEFICIENCY (GBED)

KEY POINTS

- This disorder causes muscle weakness in Quarter Horse–related breeds.
- Similar to PSSM, GBED is a glycogen storage disorder.
- The condition has been fatal in all known cases.
- The condition has been traced to a foundation Quarter Horse sire.

ETIOLOGY/PATHOPHYSIOLOGY

Glycogen branching enzyme deficiency (GBED) is an autosomal recessive form of glycogen storage disorder. The foal must be homozygous for the lethal GBED allele. Both parents are then heterozygous. Carrier frequency has been determined to be 7.1% for the Quarter Horse, 8.3% for the Paint Horse, and 26% in the Western Pleasure Horse.

CLINICAL PRESENTATION

A clinical sign in foals has included late-term abortions or stillbirths. Foals may be hypothermic and weak at birth. Foals may be less active with progressive muscle weakness. Acute deaths have been reported in foals turned out in pasture. By 18 weeks of age the condition has been fatal in all reported cases.

DIFFERENTIAL DIAGNOSIS

See the previous section on PSSM.

DIAGNOSIS MANAGEMENT

Diagnosis is based on ruling out other myopathies or conditions resulting in a weak newborn foal. Persistent elevation in muscle enzymes should be suggestive. Gross postmortem exams may overlook the diagnosis. Periodic-acid Schiff (PAS) staining of cardiac

or skeletal muscle looking for normal glycogen can be diagnostic. When suspecting GBED, skeletal and cardiac muscle should be collected and frozen at necropsy. Histopathologic and biochemical exams can be diagnostic. A test is currently available to confirm the presence of the genetic defect.

DISORDERS OF THE NEUROMUSCULAR JUNCTION

INTRODUCTION

Neuromuscular diseases in the foal are difficult to differentiate from diseases of muscle, as there are wide arrays of signs that may be seen in both disease processes. Additionally, these conditions may initially be present with a complaint of colic, neurologic disease, or musculoskeletal disease. Electrolyte disturbances may exhibit similar clinical signs to the neuromuscular disorders. Diagnosis is made subsequent to careful examination and observation. Epidemiologic factors (e.g., the geographic distribution of *C. botulinum* or the tick that causes *C. botulinum* and tick paralysis) aid the diagnosis of these conditions; however, variations in tick populations can be dramatic, with seasonal and annual variations. Botulism is typically seen in locations of heavy soil contamination. Feed contamination with *C. botulinum* or toxin can occur in any region, resulting in the sporadic case of paralysis resulting from botulism. The mechanism of both diseases includes disruption of acetylcholine at the myoneural junction.

TICK PARALYSIS

KEY POINTS

- A geographic distribution exists.
- Typical presentation is a flaccid neuromuscular paralysis.

DEFINITION/OVERVIEW

Infestation with ticks can result in a flaccid neuromuscular paralysis or muscle cramping. The disease has similarities to the condition seen in dogs and humans. There is an obvious geographic distribution (endemic tick habitats) of the disease; however, areas where the condition is not typically noted can be affected in years of unusually high tick infestation.

ETIOLOGY/PATHOPHYSIOLOGY

A variety of ticks may be involved with this condition. *Dermacento, Ixodes,* and *Otobius* spp. have been reported to be involved. Nymphs and larvae may also cause the disease. The toxin is inoculated into the host through saliva as the parasite feeds. In cases of flaccid paralysis, the toxin (neurotoxin) influences neuromuscular transmission at the motor neuron junction via alterations in acetylcholine. The toxic principle of the ear tick (*Otobius megnini*) is also likely to be related to neuromuscular junction dysfunction.

CLINICAL PRESENTATION

Typical tick paralysis results in a flaccid neuromuscular paralysis, which is often progressive and may be fatal. Clinical signs with ear tick infestation include, primarily, muscle cramping, muscle fasciculation, sweating, third eyelid prolapse, and colic.

DIFFERENTIAL DIAGNOSIS

As tick paralysis can present with neuromuscular paralysis and/or varying degrees of muscle cramping/fasciculation, conditions consistent with this variety of clinical signs must be considered. The major rule out for a foal with a flaccid neuromuscular paralysis is botulism. The major rule out for a foal with muscle stiffness is NM. Other conditions to consider are listed in *Table 66*.

DIAGNOSIS

Diagnosis is based on geographic location, season of the year (high tick population), dynamics of the tick population (excessive numbers), and identification of the offending parasite. Identification of the ear tick can be difficult; evaluation of the inner ear is necessary.

MANAGEMENT

Removal of the offending parasites plus supportive care is the treatment of choice. If paralysis is present, mortality is not infrequent. Ear tick removal often results in improvement in days to weeks.

BOTULISM

KEY POINTS

- Botulism is typically a geographic-related disease.
- An exotoxin (one of the most potent neurotoxins known) is produced by *C. botulinum*.
- Routes of infection include ingestion of preformed toxin, elaboration of toxin *in vivo*, and wound contamination with local production of toxin.
- The neuromuscular paralysis of botulism is a result of interference with the release of acetylcholine (ACh).
- Clinical signs are related to a flaccid neuromuscular paralysis.
- The CNS is not affected by the botulism toxin, therefore the botulism patient is bright and alert.
- The term "shaker foal" was derived from the muscle tremors that are frequently seen in affected foals.
- Botulism antitoxin can be beneficial in treatment.
- Botulism is a clinical diagnosis; confirmation may be provided by culturing of stool/environment or infected wounds.
- A vaccine is available and effective as a preventative.

DEFINITION/OVERVIEW

Botulism is a flaccid neuromuscular paralysis that can affect all mammals. Horses, however, are one of the most susceptible species. The disease can affect both foals and adult horses. In foals the disease has been called "shaker foal syndrome." The neuromuscular paralysis is a result of interference of ACh release at the motor endplate. The disruption of ACh release is caused by the exotoxin of the Gram-positive bacterium *Clostridium botulinum*. This exotoxin is one of the most potent neurotoxins known. Botulism occurs in horse populations throughout the world; however, the only geographic areas where non-feed contamination outbreaks are found are in the United States, where the organisms are present in high numbers in the soil. *C. botulinum* grows preferentially in neutral or alkaline soils and it grows and produces toxin in an anaerobic environment. *C. botulinum* spores have been found in 18.5% of the soils sampled in the United States. However, the distribution of spores is variable and is likely related to the geographic frequency of the disease. Type B toxin is the most common cause

of clinical botulism in horses in the United States. It is found in high concentrations in soils in central Kentucky and along the Mid-Atlantic seaboard. Shaker foal syndrome is frequently seen in central Kentucky because of the large population of susceptible foals and the prevalence of the organism. Type *C. botulinum* toxin causes disease in European countries, but is not a frequent cause of disease in the United States. Type C organisms have been found in high concentrations in soils in Florida and they were the causative organism in a California outbreak of botulism.

ETIOLOGY/PATHOPHYSIOLOGY

Three routes of botulism infection have generally been accepted to exist: ingestion of preformed toxin, toxico-infectious botulism, and wound botulism. Ingestion of preformed toxin is thought to be the most common route of infection and gives rise to the syndrome known as "forage poisoning." Toxico-infectious botulism is the elaboration of toxin within the gastrointestinal (GI) tract. Toxin is produced when spores are ingested and vegetate or when the local GI environment is favorable to an overgrowth of *C. botulinum*. The wound route of infection includes abscesses or damage to tissue that results in an anaerobic environment conducive to the growth of *C. botulinum*. Toxin is locally produced and subsequently spreads throughout the body. Infected umbilical remnants have been suggested to be a source of this type of infection in foals. Wound botulism has been reported as a consequence of castration in the horse.

The neuromuscular paralysis of botulism is a result of an interference with the release of ACh (**323**). This blockage of ACh release can occur at neuromuscular junctions, peripheral cholinergic nerve terminals in autonomic ganglia, and in postganglionic parasympathetic nerve endings. The CNS and sensory nerves are not affected. Two proposed mechanisms of toxin action include (1) interference

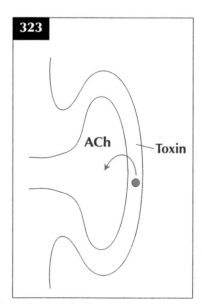

323 Inhibition of acetylcholine release at the myoneural junction. Botulism toxin interferes with the release of ACh from the motor neuron. Proposed mechanisms include interference with calcium function at the nerve terminal and blockage of exocytosis of synaptic vesicles. ACh = acetylcholine.

with calcium function at the nerve terminal thereby inhibiting the release of ACh, and (2) blockage of exocytosis of synaptic vesicles, thereby preventing the release of ACh.

CLINICAL PRESENTATION

Clinical signs of botulism are generally related to a flaccid neuromuscular paralysis. Signs may be mild to severe and are dependent on the amount of toxin ingested or elaborated (*Table 68*). The CNS is not affected by the *C. botulinum* neurotoxin, therefore the animal should be bright and alert.

The disease in foals has been reported as early as two weeks of age. The signs vary from mild to severe. Severe signs of disease may include paralysis, which has progressed to an inability to stand, or foals found dead. If the disease is mild and gradual in progression, some of the first signs noted are varying degrees of muscle weakness, spending large amounts of time lying down (**324**), and dribbling milk from the nostrils or mouth (**322**). The initial muscle weakness can appear as a stiff, stilted gait that can be difficult to differentiate from mild proprioceptive deficits. The foal may walk slowly and have difficulty keeping up with the mare. If signs progress, muscle tremors may be evident and the foal can have difficulty standing, may stand for only brief periods, or may become recumbent. Muscle weakness is evident when foals lie down, because they often collapse to the ground instead of lying down gracefully. The term "shaker foal" is derived from the severe muscle tremors that are frequently seen with the disease. Other signs of neuromuscular paralysis include poor tail, tongue (**325**), and eyelid tone, or dysphagia. Poor tongue tone results in difficulty nursing and milk dripping from the sides of the mouth. If ingestion or elaboration of toxin

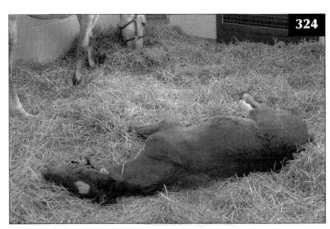

324 Foal with botulism in lateral recumbency. The foal has flaccid paralysis, which if severe, can progress to paralysis of the diaphragm.

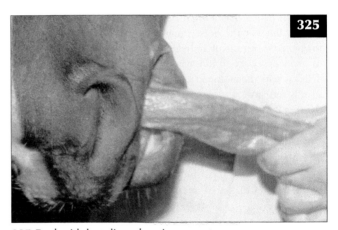

325 Foal with botulism showing poor tongue tone.

has been extensive, foals may be recumbent and in respiratory distress. Respiratory rate and effort increase and chest excursion is reduced, as evidenced by an increase in the abdominal component of breathing. Respiratory difficulties result from paralysis of intercostal and diaphragmatic musculature. Death due to botulism is a result of respiratory paralysis.

DIFFERENTIAL DIAGNOSIS

Botulism should be on the list of differential diagnoses for a foal that is recumbent and cannot stand or is found dead. Other conditions resulting in weakness, dysphagia, and progressive flaccid neuromuscular paralysis should be considered (*Tables 66* and *67*).

DIAGNOSIS

Diagnosis of botulism is based on historical evidence and clinical signs. Owners may report signs referable to a progressive muscle weakness, as described in the previous section. A failure to vaccinate or an incomplete vaccination schedule in endemic areas is a common factor in foals with botulism. FPT is another possible source of vaccine failure in endemic areas.

Table 68. Clinical signs of botulism (flaccid neuromuscular paralysis)

- Early/less severe:
  - Weakness
  - Extended periods of lying down/fatigue
  - Stumbling/stiff gait
  - Dribbling milk from mouth or nostrils subsequent to suckling/mild dysphagia
  - Walking slowly, difficulty keeping up with the mare
  - Poor tail, tongue, and eyelid tone
  - Trembling/shaking (particularly of the forelimbs)
- Progressive:
  - Muscle tremors
  - Difficulty standing
  - Collapse when attempting to lie down
  - Difficulty returning to sternal from lateral recumbency
  - Pharyngeal paresis/paralysis
  - Dysphagia
  - Dyspnea
  - Recumbency
  - Respiratory paralysis/death

When considering botulism as a diagnosis, it is helpful to remember that the CNS is unaffected, therefore the patient should be "bright and alert." This can be useful in differentiating botulism from diseases that result in CNS signs.

When the disease is slowly progressive in onset, dysphagia is often one of the first signs noted by owners. The differential diagnosis of dysphagia (*Table 69*) should include obstructive lesions in the pharynx, guttural pouch lesions, and dysphagia resulting from CNS lesions. The most common brainstem lesion resulting in dysphagia is protozoal myelitis. However, any encephalitis or encephalopathy such as leukoencephalomalacia, yellow star thistle poisoning, and rabies can result in dysphagia. Other conditions causing neuromuscular paralysis include white snakeroot toxicity, organophosphate poisoning, tick paralysis, and hypocalcemia.

Clinicopathologic abnormalities can be useful in excluding other diseases, but these are few in number and generally nonspecific in horses with botulism. Examination of CSF can be useful in differentiating inflammatory CNS diseases from botulism; the botulism patient has normal cerebrospinal fluid (CSF). In many species, but not the horse, mouse inoculation tests can identify toxin in the serum of individuals with botulism. The amount of toxin necessary to kill a horse may be so small that it is not detectable by the mouse inoculation system. In addition, the toxin spends very little time in circulation because it is rapidly bound to the motor endplate. Electromyographic evaluation during repetitive nerve stimulations has been useful in evaluating botulism in humans. However, in horses it is unreliable as a diagnostic aid and is difficult to perform.

Culturing the feces of horses suspected of having botulism can be useful to confirm a diagnosis. However, the organism is difficult to culture and few laboratories are equipped to do so. A real time PCR test for *C. botulinum* toxin genes is available. *C. botulinum* spores can be cultured from the stool of 20% of affected adult horses. Spores can be found in approximately 80% of affected foals. Spores are rarely found in the GI contents of a normal horse not at risk for botulism.

MANAGEMENT

The development and use of the polyvalent equine origin botulism antitoxin containing types A, B, C, D, and E has greatly improved the chances for survival of a horse with botulism. Before the advent of the antitoxin the mortality rate approached 90%. With the use of the antitoxin and appropriate nursing and nutritional therapy, prognosis for survival is >70% in adult horses and is higher in "shaker foals." The antitoxin is produced by hyperimmunization of horses with *C. botulinum* toxoid and is expensive. The recommended dose for the adult and foal is 400 and 200 mL, respectively. It must be used early in the course of the disease and its use does not guarantee recovery. The antitoxin is of critical importance in the severely affected animal, but horses with slowly progressive mild disease can survive without it. Clinical signs are not reversed by antitoxin and owners must be warned that patients may actually worsen after antitoxin administration. The reason for this is that antitoxin binds circulating toxin, but does not bind toxin that is already attached to the motor endplate. This bound toxin can result in a deterioration of clinical signs as it proceeds to block ACh release.

The prognosis is related to the rapidity of onset and progression of flaccid paralysis. Patients that present with a gradual onset and slow progression of signs have most likely been exposed to a small dose of toxin compared with the patient with rapid onset and progression of signs, which has most likely been exposed to a large dose of toxin. The recumbent horse (or horses) with rapid-onset disease may succumb despite the administration of antitoxin.

Broad-spectrum antibiotic therapy is advisable if aspiration pneumonia is suspected. Potassium or sodium penicillin (22,000–44,000 IU/kg i/v) should eliminate any proliferating *C. botulinum* if wound botulism is suspected. The use of oral antibiotics is controversial because they may either kill the vegetative, GI form of the bacterium, resulting in increased toxin release, or they may result in upset of the GI flora and allow overgrowth of *C. botulinum*.

The use of drugs such as neostigmine that potentiate neuromuscular transmission are contraindicated. The effect of these drugs is only transient. Patients receiving these drugs often worsen dramatically after a brief period of improvement. Ventilatory support may become necessary if respiratory paralysis develops. Adult horses are very difficult to ventilate, but foals can be successfully ventilated if the right equipment and expertise are available (**326**).

Vaccination of horses with *C. botulinum* toxoid has proven to be very successful in prevention of the disease when appropriate schedules are followed. For example, vaccination programs have

Table 69. Causes of dysphagia

- Prematurity
- Congenital oral/pharyngeal abnormalities:
  - Cleft palate
  - Subepiglottic cyst
- Congenital laryngeal abnormalities
- Dorsal displacement of the soft palate or rostral displacement of the palatopharyngeal arch
- Pharyngitis
- Hypoxic ischemic encephalopathy
- Encephalopathy, hepatic or other encephalopathy
- Meningitis
- Brainstem lesion
- Tetanus
- Equine herpesvirus infection
- Equine protozoal myelitis
- Botulism
- Hyperkalemic periodic paralysis
- Nutritional myodegeneration
- Hypocalcemia
- Megaesophagus or other esophageal disorders
- Retropharyngeal abscessation of the oral or pharyngeal region
- Tumors of the oral or pharyngeal region
- Foreign bodies

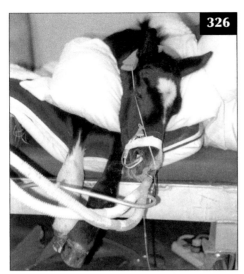

326 Foal with botulism showing respiratory difficulties being managed on a ventilator.

dramatically reduced the incidence of "shaker foals" in central Kentucky. The mare is initially given a three-dose series, with one month between doses and the last dose in the last month of gestation. This regimen provides maximal colostral antibody levels. Mares then subsequently receive a yearly booster dose during their last month of gestation. If protection is required in non-breeding stock, the initial three-dose series should be used with a yearly booster. Vaccination of horses in areas where the disease is not prevalent may not be necessary. However, vaccination of individuals maintained in endemic areas and mares that are transported to endemic areas is recommended. Vaccine breaks can occur if the initial series is incomplete, the third vaccine does not provide adequate colostral immunity, there is failure of colostral transfer, or if yearly boosters are not provided.

FURTHER READING

Bernard WV (1997) Botulism. In: *Current Therapy in Equine Practice 4* (Robinson NE, Ed.). WB Saunders, Philadelphia, PA, pp. 326–328.

Hodgson DR (1999) Diseases of muscle. In: *Equine Medicine and Surgery, Volume II*. 5th ed. (Colahan PT, Mayhew IG, Merritt AM, Moore JN, Eds.). Mosby, St. Louis, MO, pp. 1483–1486.

Katz LM, O'Dwyer S, Pollock PJ (2009) Nutritional muscular dystrophy in a four-day-old Connemara foal. *Irish Veterinary Journal* 62: 119–124.

Lofstedt J (1997) White muscle disease of foals. *Vet Clinics of North America. Equine Practice* 13: 169–185.

Schooley KE, MacLeay JM, Cuddon P et al. (2004) Atypical myotonia congenita in a foal. *Journal of Equine Veterinary Science* 24: 483–488.

Spier SS (2006) Hyperkalemic periodic paralysis: 14 years later. *Proceedings of the Annual Convention of the AAEP* 52: 347–350.

Valberg JS (2002) A review of the diagnosis and treatment of rhabdomyolysis in foals. *Proceedings of the Annual Convention of the AAEP* 48: 117–121.

Wilkins PA, Palmer JE (2002) Botulism in foals a survivable disease. *Proceedings of the Annual Convention of the AAEP* 48: 124–126.

Joint and Skeletal Disorders

12

Troy N. Trumble

INTRODUCTION

The first few months of life are one of the most vulnerable times for foals since they must adjust to their environment while still being somewhat compromised immunologically. In addition, their musculoskeletal system is growing rapidly and adjusting to the stresses applied to it due to an increasing amount of exercise. If a foal is born with, or rapidly acquires, an abnormality or disease related to the musculoskeletal system, rapid adjustments must be made in order to allow the foal to grow and respond in a fashion such that future athletic performance is minimally compromised. Therefore, problems must be identified early, requiring multiple thorough examinations so that appropriate steps can be taken. When problems are identified, treatment often entails a complex mixture of conservative therapy (e.g., exercise adjustment), medical therapy, and/or surgery.

The objective of this chapter is to summarize and discuss common musculoskeletal disorders that tend to be present or become clinically evident within the first few months to 1 year of life.

POLYDACTYLISM

DEFINITION/OVERVIEW

Polydactylism is a congenital anomaly of the skeleton where there is duplication of all or part of the digit (**327, 328**).

KEY POINTS

- Polydactylism is likely a heritable, congenital anomaly in which there is duplication of all or part of the digit.
- Polydactylism is often associated with other congenital deformities such as adactylia (absence of phalanges), arthrogryposis (multiple joint contractures), and jaw anomalies.
- Most extra digits are unilateral and originate from either metacarpus II or III on the medial aspect.
- Most extra digits have their own flexor tendons and suspensory ligament.
- Extra digits usually are not weight bearing, but they can interfere with locomotion, especially those digits originating on the medial aspect of the limb.
- Radiographs will define the extent of the anomaly.
- Treatment options should take into account the presence or absence of other anomalies. If no other anomalies are present, surgery can be performed to improve appearance, but horses should be neutered.

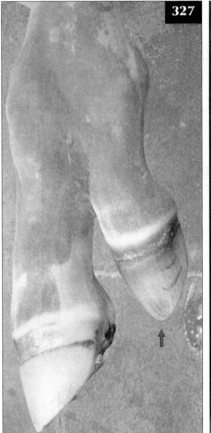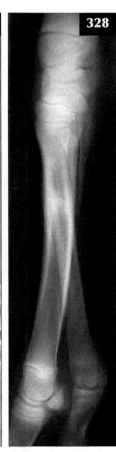

327, 328 Photograph (**327**) and lateral radiograph (**328**) of polydactylism in a foal. The extra digit originated in the carpus and extended distally on the medial aspect of the forelimb. Note that the extra digit (arrow) does not contact the ground.

ETIOLOGY/PATHOPHYSIOLOGY

There is no known cause of polydactylism, but this anomaly may be heritable since the modern horse likely originated from animals that had multiple phalanges. However, there has not been enough evidence to support a hereditary cause.

CLINICAL PRESENTATION

Most of the extra digits are unilateral and originate from either metacarpus II or III, with 80% being on the medial side of the forelimb.

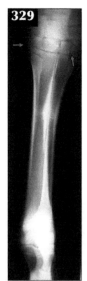

329 Dorsopalmar radiograph of the polydactyl foal in **327/328** demonstrating the presence of an extra carpal bone (arrow).

However, they can originate from the carpus, including the presence of extra carpal bones (**329**). Most of these limbs lack extensor tendons, but they do have their own superficial and deep digital flexor tendons as well as suspensory ligaments. The limbs are usually not long enough to be weight bearing, but they can interfere with normal locomotion due to their occupation of space.

DIFFERENTIAL DIAGNOSIS
Often, polydactylism is associated with other congenital deformities such as adactylia (absence of phalanges), arthrogryposis (multiple joint contractures), and jaw anomalies.

DIAGNOSIS
Radiographs are required to diagnosis the origin and extent of the polydactylism.

MANAGEMENT
Nothing has to be done on many of these horses as it is not usually a painful deformity. Surgery can be performed to improve the appearance of the limb as well as prevent any lameness or interference with normal locomotion due to its occupation of space (**330, 331**). If this anomaly is surgically manipulated, it is strongly recommended that these foals are neutered, since there may be a genetic component. Euthanasia may be elected, especially if other congenital abnormalities are present.

HOOF WALL ASYMMETRY

KEY POINTS
- Any defect in hoof wall growth in foals that results in asymmetry of the size and/or shape of the hoof wall on one limb.
- There is likely a congenital cause resulting in agenesis or hypoplasia of the middle phalanx, distal phalanx, or navicular bone. Other congenital deformities may also be present.
- The abnormal foot is usually smaller and may deviate in any direction.
- Degree of lameness is variable, with most affected foals having permanent lameness.
- Radiographs will diagnose the deformity and identify the severity.

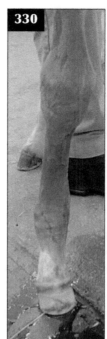
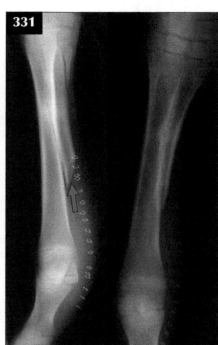

330, 331 Photograph (**330**) and radiographs (**331**) of the polydactyl foal in **327/328** following surgical removal of the distal aspect of the extra digit (arrow).

- No treatment option completely corrects the deformity, but trimming and shoeing may decrease lameness.
- For severe cases, euthanasia should be considered.

DEFINITION/OVERVIEW
Hoof wall asymmetry in the foal presents as a defect in hoof wall growth that has resulted in a noticeable asymmetry in the size and/or shape of the hoof wall on one limb (**332, 333**).

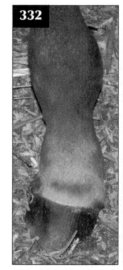
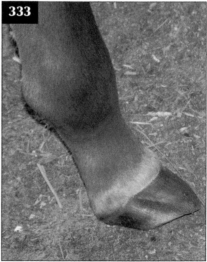

332, 333 Abnormal hoof wall in a foal. Note the medial deviation of the hoof wall (**332**) because of a linear defect on the medial aspect of the hoof wall (**333**).

ETIOLOGY/PATHOPHYSIOLOGY

There is no known cause, but many cases are congenital in origin. The most common congenital problems identified radiographically include agenesis or hypoplasia of the middle phalanx, distal phalanx (334), or the navicular bone, as well as the bipartite and tripartite navicular bones (335). It has been hypothesized that these bones may fail to form correctly due to an alteration in the vascular supply to the digit during embryogenesis.

CLINICAL PRESENTATION

Foals present with an abnormal shape and/or size, usually of one hoof, when compared with the remaining feet. The abnormal foot is usually smaller and may be deviated in any direction (332, 333). The degree of lameness is variable, but most of these foals are likely to have some degree of permanent lameness.

DIFFERENTIAL DIAGNOSIS

Other congenital deformities may also be present.

DIAGNOSIS

Radiography is usually required to diagnose definitively the deformity and determine the severity of the bone deformity present (334, 335).

MANAGEMENT

Since most of these deformities are due to a congenital deformity of one of the bones in the hoof, there is no treatment option that will correct the disorder. Most affected foals will have a permanent lameness that may or may not be controllable with a combination of corrective trimming and shoeing and appropriate medical therapies into the synovial structures. Euthanasia may be elected if the lameness is too severe or cannot be adequately controlled.

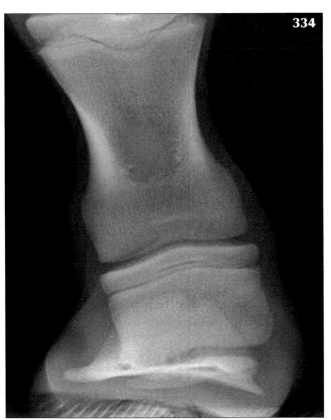

334 Dorsoplantar radiograph of the foal in **332/333** demonstrating hypoplasia of the medial aspect of the third phalanx as the underlying cause of the hoof wall deformity.

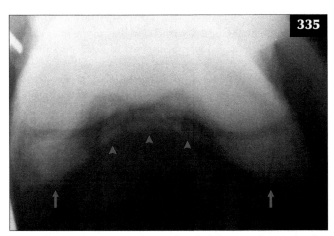

335 Palmaroproximal–palmarodistal oblique radiograph of the distal phalanx and navicular bone of a yearling demonstrating a tripartite navicular bone where the medial and lateral aspects of the navicular bone are present (arrows) but the middle of the bone is hypoplastic (arrowheads).

CONTRACTED FOAL SYNDROME

KEY POINTS

- Common congenital anomaly of the horse in which multiple different areas of the skeleton are affected including the forelimbs, cranium, and spine (rotation or lateral deviation).
- Most affected foals result in dystocia and need to be delivered via cesarean section or fetotomy.
- Severity determines prognosis and treatment.
- Most are euthanized due to multiple defects or die during parturition.

DEFINITION/OVERVIEW

Contracted foal syndrome is one of the most common congenital anomalies diagnosed in the horse. Multiple different areas of the skeleton are affected including the forelimbs, cranium, and spine.

ETIOLOGY/PATHOPHYSIOLOGY

The etiology of this congenital syndrome is unknown.

CLINICAL PRESENTATION

Because of the nature of these deformities, most affected foals result in a dystocia and need to be delivered via cesarean section or fetotomy. Often, affected foals have bilateral contracture of multiple joints on the forelimbs (336), asymmetric formation of the cranium, torticollis (rotation of the spine), and/or scoliosis (lateral deviation of the spine).

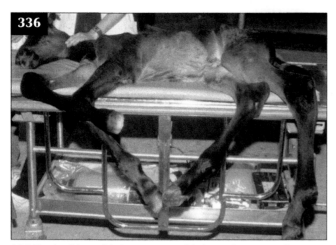

336 Foal with multiple contracted joints. (Courtesy of M. Brown)

DIFFERENTIAL DIAGNOSIS
Another congenital syndrome reported in the horse is congenital hypothyroidism dysmaturity. These foals have mandibular prognathia (underbite), flexural deformities, ruptured extensor tendons, and incompletely ossified carpal or tarsal bones.

MANAGEMENT
The severity of the condition determines the prognosis, as there are no treatments described. Because of the multiple defects, euthanasia is usually recommended.

SEPTIC ARTHRITIS AND OSTEOMYELITIS

KEY POINTS
- Septic arthritis and osteomyelitis result from inflammation and infection after bacterial invasion of synovial structures.
- Foals will often acquire a septic joint or osteomyelitis via hematogenous spread of bacteria.
- Septic joints or osteomyelitis should be considered in any lame foal less than 1 month of age.
- The first detectable clinical signs will include one or all of the following: moderate to severe synovial distension and/or heat, periarticular edema, pain from and/or restriction to passive movement, as well as focal pain on palpation of the joint or bone.
- Any joint or combination of joints can be involved, but usually the larger joints such as the stifle, hock, carpus, and fetlocks are affected.
- The presence of inflammation leads to an increase in the permeability of the vasculature of the synovial membrane, increasing both total protein as well as white blood cells (WBCs) within the synovial fluid.
- Usually, a synovial fluid total protein level of 40 g/L (>4 g/dL) is indicative of a severe inflammation that can be associated with infection. When this is combined with a synovial fluid WBC count of >30,000/μL, infection should be suspected, but a synovial fluid WBC count >100,000/μL is pathognomonic for infection.

- Obtain synovial fluid and/or synovial membrane for culture whenever possible, even if antibiotic therapy has already commenced.
- Radiography should be considered in order to determine the severity of the condition and monitor progression.
- Treatment should be aggressive and include a mixture of the following options: antibiotics (systemic and/or regional), anti-inflammatories, joint lavage, and/or debridement.
- Presence of fibrin in the joint will sequester bacteria from antibiotics.
- Overall, the prognosis for survival and successful athletic performance in foals with septic joints and/or osteomyelitis is guarded, but for the best chance of success, early and aggressive treatment using any combination of the methods described above is required.

DEFINITION/OVERVIEW
Septic arthritis and osteomyelitis are inflammation and infection of synovial structures because of invasion by bacteria.

ETIOLOGY/PATHOPHYSIOLOGY
In general, because of their immature immune system, neonates are more likely to be susceptible to infection and acquire subsequent septicemia than adult horses. A slow rise in endogenous antibodies, combined with a rapid decrease in passive antibody levels, makes foals more susceptible to infection. In addition, if the foal fails to fully absorb adequate levels of antibodies from colostrum, then sepsis is a common sequela. Generalized septicemia has a tendency to infect a foal's other tissues, such as the joints or bones, via hematogenous spread of the bacteria. In two studies examining foals with confirmed sepsis, 26% and 28%, respectively, had concurrent septic arthritis and/or osteomyelitis. However, it is important to note that foals can also get septic joints secondary to trauma. Nonetheless, the bacteria most commonly isolated from septic arthritis or osteomyelitis are the same ones that can cause the initial septicemia.

In immature bones and joints there is a rapid growth phase that requires an increased blood flow via transphyseal vessels to the metaphysis, physis, and epiphysis, as well as to the joint capsule. This physeal region is more predisposed to developing infection because the blood has a lower oxygen tension as well as a decreased flow, with pooling in sinusoids. Colonization of these vessels can result in thrombosis and ischemic necrosis of the physeal region as well as thrombosis of the vasculature of the synovial membrane. This results in impaired synovial fluid production and exchange due to increased vascular permeability. Prematurity or dysmaturity can actually maintain this vascular pattern for longer than normal, making these foals more prone to joint and bone infections. The normal production and drainage of synovial fluid becomes impaired, which in turn affects cartilage metabolism, since cartilage derives its nutrients from synovial fluid. The presence of inflammation within the joint leads to an increase in the permeability of the vasculature of the synovial membrane. This leads to an increase in both total protein as well as WBCs within the synovial fluid. The total protein levels increase quickly in response to the inflammation, but the WBC count does not obtain its greatest increase until 12–24 hours after initiation of the infection. This increased influx of serum proteins, WBCs, and proteolytic enzymes in the synovial fluid can disrupt the reparative nature of the chondrocytes and cause eventual degradation of articular cartilage. In addition, a decreased synovial fluid pH can activate the degradative enzymes, contributing to further damage to the cartilage.

CLINICAL PRESENTATION

Identification of septic arthritis or osteomyelitis can be rather difficult in young foals, especially systemically septic foals, because they are often weak and recumbent. In addition, alterations in the rectal temperature or hemogram are inconsistent and tend to correlate more with the overall systemic condition of foals. Therefore, thorough daily musculoskeletal examinations are very important. Often, the first detectable clinical signs will include one or all of the following: moderate to severe synovial distension and/or heat (**337, 338**), periarticular edema, pain from and/or restriction to passive movement, as well as focal pain on palpation of the joint or bone. Lameness takes approximately 8–24 hours to develop after sufficient bacteria have colonized the joint; however, lameness due to sepsis in the synovial cavity has been identified as early as 12 hours after parturition and should be considered in any lame foal less than 1 month of age. Any joint or combination of joints can be involved, but usually the larger joints, such as the stifle, hock, carpus, and fetlocks, are most often affected.

DIFFERENTIAL DIAGNOSIS

In foals that have joint effusion it is important to rule out developmental problems associated with delayed or abnormal ossification of cuboidal bones, osteochondrosis, and fracture of the epiphyseal region of the long bones or intra-articular bones, as well as major trauma resulting in subluxations or puncture wounds.

DIAGNOSIS

In one study, the only consistent hemogram finding in foals with septic joints was a plasma fibrinogen level >1.18 μmol/L (>40 g/dL). However, examination of the synovial fluid helps to confirm the diagnosis and monitor the effectiveness of therapy, as well as potentially identifying the causative agent, thereby directing future therapies.

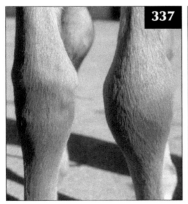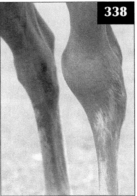

337, 338 Photographs of joint effusion in the left carpus (**337**) and left tarsus (**338**) secondary to sepsis. (Courtesy of M. Brown)

Synovial fluid should be collected aseptically to allow for evaluation of at least the total WBC count and total protein; ideally, the differential leukocyte count and pH should be analyzed as well. Serum amyloid A (an acute phase protein) in both the serum and synovial fluid has also been shown to increase from normal when a joint is infected; however, it is important to note that it might be sensitive to treatment (antibiotics or steroid administration) such that levels appear normal in spite of infection.

Usually, a synovial fluid total protein level of 40 g/L (>4 g/dL) is indicative of a severe inflammation that can be associated with infection. When this is combined with a synovial fluid WBC count of >30,000/μL, infection should be suspected, but a synovial fluid WBC count >100,000/μL is pathognomonic for infection. It is important to note that the presence of fibrin within the joint can produce falsely low WBC counts because the cells can aggregate with the fibrin clots. If a differential analysis of the leukocytes is performed, the synovial fluid in cases of septic arthritis usually has ≥80%–90% neutrophils compared with mostly mononuclear cells in normal synovial fluid. In addition, septic synovial fluid is usually acidic, with a pH as low as 6.2 compared with a normal synovial fluid pH of 7.3.

Synovial fluid should also be collected for bacterial culture in order to help select the appropriate antibiotic. The sample should be collected even if the foal has been started on antibiotics (as is typical for systemically septic foals), but it is preferable to collect the sample prior to initiation of antibiotic therapy. To maximize the chance of a positive culture, approximately 5–10 mL of synovial fluid should be collected and placed directly into blood culture medium (thioglycolate broth). This is the same medium used for systemic blood culture, and it enhances the recovery of many aerobic, microaerophilic, and anaerobic bacteria. The chances of obtaining a positive culture are partly based on the sample handling and the number and virulence of the organisms present, as well as their defense mechanisms. The reported chances of obtaining a positive bacterial culture from synovial fluid range from 64% to 89%. Additional collection of synovial membrane for culture has been shown to increase the chance for isolation of the bacteria by 10% over synovial fluid culture alone. It is not uncommon to identify multiple bacterial species in foals with septic arthritis and/or osteomyelitis. Presumptive results can also be obtained by analyzing the synovial fluid via Gram staining, which might help guide the initial therapy before the culture results come back.

When the clinical signs point toward either septic arthritis or osteomyelitis, it is important to obtain radiographs of the joints of interest as soon as possible. This is partly because infection of the joint and physeal region are closely related due to the proximity of the vascular network, making it very possible to have both problems concurrently. In fact, the relationship of septic arthritis and osteomyelitis has been classified based on clinical, radiographic, and pathologic findings. Radiographic changes such as concurrent osteomyelitis, physitis, and/or osteoarthritis have been reported to also be present in 38%–80% of foals with septic arthritis. If both the bone and joint are infected, the prognosis will be adversely affected. Identification of osteomyelitis is usually delayed when compared with septic arthritis because it takes 10–14 days to get noticeable radiographic changes (**339**). Therefore, if a set of radiographs is taken when the infection is first diagnosed (**339a**), they

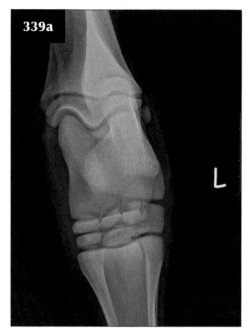
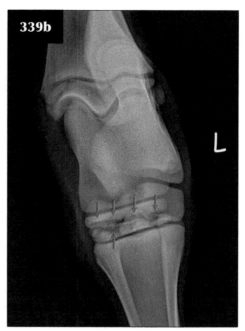

339 Radiograph of the carpus of a foal with a septic middle carpal joint and secondary osteomyelitis of the third carpal bone (arrow). **339a, 339b** Radiograph of the tarsus from a foal with a septic distal intertarsal joint at presentation (**339a**) and 9 days later (**339b**).

can be used as a baseline to determine whether there is any initial bony involvement (at the time of first examination) and whether further therapy is worth pursuing. If the foal does not respond to therapy or regresses during treatment, more radiographs should be taken (**339b**) and compared with the baseline radiographs (**339a**). In addition, since radiographs are relatively insensitive to early bone changes, other more advanced diagnostic imaging techniques could potentially be used to identify osteomyelitis prior to radiographic changes; this includes ultrasound, nuclear scintigraphy (utilizing radionucleotide-labeled leukocytes), computed tomography (CT), or magnetic resonance imaging (MRI).

MANAGEMENT

Treatment for septic arthritis in foals, especially neonates, can be very difficult because, as mentioned earlier, many have multisystemic disease. Successful outcomes on these foals are often associated with early diagnosis and aggressive treatment. No one form of treatment is necessarily better than another and, in reality, a combination of some or all probably leads to the best chance for a successful outcome. The clinical course and the economic situation must be taken into account. In addition, it is important to consider the defense capabilities of the foal, as the treatment choices may need to be altered accordingly.

Administration of systemic antibiotics should be commenced as soon as possible after the diagnosis is confirmed, or even presumed. Initial antibiotic selection will need to be chosen prior to having knowledge of the infecting organism and should be based on experience of the common regional bacterial isolates, since culture results generally take approximately 48 hours to obtain.

Broad-spectrum antibiotics should be chosen since many foals have Gram-negative organisms that inoculate the joints. Anaerobic infections can occur, but tend to be gradual in onset and

nonresponsive to appropriate aerobic therapy. When deciding on which broad-spectrum antibiotics to choose, the following needs to be taken into consideration:

- The antibiotic should ideally be bactericidal, since the immune system of many of these affected foals is already compromised.
- Many foals also have renal compromise, so the excretion/metabolism of the antibiotic needs to be considered.
- In foals, the most ideal route of administration is either intravenous, regional perfusion, or oral, not intramuscular as there is little relative muscle mass.
- The antibiotic chosen should also have the best opportunity to be delivered to the bone and synovia at adequate therapeutic concentrations.

Cephalosporins, beta-lactams, and aminoglycosides have historically been the three most effective classes of broad-spectrum bactericidal drugs used in the treatment of septic joints in foals. The cephalosporins (e.g., cefazolin or ceftiofur) and aminoglycosides (e.g., gentamicin or amikacin) are efficacious against Gram-negative organisms and the beta-lactams (penicillins) are better against Gram-positive organisms. Generally, either a cephalosporin or a beta-lactam is used in combination with an aminoglycoside, depending on the regional occurrence of the organism and the availability of the drug. The following important considerations need to be taken into account when using these antibiotics in septic joints:

- Little is known about the actual penetration of systemically administered antibiotics into inflamed joints because of the alterations in the blood supply and tissue metabolism in response to the inflammation. This becomes important when using aminoglycosides, since the bactericidal effect is proportional to the peak drug concentration obtained within the tissues.

- The acidic environment of the synovial fluid combined with the presence of purulent material can also decrease the efficacy of some antibiotics, aminoglycosides in particular. Third-generation cephalosporins (ceftiofur) have been demonstrated to have good penetration into the bone and synovial fluid in normal joints, and amikacin has been shown to be the most efficacious aminoglycoside against orthopedic pathogens.
- Bacteria rarely develop resistance to amikacin.
- Aminoglycosides such as amikacin need to be used with caution in foals due to their nephrotoxic nature.

NSAIDs can also be beneficial in these cases because of their potent anti-inflammatory properties. In addition, NSAIDs are very good at providing musculoskeletal analgesia. The combination of providing analgesia and decreasing the inflammation can be quite valuable in septic joints. This makes it possible to obtain better antibiotic penetration into the synovial fluid by decreasing the degree of vascular thrombosis within the synovial membrane and allowing better clearance of the pro-inflammatory mediators and degradative enzymes within the synovial fluid via the lymphatic system. In addition, NSAIDs are often antipyretic, presumably due to mitigation of the effect of endotoxins. The main disadvantage to NSAID use in the systemically compromised foals is their side-effects. These include gingival and gastric ulceration, hypoproteinemia, and renal papillary necrosis. The ulceration side-effects can be decreased by using anti-ulcer medication in combination with the NSAID. Even if NSAIDs are not used in these foals, a case can be made for the administration of anti-ulcer medication due to the pain as well as the stress of being constantly manipulated. Commonly used anti-ulcer medications include H_2-histamine receptor antagonists (ranitidine and cimetidine), proton pump inhibitors (omeprazole), and ulcer-binding protectants (sucralfate).

Joint lavage can also enhance the effectiveness of systemic antibiotic therapy. In essence, it decreases the number of organisms present within the synovial fluid so that the systemic antibiotic has the potential to be more effective against the decreased numbers. In addition, joint lavage allows for the actual removal of debris and inflammatory products from the synovial fluid, decreasing the likelihood of osteoarthritis development secondary to enzymatic degradation. Ideally, 1–2 liters of a balanced buffered polyionic Ringer's solution or physiologic saline is lavaged through any joint suspected of being infected. This type of lavage can be performed aseptically by placing needles into the joint of heavily sedated or anesthetized foals. Two basic techniques can be used to perform an adequate joint lavage. The first is the distension–irrigation technique. One large gauge needle (14–18 gauge) is inserted into the joint and the joint is then alternately infused to distension with the irrigating fluid and then aspirated. The second technique is the through-and-through lavage where two or more large gauge needles (14–18 gauge) are placed as far away from each other as possible in the joint (340). One needle then functions as ingress and the other needle(s) functions as egress. In general, the joint lavage will need to be repeated within 48 hours if there is no significant improvement in the amount of effusion or degree of lameness. The number of lavages that need to be performed is

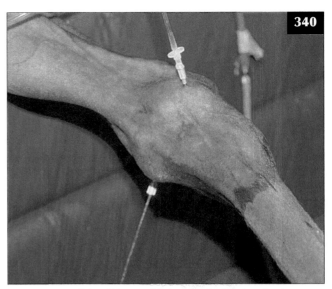

340 Lavage of the tibiotarsal joint in a foal using the ingress–egress technique.

based on the individual case. One study reported that the average number of lavages required was 3.3, with a range of 2–11. To have the most beneficial effect, lavage should be performed within the first 24–48 hours after the initiation of infection, prior to accumulation of fibrin. Once significant inflammation is present, the fibrin and debris become too big or viscous to remove adequately through the needles. At this stage, treatment needs to become more aggressive by combining debridement with lavage via an arthrotomy or arthroscopically.

One of the main reasons for treatment failure in septic joints is the inability to eliminate the causative agent. Once fibrin accumulates within the joint, which can occur as quickly as 48 hours after infection, bacteria will congregate around the fibrin aggregates, making it difficult to adequately decrease the number of organisms until the fibrin is removed. If the foal's joint has been lavaged repeatedly with little to no improvement in clinical signs, then debridement must be performed in order to have a chance of a successful outcome. If the septic joint has not been treated for more than 2 days after the initial identification of the infection, then lavage alone is going to be of limited value. In addition, if the economic value of the foal is high, arthroscopic debridement and lavage can be considered as the first treatment rather than lavage alone. When debridement of the fibrin and debris is required, either arthroscopy or an arthrotomy can be used successfully (341).

An additional approach to consider when treating septic joints is to deliver antibiotics in a greater local concentration. As mentioned earlier, alterations in tissue blood supply, pH, and metabolism can limit the amount and activity of the systemically administered antibiotic in the actual infected tissue. Therefore, delivery of a high concentration of antibiotics directly to the infected site may be critical for the success of therapy. In addition, since most septic joints are infected via hematogenous spread of bacteria, it is important to treat the surrounding vascular system as aggressively as the septic joint. This local delivery of antibiotics is referred to as regional perfusion.

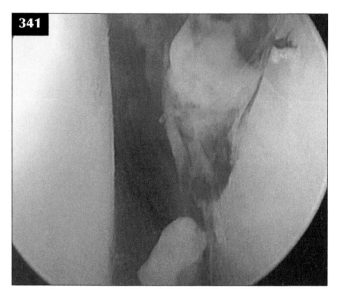

341 Arthroscopic view of fibrin (arrow) in a septic fetlock joint.

Regional perfusion has proven to be a valuable adjunctive therapy in septic orthopedic conditions. Regional perfusion can be broken down into two basic techniques. The first is commonly referred to as distal limb perfusion and is performed by delivering drugs directly into the tissue via the venous system (**342**); the second is referred to as intraosseous perfusion and the drugs are administered via the medullary cavity (**343**). In both techniques the antibiotic is administered under pressure. With distal limb perfusion, a tourniquet is placed proximal to the infected site and the antibiotic is injected directly into a vein, whereas with the intraosseous technique a small hole is drilled through one cortex of the bone proximal to the infected joint and the antibiotic is delivered directly into the medullary cavity. The presumption is that by delivering the antibiotic through a pressurized system, a high concentration of antibiotic will diffuse into the ischemic tissues and exudates. In normal tissues, both techniques have

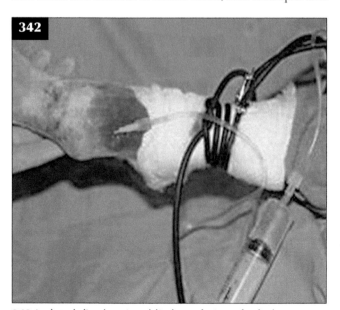

342 Isolated distal regional limb perfusion of a foal. (Courtesy of M. Brown.)

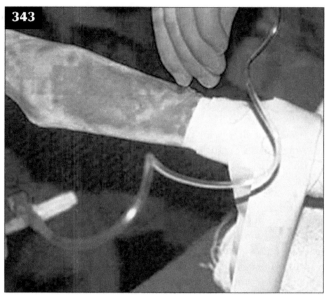

343 Intraosseous perfusion of the third metacarpal bone in a foal. (Courtesy of M. Brown.)

provided 5–50 times the recommended peak serum concentration of the antibiotic needed to produce a therapeutic effect in the synovial fluid. The ideal number of regional perfusions that should be performed to clear up septic arthritis or osteomyelitis is unknown, but repeat administration is often performed within 48 hours, especially if the joint is being lavaged again. For repeat administration, intraosseous perfusion is easier because access to the veins is often disrupted due to edema or localized hemorrhage and thrombophlebitis.

Since most of the bacterial isolates of septic joints and osteomyelitis will be Gram-negative organisms, aminoglycosides such as amikacin and gentamicin are routinely used for regional perfusion. Amikacin is generally used the most because it has demonstrated the greatest efficacy against most equine musculoskeletal disorders, with little development of bacterial resistance. There are reports of 50 mg to 1 g of amikacin or gentamicin in 10, 30, or 60 mL of LRS (dose and volume generally depends on the size of foal and area to be perfused) being administered intravenously or intraosseously. However, anecdotally, soft tissue sloughing has been reported to occur with administration of >1 g of aminoglycosides.

Additional therapies that have been reported to be of some benefit in septic joints include intra-articular (i/a) antibiotic administration and antibiotic impregnated beads, as well as indwelling drains. Initial studies on i/a administration of antibiotics suggested that they can produce a chemical synovitis, but the effect of this synovitis has been shown to be minimal, especially when compared with the deleterious effects of the infection. Intra-articular administration results in significantly higher synovial fluid concentrations than systemic routes. It can be performed whenever the joint is tapped to obtain synovial fluid or immediately after lavage/ surgery. In addition, i/a administration of antibiotics on a daily basis after lavage or surgery can also be beneficial. Antibiotics can be administered either via repeated arthrocentesis or via a continuous joint infusion kit (**344, 345**). For reasons mentioned earlier, aminoglycosides such as amikacin or gentamicin (250–500 mg per joint) are routinely used. For more refractory cases, antibiotics such

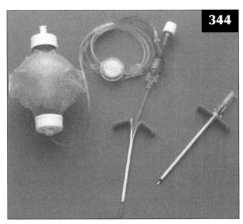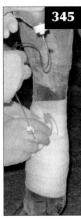

344, 345 Joint Infusion Kit (Mila International, Inc.) (**344**) and its use in a fetlock joint (**345**).

as gentamicin, impregnated in polymethyl methacrylate (PMMA) beads to allow for a more controlled and periodic sustained release, can be temporarily placed in the joint. The biggest disadvantage to the use of PMMA beads in the joint is the need for another surgery to remove them. In addition, indwelling surgical drains or closed suction drains can be placed in the joint to allow for periodic flushing and continuous drainage. In general, systemic antibiotics should be continued for 2 weeks after cessation of clinical signs, unless osteomyelitis is also present; in this case, antibiotics should be continued for 2–3 months since bacteria can survive in the bone and physeal cartilage for a long time. After the infection has been completely eliminated from the joint, hyaluronic acid can be administered either intravenously or intra-articularly to provide lubrication and aid repair of the synovial membrane.

Prognosis

The prognosis for septic joints in the foal has generally been reported to be poor to unfavorable for survival. Between 42% and 84% of foals have been reported to survive to discharge. Early diagnosis and treatment via lavage and debridement have been shown to be the most important components of obtaining a successful outcome, potentially even more so than the choice of antibiotics. Other factors that affect the prognosis include the systemic status of the foal and the number of joints involved, as well as the extent of corresponding bony lesions. If a foal is septic and has septic arthritis and/or osteomyelitis, the prognosis for survival, as well as future athletic performance, is significantly less than for those septic foals lacking joint and/or bone infections. The survival and long-term prognosis for athletic function is also less for those foals that have multiple joints affected, but it does not matter which particular joints are affected. The presence of osteomyelitis can complicate the determination of prognosis, especially if extensive debridement of the physis has been performed, since this can lead to early closure of the physis and a resultant angular limb deformity (ALD).

Overall, the prognosis for survival and successful athletic performance in foals with septic joints and/or osteomyelitis is guarded, but the best chance for success results if they are treated early and aggressively using any combination of the methods described above.

HYPEREXTENSION

Key points

- Hyperextension of one or multiple joints is due to laxity of flexor tendons often as a result of dysmaturity, prematurity, or lack of use.
- Fetlock joints are most often affected, followed by the carpal and coffin joints.
- Other bony abnormalities are rarely identified on radiographs.
- Most foals are only mildly to moderately affected and will spontaneously correct within the first few days of life as they start to move around and "strengthen" their musculotendinous units.
- If the laxity does not improve over the first few days of life, corrective trimming and shoeing of the foot should be considered.
- The heels should be lowered initially in an attempt to allow the foot to completely contact the ground, followed by heel extensions (shoes or tongue depressors).
- Bandages and splints should be avoided, if possible, because they will likely worsen the laxity.
- In foals with severe hyperextension and sloughed skin with exposed tissues, euthanasia should be considered.
- Foals with long-standing systemic illness that develop laxity from general non-use of the limbs will generally correct spontaneously as they gain the ability to ambulate normally.

Definition/overview

Laxity of the flexor tendons causes the foal to have a general lack of muscle tone and hyperextend at one or multiple joints (**346**).

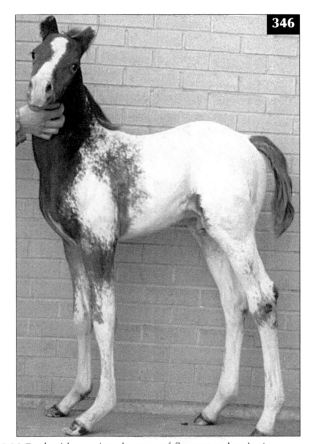

346 Foal with varying degrees of flexor tendon laxity.

Etiology/pathophysiology

Laxity in foals often presents as weakness of the flexor tendons due to dysmaturity or prematurity, causing the foal to have a general lack of muscle tone. It may be partly due to insufficient cross-linking of collagen fibrils in the flexor tendons. However, it is also common for term foals to present with laxity immediately after parturition. With flexor tendon laxity, muscular abnormalities have not been identified with either electromyography or histology. It is important to note that foals with long-standing systemic illness can develop laxity from general nonuse of the limbs.

Clinical presentation

The fetlock joint is usually affected the most, with evidence of weakness in both forelimbs, both hindlimbs, or all four limbs. Affected foals generally rock back onto the caudal portion of the hoof wall and heel bulbs such that the pastern will hyperextend, the fetlock drop, and the toe flip up into the air (**347, 348**). Abnormalities can also be present at the carpus as well as in the coffin joint (**349, 350**). Weight-bearing

radiographs can be taken to demonstrate the abnormal bony alignment, but other bony abnormalities are rarely identified.

Differential diagnosis

Radiographs are not imperative unless the foal was born normal and then developed hyperextension. In these foals the foot should be radiographed to rule out an avulsion fracture of the deep digital flexor tendon from its insertion on the third phalanx. It is also important to examine the foal's neurologic status to make sure that there are no underlying central or peripheral nervous system defects that might lead to decreased tendon reflexes and weakness.

Management

Most foals are only mild to moderately affected and will spontaneously correct within the first few days of life as they start to move around and "strengthen" their musculotendinous units. Therefore, generally nothing needs to be done to these foals unless they do not improve or get worse. If the laxity does not improve over the first few days of life, corrective trimming and shoeing of the foot should be considered. Initially, the heels should be lowered in an attempt to allow the foot to completely contact the ground. This also requires that the bedding is kept shallow so that the foot has the capability of contacting the surface of the ground. If lowering of the heels is not successful, then heel extension shoes should be placed on the foot so that the weight-bearing surface is extended caudally, thus providing more support for the fetlocks (**351–353**). This can be accomplished with commercially available shoes or with tongue depressors glued to the bottom of the foot. Most foals will demonstrate some degree of soft tissue trauma to their heel bulb region (**354**); this can be protected by applying an adherent bandage loosely around the phalanges. Thicker bandages and splints should be avoided, if possible, because they will likely worsen the laxity. When normal foals are placed in splints or casts they will generally develop laxity within 5–10 days, with younger foals developing worse deformities. Euthanasia should be considered for foals with severe hyperextension and sloughed skin with exposed tissues. Foals with long-standing systemic illness that develop laxity from general non-use of the limbs will generally correct spontaneously as their systemic status improves and they gain the ability to ambulate normally.

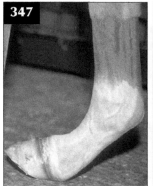 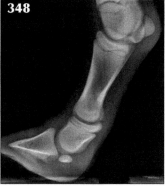

347, 348 Photograph (**347**) and radiograph (**348**) of a foal with flexor tendon laxity demonstrating hyperextension of the fetlock, pastern, and coffin joints such that the fetlock drops and the toe flips up in the air.

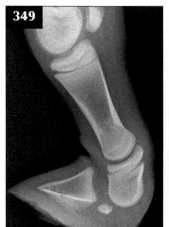 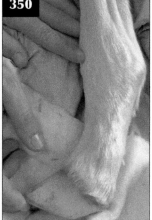

349, 350 Radiograph (**349**) and photograph (**350**) of laxity centered around the coffin joint such that the joint can be hyperextended independent of the pastern and fetlock joints.

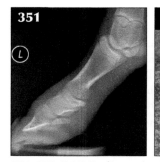 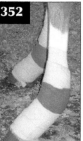 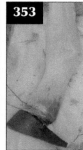

351–353 (**351**) Radiograph of a foal with flexor tendon laxity. (**352, 353**) Application of a glue-on heel extension shoe to prevent the toe from flipping in the air and decrease the degree of hyperextension at the fetlock.

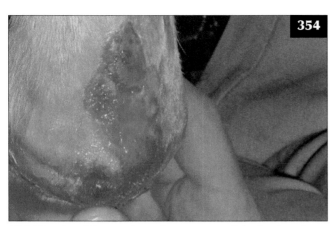

354 Skin sloughing on the palmar aspect of the heel and pastern region. This is typical for a foal with hyperextension of the limb distal to the fetlock.

CONTRACTURAL DEFORMITIES

KEY POINTS
- Contractural deformities are often referred to as contracted tendons and are described with reference to the joint that cannot be straightened.
- Generally present at birth (bilateral or unilateral), but can be acquired within 1 year of age because any source of pain in the limb (e.g., physitis) can lead to flexural deformities.
- The carpus, fetlock, pastern, coffin joint, and tarsus can all be affected, with multiple joints occasionally affected at the same time.
- When manual straightening of the limb around the affected joint is attempted, it is often unsuccessful.
- Palpation of the flexor tendons when the limb is extended can identify which tendons are affected by determining which tendons become taught.
- Radiographs of the affected joints are usually normal.
- Congenital anomalies and syndromes must be ruled out, since many can be combined with contractural deformities.
- Generally, if the neonate is able to stand on the affected limb, the foal will spontaneously improve over 4–5 days for carpal, fetlock, and coffin joint deformities.
- If the deformity is mild to moderate and where the limb is manually reducible, a combination of splinting and medical therapy is often successful.
- In general, cast material is better for the more severe deformities, as it allows for better molding of the splint to the limb.
- Medical therapy often consists of oxytetracycline (calcium channel blocker that allows the musculotendinous unit to become more lax) administration at a dose of 2 to 3 g (~40–70 mg/kg i/v in 500 mL saline) regardless of body weight.
- Oxytetracycline appears to have a transient effect clinically, therefore some foals require second or third doses 24 hours apart.
- If splinting and medical therapy does not significantly improve affected foals after 2–4 days, either surgery or euthanasia should be considered.

DEFINITION/OVERVIEW
Contractural deformities are often referred to as contracted tendons, even though there is no evidence that the tendons are shorter, or contracted, with respect to the bone. These deformities are generally described with reference to the joint that is affected (i.e., the joint that cannot be straightened). The severity is often assessed in terms of degrees of deformity from normal. For example, if the entire forelimb is considered a straight line, then a 30-degree deformity of the carpus would describe the angle of the limb distal to the carpus in a caudal direction (**355**).

ETIOLOGY/PATHOPHYSIOLOGY
Contractural deformities are a common problem in foals. They are generally present at birth, but can be acquired within 1 year of age. Congenital deformities are usually the result of external environmental factors during gestation, bone or joint malformation, or from other physiologic causes such as intrauterine malpositioning. The relative position of the fetus in the uterus with respect to the body wall and gastrointestinal (GI) tract can prevent the foal from extending its limb or limbs, resulting in a joint that cannot be straightened.

CLINICAL PRESENTATION
Contractural deformities can be either bilateral or unilateral. The carpus, fetlock, pastern, coffin, and tarsal joints can all be affected, with multiple joints occasionally affected at the same time (**355–357**). Contractural deformities are relatively straightforward in terms of diagnosis, since most of the foals have trouble standing immediately after birth. When manual straightening of the limb around the affected joint is attempted, it is often unsuccessful. Palpation of the flexor tendons when the limb is extended can identify which tendons are affected by determining which tendons become taught. Radiographs of the affected joints are usually normal, but changes can occur to the palmar aspect of the third carpal bone and radiocarpal bone. Dorsal subluxation of the proximal phalanx on the middle phalanx at the level of the pastern joint is rare, but it can occur bilaterally or unilaterally in the forelimbs (**358**). The luxation is usually not manually reducible and often has soft tissue calcification or osseous changes present on radiography. It is thought that this deformity is likely due to disruption of the distal sesamoidean ligaments. In addition, flexural deformities of the tarsus are rare because the deformity often causes a dystocia, leading to stillbirth (**359**).

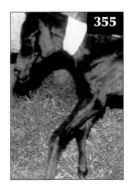
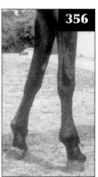
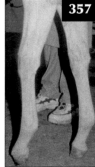

355–357 Carpal (**355**), fetlock (**356**), and coffin (**357**) joint contracture in foals and weanlings.

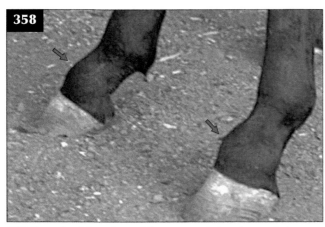

358 Dorsal subluxation of the pastern joints (arrows) due to contracture around the pastern joints in a yearling. (Courtesy of A.S. Turner.)

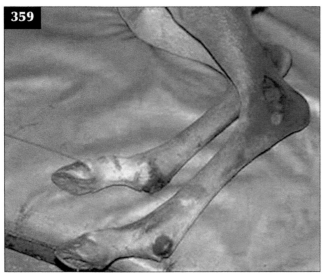

359 Contracture of the hocks preventing full extension of the limbs. (Courtesy of R. Walton.)

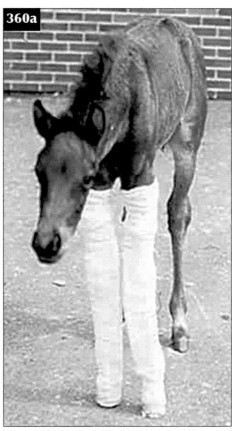

360a Foal with bilateral forelimb splint application such that the foot is not incorporated in the splint. For contracted tendons, the splint is applied on the caudal aspect of the limb, whereas for angular limb deformities the splints are applied on the lateral aspect of the limb. (Courtesy of R. Walton.).

DIFFERENTIAL DIAGNOSIS

Congenital anomalies and syndromes must be ruled out since many can be combined with contractural deformities. In addition, any source of pain in the limb (e.g., physitis) can lead to flexural deformities.

MANAGEMENT

Generally, if the neonate is able to stand on the affected limb, no therapy is required for carpal, fetlock, and coffin joint contractural deformities and the foal will spontaneously improve over 4–5 days. If the deformity is mild to moderate and the limb is manually reducible, a combination of splinting and medical therapy is often successful. A combination of bandages and splints helps apply a consistent pressure to the tendons so that the limb stays in a straightened position. This will help the musculotendinous unit to become more lax (**360a**). This relaxation presumably occurs due to a reflex inhibition of the respective muscles. Either polyvinyl chloride (PVC) pipe or fiberglass cast material can be used successfully to create a splint. In general, cast material is better for the more severe deformities, as it allows for better molding of the splint to the limb. Care must be taken with any splint with regards to protecting the underlying soft tissues. The splints generally need to be replaced every day or every other day.

Medical therapy consists of symptomatic and supportive care via analgesia and controlled exercise, as well as pharmaceutical intervention with oxytetracycline. Most foals with contractural deformities require assistance with standing and nursing. Any source of pain in the limb can lead to flexural deformities; therefore, analgesics (e.g., NSAIDs) may be required to eliminate the source of the pain. Oxytetracycline is a calcium channel blocker that allows the musculotendinous unit to become more lax, as demonstrated with marked alterations in the fetlock and coffin joint angles of mild to moderately contracted deformities, as well as in clinically normal foals. The most commonly reported dose of oxytetracycline for flexural deformities is 3 g (~60–70 mg/kg i/v in 500 mL saline) regardless of body weight, which is much higher than the antimicrobial dose (5–20 mg/kg). However, 2g (~40–50mg/kg i/v) has proven to have similar effects in neonates. (*Note:* Foals that are candidates for treatment should have a complete hematologic examination performed prior to administration, since acute renal failure can occur secondary to nephrotoxicosis, especially with pre-existing renal insufficiency; however, the 3 g dose has been shown to be safe in foals with normal renal function.) Oxytetracycline appears to have a transient effect clinically as well as *in vitro*. Therefore, some foals require second or third doses 24 hours apart. This tends to occur mostly with carpal deformities and in deformities involving both the superficial and the deep digital flexor tendons. The only adverse effect noticed in foals that received two doses was soft feces 24 hours after the last administration. Overcorrection secondary to oxytetracycline administration has been reported (**360b**), and if it does occur, the foals tend to resolve spontaneously within 5–10 days.

If splinting and medical therapy does not significantly improve affected foals after 2–4 days, either surgery or euthanasia should be considered. For foals with a flexural deformity of just the coffin joint, an inferior check ligament desmotomy may be performed with a reasonable chance for success. However, in more moderate cases involving the fetlock, both the inferior and superior check ligaments often need to be transected; in the most severe cases,

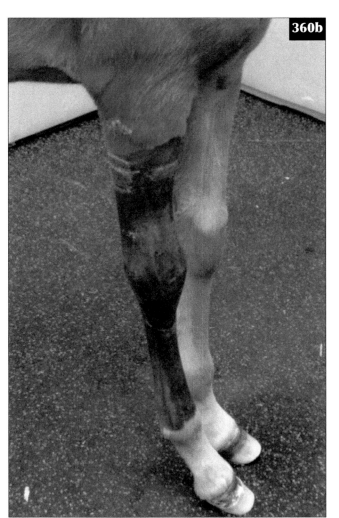

360b Laxity at the level of the right carpus following prolonged bandaging and splinting.

a suspensory ligament desmotomy must also be performed. For severe carpal deformities the palmar carpal structures may need to be transected. In general, if surgery is performed, the foals are being salvaged for breeding or light riding. However, when the suspensory and both check ligaments are transected, the prognosis for an athlete is poor. The treatment for dorsal subluxation of the proximal phalanx on the middle phalanx at the level of the pastern joint is surgical realignment and arthrodesis of the pastern joint. The prognosis for soundness is fair, but better if the condition is unilateral.

COMMON DIGITAL EXTENSOR RUPTURE

KEY POINTS
- Common digital extensor rupture is tearing of the common digital extensor tendon in its sheath on the dorsal surface of the carpus.
- Affected foals have a relatively large, nonpainful effusion of the common digital extensor tendon sheath on the dorsal lateral aspect of the carpus.
- Some foals will have a buckled appearance to the carpus when standing that needs to be distinguished from contracture of the flexor tendons.
- In general, most foals do not have a gait abnormality until they move quickly and the fetlock buckles.
- There is no need for surgical intervention to repair the torn extensor tendon in foals because the ends will re-appose naturally over about 6 months and with minimal swelling.
- Bandages and splints may be required for foals that continually buckle forward at the fetlock; however, external coaptation is generally only required if flexor tendon contracture is present.

DEFINITION/OVERVIEW
Common digital extensor rupture is tearing of the common digital extensor tendon in its sheath on the dorsal surface of the carpus. This may cause the foal to buckle forward at its carpus.

ETIOLOGY/PATHOPHYSIOLOGY
Rupture of the common digital extensor tendon is a common problem that has been related to flexor tendon contraction. It can also occur independently of flexor tendon contracture. The cause is unknown, but it has been postulated that the contraction of the flexor tendons places too much tension on the extensor tendon so that it eventually ruptures in its sheath.

CLINICAL PRESENTATION
Affected foals have a relatively large, nonpainful effusion of the common digital extensor tendon sheath on the dorsal lateral aspect of the carpus (**361**). The ruptured ends of the common digital extensor tendon can often be palpated within the sheath. The clinical picture varies depending on what other problems exist in the foal. Some foals will have a buckled appearance to the carpus when standing that needs to be distinguished from contracture of the flexor tendons (**362**). In general, most foals do not have much of a gait abnormality unless they move quickly and the fetlock buckles.

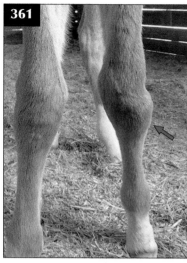 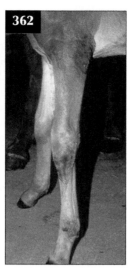

361, 362 Rupture of the common digital extensor tendon. (**361**) Foal demonstrating a swelling in the extensor sheath on the dorsolateral aspect of the carpus (arrow) and (**362**) a foal showing the common degree of buckling that may occur at the level of the carpus.

DIFFERENTIAL DIAGNOSIS

This condition is often present in association with flexor tendon contraction.

MANAGEMENT

There is no need for surgical intervention to repair the torn extensor tendon in foals because the ends will re-appose naturally over about 6 months and with minimal swelling. Bandages and splints may be required for foals that continually buckle forward at the fetlock; however, external coaptation is generally only required if flexor tendon contracture is present.

ANGULAR LIMB DEFORMITIES

KEY POINTS

- ALDs are conformational deviations that are described in the frontal plane based on the relationship of the limb distal to a particular joint.
- ALDs are most often from congenital causes, but they can also result in response to pathology (abnormal weight bearing on support limb or delayed ossification of cuboidal bones).
- Most common ALDs encountered in foals include carpal and/or tarsal valgus as well as fetlock varus.
- Rotation of the limb is often associated and coupled with ALDs. Therefore, when examining a limb for an ALD, it is very important to be directly lined up in front of the limb and not just in front of the foal.
- Picking up and flexing the limb will often help alleviate some of the perceptual problems that can be encountered from rotation of the limb.
- Picking up and manipulating the limb in a medial to lateral direction allows the examiner to determine whether the limb can be manually straightened or not. If the limb can be

manually straightened, it is highly likely that the deformity is centered within the joint. If the limb cannot be straightened, the deformity likely originates at the physeal region.

- Watching the foal walk is often very useful in distinguishing how much of the ALD is a component of ligamentous laxity, since this will tend to show more exaggerated movements around the joint.
- Radiographs are not required unless radical changes have occurred between examinations or it is the first time an older foal (2 months of age) is examined.
- Foals with laxity of the soft tissues, but normal ossification, require a gradual increase in exercise to strengthen the muscles and soft tissues.
- Most foals with delayed ossification require strict stall rest and splinting to prevent the development of osteoarthritis as well as further damage to the cuboidal bones.
- When splinting an ALD, the foot should not be incorporated in the splint. This is to allow strengthening of the periarticular soft tissues while maintaining a correct vertical limb axis and limb loading.
- In general, for physeal origin ALDs, allowing the foal to correct on its own with minimal intervention should be the preferred method of therapy.
- In severe cases of ALD, loading becomes static, bone growth stops, and the angulation tends to get worse and requires surgical intervention.
- To balance the hoof, the outside wall of the foot needs to be trimmed with valgus deformities and the inside wall needs to be trimmed for varus deformities.
- All improvements should be made within the time frame for maximal growth for each particular growth plate (2 months for the metacarpal/metatarsal bones, 4 months for the tibia, and 6 months for the carpus) so that the bone can still respond.

DEFINITION/OVERVIEW

ALDs are defined as conformational deviations in the frontal plane. They are axial deviations based on the relationship of the limb distal to a particular joint. For example, a carpal valgus deformity is defined as a lateral deviation of the limb distal to the carpus when compared with the limb proximal to the carpus (**363a**), and a fetlock varus is a medial deviation of the limb distal to the fetlock joint when compared with the limb proximal to the fetlock.

ETIOLOGY/PATHOPHYSIOLOGY

ALDs in foals are most often from congenital causes such as abnormal uterine positioning (**363b**) and chemical insults while *in utero*, as well as hormonal or nutritional imbalances. However, ALDs in foals can also result as a response to pathology. Foals that must bear an abnormal amount of weight on one limb due to injury of the contralateral limb are more prone to develop an ALD on the support limb. In addition, injuries or inflammation of the physis can result in an asymmetrical early closure of either the medial or lateral aspect of the physis, resulting in an ALD. ALDs can also be a complicating component of prematurity or immaturity in foals. This is usually directly related to bone immaturity and delayed ossification

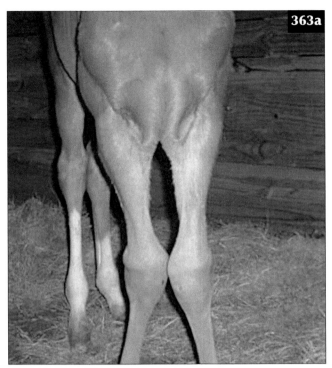

363a Foal with bilateral carpal valgus.

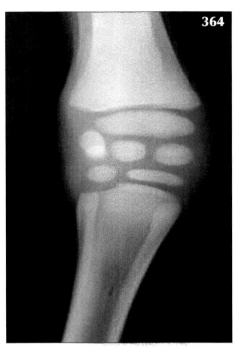

364 Dorsopalmar radiograph of a premature foal demonstrating incomplete ossification of the cuboidal bones of the carpus.

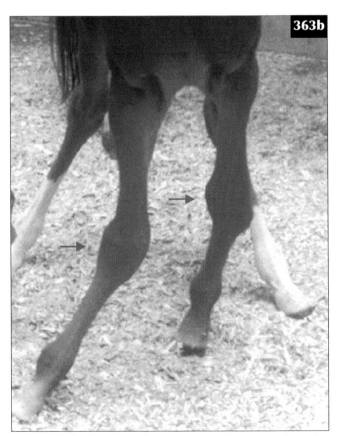

363b Foal that has a windswept ALD at the carpus; the right carpus is valgus, while the left carpus is varus.

of the cuboidal bones (**364**). The cuboidal bones of the carpus and tarsus undergo articular ossification during the last 2–3 weeks of gestation. Therefore, if the foal was born premature or is weak and immature for its age, then some of the cuboidal bones may be incompletely ossified and will effectively be crushed when the foal bears weight across these bones, thus causing an ALD.

CLINICAL PRESENTATION

The most common ALDs encountered in neonatal foals include carpal and/or tarsal valgus as well as fetlock varus. In general, examination of the foal for ALDs should start as close to birth as possible, then every week until 1 month of age, as this is a critical time in which many changes can occur in response to growth and exercise demands. Examinations should then be continued on a monthly basis until 6 months of age. A complete examination entails examination of the limb of interest in a standing as well as in a flexed position, followed by exercise and radiography. (*Note:* When examining foals for ALDs, correct conformation for the foal is not the same as correct conformation for the adult.)

When examining the limb standing, rotation of the limb can make interpretation of the degree of ALD more difficult, especially distal to the fetlock. Rotation of the limb or torsion around the weight-bearing axis of the limb is often associated and coupled with ALDs. Therefore, when examining a limb for an ALD, it is very important to be directly lined up in front of the limb and not just in front of the foal (**365**). Being directly lined up in front of the limb will give a more accurate assessment of the ALD, especially when there is also a rotational component to the limb. For example, for the novice clinician who stands directly in front of the foal, but not in front of the limb, the limb often looks like it has a fetlock valgus. However, when the examiner looks directly in front

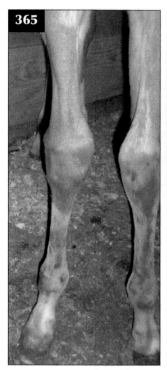
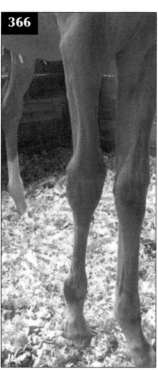

365, 366 Views from directly in front of (**365**) and directly in front of the right forelimb (**366**) of the same foal. When external rotation is present, as is the case on the right forelimb of this foal, it is important for the examiner to line up in front of the limb instead of the foal because otherwise a slight fetlock varus (**366**) can be mistaken as a slight fetlock valgus (**365**).

of the limb, it is often noticed that the fetlock is actually straight or varus with an external rotation of the limb (toed out) (**366**). This usually happens because the rotation originates high up in the limb, rotating the entire limb, thus making it pertinent to line up straight with the limb. Most foals have some degree of external (toed out) rotation that will generally improve with age as the chest broadens and pushes the elbow outward.

Picking up and flexing the limb will often help alleviate some of the perceptual problems that can be encountered from rotation of the limb. Flexion of the limb around the joint of interest allows the examiner to compare the relative position of the distal limb to the proximal limb by putting them in closer proximity to each other. In addition, it helps to distinguish some of the more complicated cases in which there are ALDs involving both the carpus and fetlock. Picking up and manipulating the limb in a medial to lateral direction also allows the examiner to determine whether the limb can be manually straightened or not. If the limb can be manually straightened, it is highly likely that the deformity is centered within the joint and results from delayed ossification of the cuboidal bones or laxity of the periarticular soft tissues. If the limb cannot be straightened, the deformity likely originates at the physeal region. Watching the foal walk is often very useful in distinguishing how much of the ALD is a component of ligamentous laxity. Ligamentous laxity will tend to show more exaggerated

movements around the joints of interest, making the ALD more pronounced. In these foals it is important to note the age and exercise level of the foal in order to know what is the best treatment for correcting the laxity; this way a better evaluation of the ALD can be made. For example, neonates are often very lax and require more exercise, whereas older foals that have exercised rigorously need to be stall confined for a few hours for the laxity to improve.

If foals are examined on a regular basis, radiographs are not necessarily required unless radical changes have occurred between examinations. However, if it is the first time the foal is examined for an ALD, especially in older foals, radiographs are very useful for determining the cause. Only dorsopalmar and lateral radiographic views are required unless there is evidence of problems within the joint, then oblique views should be added. The radiographs should be centered over the joint of interest and include the mid-diaphysis of the proximal and distal long bones. These views allow identification of the "pivot point" of the ALD by drawing lines down the middle of the long bones on the dorsopalmar view.

Where the lines bisect is where the deformity originates (**367**). Radiographs are also useful in identifying any congenital abnormalities, such as more distinct ulnas or fibulas or abnormal shapes to or fractures of the cuboidal bones, as well as infection of the physis.

DIFFERENTIAL DIAGNOSIS
Physitis, contralateral limb injury, prematurity/immaturity.

MANAGEMENT
The treatment of foals in which the ALD originates at the joint itself (e.g., as with delayed ossification of the cuboidal bones or laxity of periarticular soft tissues) is very different from the treatment of ALDs that originate from the physeal region. Foals with laxity of the soft tissues, but normal ossification, require a gradual increase in exercise (5–10 minutes daily) to strengthen the muscles and soft tissues. However, foals with delayed ossification require strict stall rest to prevent the development of osteoarthritis as well as further damage to the cuboidal bones. Permanent deformation of the cuboidal bones will occur after 3–4 weeks of angulation. Since the limb can be manually straightened at the level of the joint, these foals can be placed in splints (**360a**). The type of splint used is not all that important, but the placement is (i.e., regardless of whether commercial splints or splints made out of cast material or PVC pipe are used, the foot should not be incorporated in the splint). Splinting allows the foal to strengthen the periarticular soft tissues while maintaining a correct vertical limb axis and limb loading. The goal of the splint is to maintain the limb in the correct vertical limb axis so that normal ossification can proceed concentrically around the cartilaginous cuboidal bone. Radiographs should be taken every 10–14 days to determine the progress of the ossification.

It is important for the practitioner to know what treatment options are available for physeal origin ALDs and to understand how to determine when and if treatment needs to be performed. In general, allowing the foal to correct on its own with minimal intervention should be the preferred method of therapy. Trimming of the hoof is another way to attempt to balance the compressive forces across the physis so that the loads remain in

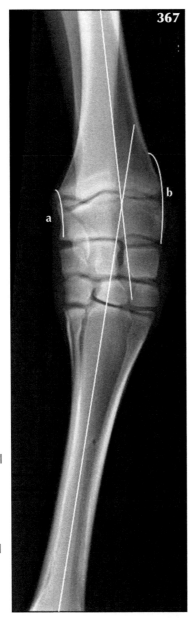

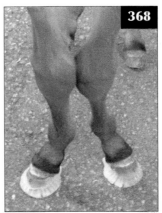 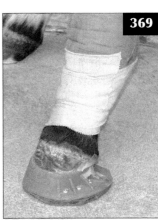

368, 369 Application of medial (**368**) and lateral (**369**) hoof extension shoes for fetlock valgus (**368**) and fetlock varus (**369**) deformities.

367 Dorsopalmar radiograph of a foal with a valgus ALD. Bisecting lines are placed on the distal radius and proximal third metacarpus. Where those lines overlap (distal radial physis) is a rough estimate of where the ALD originates. The lateral aspect of the physeal region (**a**) is the concave surface, and the medial physeal region (**b**) is the convex surface.

physiologic limits and changes can occur naturally. However, in more severe ALDs where the foal is windswept (**363b**), loading has become static, bone growth stops and the angulation tends to get worse. Surgical intervention is usually required in these cases. Hemicircumferential periosteal transection and elevation (HPTE) is performed on the concave surface of the metaphysis in an attempt to reduce the static compression and allow bone growth to start up again, whereas transphyseal bridging is performed on the convex surface in order to create a static compression so that bone growth is retarded on that side (**367**).

General approaches to management of ALDs in foals have been well described and some basic general concepts are worth discussing. If the ALD remains stagnant or becomes worse over a 2–3 week period, a change in the exercise protocol should be considered. For most foals this will require exercise to become more restricted. However, for a few foals an increase in exercise will actually provide appropriate loading to the bone so that the limb will begin straightening. In addition, balancing of the foot at this time may also prove to be effective in balancing the forces across the growth plate. This is especially true for fetlock ALDs, but also works for some carpal ALDs. To balance the hoof, the outside wall of the foot needs to be trimmed with valgus deformities and the inside wall needs to be trimmed for varus deformities. If trimming does not improve the foal within 2 weeks, foot extensions (medial extension for valgus and lateral extension for varus) can be applied to the foot in an attempt to increase the weight-bearing surface of the foot (**368, 369**).

All improvements should be made within the time frame for maximal growth for each particular growth plate so that the bone can still respond. The maximal growth in the distal physes is over after 2 months for the metacarpal/metatarsal bones, after 4 months for the tibia, and after 6 months for the carpus. HPTE should be considered during this time if the conservative management described above is not improving the foal in a timely fashion for the intended use of the horse, or if the philosophy of the farm management dictates it. Transphyseal bridging should be considered for all severe ALDs in foals less than 3 months of age, as well as those not responding at or near the end of the rapid growth phase for each particular physis.

PHYSITIS

KEY POINTS
- Physitis is inflammation of the physeal region (growth plate) of immature bone, causing bone remodeling.
- Inflammation around the physis tends to occur when newly forming bone is not able to withstand the load being placed on it (i.e., normal bone has too great a load being placed on it as a result of exercise, weight, or conformation, or the bone itself is abnormal and cannot withstand normal loads).
- In cases where the cause of the physitis is due to the level of exercise or the amount of weight, the physitis is symmetrical

(i.e., involves medial and lateral aspect of physis), whereas for those that are due to conformation or cartilage retention, the physitis is asymmetrical (i.e., involves only part of the physis, either medial or lateral).

- In general, the physis at the distal metacarpus/metatarsus and proximal physis on the proximal phalanx are most often affected in foals, since they have the most active growth for the first 3 months of life.
- Most of the time, physitis is not much of a clinical problem until most of the physes start to close around 4–8 months of age.
- Clinical signs are variable, but usually include a stiff gait with a shortened cranial phase to the stride, increased time lying down, trembling when standing, or buckling forward at the carpus or fetlock.
- Pain can usually be elicited when pressure is applied across the growth plate of interest.
- Radiographs usually indicate a combination of lysis, directly in the physis, and sclerosis surrounding the physis.
- Treatment of physitis in foals needs to incorporate treatment of the symptoms (i.e., pain), but also needs to treat the source (i.e., if an ALD is present, this should be treated appropriately, or if the foal is getting too much exercise, this should be reduced, but not eliminated).

DEFINITION/OVERVIEW

Physitis is inflammation of the physeal region (growth plate) of immature bone, causing bone remodeling.

ETIOLOGY/PATHOPHYSIOLOGY

The metaphysis provides much of the longitudinal growth in the foal and is therefore more prone to inflammation from repetitive loading than the epiphysis. In young foals, inflammation around the physis tends to occur when this newly forming bone is not able to withstand the load being placed on it. This is usually because either the normally growing bone has too great a load being placed on it as a result of exercise, weight, or conformation, or because the bone itself is abnormal and cannot withstand normal loads. In cases where the cause of the physitis is due to the level of exercise or the amount of weight, the physitis is symmetrical (i.e., involves medial and lateral aspect of physis), whereas for those that are due to conformation or cartilage retention, the physitis is asymmetrical (i.e., involves only part of the physis, either medial or lateral). In addition, one of the most common examples and reasons young foals develop physitis is because of a lack of exercise due to disease. If a foal spends the first few weeks of its life recumbent, the bone needs to adapt to the loads placed on it when the foal is standing. If the exercise level increases dramatically in this time frame, adaptation of the bone will not occur quickly enough, resulting in some degree of clinical physitis. Therefore, careful control of exercise is important in these particular foals.

CLINICAL PRESENTATION

In general, the physis at the distal metacarpus/metatarsus and proximal physis on the proximal phalanx are most often affected in foals, since they have the most active growth for the first 3 months of life. However, most of the time physitis is not much of a clinical

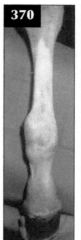
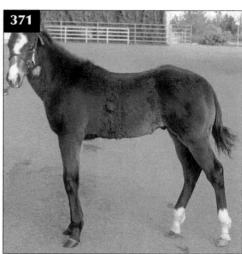

370, 371 Typical appearance of foals with physitis of the distal metacarpal/metatarsal physis. The physis is often enlarged (**370**) and sensitive to palpation and the foal will often stand with the fetlocks buckled forward (**371**).

problem until most of the physes start to close around 4–8 months of age. The clinical signs in young foals are variable, but usually include an enlarged physis, a stiff gait with a shortened cranial phase to the stride, increased amount of time lying down, and trembling when standing, potentially buckling forward at the carpus or fetlock (**370, 371**). These clinical signs are directly related to pain at the physis and can therefore result in a progressive increase in muscle tension that can lead to contraction of the flexor tendons. Pain can usually be elicited when pressure is applied across the growth plate of interest. Radiographs usually indicate a combination of lysis, directly in the physis, and sclerosis surrounding the physis (**372**).

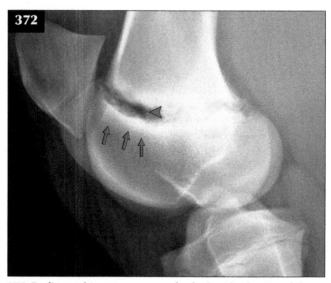

372 Radiographic appearance of a foal with physitis of the distal femur demonstrating the combination of lysis (arrowhead) and sclerosis (small arrows).

DIFFERENTIAL DIAGNOSIS
Contracted tendons, ALDs.

MANAGEMENT
Treatment of physitis in young foals needs to incorporate treatment of the symptoms (e.g., pain), but also needs to treat the source (i.e., if an ALD is present, this should be treated appropriately, or if the foal is getting too much exercise, this should be reduced but not eliminated). NSAIDs can be administered in low doses every other day to help with the inflammatory pain. Care must be taken to protect the GI tract during this treatment period.

FRACTURES

KEY POINTS
- A fracture is a break in a bone that results in the foal being unable to bear weight on the injured limb.
- Most commonly, a fracture is a direct result of trauma such as being stepped on or kicked by the mare or overzealous assistance during parturition.
- The weakest area in a long bone is generally the physis, since it has a cartilaginous portion that extends across the bone.
- Each fracture, whether it is physeal or mid-diaphyseal, should be assessed based on the clinical signs, the severity of injury, the degree of contamination, and the economic value of the foal.
- Depending on the assessment, the initial management can include internal fixation, external coaptation, stall confinement, or euthanasia.
- Repair of physeal fractures often results in premature closure of the physis, which can result in an ALD.
- In general, uncomplicated fractures of the mid-diaphysis of foals can be easily reduced and internally fixated, allowing for satisfactory healing.

DEFINITION/OVERVIEW
A fracture is a break in a bone that results in the foal being unable to bear weight on the injured limb (373). Fractures are classified according to their character and location.

ETIOLOGY/PATHOPHYSIOLOGY
Most commonly, a fracture is a direct result of trauma such as being stepped on or kicked by the mare or overzealous assistance during parturition. In young foals the tendinous structures tend to be stronger than the bone. Therefore, the bone tends to fracture before injury occurs to the tendon or tendon–bone interface. The weakest area in a long bone is generally the physis, since it has a cartilaginous portion that extends across the bone. The physes most often fractured in foals are the pressure physes or those that contribute to longitudinal growth and are subjected to compressive forces, as opposed to traction physes that are associated with muscle attachments.

CLINICAL PRESENTATION
Foals are typically nonweight bearing on the fractured limb. Soft-tissue swelling around the fracture site is usually easy to identify and the foal will resent palpation/manipulation of the area. It is prudent to see if there is any break in the skin as foal skin is relatively

thin, making it relatively easy for fractures to poke through, contaminating the site. In general, fractures in foals are more simple (transverse or oblique) than adults, but comminution can occur (374). The types of fractures that occur at the growth plate have been well described and are based on the relationship of the fracture to the physis itself as well as to the epiphysis and metaphysis (375).

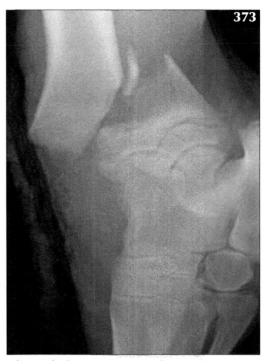

373 Radiograph demonstrating a Salter–Harris type II fracture of the distal tibia in a weanling.

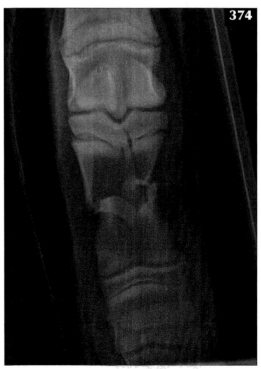

374 Comminuted fracture P1.

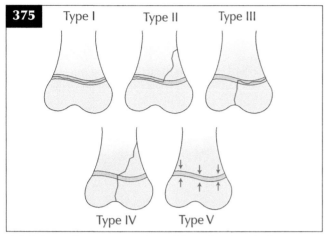

375 Schematic representation of the Salter–Harris fracture classification. Type I fractures extend through the physis only. Type II fractures extend through the physis and up into the metaphysis. Type III fractures extend through the physis and the epiphysis. Type IV fractures extend through the epiphysis, physis, and metaphysis. Type V fractures are compression fractures of the physis.

It has been reported that 27% of physeal fractures in foals are in animals ≤1 month of age. The most common fracture type to occur in young foals is the Salter–Harris type II fracture, where the fracture goes through the physeal cartilage as well as part of the metaphysis (**373, 375**), followed by the Salter–Harris type I fracture, where the fracture only goes through the physeal cartilage (**375**). Each fracture, whether it is physeal or mid-diaphyseal due to trauma from the mare standing on the foal, should be assessed based on the clinical signs, the severity of injury, the degree of contamination, and the economic value of the foal.

DIFFERENTIAL DIAGNOSIS
Ligamentous injury, neuromuscular injury.

MANAGEMENT
Depending on the assessment, the initial management can include internal fixation, external coaptation, stall confinement, or euthanasia. The prognosis for a straight, functional, pain-free limb is better with a lower Salter–Harris classification (e.g., a type I fracture has better prognosis than a type V fracture). However, even though 54% of physeal fractures have been shown to heal, only 25% have resulted in a sound horse. Repair of physeal fractures often results in premature closure of the physis, which can result in an ALD, but obtaining healing overshadows this potential growth retardation. In general, uncomplicated fractures of the mid-diaphysis of foals can be easily reduced and internally fixated, allowing for satisfactory healing (**376, 377**). Foals with comminuted fractures (**374**) usually heal better than adults with the same fractures due to their size, their rapid healing capacity, and the fact that they lay down for a large portion of the day. However, they are still prone to many complications (ALD on opposite limb, cast sores, infection, implant loosening, laxity due to prolonged cast application) that need to be considered prior to surgery.

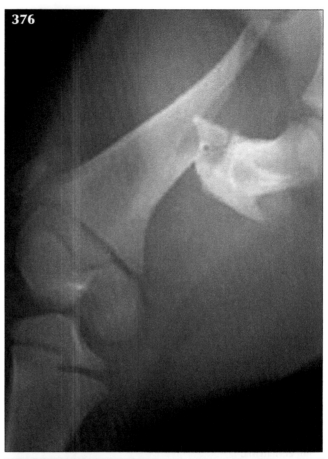

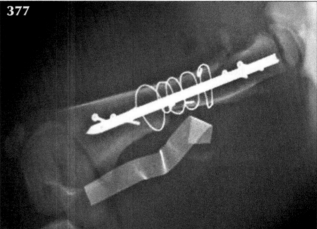

376, 377 Radiographs of a long oblique fracture of the proximal femur (**376**) and repair using an interlocking intermedullary pin (**377**) in a miniature foal.

DEVELOPMENTAL ORTHOPEDIC DISEASES

KEY POINTS
- Developmental orthopedic diseases (DODs) are abnormalities in the normal developmental process at the subchondral bone and cartilage interface.
- Osteochondrosis (OC) is a DOD that is caused by failure of normal endochondral ossification resulting in a persistence

of thickened hypertrophied cartilage. Subsequent physical stresses can give rise to fissures leading to dissecting osteochondral fragments called osteochondritis dissecans (OCD).

- Subchondral bone cysts are cystic lesions in the epiphysis with an overlying cartilage defect on the articular surface.
- The etiology of DOD is unknown, but is likely multifactorial. Suspected causes include rapid growth, dietary mismanagement, genetic predisposition, endocrine factors, and trauma.
- Clinical signs of DOD are most commonly seen between 4 months and 2 years of age.
- Joint effusion is usually present and the degree of lameness is often low grade (<2/5 on the American Association of Equine Practitioners [AAEP] grading scale).
- Diagnosis is often based on a physical and lameness examination combined with radiography, since most DOD lesions are in site-specific locations.
- In general, surgical management is recommended for foals destined for demanding athletic careers, since inflammation and effusion will perpetuate a lameness.

DEFINITION/OVERVIEW

DODs are abnormalities in the normal developmental process at the subchondral bone and cartilage interface. OC is a DOD that is caused by failure of normal endochondral ossification resulting in a persistence of thickened hypertrophied cartilage. Subsequent physical stresses can give rise to fissures leading to dissecting osteochondral fragments called osteochondrosis dissecans (syn: OCD, marginal OC, peripheral dissecting lesions) (**378**). Subchondral

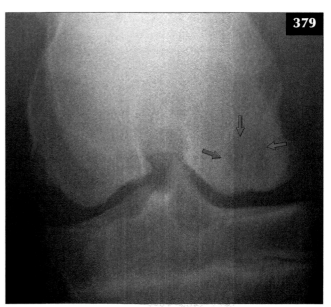

379 Plantar–dorsal radiograph of the stifle of a yearling demonstrating the presence of a large subchondral bone cyst on the distal aspect of the medial femoral condyle (arrows).

bone cysts (syn: osseous cyst-like lesions, non-marginal OC, central cystic lesions) are cystic lesions in the epiphysis with an overlying cartilage defect on the articular surface (**376, 379**).

ETIOLOGY/PATHOPHYSIOLOGY

The etiology of DOD is unknown, but is likely multifactorial. Suspected causes include rapid growth, dietary mismanagement, genetic predisposition, endocrine factors, and trauma. Large-framed foals anecdotally appear to be more at risk; however, this has been disputed by controlled nutritional studies. Excess digestible energy alone or in combination with calcium/phosphorus or trace mineral (zinc excess or copper deficiencies) imbalances may be one of the leading causes. There may also be a genetic predisposition. Hormonal imbalances have been examined as well as high glucose and insulin levels after feeding (insulin promotes chondrocyte survival). Trauma also appears to play a role in DODs, as there is apparent site vulnerability.

The pathogenesis of DOD is also not completely understood. OC is the failure of endochondral ossification due to disruption in normal differentiation of chondrocytes. Resting cells proliferate, but instead of forming organized columns the cells are randomly arranged and fail to mature and form matrix vesicles. Capillary buds do not penetrate into these disorganized columns of cartilage and the cartilage matrix fails to ossify. Cartilage resorption ceases, as does cartilage conversion into bone. The net result is necrosis in the basal layers due to lack of nutrition. This leaves an area of thickened hypertrophied cartilage that does not turn into bone. Subsequent physical stresses can give rise to fissures in this thickened cartilage, possibly leading to dissecting osteochondral (cartilage and bone) fragments called OCD. The pathogenesis of subchondral bone cysts is even less well understood. There is some thought that they may be caused by OC combined with abnormal stresses applied across a joint, leading to greater necrosis of the

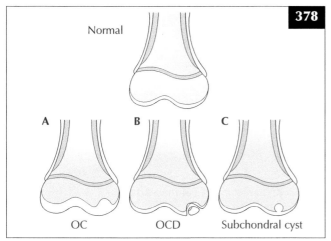

378 Schematic representation of the differences between normal endochondral ossification and the developmental orthopedic diseases. The black regions represent bone and the white regions represent cartilage. (**a**) In osteochondrosis there is failure of normal endochondral ossification such that there is a retained area of cartilage that is thicker than the rest and does not turn into bone. (**b**) In osteochondritis dissecans, stresses placed across the thicker region of cartilage cause osteochondral fragmentation. (**c**) In subchondral bone cysts, stresses placed across the joint lead to necrosis of the subchondral bone leading to development of a cyst.

subchondral bone, and are thus a form of DOD. However, there is also plenty of evidence that supports the formation of subchondral bone cysts in normal joints following articular trauma.

CLINICAL PRESENTATION

Clinical signs of DOD are most commonly seen between 4 months and 2 years of age. Joint effusion is usually present, especially in the tibiotarsal, femoropatellar, and fetlock joints, but the degree of effusion is quite variable. The degree of lameness is often variable as well, with most being low grade (<2/5 on the AAEP grading scale).

DIFFERENTIAL DIAGNOSIS

Joint inflammation or sepsis.

DIAGNOSIS

Diagnosis is often based on a physical and lameness examination combined with radiography (**380**). Most DOD lesions are in site-specific locations (*Table 70*).

MANAGEMENT

Most DOD lesions in foals are treated either surgically or medically. In general, surgical management is recommended for foals destined for demanding athletic careers, since the inflammation and effusion will always perpetuate a lameness. Surgical therapy usually consists of arthroscopic debridement and lavage of the joint. In rare cases in which the fragments are large, an arthrotomy

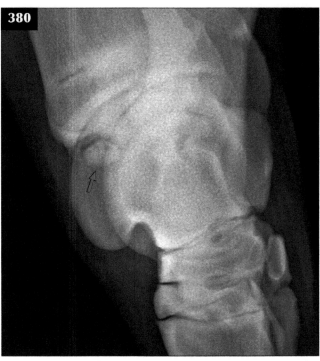

380 Radiograph of the tarsus of a yearling demonstrating the presence of an osteochondritis dissecans lesion on the distal intermediate ridge of the tibia (arrow).

Table 70. Common sites of occurrence of osteochondrosis in the horse

Joint	Osteochondrosis dissecans	Subchondral cystic lesions
Femoropatellar	*Lateral trochlear ridge* Medial trochlear ridge Patella	*Medial femoral condyle* Lateral femoral condyle Proximal tibia Patella
Tibiotarsal	*Distal intermediate ridge of the tibia* *Lateral trochlear ridge of the talus* Medial and lateral malleoli of the tibia Medial trochlear ridge of the talus	
Shoulder	Glenoid *Humeral head*	Glenoid
Fetlock	Dorsal sagittal ridge	Distal III metacarpus or metatarsus Proximal first phalanx
Carpus	Distal radius	Distal radius Carpal bones
Pastern		Distal first phalanx Proximal second phalanx
Coxofemoral	Femoral head	Acetabulum
Distal interphalangeal		Third phalanx Navicular bone
Cervical spine	Articular facets	

Note: Sites in italics are the most common sites for occurrence within each joint.

may still be performed. Medical treatment consists of one or any combination of the following: rest, controlled exercise, NSAIDs, joint injections (e.g., steroids, hyaluronic acid), or nutraceuticals.

GASTROCNEMIUS RUPTURE

KEY POINTS
- Gastrocnemius rupture is a tearing of either the gastrocnemius muscle or the tendon of the gastrocnemius muscle, resulting in an inability for the foal to stand on the injured limb.
- Rupture of the gastrocnemius muscle has been observed in foals during parturition, especially in assisted deliveries when the stifle is forced into extension during delivery while the hock is flexed.
- Diagnosis of a ruptured gastrocnemius muscle can be confirmed by palpation of the muscle and flexion of the hock when the stifle is extended.
- Ultrasonography usually demonstrates a large amount of hemorrhage within the muscle belly of the gastrocnemius. The gastrocnemius tendon is usually unaffected in neonates.
- Most cases are unilateral, but the occasional bilateral rupture occurs.
- Management of gastrocnemius ruptures includes complete stall rest and external coaptation.
- Some foals can get abscessation of the hematoma, presumably from hematogenous bacteria.

DEFINITION/OVERVIEW
Gastrocnemius rupture is a tearing of either the gastrocnemius muscle or the tendon of the gastrocnemius muscle, resulting in an inability for the foal to stand on the injured limb.

ETIOLOGY/PATHOPHYSIOLOGY
Rupture of the gastrocnemius muscle at the level of its fossa in the femur has been observed in foals during parturition, especially in assisted deliveries. Rupture may occur if the stifle is forced into extension during delivery while the hock is flexed.

CLINICAL PRESENTATION
The gastrocnemius, in combination with the superficial flexor tendon, supports the hock in a standing position and is the main extensor of the hock. Therefore, when the gastrocnemius muscle is ruptured, moderate hyperflexion of the hock occurs (381). Diagnosis of a ruptured gastrocnemius muscle can be confirmed by palpation of the muscle (382) and flexion of the hock when the stifle is extended. Ultrasonography usually demonstrates a large amount of hemorrhage within the muscle belly of the gastrocnemius muscle, along with fluid and edema at its fossa. The gastrocnemius tendon is usually unaffected in cases of gastrocnemius rupture. Most cases are unilateral, but the occasional bilateral rupture occurs.

DIFFERENTIAL DIAGNOSIS
Ruptured peroneus tertius (which may occur alone or in combination with rupture of the gastrocnemius muscle), fractures, septic joints.

MANAGEMENT
Management of gastrocnemius ruptures has included complete stall rest and external coaptation (383, 384, 385).

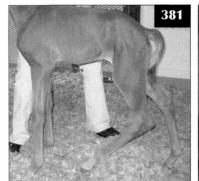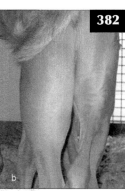

381, 382 A 1-day-old foal with rupture of the gastrocnemius muscle. Note the inability of the foal to stand on and place weight on the left hindlimb (381), as well as the swelling of the gastrocnemius muscle in the left hindlimb (382).

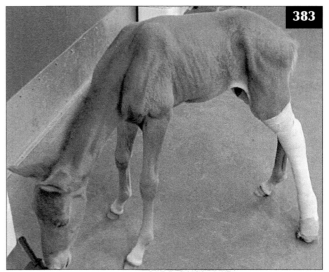

383 The foal in 381, 382 with a full-limb cast applied to the left hindlimb to allow the foal to ambulate.

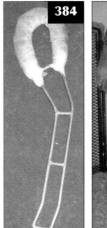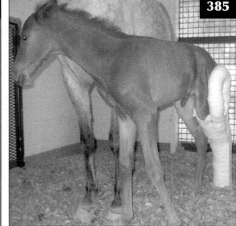

384, 385 The foal in 381, 382 with a modified Thomas–Schroeder splint (384) applied to the left hindlimb (385) to decrease the weight of a cast and allow ambulation.

In general, if the foal can bear weight, then stall rest without any external support is recommended; however, if the hock is severely dropped, a full-limb cast should be applied with the limb in a normal weight-bearing position. Some foals can get abscessation of the hematoma, presumably from hematogenous bacteria. The prognosis is favorable for future athletic soundness.

PATELLA LUXATION

KEY POINTS
- Patella luxation is a displacement of the patella from its normal location, resulting in an abnormal stance and function of the limb.
- Lateral luxation of the patella is most common, with some foals having hypoplasia of the lateral trochlear ridge of the femur, resulting in intermittent lateral luxation.
- Foals stand in a squatting position because the quadriceps act as flexors to the limb when the patella is displaced.
- The foal can be either unilaterally or bilaterally affected.
- Radiographs should be taken to identify whether the foal has hypoplasia of the lateral trochlear ridge of the femur.
- The prognosis for athletic soundness is guarded, but surgery can be attempted to reposition and maintain the position of the patella.

DEFINITION/OVERVIEW
Patella luxation is a displacement of the patella from its normal location, resulting in an abnormal stance and function of the limb.

ETIOLOGY/PATHOPHYSIOLOGY
Lateral luxation of the patella is another potentially heritable, congenital abnormality in foals. Some of these foals can have hypoplasia of the lateral trochlear ridge of the femur, resulting in intermittent lateral luxation.

CLINICAL PRESENTATION
The clinical presentation is of a foal in a squatting position because the quadriceps act as flexors to the limb when the patella is displaced. The foal can be either unilaterally or bilaterally affected, and the degree of squatting position obtained depends on the severity of the luxation. Radiographs should be taken to identify whether the foal has hypoplasia of the lateral trochlear ridge of the femur.

DIFFERENTIAL DIAGNOSIS
Gastrocnemius rupture.

MANAGEMENT
Surgery can be performed to reposition the patella by releasing the soft tissues on the lateral side, including part of the lateral patellar ligament, and/or performing a medial imbrication. In foals that have hypoplastic lateral trochlear ridges, a trochleoplasty may need to be performed to keep the patella in the trochlear grooves. Regardless of the treatment, the prognosis for athletic soundness is guarded.

SUMMARY

A wide variety of orthopedic disorders can be present in the neonatal foal. A rapid and accurate diagnosis of these conditions is imperative so that the best future athletic potential can be achieved.

FURTHER READING

Auer JA, Stick JA (Eds.) (2012) *Equine Surgery*, 4th ed. Elsevier Saunders, St. Louis, MO.

Ross MW, Dyson SJ (Eds.) (2011) *Diagnosis and Management of Lameness in the Horse*, 2nd ed. Elsevier Saunders, St. Louis, MO.

Sanchez LC (Guest Ed.) (2005) Neonatal medicine and surgery. *Veterinary Clinics of North America: Equine Practice* August 21: 2.

Baxter GM (Ed.) (2011) *Adams and Stashak's Lameness in Horses*, 6th ed. Wiley-Blackwell, Ames, IA.

Ophthalmologic Disorders

13

Mary Lassaline and Claire Latimer

INTRODUCTION

A complete ocular examination of the neonate allows for identification of congenital abnormalities, which may be inherited or acquired, and for determining the prognosis and treatment of such abnormalities. Neonatal foals in intensive care often have ocular disease as well as multiple systemic problems associated with septicemia, prolonged recumbency, and dehydration. In one survey, 21% (52/248) of neonatal foals admitted to an ICU between 1989 and 1992 had ulcerative keratitis and 19% (48/248) had entropion.

This chapter will begin with a review of normal ocular anatomy, vision, and reflexes, followed by an outline of a routine ocular examination and diagnostic procedures. Clinical ocular disorders are divided into congenital and acquired where appropriate, and are ordered within each section from the front to the back of the eye. Drugs commonly used in ophthalmic examination and treatment are listed in *Table 71*.

Table 71. Drugs commonly used in ophthalmic examination and treatment

Drug	Dosage	Comments
Anesthetics		
Lidocaine	2% s/c	Local anesthesia and akinesia
Mepivicaine	2% s/c	Local anesthesia and akinesia
Proparacaine	0.5% topically	Topical anesthesia; may induce minor superficial corneal irregularities; may decrease tear production
Tetracaine	0.5% topically	Topical anesthesia; may induce minor superficial corneal irregularities; may decrease tear production
Antibiotics		
Amikacin	15 mg/kg i/v q24h	Bactericidal aminoglycoside; good against Gram-negative bacilli
Bacitracin–neomycin–polymyxin B	o/o topically q2–8h	Broad-spectrum bactericidal
Chloramphenicol	1% o/o topically q2–8h	Gram-positive spectrum
Ciprofloxacin	0.3% o/s topically q2–8h	Broad-spectrum bactericidal fluoroquinolone; reserve for treatment of severe infections by sensitive organisms
Doxycycline	10 mg/kg p/o q12h	Bacteriostatic, broad spectrum; good against *Leptospira* spp.
Gatifloxacin	0.3% topically q2–8h	Fourth-generation fluoroquinolone
Gentamicin	6.6 mg/kg i/v q24h;	Bactericidal aminoglycoside;
	0.3% o/s topically q2–8h	Gram-negative spectrum, also Gram-positive aerobes; nephrotoxic, ototoxic
Minocycline	4 mg/kg p/o q12h	Broad-spectrum antibiotic with anti-inflammatory activity

(Continued)

Table 71. (*Continued*) Drugs commonly used in ophthalmic examination and treatment

Drug	Dosage	Comments
Moxifloxacin	0.5% topically q2–8h	Fourth-generation fluoroquinolone
Ofloxacin	0.3% o/s topically q2–8h	Broad-spectrum antibiotic with better Gram-positive coverage and less topical irritation than ciprofloxacin
Potassium penicillin G	22,000 IU/kg i/v q6h	Bactericidal; Gram-positive spectrum
Procaine penicillin G	22,000 IU/kg i/m q12h	Bactericidal; Gram-positive spectrum
Tobramycin	0.3% o/s topically q2–8h	Gram-negative spectrum; restrict use to severe corneal infections, particularly *Pseudomonas aeruginosa*
Trimethoprim/ sulfamethoxazole	5 mg/kg p/o q12h	Bacteriostatic, broad spectrum
Anticollagenolytics		
Acetylcysteine	10% o/s topically q1–4h	
EDTA	0.05% o/s topically	
Anticollagenolytics		
Serum	Topically q2–6h	Contains α-macroglobulins; inhibits matrix metalloproteases, serine proteases; collect new autogenous sample every 7 days
Antifungals		
Amphotericin B	1.5% o/s topically	Broad-spectrum polyene; poor intraocular penetration when given parenterally; poor corneal penetration topically
Fluconazole	0.2% o/o topically q4–8h; 1 mg/kg p/o q12h	Imidazole
Itraconazole	1% o/o topically q4–8h; 3 mg/kg p/o q12h	Imidazole; high corneal concentration; compounded in ointment with 30% DMSO
Miconazole	1% o/s topically q4–8h	Imidazole, excellent corneal penetration; also active against Gram-positive cocci
Natamycin	5% o/s topically q4–8h	Only commercially available antifungal
Povidone-iodine	2% solution topically	Also antibacterial, antiviral, antiprotozoal
Voriconazole	1% o/s q4–8h	Triazole; effective against *Aspergillus*
Anti-inflammatories		
Dexamethasone	0.05–0.1 mg/kg i/v q24h; 0.1% o/o or o/s topically	Corticosteroid
Diclofenac	0.1% o/s topically	Nonsteroidal
Dimethylsulfoxide	30% o/o topically	Topical ointment compounded with itraconazole
Flunixin meglumine	1 mg/kg i/v or p/o q12–24h	Nonsteroidal; can cause GI ulceration
Flurbiprofen	0.03% o/s topically	Nonsteroidal
Phenylbutazone	2 mg/kg p/o q12–24h	Nonsteroidal; can cause GI ulceration
Prednisolone acetate	1% o/s topically	Corticosteroid

(*Continued*)

Table 71. (*Continued*) Drugs commonly used in ophthalmic examination and treatment

Drug	Dosage	Comments
Mydriatic/cycloplegics		
Atropine	1% o/o or o/s topically	Parasympatholytic mydriatic, cycloplegic; use q8–12h until pupil dilates then according to circumstances; monitor for signs of colic
Tropicamide	1% o/s topically	Shorter duration than atropine
Tranquilizers		
Butorphanol	0.005 mg/kg i/v	Opioid; also provides analgesia; add to alpha-agonist as needed
Detomidine	0.005–0.02 mg/kg i/v	Long-acting alpha-1 agonist; analgesic
Diazepam	0.1 mg/kg i/v	Muscle relaxant
Xylazine	0.3 mg/kg i/v	Also provides analgesia; short-acting alpha-agonist

Note: o/o = ophthalmic ointment; o/s = ophthalmic solution.

NORMAL FOALS

NORMAL ANATOMY

Horses are grazing animals with a strong flight instinct, and their ability to survive in the wild depends in part on successfully detecting and running away from predators. Several anatomic structures serve an important function in this respect. For example, lateral globe placement and a horizontally rectangular pupil provide a wide field of view, while vibrissae allow tactile detection of objects too close to see.

The ocular anatomy of horses is similar to other domestic animals. Like other domestic animals, horses have vibrissae and cilia; however, most horses lack inferior cilia. They have a nictitans, which produces tears and rapidly sweeps the surface of the cornea following globe retraction in response to pain. The equine cornea, like other grazing animals, is taller medially than laterally. The gray line visible at the limbus represents the iridocorneal angle, which (unlike that of dogs) is easily evaluated without special lenses. The equine iris is normally brown, but heterochromia (where all or a portion of one iris is blue) may occur, most often in color dilute horses (**386**). The corpora nigra are exaggerations of the pupillary ruff. These structures are found in all grazing animals and are thought to serve as protection against actinic damage to the lens and retina. The normal lens is clear, but sutures may be visible. The foal fundus is like that of adult horses, with a salmon-colored oval optic disk located in the nontapetal fundus (**387, 388**). The tapetum is usually green, but it may vary from yellow to blue depending on coat color. The nontapetal fundus is usually brown. Some horses, particularly color dilute horses or horses with blue irides, may have no tapetum or lack pigment in the nontapetal retina such that choroidal vessels are visible, resulting in a tigroid fundus. The vascular pattern of the equine retina (unlike other grazing animals including cattle, sheep, and goats) is paurangiotic, with 50–80

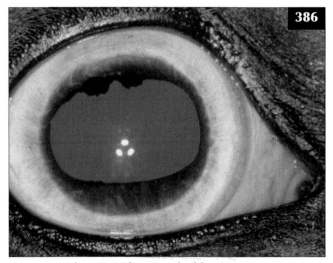

386 Heterochromia iridis. Note the blue iris.

small retinal arterioles and venules extending only a short distance from the edge of the optic disk. The ventral portion of the optic disk is not perfused by retinal vessels. Choroidal capillaries can be seen end-on as small dots distributed throughout the tapetum; these are called "Stars of Winslow."

VISION

Relative to other species, horses have lateral globe placement and a horizontal pupil. This provides a wide monocular field of view (190% horizontal and 178% vertical), a binocular field of only 65%, with a total field of view (monocular and binocular) of >350%. The equine retina has an "area centralis" with two parts: the area centralis rotunda (small circular region dorsotemporal to the optic disk),

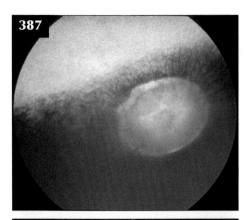

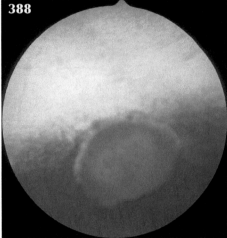

387, 388 Equine fundus. (**387**) Normal equine fundus. (**388**) Normal variant seen in a Paint Horse.

the region with the highest ganglion cell density; and the area centralis stratiformis, or visual streak (horizontal band dorsal to the optic disk, medial to the area centralis rotunda). Most horses have refractive errors within 1 diopter of emmetropia, with retinoscopy indicating minimal refractive errors (a mean of 0.33 D, and a range of –3 to 3 D).

Visual acuity is the ability to see detail. Horses have fewer cones than rods, which suggests that they are adapted for night vision and motion detection rather than detailed color vision. Even so, visual acuity in horses is estimated as being better than in dogs and cats, but not as good as that of humans. Therefore, if normal human vision is 20/20, horses would have 20/33 (i.e., the horse has the same acuity at 20 feet from an object that a person has at 33 feet). Behavioral experiments have demonstrated color discrimination ability in horses. Horses have two spectrally different cone types, which serve as the photopigment basis for dichromatic color vision. Based on analogy to human dichromats who have inherited red-green color vision defects, it is believed that horses "see" yellow and blue best, but have trouble with red and green. Wavelengths of light outside the yellow or blue ranges are perceived either as achromatic (white or gray) or as a desaturated version of yellow or blue. Rods outnumber cones throughout the retina, but cone density is highest in the area centralis, suggesting that this is the area of maximal acuity. Visual stimulation during neonatal life is thought

to be critical for proper development of central visual pathways such that lack of, or blurred, vision (i.e., with congenital cataracts) may compromise future vision. Although the critical time for the development of vision in horses is unknown, experiments with kittens deprived of visual stimulation suggest that there is a critical period. Young kittens that had one eye sutured closed for various periods of time after birth acted blind when the previously sutured eye was opened and the previously undeprived eye was covered, and neurons in the visual cortex of these kittens did not respond to stimulation of the previously deprived eye. The critical period for visual deprivation in kittens was 4–8 weeks. Taking into account this research with kittens, there may be some urgency to correct visual deprivation in foals, as occurs with cataracts.

EVALUATING LIGHT RESPONSES AND VISION

Normal foals are born with their eyes open and with functional vision, but there are some differences between foals and adults. There is a widely held belief that in foals the pupil has a sluggish pupillary light reflex and is more round than the adult pupil, becoming more horizontally oval within the first week of life. The pupillary light reflex may seem sluggish if the light source is not sufficiently brighter than ambient light. Also, in a neonate inexperienced with people and bright lights, the pupils may appear round and slow to dilate due to sympathetic override of a normal reflex. The pupillary light reflex requires a functional retina, optic nerve, optic chiasm, and oculomotor nucleus in the midbrain, oculomotor nerve, and pupillary constrictor muscle. This reflex is not affected by lesions involving the visual cortex (i.e., a centrally blind foal can have a positive pupillary light reflex). The menace response, defined as a blink or head movement in response to a threatening gesture, is most commonly used to assess vision in nonverbal animals. The menace response is learned and requires a functional optic nerve, optic chiasm, visual cortex, facial nucleus, and orbicularis oculi muscle. The menace response has been reported to take from days to weeks to develop. In one study of 26 Dutch Warmblood foals, although all the foals had a positive pupillary light reflex when examined within the first 24 hours post partum, some foals did not have a menace response until several days to a week after birth. All the foals had a menace response by day 9. In that study, the menace response developed incrementally, with a partial blink preceding a compete blink, and asymmetrically, often with a menace in one eye before the other. An absent menace response may indicate facial nerve paralysis, cerebellar disease, or lack of experience.

CORNEAL SENSITIVITY

Corneal sensitivity is important in tear production, in the blink reflex, and in corneal healing, as corneal nerves have a trophic effect on the corneal epithelium. The corneal touch threshold, a measure of corneal sensitivity that indicates the degree of corneal surface stimulation necessary to cause a blink reflex, has been measured in adult horses and foals. Foals have a lower corneal sensitivity than adults, and sick foals have a lower sensitivity than healthy foals.

TEAR PRODUCTION

Tears are important for corneal protection and healing. Tear production in adult horses appears to be widely variable, but is not affected by signalment, housing, season, or time of day. In a study of tear production in healthy and sick foals, both groups of foals had lower tear production than adults, but there was no difference between healthy and sick foals. Tear production is most commonly measured with the Schirmer tear test (STT). In this study, the mean STT values were 14.2 ± 1.0 mm, 12.8 ± 2.4 mm, and 18.3 ± 2.1 mm wetting/minute in sick foals, healthy foals, and adults, respectively. Tear augmentation may be warranted in recumbent neonates.

OPHTHALMIC EXAMINATION AND DIAGNOSTIC TESTS

A complete ophthalmic examination typically begins with an assessment of vision. Observation of the foal at liberty and evaluation of the presence of a menace response in all parts of the visual field normally allows adequate assessment of age-appropriate behavior. Navigation in a more complex environment can be observed if vision is questionable, with care being taken to avoid injury. Light perception is evaluated by testing for the presence of the dazzle and pupillary light reflexes. Facial symmetry, including globe position and lid carriage, can be assessed by visual inspection.

The remainder of the examination is facilitated by adequate restraint and sedation, determined by the temperament and condition of the foal. Intravenous sedation, topical corneal anesthetic, and local eyelid paralysis or anesthesia may be necessary. Closure of the eyelids is produced by the orbicularis oculi muscle, which is innervated by the palpebral nerve, a branch of the facial nerve (cranial nerve [CN] VII). The upper eyelid, which moves much more than the lower eyelid, can be paralyzed by injecting 1–2 mL of 2% lidocaine or 2% mepivicain subcutaneously, adjacent to the palpebral nerve, where it can be palpated at the dorsal border of the zygomatic arch. Sensation to the upper eyelid is provided by the supraorbital nerve medially and centrally and the lacrimal nerve laterally. Both of these nerves arise from the ophthalmic branch of the trigeminal nerve (CN V). The medial part of the upper lid can be anesthetized by injecting 1–2 mL of 2% lidocaine with a 25 gauge 5/8 in needle into the supraorbital foramen, which can be palpated along the supraorbital process of the frontal bone, medial to its most narrow aspect. A line block along the lateral third of the dorsal orbital rim anesthetizes the lacrimal nerve. Sensory innervation to the lower lid is by the infratrochlear nerve medially and the zygomatic nerve laterally. These nerves can be anesthetized as they cross the rim of the orbit, at the medial (infratrochlear) and ventral (zygomatic) aspects of the orbital rim. General anesthesia may be necessary for a complete examination of extensive orbital and ocular injuries in foals.

Corneal culture for bacterial or fungal infection must be collected and tear production measured prior to instillation of any solutions onto the surface of the eye. The integrity of the corneal surface is evaluated with fluorescein staining to detect ulcers or abrasions and, possibly, with Rose Bengal staining to detect devitalized epithelial cells. Rose Bengal is a nonspecific stain for any corneal condition in which epithelial cells are nonviable, including early fungal keratitis, viral keratitis, and dry eye. Interpretation of positive Rose Bengal staining must be done with caution, as Rose Bengal may stain the area of the cornea recently contacted by a STT strip or a tonometer. Intraocular pressure (IOP) is measured with an applanation tonometer (the Tonopen is the one most widely available). Slit lamp biomicroscopy allows evaluation of the cornea, anterior chamber, iris, and lens. The posterior segment is examined using ophthalmoscopy (direct, indirect, or panoptic ophthalmoscopes can be used). Ultrasound examination may be indicated when the ocular media (cornea, aqueous humor, lens and vitreous) are not clear. Ultrasonography can identify lens luxation, persistent hyperplastic primary vitreous, retinal detachment, and space-occupying lesions in the globe and orbit. It is performed most commonly in foals prior to cataract surgery. An electroretinogram is performed to evaluate retinal function, again most commonly in foals prior to cataract surgery.

CONGENITAL DISORDERS

INTRODUCTION

The prevalence of congenital ocular anomalies is low in horses, and it can be difficult to determine whether lesions are inherited or acquired. Breeding mares that have congenital ocular anomalies, or have produced foals with such, is at the discretion of the breeder, but not recommended if said anomalies maybe inherited. Ocular defects are reported to represent 3% of all congenital defects in horses, and ocular defects occur in 0.5% of foals. The most common defects are cataracts and microphthalmia, both of which are discussed in more detail later. Multiple congenital ocular defects, with or without microphthalmia, have been observed in foals, often related to the role of the lens in induction and maturation of the structures of the anterior segment. For example, one Thoroughbred foal had bilateral, asymmetric anomalies. One eye was microphthalmic and the other had an anterior staphyloma, but both conditions could be accounted for by a fractional difference in the time at which a single insult affected each eye. Bilateral multiple congenital ocular defects, including optic nerve colobomas, have been observed in Quarter Horse foals, but it is not known whether these were inherited or acquired.

ANTERIOR SEGMENT DYSGENESIS

Anterior segment dysgenesis refers to a collection of ocular anomalies, typically including megalocornea, iris hypoplasia, and congenital miosis (resistant to dilation with mydriatics). It has been reported in a number of breeds including the Kentucky Mountain Saddle Horse, the Mountain Pleasure Horse, and pony and miniature breeds. Anterior segment dysgenesis has been documented in a survey of 514 Rocky Mountain Horses. It most commonly affects horses with a chocolate coat color and a white or flaxen mane and tail, although horses with other coat, mane, and tail colors have been affected. The genetic mutation responsible for the ocular anomalies is linked to the silver dapple gene. Mildly affected animals had only uveal or peripheral retinal cysts, whereas more severely affected animals exhibited multiple anomalies, including miosis, iris hypoplasia, megalocornea, cataract, uveal and retinal cysts, retinal detachments, and retinal dysplasia.

GLOBE AND ORBIT

ANOPHTHALMIA AND CYCLOPIA
Anophthalmia and cyclopia (true absence of an eye, or the presence of only a single eye) have been reported in other species, but not in the horse. Affected animals are typically afflicted with other ophthalmic and systemic malformations.

MICROPHTHALMIA
DEFINITION/OVERVIEW
Microphthalmia, or a congenitally small globe, is perhaps the most common congenital anomaly seen in foals, and Thoroughbred foals appear to be at increased risk. The condition may be unilateral or bilateral.

ETIOLOGY/PATHOPHYSIOLOGY
Microphthalmia can be idiopathic or due to infection, a teratogen, or a toxin. It is believed that microphthalmic globes often result from dysplastic development, because the lens, ciliary processes, and retina are often found histologically.

CLINICAL PRESENTATION
Microphthalmia varies from a slightly small but perfectly formed globe (**389**) to a very small and dysplastic globe (**390**). Most microphthalmic globes are nonvisual and are often accompanied by a small palpebral fissure, a prominent nictitans, entropion, and possibly secondary ulcerative keratitis. The skull may develop abnormally on the side of a severely microphthalmic globe.

MANAGEMENT
Treatment for microphthalmia is unnecessary unless desired for hygienic or cosmetic reasons or there is secondary ulcerative keratitis or entropion, leading to discomfort. Enucleation, with or without placement of an intraorbital prosthesis, is then indicated. A prosthesis should not be placed in young animals, as the orbit may change size with development and therefore its size will not be cosmetic in the adult.

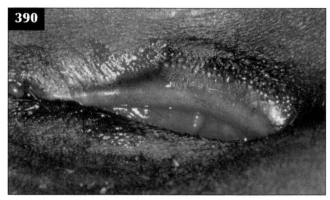

390 Microphthalmia, with a very small dysplastic globe, inapparent without careful examination.

GLAUCOMA

DEFINITION/OVERVIEW
Glaucoma has been defined as an elevation in IOP incompatible with the health of the retina and optic nerve, often leading to blindness.

ETIOLOGY/PATHOPHYSIOLOGY
Glaucoma is rare in foals. It can be congenital or acquired, and primary or secondary. Congenital glaucoma is thought to be caused by abnormalities in the development of the iridocorneal angle. Glaucoma can occur secondary to uveitis, when inflammatory proteins and cells occlude the iridocorneal drainage and impair the normal outflow of aqueous humor. Secondary glaucoma may resolve with treatment to reduce the IOP and inflammation.

CLINICAL PRESENTATION
Clinical signs may include ciliary flush, corneal edema, a dilated pupil, and aqueous flare (**391**). The IOP measured with a Tonopen applanation tonometer in the horse ranges from 7 to 37 mmHg, with a mean IOP of 23.3 ± 6.9 mmHg. While there

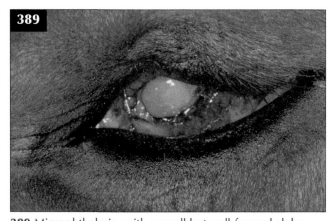

389 Microphthalmia, with a small but well-formed globe.

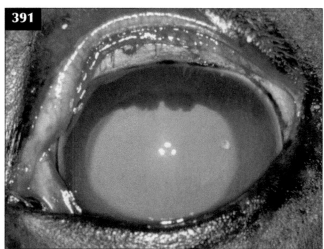

391 Glaucomatous eye with ciliary flush, corneal edema, and a dilated pupil. The IOP was 40 mmHg.

do not seem to be significant diurnal changes in IOP in the horse, the IOP in the afternoon was slightly higher than in the morning in one study.

In one case report, a 1-week-old Thoroughbred filly was affected with bilateral glaucoma with posterior lens luxation in one eye and subluxation in the other. Both globes were buphthalmic (enlarged) and the pupils were mydriatic and poorly responsive to light. The filly was euthanized.

In a case of unilateral congenital buphthalmia in a Thoroughbred filly, the foal showed neurologic signs including incoordination, abnormal suckling, and head tilt, and was diagnosed with neonatal maladjustment syndrome (NMS). Ophthalmic examination revealed typical signs of glaucoma in one eye, including an enlarged globe, increased IOP, Haab's striae, a dilated unresponsive pupil, corneal edema, pain, persistent pupillary membranes attached to the cornea, and a pale elongated optic disk. This filly was also euthanized. On gross examination, there were posterior synechiae, a lens coloboma at 10 o'clock, iris hypoplasia, absent corpora nigra, and a closed iridocorneal angle with absent pectinate ligaments and trabecular meshwork. Histologically, iris sphincter and dilator muscles were present, the ciliary processes were thin, the optic disk was cupped, and the inner retinal layers were atrophied. Buphthalmos, retinal atrophy, and optic nerve cupping are all thought to be secondary to elevation of IOP caused by iridocorneal angle abnormalities.

MANAGEMENT

Congenital glaucoma is typically not responsive to therapy, but when attempted, therapy is directed at decreasing the amount of aqueous humor produced and increasing the outflow. If therapy is not attempted, the remaining options include enucleation or euthanasia.

STRABISMUS

Strabismus, or deviation of the globe from its normal position, is rare in horses. Strabismus has been reported in mules and in Appaloosas, in which it may be associated with congenital stationery night blindness. Surgical correction of strabismus involves transposing extraocular muscle insertions in order to alter the globe position. Surgical correction should theoretically occur before cortical cells atrophy in response to lack of stimulation of both eyes, but the time point in foal development at which this atrophy might occur is unknown.

ADNEXA

ANKYLOBLEPHARON

Ankyloblepharon, or fusion of the eyelids, has been reported in a Shetland foal. Treatment of ankyloblepharon requires mechanical separation of the fused lids, either manually or surgically.

VITILIGO

Vitiligo has been reported in Arabian horses 6–24 months of age. The condition is also known as Arabian fading syndrome, juvenile Arabian leukoderma, or "pinky" syndrome. Skin at mucocutaneous junctions, including the eyelids, becomes temporarily or permanently depigmented. The condition is believed to be inherited. The etiology is unknown and there is no treatment.

NASOLACRIMAL SYSTEM

NASOLACRIMAL DEFECTS

Congenital nasolacrimal defects are often not recognized for months, when the young horse develops significant mucopurulent discharge. Affected horses usually present as weanlings or yearlings.

CLINICAL PRESENTATION

Nasolacrimal duct atresia and obstruction both appear clinically as a unilateral or bilateral, chronic mucoid or mucopurulent ocular discharge associated with dacryocystitis.

DIAGNOSIS

Nasolacrimal duct atresia is often diagnosed by noting the absence of the distal opening within the nares at the mucocutaneous junctions. It is theoretically possible for both the eyelid and the nasal punctum to be present, but the duct itself to be incomplete (nasolacrimal duct agenesis), or for the proximal openings on both upper and lower lids at the medial canthus to be absent (eyelid punctal atresia); however, these conditions are not commonly seen. Diagnosis can be confirmed with contrast dacryocystorhinography.

MANAGEMENT

Creation of a new puncta or duct can be accomplished by instillation of a catheter, which should remain in place for several weeks in order to allow the new punctum or duct to epithelialize and any dacryocystitis to resolve.

CORNEA

MICROCORNEA/MEGALOCORNEA

Microcornea, a congenitally smaller than normal cornea, and megalocornea, a congenitally larger than normal cornea, are both rare in horses. Megalocornea is associated with anterior segment dysgenesis in Rocky Mountain Horses (discussed previously). There is no treatment for either of these conditions.

DERMOIDS

Dermoids are a form of choristoma (congenital masses of tissue in an aberrant location) with skin, either with or without hair, located on the conjunctiva, third eyelid, or cornea. Dermoids have been seen in combination with aniridia in Belgians and Quarter Horses (see below). Treatment is by surgical excision of those masses causing irritation, but caution must be taken to make certain that the cornea underlying the dermoid is normal before attempting excision in order to prevent inadvertent entry into the anterior chamber.

IRIS

ANIRIDIA

DEFINITION/OVERVIEW
Aniridia, although technically referring to a complete absence of iris tissue, is a term commonly used to describe a vestigial iris with only a narrow rim of tissue at the area of the iris root.

ETIOLOGY/PATHOPHYSIOLOGY
Aniridia is an embryologic defect caused by abnormal migration of the optic cup after formation of the lens vesicle or abnormal mesodermal development inhibiting iris formation.

CLINICAL PRESENTATION
Vestigial iris was first described in horses in a Belgian stallion and 65 of his offspring, transmitted as an autosomal dominant trait. Some of the offspring also had dorsal pannus and limbal dermoids. Aniridia, cataracts, pannus, and dermoids have been reported in Quarter Horses, also inherited in an autosomal dominant pattern. Aniridia, pannus, and cataract were reported in a Welsh–Thoroughbred cross. The filly was visual, responded to bright light, and was able to navigate a maze. Anterior cortical cataracts were bilateral and progressed over the first year.

MANAGEMENT
There is no treatment for this condition.

HYPOPLASIA

Hypoplasia of the iris can be mild to extreme (**392**). In cases of severe iris stromal hypoplasia, the stroma is so thin that the iris protrudes anteriorly, giving the appearance of a cyst or mass within the iris. This is most often seen dorsally, and has been reported

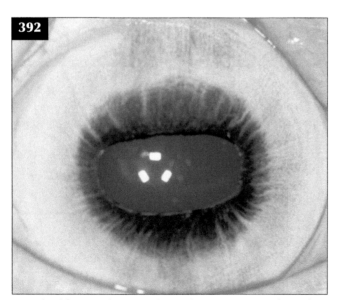

392 This blue iris shows iris hypoplasia, a congenital condition in which the stroma is abnormally thin. Light transilluminated through the pupil and reflecting off the tapetum can be seen through the iris as well as through the pupil.

most commonly in Welsh ponies. There is no treatment necessary or available for this condition. Iris hypoplasia rarely affects vision or performance. In some cases the anteriorly protruding iris can occupy the anterior chamber and contact the corneal endothelium, which may obstruct vision or cause discomfort. Short-acting topical mydriatics (e.g., tropicamide) may improve vision in these cases by opening up the pupil. Full-thickness defects are colobomas, which are classified as "typical" if they occur at the 6 o'clock position (ventral), the site of closure of the optic fissure, or "atypical" if they are not ventral. Both types of coloboma are rare in horses.

HETEROCHROMIA

Heterochromia of the iris is usually a normal variant related to coat color (**386**). "Lethal whites" (foals afflicted with a syndrome referred to as congenital intestinal aganglionosis) are born of Paint parents, most often but not always Overos, that have a white coat, blue irides, and intestinal defects that are incompatible with life.

IRIS CYSTS

DEFINITION/OVERVIEW
Iridociliary cysts appear clinically as brown thin-walled cystic structures protruding through the pupil. They may attach anywhere along the pupillary margin, but are seen most commonly along the dorsal pupil margin along with the corpora nigra. They rarely affect performance and treatment is only warranted when performance is affected.

ETIOLOGY/PATHOPHYSIOLOGY
Corpora nigra or ciliary epithelial cysts originate from the corpora nigra or from the posterior pigmented epithelium of the iris and are likely developmental in origin.

CLINICAL PRESENTATION
Iris cysts can be variably pigmented; however, they can be distinguished from solid masses by transillumination with a focal light source (**393**). Corpora nigra or ciliary cysts only become problematic if they become large enough to impair vision or obstruct the drainage angle, causing secondary glaucoma.

MANAGEMENT
Iris cysts that are impairing vision or causing undesired spooking behavior can be ablated via laser treatment, but this carries with it the risk of deposition of cyst debris in the angle and the development of secondary glaucoma.

PERSISTENT PUPILLARY MEMBRANES

Persistent pupillary membranes are strands of tissue extending from the iris collarette to another portion of the iris, to the lens, or to the cornea, or free floating in the anterior chamber. These strands of tissue result from incomplete resorption of embryonic vasculature. This mesenchymal tissue normally atrophies near the end of gestation, but remnants may be seen in neonatal foals. Persistent pupillary membranes are of no clinical significance unless they cause lens or corneal opacities. Mydriatic therapy to improve vision impaired

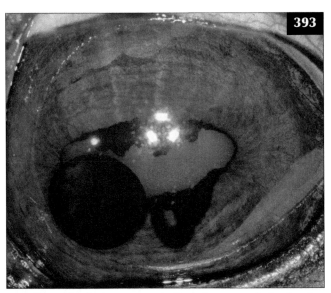

393 This iridociliary cyst was believed to cause behavioral changes including spooking that were potentially associated with impaired vision. Cyst ablation led to an improvement in behavior.

by axial persistent pupillary membranes is not recommended, as dilating the pupil may induce tension on the cornea or lens.

LENS

MICROPHAKIA

Microphakia is a congenital condition in which the lens is smaller than normal; therefore, the lens zonules can be seen when the pupil is dilated. It is often associated with other ocular anomalies. If microphakia is the only ocular anomaly, vision is often not significantly affected and no treatment is necessary.

LENTICONUS/LENTIGLOBUS

Lenticonus is a condition in which the lens is more conically shaped than normal, with the conical portion of the lens most often posterior. Lentiglobus is a condition in which the lens is more round from anterior to posterior than normal. These conditions only significantly affect vision if accompanied by cataract formation. As such, treatment is usually not necessary. Mydriatic therapy to provide a visual window around the axial opacity may improve vision.

VITREOUS

PERSISTENT HYALOID ARTERY

DEFINITION/OVERVIEW

The hyaloid artery (a branch of the embryologic dorsal ophthalmic artery) traverses the vitreous from the optic disk to the anterior and posterior surface of the developing lens (as the anterior and posterior tunica vasculosa lentis, respectively) and provides it with nutrition. The tunica vasculosa lentis regresses before birth, but a hyaloid remnant remains.

ETIOLOGY/PATHOPHYSIOLOGY

The hyaloid artery was present in all foals less than 24 hours old in one study, but regressed or was less prominent in older foals. In another survey, over 80% of neonates less than 96 hours old had some part of the hyaloid artery present bilaterally, with the presence and completeness of the structure related to the age of the foal. Remnants may be attached to the lens capsule (Mittendorf's dot) or the optic disk (Bergmeister's papilla). Atrophy of the hyaloid apparatus usually occurs by 3–4 months of age and remnants in horses, unlike in humans, rarely cause visual deficits. A persistent hyaloid apparatus may be associated with a cataract, but these rarely progress or have a significant effect on vision unless they are large.

CLINICAL PRESENTATION

A persistent hyaloid artery appears as a linear streak from the axial posterior lens to the optic disk. It may contain blood, but is more often gray in appearance. Over one-third of the foals less than 96 hours old in the previously mentioned survey had a hyaloid artery containing blood.

MANAGEMENT

There is neither treatment nor cure for this condition.

RETINA AND OPTIC NERVE

Congenital anomalies of the foal fundus are uncommon.

COLOBOMA

A coloboma is the absence of tissue that is normally present. Optic nerve colobomas, which are excavations of the optic disk containing retinal vessels, glial tissue, and a paucity of neural tissue, are typically an incidental finding, with cause unknown, no treatment, and often no apparent effect on performance unless they are large. Typical colobomas, which occur at the 6 o'clock position, are related to incomplete closure of the optic fissure during embryologic development. Central colobomas have been seen in Appaloosas with night blindness, but they are not a characteristic finding in these horses. Bilateral optic disk colobomas have been reported in a Quarter Horse filly.

OPTIC NERVE HYPOPLASIA

Optic nerve hypoplasia is uncommon in foals. It may be unilateral or bilateral. The condition appears clinically as a small optic disk, with slow pupillary light reflexes. The degree of vision depends on the degree of hypoplasia. Completely atrophic (or severely hypoplastic) disks appear pale, without retinal vessels, and affected animals are blind, with fixed, dilated pupils.

CONGENITAL STATIONARY NIGHT BLINDNESS

DEFINITION/OVERVIEW

Congenital stationary night blindness is a nonprogressive retinal disorder characterized by abnormal rod function, leading to good daytime vision but functional blindness in dim light conditions or at night. This condition has been reported most commonly in the Appaloosa, in which it is believed to be inherited as a recessive trait. The condition is present at birth and persists, but is not progressive.

CLINICAL PRESENTATION

Clinically, affected horses have difficulty seeing in conditions of reduced light and after transition from dark to light and light to dark, but day blindness has also been reported. Severely affected foals may show stargazing, head tilt, and bilateral dorsomedial strabismus, whereas less severely affected foals may just appear clumsy or awkward, disoriented at night, and sustain frequent injuries at night.

DIAGNOSIS

There are no ophthalmoscopic lesions with this disease; therefore, diagnosis requires an electroretinogram showing dominance of the A-wave (contributed by the photoreceptors in the retina) and absence of the B-wave (which is contributed by the bipolar cells).

MANAGEMENT

There is no treatment for this condition.

RETINAL DYSPLASIA

Retinal dysplasia, which is not well documented in the horse, appears clinically in other species as single or multiple, linear or geographic regions that are depigmented in the nontapetal fundus or hyperpigmented in the tapetal fundus. The clinical change in pigment corresponds histologically to regions of retina that are folded on themselves. Retinal dysplasia may be developmental or postinflammatory and in horses is most often associated with other ocular anomalies. It has been noted in Rock Mountain Horses. There is no treatment for this condition.

ACQUIRED DISORDERS

ORBITAL TRAUMA

DEFINITION/OVERVIEW

Orbital trauma, commonly resulting from a kick from a mare, can result in orbital fractures or globe rupture (394–396).

ETIOLOGY/PATHOPHYSIOLOGY

Sharp or blunt trauma can cause globe rupture. Even if the globe is not perforated directly, trauma to the globe can result in a rapid increase in IOP, leading to corneal or scleral rupture. In blunt trauma, globe rupture occurs most frequently at the limbus.

CLINICAL PRESENTATION

Clinical signs of orbital trauma include blepharedema, lid and intraorbital hemorrhage, and enophthalmos (395) or exophthalmos. Subcutaneous emphysema resulting from an orbital fracture is shown in 394.

DIAGNOSIS

Skull radiography is indicated in cases of orbital trauma, but a physical examination is often the most useful diagnostic aid; facial asymmetry (396), epiphora, crepitus, pain on palpation, and epistaxis suggest the presence of a periorbital fracture even if radiographic abnormalities are not observed or are difficult to interpret.

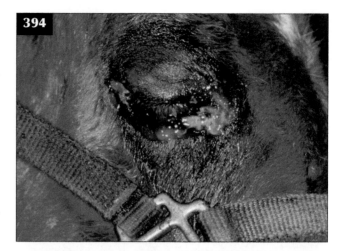

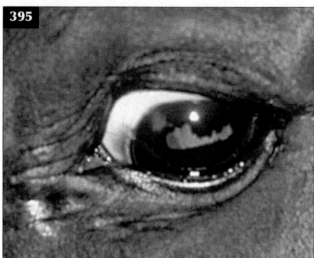

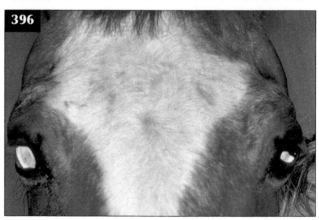

394–396 Orbital trauma. (394) Subcutaneous emphysema resulting from a periorbital fracture. (395) Enophthalmos secondary to a orbital fracture. (396) Facial asymmetry apparent with an orbital fracture.

MANAGEMENT

If the maxillary or paranasal sinuses are involved (evidenced by a fluid line on radiography), systemic antibiotic therapy is indicated, as the fracture is considered "open." Closed fractures are typically also treated with systemic antibiotics. Surgical correction is required if fracture fragments are displaced, threatening, or displacing the globe. Treatment of minimally displaced orbital fractures includes topical and systemic anti-inflammatories (including flunixin and dexamethasone) to reduce pain and lid swelling. If the optic nerve is obviously severed or the globe is severely damaged, enucleation is warranted.

ADNEXA

ENTROPION

Entropion is a condition in which the eyelid margin rolls in, potentially contacting the cornea and causing corneal ulceration. Entropion occurs in healthy neonates, but is more common in poor-doing foals and maybe associated with decreased tear production, prolonged recumbency, a poor blink reflex, and dehydration. In a survey of foals admitted to the University of Florida from 1989 to 1992, 48/248 (19%) had entropion, 27 of which (56%) had ulcerative keratitis. Surgical correction, in the form of excision of a crescent of skin along the lid margin corresponding to the entropic area, is rarely required, as entropion often corrects itself following resolution of the systemic disease. Temporary tacking using mattress tension sutures to retract the lid (397) may alleviate corneal pain and allow secondary corneal ulcers to heal. Entropion secondary to a scar formed by a lid laceration can occur and will require surgical correction (398).

BLEPHARITIS

Blepharitis, or inflammation of the eyelids, can affect foals as well as adult horses and is often associated with fly-bite dermatitis, dermatophytosis, and *Dermatophilus* and staphylococcal folliculitis.

EYELID LACERATIONS

Lid lacerations are common in horses of all ages. Prompt repair is important in order to maintain the viability of all possible tissue. Eyelids have a good blood supply and usually heal well, so minimal debridement is necessary. Excision of the avulsed eyelid is contraindicated in order to avoid being left without enough tissue to repair the laceration and maintain adequate lid closure. Surgical repair should accurately re-appose all layers of the eyelid (399, 400).

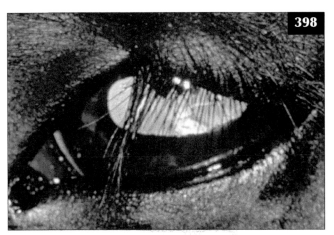

398 Cicatricial entropion secondary to a lid laceration.

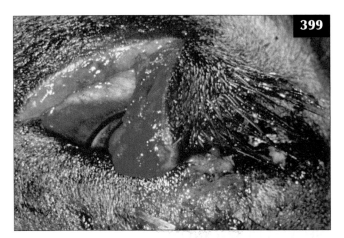

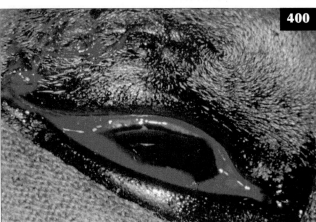

399, 400 (**399**) Preoperative view; (**400**) postoperative view.

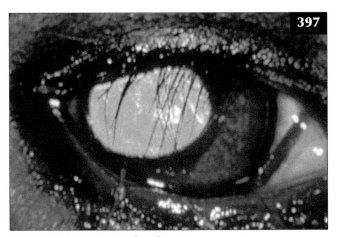

397 Entropion corrected with temporary mattress sutures.

CONJUNCTIVA

CONJUNCTIVITIS

Conjunctivitis in foals can be caused by systemic disease (e.g., viral or bacterial pneumonia), local infection, or environmental irritants. It appears clinically as excessive tear production, ocular discharge (either mucoid or mucopurulent), and conjunctival hyperemia.

Recumbent foals are particularly at risk for conjunctival irritation by bedding, feed material, dirt, or ammonia from urine-soaked bedding. Conjunctivitis is also common with corneal ulceration, ocular trauma, and uveitis. Conjunctival cytology and culture can be used to identify an infectious component. Treatment involves flushing accumulated debris and discharge from the conjunctival fornix and application of broad-spectrum antibiotic ointments if indicated.

SUBCONJUNCTIVAL HEMORRHAGE

Subconjunctival hemorrhage can result from trauma associated with parturition. It typically resolves in 7–10 days. No treatment is necessary. Foals with hypoxic ischemic encephalopathy (HIE) may show scleral hemorrhage, which usually resolves with resolution of the systemic disease.

NASOLACRIMAL SYSTEM

Nasolacrimal duct obstruction is rare in neonates. A negative Jones test, in which fluorescein instilled on the cornea fails to appear at the nasal puncta, may be indicative of a nasolacrimal duct obstruction. Treatment with a solution or ointment containing antibiotic and steroid is typically warranted to prevent repeated obstruction.

CORNEA

NEOVASCULARIZATION

Neovascularization of the cornea may be observed in the neonate, possibly related to corneal inflammation *in utero* that develops in response to either blood-borne or transamniotic bacterial or viral infection. The blood vessels may be superficial or deep, with the depth giving an indication of the level of the inciting process. Neovascularization is often associated with septicemia and accompanying uveitis (see p. 263[L1]) and it typically resolves with systemic improvement. Treatment is dictated by the presence of corneal ulceration and uveitis.

ULCERATIVE KERATITIS

DEFINITION/OVERVIEW

Ulcerative keratitis is common in healthy foals, as it is in any age group. In a study of neonates admitted to an intensive care facility, 21% (52/248) had ulcers. Of those, 34 of the cases resolved with medical treatment; the remaining 18 were euthanized or died for reasons other than ocular disease.

ETIOLOGY/PATHOPHYSIOLOGY

The cause of most ulcers is unknown, but possible causes include entropion and trauma. Bacterial or fungal infections are complications of corneal ulcers (**401**).

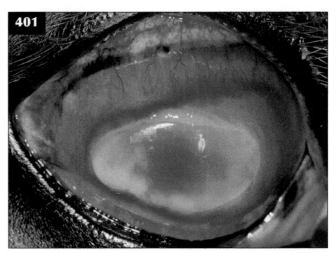

401 Fungal ulcer.

CLINICAL PRESENTATION

The clinical signs of corneal ulceration in otherwise healthy foals may include increased tear production, ocular discharge, blepharoedema, squinting, conjunctival hyperemia, corneal edema and corneal infiltrate. The clinical signs of corneal ulcers in sick neonatal foals may not be as obvious as in older foals or adults due to decreased corneal sensitivity, yet this decreased sensitivity may predispose sick neonates to ulceration and impaired healing. Often, the most easily identified sign of corneal ulceration in foals is a difference in the angle of the eyelashes, with the upper lid of the affected eye pointing down further than the unaffected eye.

DIAGNOSIS

The diagnostic workup of a corneal ulcer should include corneal cytology and culture and fluorescein staining. Often, an area that appears nonulcerated may take up stain, and one that looks like an ulcer may actually prove to be a fluorescein-negative scar.

MANAGEMENT

Infected ulcers can rapidly progress to keratomalacia (melting cornea, **402–405**), corneal rupture, and iris prolapse (**406, 407**). Therefore, any ulcer that progresses in the face of treatment should be considered an emergency. Medical treatment of corneal ulcers is based on clinical signs and cytology and culture results. Topical antibiotics, antifungals, mydriatics, anticollagenases, and systemic anti-inflammatories may all be indicated. NSAIDs should be used with caution in foals due to the risk of inducing gastric ulceration; a gastroprotectant should be administered along with the NSAID. (Chapter 5, Alimentary Tract Disorders, p. 84–86). Surgical treatment of corneal ulcers is warranted if the ulcer progresses rapidly in the face of appropriate medical therapy such that the structural integrity of the globe is at risk. Surgical options include conjunctival flaps (**408, 409**), corneal transplants for deep or full thickness lesions with missing tissue, or grafts of other biomaterials designed to support the cornea and facilitate healing (e.g., amniotic membrane).

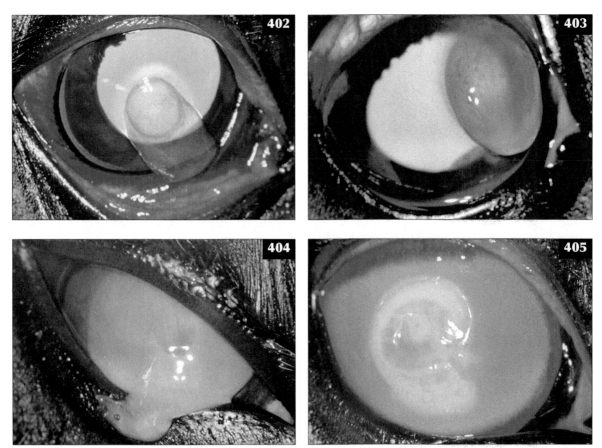

402–405 Melting ulcers. (**402**) Foals with melting corneal ulcers may appear comfortable with little appreciable uveitis. Melting is confined to a relatively small region. (**403**) In this large corneal melt, the affected cornea is very thin, with very little stroma remaining, such that the melting region is actually an outpouching filled with aqueous humor. (**404**) This melting ulcer is associated with severe diffuse corneal edema, making examination of intraocular structures difficult. The eye is painful, with a miotic pupil and hypopyon present. There is a very deep region in the center of the affected cornea, which is seen clinically as a dark spot through which a tapetal reflection can be appreciated. (**405**) This corneal ulcer shows characteristics often associated with fungal infection, including a yellow stromal infiltrate arranged in a ring with a deep furrow surrounding the more intensely yellow area, as well as dense corneal vascularization extending from the limbus axially toward the lesion.

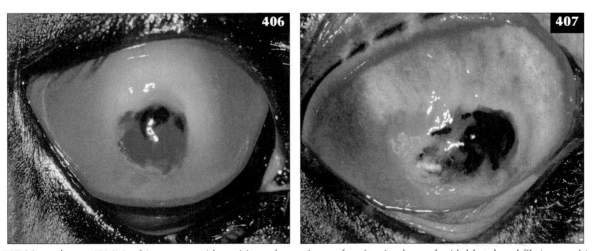

406, 407 Iris prolapse. (**406**) In this cornea with an iris prolapse the perforation is plugged with blood and fibrin, resulting in a relatively comfortable eye. Minimal vascularization is noted in the cornea, associated in this case with prior topical steroid use. (**407**) This chronically painful eye shows a large axial iris prolapse with a collapsed anterior chamber, evidenced by the presence of the iris directly apposing the corneal endothelium. The yellow color of the iris is a result of chronic uveitis in a previously blue iris.

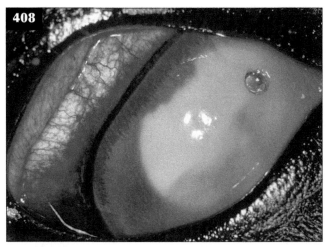

408 Deep ulcer, before conjunctival flap placed.

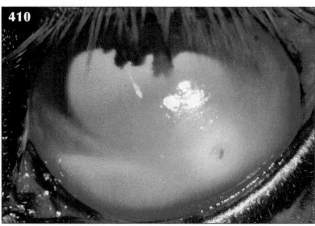

410 Corneal puncture. Fibrin and hypopyon are present in the anterior chamber of this eye with no history of trauma. A puncture wound was noted inferiotemporally. This wound was likely a micropuncture associated with environmental debris that seeded a deep infection.

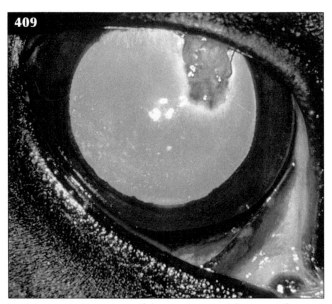

409 Postoperative view of the conjunctival flap over the fungal ulcer in the foal in **408**.

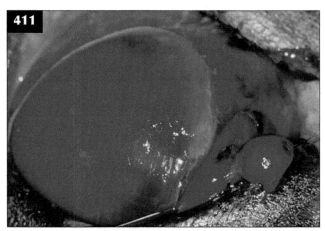

411 The limbus, which is the junction of the cornea and the sclera, is a point at which the globe may rupture when associated with blunt trauma such as that delivered by a kick.

CORNEAL TRAUMA

Corneal trauma resulting in globe perforation occurs in young foals and is associated with either blunt trauma (e.g., a kick from another mare) or sharp trauma (**410**). Blunt trauma causing globe rupture often leads to irreparable rupture at the limbus, with expulsion of the intraocular contents, but repair may be attempted. The prognosis for retention of the globe and vision following surgical repair of iris prolapse is better for wounds less than 15 mm in length and for wounds not involving or crossing the limbus (**411**). Traumatic iris prolapse carries a better prognosis for successful repair than ulcerative iris prolapse.

CORNEAL STROMAL ABSCESS

A corneal stromal abscess is a complication of corneal ulceration or trauma in the horse. Stromal abscesses may develop when epithelial cells migrate over a corneal defect and trap infectious agents or foreign bodies in the corneal stroma. Deep stromal abscesses are often fungal in origin. Stromal abscesses do not take up fluorescein stain and they typically appear as yellowish-white stromal infiltrates, with corneal edema and iridocyclitis (**412**). Initial intensive medical treatment of stromal abscesses includes topical mydriatic/ cycloplegics, topical and systemic antibiotics and NSAIDs, and topical antifungals. If significant improvement does not occur, surgical treatment in the form of a lamellar keratoplasty may be indicated.

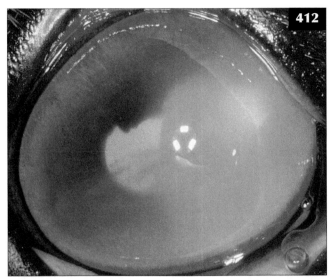

412 The faint yellow opacity in the superionasal cornea of this eye is a stromal abscess, which in this case is associated with a profound accumulation of fibrin in the anterior chamber.

IRIS

ETIOLOGY/PATHOPHYSIOLOGY

Iridocyclitis, or anterior uveitis, in neonates is most often associated with sepsis, including infection with *Salmonella* spp., *Rhodococcus equi*, *Escherichia coli*, and *Streptococcus equi* (413). Iridocyclitis often resolves when the systemic disease that underlies the condition is successfully treated.

CLINICAL PRESENTATION

Clinical signs of anterior uveitis in foals are similar to those in adults and include increased tear production, squinting, light sensitivity, corneal edema, conjunctival hyperemia, aqueous flare, hypopyon, hyphema (414), fibrin in the anterior chamber, and miosis.

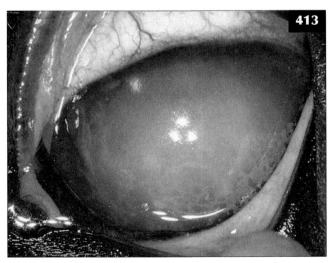

413 Profound fibrin in the anterior chamber secondary to *Rhodococcus equi* infection.

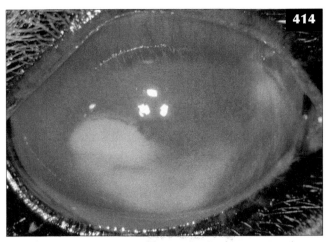

414 The massive amount of hypopyon in the anterior chamber of this eye was associated with endophthalmitis in a foal with *Rhodococcus equi* infection.

MANAGEMENT

Treatment must include directed therapy for the underlying disease (typically systemic antibiotics) and supportive treatment for the secondary anterior uveitis. This may included topical atropine and NSAIDs, as well as a systemic NSAID. If the underlying condition is immune-mediated, systemic corticosteroids may be indicated. Topical corticosteroids must not be used in the face of corneal ulceration and are potentially dangerous to use in recumbent sick animals.

LENS

LENS LUXATION

Lens luxation is a condition in which the lens is malpositioned due to the loss of zonular attachment because of malformed or ruptured lens zonules. Luxation may be anterior (in front of the iris), requiring surgical extraction to prevent corneal damage and secondary glaucoma, or posterior (into the vitreous), often requiring no treatment (415). Partial loss of zonular attachment allows the lens to shift from its normal position exposing the lens equator and

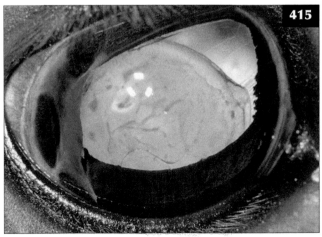

415 Lens luxation and cataract.

an aphakic crescent within the dilated pupil. Surgical extraction for anterior lens luxation requires a large corneal incision and runs the risk of severe postoperative uveitis as well as retinal detachment associated with anterior movement of the vitreous and retina. Lens luxation is often accompanied by other ocular defects and has been observed with bilateral glaucoma.

CATARACTS

DEFINITION/OVERVIEW
Cataracts are opacities in the lens, which may be inherited or acquired. In at least one report, cataracts were the most common congenital ocular defect seen in horses.

ETIOLOGY/PATHOPHYSIOLOGY
Congenital cataracts are seen sporadically in all breeds. They are seen in Rocky Mountain Horses with anterior segment dysgenesis, and have been associated with aniridia in Belgians. Congenital nuclear cataracts reported in Morgan horses were assumed to be heritable, but they occurred without other ocular defects and with no significant effect on vision.

CLINICAL PRESENTATION
Cataracts are commonly classified by stage of progression and by location within the lens. Incipient cataracts involve an insignificant portion of the lens (i.e., less than 15%) and typically do not significantly limit vision. Immature cataracts involve more than 15% but less than 100% of the lens area (**416, 417**), whereas mature cataracts involve the entire lens. Hypermature cataracts have progressed to the point that lens proteins are dissolving, causing capsular wrinkling (as the lens cortex decreases in volume) and a sparkling appearance to the lens and, possibly, resulting in an improvement in vision as a portion of the lens clears (**418**).

MANAGEMENT
The treatment for cataracts that significantly affect vision is surgical, but vision may be improved with mydriatics, when clearer areas of the lens are exposed by papillary dilation. Cataracts are often associated with some degree of lens-induced uveitis, which

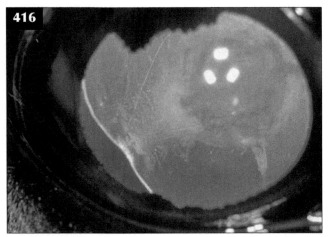

416 Immature cataract and lens coloboma.

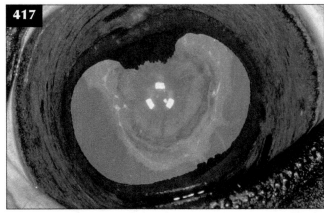

417 Immature cortical cataract.

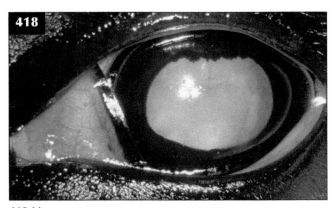

418 Hypermature cataract.

is usually treated with topical and systemic NSAIDs. Foals with mature or complete cataracts have visual disability and may be surgical candidates. A mature cataract before and after cataract surgery is shown (**419, 420**). Embryonal and fetal nuclear cataracts involve focal central opacities and are usually nonprogressive, even decreasing relatively in size as the foal grows. Cataracts may also be equatorial, floriform (or petal-shaped), or located along suture lines. While nuclear cataracts are least likely to progress and equatorial or cortical cataracts are most likely to progress, it is important to remember that all cataracts may progress.

Candidates for cataract surgery should be evaluated not only based on ocular factors (e.g., the health of the cornea and retina, the stage of progression of the cataract, and the visual status and degree of lens-induced uveitis), but also on age of the foal (particularly as related to development of the visual cortex, which requires adequate visual stimulation during a critical period of development), its temperament, its ability to be handled and treated, its systemic health, and the intended use of the foal. Foals with unilateral cataracts may or may not be good surgical candidates. It depends on how well they have adapted to unilateral vision. Taking a foal with one visual eye and one blind eye and surgically changing the blind eye into a visual but aphakic eye may not result in functional improvement in vision for that foal.

Preoperative diagnostics to increase the likelihood of vision postoperatively should include ocular ultrasonography to rule out retinal detachment and an electroretinogram to assess retinal

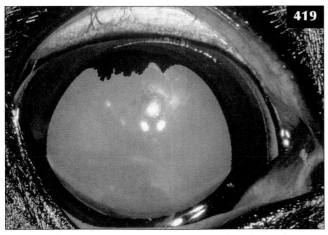

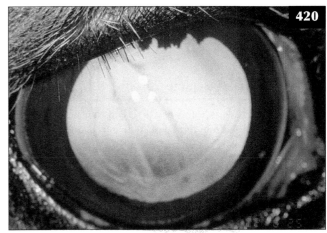

419, 420 Mature cataract. (**419**) Preoperative view of a mature congenital cataract in a Thoroughbred foal. There is minimal uveitis associated with the cataract. (**420**) Following cataract surgery, the dilated pupil (resulting from atropine administration) allows a view of the lens capsule, with a circular opacity representing the intraoperatively controlled anterior capsular tear performed to allow surgical access to the lens. Strands of vitreal fibrin can be viewed through the dilated pupil.

function. Cataracts are most commonly removed by phacoemulsification, a process by which lens material is emulsified with an ultrasonic hand piece and aspirated from inside the lens capsule.

Cataract surgery in horses is not without complication. In one study of 36 horses with 51 cataractous eyes, useful vision was restored in 30 of the horses (83%) after surgery. Reasons for poor vision in the remaining 6 horses included optic nerve atrophy, intraocular hemorrhage, posterior capsular opacities, glaucoma, and endophthalmitis. The most frequent intraoperative complication was a posterior lens capsular tear and the most frequent postoperative complication was superficial corneal ulceration. One year after surgery, 16/19 horses (84%) that had cataract surgery for which follow-up information was available were still visual, and 5 years after surgery, all 3 horses for which follow-up information was available were still visual. Overall, phacoemulsification can give good visual results, but there is more risk for complications and blindness than in other species.

Intraocular lenses have been developed for placement within the lens capsule after the cataract has been removed. These lenses are designed to leave foals emmetropic, but in foals, refraction changes as the eye elongates with age. Therefore, under correcting at the time of cataract surgery may result in emmetropia in the adult horse.

The performance of aphakic horses remains unclear, and many horses develop posterior capsular opacification at some point following cataract extraction. One study of 12 cases post phacoemulsification indicates that they perform well even though vision must be blurred due to a refractive error of +8 to 10 D.

VITREOUS

Vitritis, or hyalitis, is inflammation of the vitreous, most typically seen in septicemic foals with uveitis. Treatment, as with other manifestations of uveitis, is directed at the systemic disease and includes NSAIDs.

RETINA AND OPTIC NERVE

Some reports claim that most pathology in the equine fundus is ventral to the tapetum, and this is consistent with the phenomenon of "tapetal sparing" that has been confirmed histologically; however, this may be influenced by the ease with which lesions in this region are observed ophthalmoscopically.

RETINAL DETACHMENT

Foals with a retinal detachment (**421**) typically present with a dilated pupil, allowing observation of a veil-like retina floating in the vitreous, attached only at the optic disk. In many foals with retinal detachments the cause is unknown, but it may be

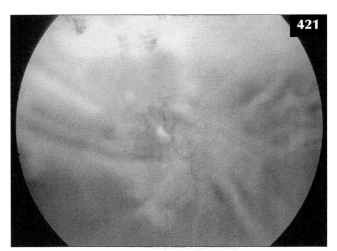

421 Retinal detachment. White streaks radiating from the axial fundus represent folds of retina formed by this completely detached retina. The view of the optic disk is obscured by the retinal folds, and the tapetum appears hyperreflective in spots.

developmental, traumatic, or inflammatory. Complete retinal detachment results in blindness. Treatment has not been reported and the prognosis for return of vision is grave.

RETINAL HEMORRHAGE

Retinal hemorrhage is a nonspecific lesion that may be associated with inflammation, retinal detachment, neoplasia, trauma (including from parturition), or a clotting disorder. It is seen in foals with HIE (dummy foal or NMS). Retinal hemorrhages can be localized by their appearance as preretinal (appearing as a keelboat), intraretinal (a dot-blot), or occurring at the nerve fiber layer (flame hemorrhages). If traumatic in origin, they are most often associated with blunt injury. Larger hemorrhages may be vitreal, arising from the uveal tract. If retinal hemorrhages are associated with inflammation, anti-inflammatory treatment should be instituted. Many retinal hemorrhages resolve without treatment. Retinal hemorrhages may take weeks to months to resolve, although in one survey all resolved within 10 days and they had no short- or long-term ocular or neurologic effects.

CHORIORETINITIS

Chorioretinitis is most often observed in foals in association with systemic disease. Acute lesions are exudative, but with time they may become bullet-hole scars, which are common in adult horses and simply indicate past inflammation. These scars may or may not significantly affect vision. Inactive lesions, or scars, have well-defined depigmented areas, often containing hyperpigmented foci. The significance of chorioretinal scars can be determined by looking for other signs of uveitis (corneal neovascularization, iris hyperpigmentation, posterior synechiae, cataract, vitritis) (**422, 423**).

RETINAL DEGENERATION

Retinal degeneration, not commonly seen in foals, appears as areas of hyperreflectivity in the tapetal fundus and depigmentation in the nontapetal fundus (**424**).

OPTIC NEURITIS

Optic neuritis is most commonly seen with uveitis and chorioretinitis. The major clinical feature that indicates optic neuritis, with or without chorioretinitis, is blindness not attributable to some other cause. Optic neuritis is usually seen in severe sepsis, may progress to endophthalmitis, and carries a grave prognosis for life. Treatment, as with other manifestations of uveitis, is anti-inflammatory, as well as directed at resolution of systemic disease.

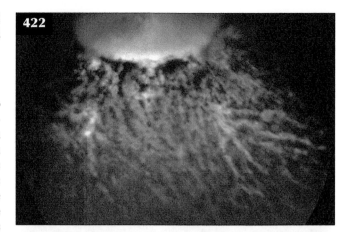

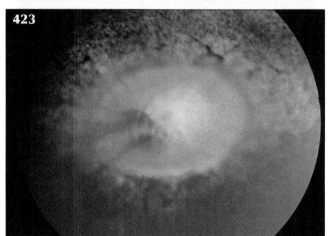

422, 423 Chorioretinitis. (**422**) Streaks of intense white sclera can be seen through the degenerated retina, surrounded by hyperpigmented areas. Depigmentation surrounded by hyperpigmentation is a characteristic associated with chronic chorioretinitis. (**423**) "Pigment bars" (or clumps of pigment associated with chronic chorioretinitis) can be seen in both the tapetal and nontapetal fundus in this eye.

TRAUMA

Head trauma can result in acute blindness, but fundic lesions may not be detected if damage to the optic nerve is retrobulbar. Optic nerve damage may lead to atrophy (**425**). Foals that have sustained head trauma will often present with bilaterally dilated pupils and blindness, and initially the optic nerve will look normal. If nerve damage is severe, the optic nerve will become atrophied in appearance and blindness will be permanent. Without or without traumatic lesions, acutely blind foals that have potentially sustained head trauma should be treated aggressively with anti-inflammatories (including NSAIDs and steroids).

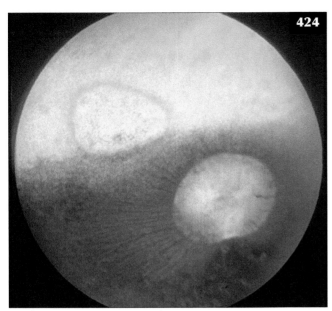

424 Focal retinal degeneration. The focal region of tapetal hyperreflectivity located just dorsal to the tapetal–nontapetal junction in the tapetal fundus of this eye, which is approximately one disk diameter in size, was noted following cataract surgery and was potentially associated with phototoxicity induced by the operating microscope.

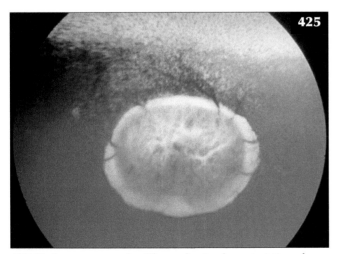

425 Optic nerve atrophy. Three classic characteristics of retinal degeneration (optic nerve atrophy, retinal vascular attenuation, and tapetal hyperreflectivity) can be seen in this fundus.

FURTHER READING

Barsotti G, et al. (2013) Ocular abnormalities in healthy Standardbred foals. *Veterinary Ophthalmology* 16(4): 245–250.

Beech J, Zappala RA, Smith G, et al. (2003) Schirmer tear tests in horses and ponies. *Veterinary Ophthalmology* 6: 251–254.

Brooks DE (2007) Equine ophthalmology. In: *Veterinary Ophthalmology*, 4th ed. (Gelatt KN, Ed.). Blackwell Publishing, London, UK, pp. 1165–1274.

Brooks DE, Clark CK, Lester GD (2000) Cochet-Bonnet aesthesiometer-determined corneal sensitivity in neonatal foals and adult horses. *Veterinary Ophthalmology* 3: 133–137.

Crispin SM (2000) Developmental anomalies and abnormalities of the equine iris. *Veterinary Ophthalmology* 3: 93–98.

Czerwinski SL, Brooks DE (2014) How to diagnose and treat common ophthalmic diseases in the neonatal foal. In *AAEP Proceedings*, vol. 60, pp. 26–31.

Enzerink E (1998) The menace response and pupillary light reflex in neonatal foals. *Equine Veterinary Journal* 30: 546–548.

Joyce JR, Martin JE, Storts RW, et al. (1990) Iridial hypoplasia (aniridia) accompanied by limbic dermoids and cataracts in a group of related Quarter Horses. *Equine Veterinary Journal* 22: 26–28.

Labelle AL, et al. (2011) Ophthalmic lesions in neonatal foals evaluated for nonophthalmic disease at referral hospitals. *Journal of the American Veterinary Medical Association* 239(4): 486–492.

Leiva M, Peña T, Monreal L (2011) Ocular findings in healthy newborn foals according to age. *Equine Veterinary Education* 23(1): 40–45.

Leiva M, et al. (2010) Uveal inflammation in septic newborn foals. *Journal of Veterinary Internal Medicine* 24(2): 391–397.

Leiva M, Pena T (2017) Ophthalmic diseases of foals. In *Equine Ophthalmology*, 3rd ed. (Gilger BC, Ed.). Wiley Blackwell, Hoboken, NJ, pp. 112–150.

Millichamp NJ, Dziezyc J (2000) Cataract phacofragmentation in horses. *Veterinary Ophthalmology* 3: 157–164.

Munroe G (1997) Congenital ocular disease. In: *Current Therapy in Equine Medicine*, 4th ed. (Robinson NE, Ed.). WB Saunders, Philadelphia, PA, pp. 355–359.

Munroe G (2000) Survey of retinal haemorrhages in neonatal thoroughbred foals. *Veterinary Record* 146: 95–101.

Munroe G (2000) Study of the hyaloid apparatus in the neonatal thoroughbred foal. *Veterinary Record* 146: 579–584.

Ramsey DT, Ewart SL, Render JA, et al. (1999) Congenital ocular abnormalities of Rocky Mountain Horses. *Veterinary Ophthalmology* 2: 47–59.

Timney B, Macuda T (2001) Vision and hearing in horses. *Journal of the American Veterinary Medical Association* 218: 1567–1574.

Turner AG (2004) Ocular conditions of neonatal foals. *Veterinary Clinics of North America: Equine Practice* 20: 429–440.

Wilkes EJA, et al. (2015) Successful management of multiple extra-pulmonary complications associated with *Rhodococcus equi* pneumonia in a foal. *Equine Veterinary Education* 28(4): 186–192.

Dermatologic Disorders 14

William V. Bernard

INTRODUCTION

Although not common, there are numerous congenital and developmental skin conditions that can affect the foal. Many of these conditions are rare; however, they can be catastrophic when present. Congenital conditions are present at birth, but developmental conditions may progress from as early as a few days of age. Foal skin diseases may be self-limiting, respond to therapy, or be life threatening. Congenital conditions may be genetically influenced. Developmental conditions in the newborn foal are primarily immune mediated or allergic. Infectious diseases, parasitic diseases, nutritional conditions, and insect bites/allergies can all affect the pediatric equine patient. The reader should consult a more detailed dermatologic text for information regarding the numerous etiologies and therapies of equine skin disease.

CYSTS

KEY POINTS
- Cysts are fluctuant or firm, usually nonpainful swellings.
- Cysts can be developmental or congenital.
- The majority of cysts are found on the head region.
- Cytology may be useful diagnostically.
- Histopathology is diagnostic.
- Surgical removal is usually possible.

DEFINITION/OVERVIEW
Various forms of cysts are seen in the foal as congenital or developmental conditions. These include epidermoid, dermoid, dentigerous, and conchal cysts. These cysts appear as swellings that are usually nonpainful and may or may not be fistulated. Cysts are classified according to their location. There is no breed predilection.

ETIOLOGY/PATHOPHYSIOLOGY
Cysts may be present at birth (congenital) or develop over time (developmental) and likely result from abnormal location of germinal tissue. Dentigerous cysts arise from germinal tooth tissue. Dermoid cysts are thought to be a result of displacement of ectoderm into the subcutis.

CLINICAL PRESENTATION
Epidermoid cysts, also known as atheromas or nasal inclusion cysts, are solitary, firm to fluctuant, freely moveable nodules that most typically occur in the head region. The most common location is at the distal limit of the false nostril. Epidermoid cysts may remain unchanged over time. They contain fluid that ranges from a clear yellow to a thin cheesy appearance.

Dermoid cysts are cutaneous cysts that are most commonly identified on the dorsal midline. They may contain hair, are often cheesy in consistency, and may be individual or multiple.

Dentigerous cysts (426) are usually found between the ear and the eye, but can occasionally be found in a sinus cavity. They may have a fluidy persistent discharge. There can be remnants of dental tissue associated with a dentigerous cyst. The dental tissue remnant may be fixed or freely moveable.

Conchal cysts are located at the base of the ear and may be fistulated, with the fistula involving the pinna of the ear (lower one-third). These cysts are not of germinal tooth tissue origin.

DIFFERENTIAL DIAGNOSIS
The differential list includes a variety of conditions that can cause swelling anywhere on the patient's body (*Table 72*).

DIAGNOSIS
Diagnosis of the various cysts is based clinically on the typical location and by ruling out other possible conditions. The diagnosis can be supported by determination of cell types when aspirates are feasible. Inflammatory cells indicate an infectious process. Identification of stratified squamous epithelial cells suggests a dermoid cyst; the dermoid cyst is lined with keratinized epithelium. Histopathology may confirm diagnosis of a cyst. The dental tissue of dentigerous cysts may be identified radiographically or ultrasonographically.

MANAGEMENT
Surgical removal of the cyst and fistula (if present) is the appropriate therapy. This can be a difficult procedure when treating a dentigerous cyst (427).

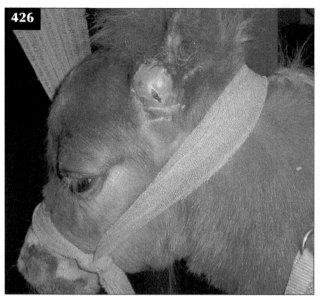

426 Dentigerous cyst (below and in front of the base of the ear) in a 4-week-old foal.

Table 72. Differential list for when a cyst is being considered as the cause of a swelling on the skin

- Foreign body reaction
- Sarcoid
- Hypodermiosis
- Other cystic structures
- Abscess
- Neoplasia
- Chronic fistulas
- Otitis (conchal cysts)

HYPOTRICHOSIS

KEY POINTS
- Hypotrichosis is a lack of, or thinning, of hair.
- Most common in the Arabian breed.
- Most common around the eyes and muzzle.

DEFINITION/OVERVIEW
Hypotrichosis is a permanent thinning (or lack) of hair in various areas of the body. The condition is most common in the Arab breed and is most common around the eyes or muzzle.

ETIOLOGY/PATHOPHYSIOLOGY
Hypotrichosis appears to be hereditary in the Arab breed. A congenital lack of hair in other breeds (Percheron foal) is rare, but may be seen in patchy locations. The etiology is unknown. Hypotrichosis is not associated with hair color.

CLINICAL PRESENTATION
A lack of hair, or a thinning of hair, particularly around the eyes and muzzle (**428**).

DIFFERENTIAL DIAGNOSIS
Deficiencies and excess of micronutrients in the diet can result in chronic hair loss.

DIAGNOSIS
Skin biopsy identifies absent or reduced hair follicles.

MANAGEMENT
None, as the condition involves an absence or reduction in the number of hair follicles.

---

427 Intraoperative appearance of the dentigerous cyst shown in **426**.

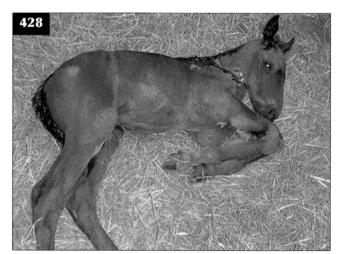

428 Severe Hypotrichosis with hair loss/thinning over large parts of the body in a 3- to 4-week-old foal.

EPIDERMOLYSIS BULLOSA

KEY POINTS
- Most common in the Belgian breed.
- Lesions may be seen at birth.

DEFINITION/OVERVIEW
Epidermolysis bullosa is a mechanobullous disease. It is seen in the Belgian breed and, rarely, in non-Belgian breeds. In other breeds it is considered a differential for other bullous diseases.

CLINICAL PRESENTATION
Mild trauma results in blister formation. Involvement of muco-cutaneous junctions, oral mucosa, and other regions of the body (particularly the limbs) may be seen at birth.

DIFFERENTIAL DIAGNOSIS
Other conditions to be considered include bullous pemphigoid, pemphigus foliaceus, and sepsis.

DIAGNOSIS
Diagnosis is based on histopathology.

MANAGEMENT
No treatment is available.

HYPERELASTOSIS CUTIS/EHLERS-DANLOS-LIKE SYNDROME (EDLS)

KEY POINTS
- Is an inherited defect of connective tissue.
- Clinically appears as loose, wrinkly, fragile skin.
- A condition of the Quarter and other horse breeds.

DEFINITION/OVERVIEW
Hyperelastosis is a disease of Quarter horses and other breeds involving connective tissue. It is an inherited autosomal reces-sive trait in the Quarter and has been named hereditary equine regional dermal asthenia (HERDA). In other breeds similar EDLS has been identified. These include the Thoroughbred, draft horse Arabians and Warmbloods. In Warmbloods the condition is called Warmblood fragile foal syndrome (WFFS).

ETIOLOGY/PATHOPHYSIOLOGY
Ehlers-Danlos syndrome, HERDA, and WFFS have been asso-ciated with an inherited genetic disorder. The genetic mutation results in an inherited decrease in connective tissue (collagen) with fiber fragmentation and disorientation.

CLINICAL PRESENTATION
Affected areas vary in appearance from loose, wrinkly skin to fragile, easily damaged skin (skin hyperelasticity) and loss of hoof capsule. Infections may ensue. Skin repair is slow and scar formation is frequent. Lesions may be seen on the back, flanks, shoulders, and legs. Scar formation and poor skin healing may be noted. The condition may result in *in-utero* embryonic loss or abortion.

DIAGNOSIS
Histopathology has not been well documented. Various changes in the dermis and collagen are noted. Genetic testing is available for confirmation of both HERDA and WFFS.

MANAGEMENT
Treatment involves minimizing trauma and undertaking wound management when necessary.

EPITHELIOGENESIS IMPERFECTA

KEY POINTS
- An inherited lack of epidermis (skin).
- Presents clinically as patches of skin loss.
- Most commonly seen in the limbs.

DEFINITION/OVERVIEW
Epitheliogenesis imperfecta is a cutaneous defect, likely inherited, which presents as a lack of skin. The condition is rare.

ETIOLOGY/PATHOPHYSIOLOGY
There is an inherited lack of epidermis.

CLINICAL PRESENTATION
The condition presents as areas of complete loss of epidermis that can be seen in any body region, but are most common on the appendages and particularly distal to the carpi and tarsi. Infection, accompanied by septicemia and hemorrhage, is a common sequela.

DIAGNOSIS
Diagnosis is based on the typical loss of skin, which is unlike other skin diseases. Biopsy can confirm the lack of epidermis.

MANAGEMENT
Grafting or primary closure may be useful in small defects. Larger defects result in a guarded prognosis.

PEMPHIGUS FOLIACEUS

KEY POINTS
- Pemphigus foliaceus is an immune-mediated skin disease with cell separation at the level of the dermis.
- Vesicles may be followed by crusting, scaling, and exudation.
- Head, neck, and limbs are frequently involved.

DEFINITION/OVERVIEW
The skin of the foal, as in the adult horse, can be influenced by immune-mediated inflammatory lesions. Numerous lesions/diseases such as urticaria, atopy, pemphigus, vasculitis, alopecia, drug contact, insect hypersensitivities, and folliculitis can be seen in the pediatric patient. The reader is referred to other texts for detailed descriptions of these diseases. Pemphigus foliaceus is an immune-mediated disease that can be observed in the neonate.

ETIOLOGY/PATHOPHYSIOLOGY
Pemphigus foliaceus is an autoimmune disease. Autoantibodies are produced against intercellular aspects (cement) of the epidermis.

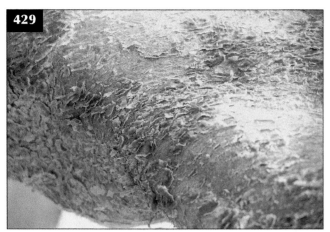

429 Pemphigus foliaceus in a foal.

This type II hypersensitivity mechanism results in cell separation (acantholysis) at the level of the epidermis.

CLINICAL PRESENTATION

There may be early pustule and vesicle formation. This is followed by crusting, scaling, and exudation (**429**). The head, neck and limbs are often involved. Some patients may have only coronary band involvement. Edema may be associated with areas of crusting and scaling.

DIFFERENTIAL DIAGNOSIS

Dermatophytosis, dermatophilosis, bacterial folliculitis, vasculitis, and hypersensitivities may appear clinically similar to pemphigus foliaceus.

DIAGNOSIS

Other skin conditions that are similar in appearance are more common in the adult than in the foal, therefore a scaling/crusting disease in the foal should be highly indicative of pemphigus foliaceus. Biopsy is the diagnostic test of choice; histopathology changes are definitive. Direct immunofluorescence with deposition of immunoglobulin G (IgG) in intracellular spaces presumes a diagnosis. The clinician should be cautioned that false-negative and false-positive results have been seen.

MANAGEMENT

The juvenile form of pemphigus foliaceus is usually successfully treated and may be self-limiting. Steroid therapy with either prednisolone or dexamethasone has been used as the therapy of choice (prednisolone at 1–2 mg/kg or dexamethasone at 0.1 mg/kg p/o q24h or q12h). The dosage can then be progressively decreased depending on response to therapy. Long-term, low-dose therapy of several weeks duration may be necessary.

ULCERATIVE DERMATITIS/ THROMBOCYTOPENIA

DEFINITION/OVERVIEW

Recently, a syndrome that includes ulcerative dermatitis, thrombocytopenia, and neutropenia has been reported. The syndrome occurs in neonates and has responded to therapy. Clinical signs of thrombocytopenia are often present. Infection (septicemia) may be present, but it may not be a primary entity. The condition has repeated in one mare's offspring.

ETIOLOGY/PATHOPHYSIOLOGY

The precise etiology/pathophysiology has not been determined. Colostrum antiplatelet antibodies or some other factor in colostrum are suspected as the possible cause. This is supported by the fact that one mare who had produced two affected foals did not produce a third when colostrum was withheld. The skin lesions may be related to the fact that antibody is directed against vascular or dermal structures or to antigen–antibody deposition.

CLINICAL PRESENTATION

Thrombocytopenia is recognized clinically as petechiation and/or ecchymosis or bleeding tendencies. The ulcerative dermatitis is most commonly identified at cutaneous junctions (i.e., mouth, eyes, anus). Lingual ulcerations have been reported. The dermatitis can be seen in parts of the trunk or neck. The thrombocytopenia may be severe. A neutropenia is usually seen in conjunction with the thrombocytopenia and dermatitis and clinical signs of septicemia may be present.

DIFFERENTIAL DIAGNOSIS

The differential diagnosis would include other causes of thrombocytopenia (see Chapter 4, Immunologic and Hematologic Disorders, p. 71) or similar lesions. Pemphigus foliaceus would be the primary skin lesion to consider.

DIAGNOSIS

The combination of skin lesions with a thrombocytopenia is suggestive of the condition. Histopathology of the skin lesions has revealed dermal hemorrhage, epidermal clefting, and superficial papillary necrosis. Testing for platelet antibodies should be considered.

MANAGEMENT

If thrombocytopenia is severe, or is associated with bleeding tendencies, then treatment with platelet-rich plasma or whole blood may be required. Corticosteroids (see Chapter 17, Pharmacology, p. 297) can be used until platelet counts return to normal. In some cases, prolonged therapy may be necessary. Broad-spectrum antimicrobial therapy is warranted as secondary infection is possible.

FURTHER READING

Giguere S, Polkes AC (2005) Immunologic disorders in neonatal foals. *Veterinary Clinics of North America: Equine Practice* 21: 241–272.

Monthoux C, de Brot S, Jackson M, et al. (2015) Skin malformations in a neonatal foal homozygous for Warmblood fragile foal syndrome. *BMC Veterinary Research* 11: 12.

Rees CA (2004) Disorders of skin. In: *Equine Internal Medicine* (Reed SM, Bayly WM, Sellin DS, Eds.). WB Saunders, Philadelphia, PA, pp. 667–720.

Endocrine and Metabolic Disorders

William V. Bernard

15

HYPOCALCEMIA

KEY POINTS

- Calcium plays a critical role in numerous physiologic functions; however, clinical signs of hypocalcemia are related to the musculoskeletal and/or nervous system.
- Hypocalcemia is a medical emergency that can be life threatening.
- The most likely causes of hypocalcemia in the foal are primary hypoparathyroidism or a failure of renal reabsorption of calcium.
- The clinical signs of hypocalcemia can be variable; however, typically there is a tetany with abnormal facial expressions/trismus, muscle spasms/fasciculations, hyperhidrosis, and/or synchronous diaphragmatic flutter.
- Diagnosis is based on measurements of serum total or ionized calcium.
- Serum ionized calcium is a more precise indicator of hypocalcemia.
- Slow intravenous administration of calcium is the treatment of choice.

DEFINITION/OVERVIEW

Hypocalcemia is not a common abnormality in the foal; however, calcium plays a vital role in numerous cell functions including membrane excitability, muscle contraction, hormone release, bone formation, enzyme activity, and blood coagulation. Clinical signs of hypocalcemia are typically related to the musculoskeletal and/or nervous system. Hypocalcemia is an uncommonly diagnosed metabolic disorder. The condition is more commonly seen in adults than in foals. Hypocalcemia can be exacerbated by metabolic or electrolyte abnormalities. Respiratory or metabolic alkalosis alters the protein binding of calcium. In the presence of alkalosis, clinical signs of hypocalcemia may be present, with low normal calcium values. Clinically, the initial presentation of a foal with hypocalcemia can be difficult to differentiate from other conditions. Hypocalcemia is a metabolic emergency that can be life threatening.

ETIOLOGY/PATHOPHYSIOLOGY

The causes of hypocalcemia that must be considered include dietary deficiency, inadequate absorption from the gastrointestinal (GI) tract, primary hypoparathyroidism, parathyroid hormone (PTH) resistance, chronic renal or liver disease, failure of renal reabsorption of calcium, pancreatitis, and toxicosis such as blister beetle toxicosis (*Table 73*).

Dietary deficiency can be ruled out in the suckling foal if milk production is adequate. It is considered rare to impossible for milk to contain insufficient quantities of absorbable calcium. Failure of calcium absorption has not been documented in the foal. The causes of hypocalcemia in the foal are most likely either primary hypoparathyroidism (inadequate levels of circulating PTH) or a failure of renal reabsorption of calcium. Hypoparathyroidism has been suggested to occur in foals with low PTH values and in which necropsy has failed to identify parathyroid tissue. Parathyroid tissue can be difficult to identify, therefore its absence is not conclusive of hypoparathyroidism. A renal tubular receptor abnormality has been documented in humans. In this condition, PTH fails to act through the receptor site to stimulate reabsorption of calcium and calcium is excreted (lost) in the urine in the face of peripheral hypocalcemia. This defect has not been documented in the horse; however, cases of hypocalcemia (in foals) have been seen with normal PTH levels and increased fractional excretion of calcium, suggesting a failure of renal response to PTH.

Ionized calcium is the metabolically active fraction of calcium. Ionized calcium is highly protein bound and the protein binding of calcium is highly influenced by acid–base status. Alkalosis can significantly increase the protein binding of calcium to a point where, in combination with marginal calcium values, clinical signs of hypocalcemia may be seen. The causes of alkalosis may be respiratory or metabolic. Examples of respiratory alkalosis include the

---

Table 73. Causes of hypocalcemia

- Dietary deficiency
- Inadequate absorption
- Primary hypoparathyroidism
- Parathyroid hormone resistance
- Chronic renal or liver disease
- Failure of renal reabsorption of calcium
- Pancreatitis
- Toxicosis, blister beetle

430

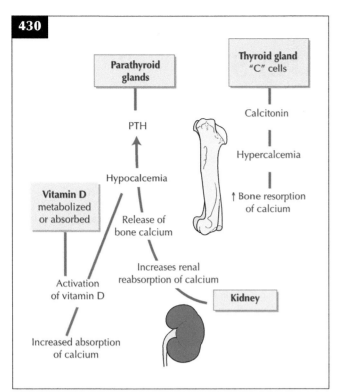

430 Schematic diagram illustrating the mechanism of calcium homeostasis.

431

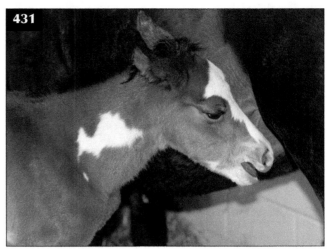

431 Foal with hypocalcemia showing an abnormal facial expression, trismus, and a sardonic grin.

tachypnea/hyperventilation of pain, heat and/or humidity, and excessive exercise. An example of metabolic alkalosis is excessive losses of gastric fluid contents (reflux). Excessive exogenous bicarbonate therapy can result in an iatrogenic alkalosis. Electrolyte abnormalities (hypokalemia/hypochloremia) can contribute to, or accompany, hypocalcemia. Excessive sweat loss can also result in such electrolyte abnormalities.

Calcium homeostasis is highly integrated via calcitonin, PTH, and vitamin D (**430**). PTH is produced in the two pairs of parathyroid glands. Calcitonin is produced in the "C" cells of the thyroid. Vitamin D is ingested or produced *in vivo*. Calcitonin responds to hypercalcemia through increased bone deposition of calcium. Vitamin D increases GI absorption of calcium. Parathyroid hormone responds to hypocalcemia through influences on bone metabolism, kidney reabsorption, and intestinal absorption. PTH causes release of bone calcium, decreases renal excretion (promotes reabsorption), and activates vitamin D.

CLINICAL PRESENTATION

The neurologic component of hypocalcemic tetany includes primarily tonic spasms; however, the signs can be variable and include increased muscle tone, a stiff stilted gait, hindlimb ataxia, seizures, muscle fasciculations, trismus, abnormal facial expressions (grimace or sardonic grin) (**431**), anxiety, sweating, tachypnea with flared nostrils, dyspnea, laryngospasm, fever, hypomotility, normal pupillary light reflex, tachycardia, synchronous diaphragmatic flutter, cardiac arrhythmias, convulsions, coma, and death (*Table 74*). Handling or excitement may exacerbate signs; loud noises do not.

Table 74. Clinical signs of hypocalcemia

- Tetany or tonic spasms
- Increased muscle tone
- Stiff/stilted gait
- Ataxia
- Muscle fasciculations
- Trismus
- Abnormal facial expressions (grimace or sardonic grin)*
- Anxiety
- hyperhidrosis*
- Tachypnea
- Tachycardia
- Flared nostrils
- Synchronous diaphragmatic flutter*
- Dyspnea
- Laryngospasm
- Fever
- Hypomotility
- Normal pupillary light reflex
- Cardiac arrhythmias
- Convulsion
- Coma
- Death

* These signs are highly suggestive of hypocalcemia.

DIFFERENTIAL DIAGNOSIS

A very large list of differentials (*Table 75*) must be considered when faced with the array of clinical signs mentioned in the preceding section. Neuromuscular disease (tetanus, tick paralysis), colic, musculoskeletal disorders, pheochromocytoma, and other electrolyte abnormalities must be considered.

DIAGNOSIS

The presence of facial trismus or grimace, hyperhydrosis, and/or synchronous diaphragmatic flutter is highly suggestive of hypocalcemia.

Diagnosis is based on identification of a serum total calcium concentration of <2 mmol/L (8 mg/dL) or, more accurately, a serum ionized calcium concentration of <1.0–1.25 mmol/L (4–5 mg/dL). These values may vary depending on laboratory reference values. Serum total calcium is dependent on serum total protein. Extracellular calcium is divided into two fractions: non-diffusible (protein bound) and diffusible. Diffusible extracellular calcium is an ionic state or complexed with other molecules such as citrate, carbonate, or phosphate. Neuromuscular activity is responsive only to the ionized fraction, which diffuses across cell membranes. The ionized fraction is approximately 50% of the total plasma calcium. When assessing calcium-related disorders, the ionized fraction should be evaluated as it is this fraction that is related to clinical signs. When evaluating calcium status, other metabolic conditions such as acid–base status and serum protein must be considered. Alkalosis decreases the solubility of calcium salts; therefore, an alkalotic horse could show signs of hypocalcemia with normal total serum calcium, increased protein-bound fraction, and a low ionized fraction. Additionally, in conditions of hypoproteinemia, the protein-bound calcium fraction is lower, with a normal ionized fraction and low total serum calcium.

Once hypocalcemia has been documented, then PTH and the activated forms of vitamin D (cholecalciferol) can be measured to assess the presence of PTH and its role in the activation of vitamin D. Availability of this testing is limited. Interpretation of results is difficult due to the lack of normal information. Determination of urinary excretion of calcium (fractional excretion) evaluates the role of renal reabsorption in hypocalcemic states. Possible contributions of liver or renal disease can be evaluated with complete blood chemistries.

MANAGEMENT

A slow intravenous administration of intravenous calcium is the treatment of choice for acute episodes of hypocalcemia. Standard commercial solutions of calcium are generally 20% solutions. Infusion of 0.5–1.0 mL/kg is usually sufficient to ameliorate signs of hypocalcemia. Monitoring heart rate and rhythm during infusions is recommended. An additional dose of 0.5–1.0 mg/kg may be necessary to resolve acute hypocalcemia. Continued treatment is necessary if the underlying problem is not resolved. PTH, oral calcium, or vitamin D supplementation has not been successful in the treatment of idiopathic cases of persistent progressive hypocalcemia in foals.

HYPOTHYROIDISM

KEY POINTS

- Thyroid dysfunction in foals is uncommon.
- The presence of goiter (palpable thyroid hyperplasia) in the absence of other clinical signs does not include hypo- or hyperthyroidism.
- The two recognized but poorly defined syndromes of hyperthyroidism are metabolic syndrome and multiple congenital musculoskeletal disorders.
- Clinical presentation includes weakness, hypothermia, musculoskeletal disorders, and goiter.
- The diagnosis is problematic.
- Individual measurements of thyroid values are reliable.
- Response to stimulation tests is variable.
- Treatment includes supportive care with thyroid supplementation when hypothyroidism has been documented.
- The prognosis is poor/guarded, particularly when musculoskeletal defects are present.

DEFINITION/OVERVIEW

The thyroid hormones thyroxin (T_4) and triiodothyronine (T_3) are involved in cellular growth and metabolism. These hormones regulate growth and energy metabolism *in utero* and throughout life. Thyroid dysfunction in foals is uncommon. Two "hypothyroid syndromes" have been recognized in the foal, one being a hypometabolic state and the other characterized by multiple congenital musculoskeletal disorders. Low levels of thyroid hormones are present in each syndrome. Thyroid hyperplasia (goiter) is often visibly or palpably present; however, clinically normal foals born with goiter are usually not hyperthyroid. Thyroid hormones are synthesized in the thyroid glands initially as thyroglobulin (a glycoprotein, prohormone). Thyroglobulin is stored in the thyroid gland. The thyroid gland also collects iodine from the systemic circulation and subsequently iodinates thyroglobulin to the thyroid

---

Table 75. Differential diagnosis of hypocalcemia

- Neurologic diseases causing seizures, ataxia, stiff/stilted gait, trismus, or abnormal facial expressions:
  - Spinal cord disease (stiff/stilted gait, ataxia)
  - Central nervous system disease:
    - Meningitis (fever, hyperhydrosis, trismus, abnormal facial expression, anxiety)
- Neuromuscular disease:
  - Tetanus
  - Tick paralysis
- Colic
- Electrolyte abnormalities
- Pheochromocytoma

hormones T_4, T_3, and reverse T_3 (rT_3). The T_4 and T_3 that are released into the circulation are highly protein bound (>99%). The circulating protein-bound T_3 and T_4 maintain a constant source of free (nonprotein-bound, active form) of T_3 and T_4. Circulating T_4 can also be converted to T_3 (liver metabolism). Cellular thyroid hormones influence growth/metabolism through thyroid hormone receptors and alteration of messenger RNA and protein synthesis. Blood thyroid hormone concentrations are regulated through the hypothalamic–hypophyseal–thyroid axis; thyroid stimulating hormone (TSH) and thyroid releasing factor (TRF) are integrally involved.

ETIOLOGY/PATHOPHYSIOLOGY

The neonatal hypothyroidism that is manifested as a hypometabolic state is a result of excessive iodine intake (by the mare) during gestation. It may also occur when mares are fed exclusively low-iodine feeds. In both etiologies, very low T_3 and T_4 levels are present at birth. Iodine-deficient diets eventually produce a feedback stimulation of thyroglobulin (increased thyroid gland storage of thyroglobulin) that results in thyroid hyperplasia (goiter). Iodine-excessive diets interfere (limit the generation of iodine within the thyroid gland) with the synthesis of T_3 and T_4. A resulting feedback leads to increased production of thyroglobulin and sequential hyperplasia (goiter). The mustard plant has been associated with goiter in the horse. Excessive iodine uptake has been associated with kelp supplementation. The adult is able to regulate the high iodine uptake; however, the foal is unable to regulate the high amount of iodine crossing the placental border. The fetal thyroid gland is inhibited resulting in congenital goiter and hypothyroidism. The syndrome of hypothyroidism that has been reported in Western Canada and areas of the Northern United States does not have a definitively established etiology; however, it is suspected that low or marginally available dietary iodine may be involved. These foals are born with low T_4 and T_3 levels and do not respond to stimulation testing. Mares experimentally fed endophyte-infected fescue may have a prolonged gestation and deliver foals that are dysmature and weak. These foals have low T_3 values, but normal T_4 and rT_3 values.

CLINICAL PRESENTATION

Hypothyroid metabolic disorder and the musculoskeletal syndrome can share clinical signs. Incoordination, weakness, musculoskeletal abnormalities, poor suckle, hypothermia, and goiter are typical. The more usual clinical signs with the musculoskeletal syndrome (Pacific Northwest), as the name implies, are musculoskeletal disorders; however, prolonged gestation and dysmaturity are often seen in addition to the musculoskeletal abnormalities, which include failure of tarsal or carpal cuboidal bone ossification, goiter, and mandibular prognathism. Most of these individuals are euthanized or die within the first few weeks of life.

DIFFERENTIAL DIAGNOSIS

Hypothyroidism should be considered when goiter (thyroid hyperplasia) is identified in foals with compatible clinical signs. Intrauterine growth retardation secondary to placental or other abnormalities can result in dysmature, weak foals with musculoskeletal abnormalities. Fescue toxicity can result in prolonged gestation and dysmaturity. Foals may be born with musculoskeletal defects and no other sign of hypothyroidism; the etiology of these musculoskeletal abnormalities is not known.

DIAGNOSIS

Diagnosis of hypothyroidism can be problematic as thyroid levels change rapidly and dramatically after birth and responses to stimulation tests can be very variable. Individual measurements of thyroid hormone values are not a reliable indication of hypothyroidism. There are numerous factors other than primary thyroid disease that influence thyroid hormone values including diet, age, exercise, and drug therapy. To accurately diagnose hypothyroid states, the hypothalamic–pituitary–thyroid axis must be evaluated. If the hormonal axis is normal, the patient is not considered to be primarily hypothyroid. To distinguish primary from secondary hypothyroidism, TSH concentrations should be measured. Unfortunately, commercial TSH assays are not readily available, therefore TSH or TRF stimulation tests are the definitive test of choice. The commercial availability of TSH is variable. Administration of TRF intravenously should double baseline T_3 and T_4 levels within 2–4 hours. Some authors have suggested that post stimulation T_3 measurements are more reliable than T_4 measurements.

MANAGEMENT

The treatment of hypothyroid foals is based on correction of the underlying cause when possible, correcting the mares diet if necessary. Foals born with significant musculoskeletal problems frequently do not recover. The severity of musculoskeletal abnormalities should be determined before treatment is considered. Supplementation cannot reverse permanent lesions that occurred during periods of hypothyroidism. Supportive care with adequate nutrition may be sufficient in foals born in the hypometabolic state. Oral supplementation with synthetic thyroxine (0.02 mg/kg) can be used, dosages are not well established. A combination of T_3 and T_4 should be used. Thyroid hormone levels should be monitored. Exercise restriction should be considered in foals with cuboidal bone abnormalities.

HYPOGLYCEMIA

KEY POINTS

- Hypoglycemia is a common metabolic disorder in foals.
- Low glycogen stores at birth make the neonate particularly susceptible to hypoglycemia.
- The liver plays a key role in gluconeogenesis. Foals with acute liver disease are often hypoglycemic.
- Foals with hypoglycemia may be lethargic, weak, and/or disoriented.
- Seizures secondary to hypoglycemia are more common in the older foal than the neonate.
- Diagnosis is based on finding of low blood glucose levels.
- Treatment of choice is intravenous administration of a glucose solution.

DEFINITION/OVERVIEW

Hypoglycemia (low blood glucose) is a common metabolic disorder in the neonate; it is less commonly identified in the older foal. Neonates generally have low glycogen stores and are susceptible to conditions that interrupt glucose metabolism. Hypoglycemia should be addressed rapidly as prolonged severe hypoglycemia can lead to cell damage and death. Clinical signs may vary from depression to seizures and coma.

ETIOLOGY/PATHOPHYSIOLOGY

The newborn foal, and particularly the premature foal or the foal that undergoes significant stress at birth, has limited glycogen stores and a limited gluconeogenic capacity. Perinatal stress, hypoxia, sepsis, infection, delayed standing to suckle, and inadequate milk supply or intake can increase glucose utilization in a situation where limited gluconeogenic capacity is present. These combinations of factors can result in hypoglycemia. If the hypoglycemia is pronounced/prolonged, then the hypoglycemia itself can further influence gluconeogenesis and hypoglycemia. Foals that are premature or immature may have an immaturity of metabolic pathways (enzymatic induction) contributing to hypoglycemia. Any age foal suffering from shock (involving decreased peripheral blood flow) may develop hypoglycemia. The liver plays a critical role in gluconeogenesis; hepatic disease in neonates or foals can result in marked hypoglycemia.

CLINICAL PRESENTATION

Clinical signs can vary considerably. Foals may be lethargic, depressed, weak, disoriented, or hypothermic. Affected foals may collapse, have difficulty rising or be unable to rise, and, rarely, may exhibit seizures. Seizures secondary to hypoglycemia are uncommon and are more frequent in older foals than in adults. Foals with low blood glucose levels do not invariably exhibit clinical signs of hypoglycemia.

DIFFERENTIAL DIAGNOSIS

The differential diagnosis should include a wide variety of conditions that could result in nonspecific signs of depression and weakness. Disease of the central nervous system (CNS) (see Chapter 10, Neurologic Disorders) should be considered if seizures, disorientation, or coma are present.

DIAGNOSIS

Laboratory diagnosis of hypoglycemia is based on a blood glucose level of <2.2 mmol/L (40 mg/dL) in a pre-suckle foal and <4.4 mmol/L (80 mg/dL) in a post-suckle foal. Blood glucose is most accurately determined in the laboratory; however, reagent strips (when used appropriately) can be useful and fairly accurate. Glucometers (reagent strips with a metered reading) are now readily available and inexpensive. If collected samples are to be delayed in interpretation, then red cells must be separated from serum; otherwise, collection tubes containing reagents that inhibit glycolysis (sodium citrate) should be used.

MANAGEMENT

Severe hypoglycemia can be treated with boluses of intravenous glucose, but the most efficacious therapy is a continuous intravenous infusion. Boluses of dextrose solutions can result in hyperglycemia, diuresis, potentially cerebral edema, and/or rebound hypoglycemia. An appropriate bolus solution of dextrose is 100 mL of a 10% solution. The continuous infusion dose of dextrose is 5–10 g/kg/day, or 200–400 mL/h, of a 5% solution to a 50 kg foal. When lesser volumes of fluid are required, higher concentrations of dextrose solution (10%–50%) can be used. These solutions should be infused continuously and preferably with infusion pumps or microdrip sets. Glucose therapy must be monitored frequently. Blood glucose can be evaluated by the means mentioned above. Blood glucose levels are preferably maintained at >5.6 mmol/L (100 mg/dL) and <11.1 mmol/L (200 mg/dL). The renal threshold for glucose is in the range of 11.1–13.9 mmol/L (200–250 mg/dL). Urine dipsticks can be used to monitor therapy; if glucose is present in the urine, then excessive glucose is being administered. Subsequent to treatment of hypoglycemia, the underlying factors contributing to the metabolic disorder need to be addressed.

FURTHER READING

Breuhaus B (2011) Disorders of the equine thyroid. *Veterinary Clinics of North America: Equine Practice* 27: 115–128.

Frank N, Sojka J, Messer NT (2002) Equine thyroid dysfunction. *Veterinary Clinics of North America: Equine Practice* 18: 305–320.

Johnson AL, Gilesan WF, Palmer JE (2012) Metabolic encephalopathies in foals—Pay attention to serum biochemistry panel. *Equine Veterinary Education* 24: 233–235.

Loftedt J (1997) White muscle disease of foals. *Veterinary Clinics of North America: Equine Practice* 13: 169–185.

Naylor JM (1997) Hyperkalemic periodic paralysis. *Veterinary Clinics of North America: Equine Practice* 13: 129–144.

Schwarz B, van den Hoven R (2012) Seizures in an Arabian foal due to suspected prolonged transient neonatal hypoparathyroidism. *Equine Veterinary Education* 24: 225–231.

Toribio RE (2004) Disorders of the endocrine system. In: *Equine Internal Medicine* (Reed SM, Bayly WM, Sellon DC, Eds.). WB Saunders, Philadelphia, PA, pp. 1295–1365.

Toribio RE (2011) Endocrine dysregulation in critically ill neonates. *Veterinary Clinics of North America: Equine Practice* 27: 129–147.

Neoplasia

Bonnie S. Barr

INTRODUCTION

Neoplasia is a rare clinical problem in the equine pediatric patient. There are a few reports in the literature and most of the neoplasms described in this chapter are based on these reports. Some of the information has been extrapolated from the human literature.

NASOMAXILLARY FIBROSARCOMA

KEY POINTS
- Locally invasive tumor of the upper respiratory tract (URT).
- Facial deformity or respiratory signs.
- Diagnosis is based on histopathologic evaluation.
- Surgical excision is the best treatment.

DEFINITION/OVERVIEW
A nasomaxillary fibrosarcoma can develop at an early age, even as a congenital lesion. The tumor is considered to be locally invasive and nonmetastatic.

ETIOLOGY/PATHOPHYSIOLOGY
Unknown.

CLINICAL PRESENTATION
Clinical presentation of a nasomaxillary fibrosarcoma includes facial deformity, unilateral nasal discharge, respiratory stridor, or respiratory distress.

DIFFERENTIAL DIAGNOSIS
Differential diagnosis of fluid- or tissue-dense structures in the nasal maxillary region includes cyst-like lesions, polyps, neoplasia, inflammatory or septic conditions (abscess), and progressive ethmoid hematomas.

DIAGNOSIS
Physical examination may reveal facial deformity and decreased air movement from a nostril. Radiographs of the skull reveal a soft tissue mass within the maxillary sinus. A definitive diagnosis of a fibrosarcoma is made on histopathology.

MANAGEMENT
The best treatment is surgical excision. Cytoreductive surgery was successful in one of the documented cases. If a diagnosis is made at an early stage of the tumor growth, the prognosis is good, although radiographic monitoring may need to be periodically performed.

LEUKOPROLIFERATIVE DISORDERS

KEY POINTS
- Neoplasia of the hematopoietic system.
- Includes lymphoproliferative and myeloproliferative disorders.
- Clinical signs are often vague and nonspecific.
- No effective treatment.

DEFINITION/OVERVIEW
Leukoproliferative disorders are rarely reported in horses and almost never reported in foals. These disorders can be divided into lymphoproliferative disorders and myeloproliferative disorders.

ETIOLOGY/PATHOPHYSIOLOGY
Lymphoproliferative disorders include lymphoma (lymphosarcoma), lymphocytic leukemia, and plasma cell myeloma. Myeloproliferative disorders include diseases of granulocytes, monocytes, eosinophils, erythrocytes, and megakaryocytes. Leukemia is neoplasia of one or more hematopoietic cell lines in the bone marrow, which may include the myeloproliferative and the lymphoproliferative disorders. Leukemia is characterized by the cell line of origin and the number of neoplastic cells in the peripheral blood. Lymphoma, which is also referred to as lymphosarcoma, is the most common neoplasm of the hematopoietic system and the most common malignant neoplasm in horses. (See Lymphoma/lymphosarcoma for information on lymphoma.) An eosinophilic myeloproliferative disorder has been reported in a 10-month-old colt.

CLINICAL PRESENTATION
In general, clinical signs of leukoproliferative disorders are often vague and nonspecific. The most common signs include depression, anorexia, fever, and weight loss. There may also be evidence of limb edema, petechiation, episcleral hemorrhage, or epistaxis. Often, secondary infections of body systems such as the respiratory system are present.

DIFFERENTIAL DIAGNOSIS
Differential diagnosis for lymphoproliferative disorders includes immune-mediated diseases, infectious diseases, coagulation disorders, vasculitis, septicemia, and other neoplasms.

DIAGNOSIS
Hematologic features generally include anemia, thrombocytopenia, and neutropenia. Atypical cells may be found in the peripheral

blood and frank leukemia (granulocytic, myelomonocytic, or eosinophilic) may be noted. Bone marrow aspiration or biopsy may reveal atypical ratios in the precursor cells.

MANAGEMENT
The prognosis is guarded. The only treatment is supportive.

LYMPHOMA/LYMPHOSARCOMA

KEY POINTS
- Most frequently encountered malignant neoplasm in horses.
- Classification is based on body system involved.
- Definitive diagnosis is based on histopathology.
- Cutaneous lymphoma is the only treatable form.

DEFINITION/OVERVIEW
Lymphoma, which is also referred to as lymphosarcoma, rarely occurs in the foal but it is the most frequent malignant neoplasm encountered in horses. It has been noted in an aborted fetus and in a few foals. It is a neoplasia of the lymphoid tissue with occasional involvement of the hematopoietic system. Equine lymphoma is classified into four categories on the basis of distribution: alimentary, thymic, multicentric, and cutaneous forms.

ETIOLOGY/PATHOPHYSIOLOGY
The etiology is unknown.

CLINICAL PRESENTATION
Clinical signs of alimentary lymphoma include weight loss, diarrhea, and colic. The clinical signs of thymic/thoracic lymphoma include fever, peripheral lymphadenopathy, tachypnea, and pleural effusion. Multicentric lymphoma commences in the lymph nodes and then may also invade the liver, spleen, intestine, kidney, and bone marrow; therefore, the clinical presentation depends on the degree of organ involvement and the specific organs involved. Other tissues such as the larynx, pharynx, nasal cavity, brain, spinal cord (**432, 433**), heart, ovary, and retrobulbar tissues may also be involved. Nonspecific clinical signs include ventral edema, weight loss, lymphadenopathy, intermittent fever, intermittent colic, and respiratory disease. Clinical signs of the cutaneous form include solitary or multiple, nonpainful, well-circumscribed, dermal, or subcutaneous masses (**434**). The lesions are commonly found on the shoulder, perineum, axilla, and trunk, but cutaneous lymphosarcoma lesions can develop anywhere on the integument. Recognition of cutaneous lesions should warrant an extensive examination for evidence of internal disease.

DIFFERENTIAL DIAGNOSIS
For the alimentary form, differentials include infectious diseases, inflammatory diseases, gastrointestinal (GI) parasites, and GI abscesses. For the thymic form, differentials include viral pneumonia and bacterial pneumonia. Differentials for the cutaneous form include plaques of urticaria, sarcoid, and multiple insect bite reactions.

DIAGNOSIS
Definitive diagnosis is by biopsy and histopathology of the mass or tumor or by identification of neoplastic cells in the bone marrow.

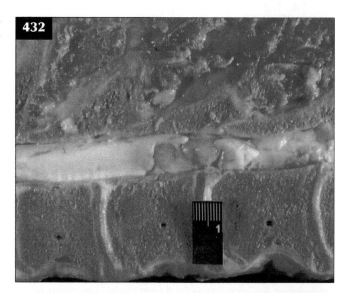

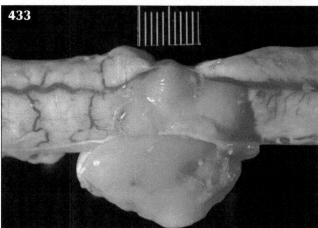

432, 433 Lymphoma. (**432**) *In-situ* spinal cord mass in a 5-month-old foal. (**433**) The spinal cord of the foal in **432** after it had been dissected out. (Courtesy of S. Reed.)

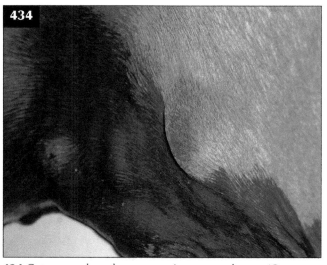

434 Cutaneous lymphosarcoma in a young horse. (Courtesy of U. Bryant.)

MANAGEMENT

The prognosis is guarded. The only treatment is supportive. Treatment for cutaneous lymphoma includes administration of systemic corticosteroids (prednisolone, 1 mg/kg q24h, or dexamethasone, 0.2–0.4 mg/kg q24h). In addition, chemotherapeutic agents such as asparaginase and cyclophosphamide have been used successfully.

MULTIPLE MYELOMA

KEY POINTS

- Involves plasma cells of the bone marrow.
- Clinical signs are vague.
- Definitive diagnosis requires examination of a bone marrow aspirate.
- Treatment with steroids and chemotherapy may prolong life.

DEFINITION/OVERVIEW

Multiple myeloma (or plasma cell myeloma) is defined as a malignant proliferation of plasma cells or lymphocytoid plasma cells that involves principally the bone marrow. Uncontrolled proliferation of a clone of B lymphocyte-derived plasma cells, which normally synthesize and secrete immunoglobulin (Ig), results in overproduction of complete Ig (monoclonal gammopathy) and Ig fragment (M protein or paraprotein). There are only a few reports of this disease in the foal.

ETIOLOGY/PATHOPHYSIOLOGY

The etiology is unknown.

CLINICAL PRESENTATION

Common clinical signs include weight loss, anorexia, fever, limb edema, lameness, and lymphadenopathy. Chronic anemia and recurrent infections are often present due to progressive bone marrow suppression. A few of the reported cases had evidence of hemorrhagic diathesis and renal failure.

DIFFERENTIAL DIAGNOSIS

Differentials to consider include bacterial infections of any organ system, other neoplasia (lymphoma), and renal failure.

DIAGNOSIS

Definitive diagnosis requires histologic examination of a bone marrow aspirate or biopsy (sternum, rib, or wing of ilium) detecting abnormal, atypical, or immature plasma cells. In addition, serum or urine monoclonal paraproteins must be identified.

MANAGEMENT

Treatment with prednisolone and chemotherapy may prolong life, but overall the prognosis is grave.

MELANOCYTIC TUMORS

KEY POINTS

- Tumors arising from melanotic cells.
- Melanocytic nevi tumors located on atypical sites of the integument.
- Diagnosis is based on histopathology.
- Several medical and surgical approaches for treatment.

DEFINITION/OVERVIEW

Melanocytic tumors are commonly reported dermal tumors that typically develop in older adults. Melanocytic tumors that affect younger animals are termed melanocytic nevi (melanocytoma), which is a term that has been adapted from the human literature. Unlike the "classic" melanocytic tumor of aged gray horses, melanocytic nevi occur in both gray and non-gray animals. In addition, they are located on atypical sites on the integument and are usually solitary, discrete, and superficial masses.

ETIOLOGY/PATHOPHYSIOLOGY

Melanocytic tumors are neoplasms arising from melanotic cells, the melanin-producing cells found within the epidermis at the epidermal–dermal junction. Melanotic cells are also found in other tissues such as the choroids, retina, ciliary processes, and meninges. The exact etiology is unknown, but in the human literature there is a report of metastatic spread of malignant melanoma to the infant *in utero*.

CLINICAL PRESENTATION

Melanocytic nevi are found on atypical sites on the integument. Common sites at which this tumor develops include the limbs, the neck, and the trunk. They are usually solitary masses located in the superficial dermis or at the dermoepidermal junction. Ulceration of the overlying epidermis is fairly common. They seldom metastasize.

DIFFERENTIAL DIAGNOSIS

A cutaneous abscess and other cutaneous neoplasms should be considered as differentials.

DIAGNOSIS

Diagnosis is based on biopsy and histopathologic examination of the cutaneous nodule.

MANAGEMENT

Small tumors may regress spontaneously and require no treatment. Otherwise, surgical excision with wide margins is necessary. If wide margins are not obtained, the tumor may recur. Cryonecrosis may be used in conjunction with surgical excision for those tumors that cannot be completely removed, although the tumors tend to regrow at sites treated with cryonecrosis. Intralesional BCG injections may cause an inflammatory response, but often are not effective. Intralesional cisplatin injections can be effective in the treatment of smaller lesions or lesions in which wide, complete margins cannot be obtained with surgical excision. More recently, implantation of cisplatin-containing biodegradable beads, with or without tumor debulking, has been found to be an effective treatment. Cimetidine has been advocated in the treatment of melanocytic tumors based on research done in humans. The antitumor activity attributable to cimetidine is associated with general enhancement of the immune system. Cimetidine (doses range from 2.5 mg/kg q8h to 1.6 mg/kg q24h) may enhance immunity by antagonizing the stimulating effect of histamine on suppressor T cells. There are variations in the response seen with cimetidine treatment. The best results have been noted with the higher dose rate and in rapidly growing tumors. The length of treatment has not been documented, but if a favorable response is not seen within 3 months, treatment should probably be discontinued. Immunomodulatory agents have been used with some success as a postsurgical treatment in the management of melanomas in humans. There are also reports that the use of a whole-cell melanoma vaccine has been successful in managing equine melanomas.

LEIOMYOSARCOMA

KEY POINTS

- Malignant tumor originating from smooth muscle.
- Clinical signs depend on organ system involved.
- Diagnosis depends on histologic examination of a biopsy specimen.
- Surgical excision is the best treatment.

DEFINITION/OVERVIEW

Leiomyosarcoma is a rare malignant tumor originating from smooth muscle. These tumors usually develop in areas that contain abundant smooth muscle, such as the reproductive tract and GI tract. They have also been detected in the retroperitoneal space, kidneys, skeletal muscle, and the head and neck region.

ETIOLOGY/PATHOPHYSIOLOGY

The etiology is unknown. It has been speculated that leiomyosarcomas of the head and neck region arise from vascular smooth muscle or undifferentiated mesenchymal cells.

CLINICAL PRESENTATION

The clinical signs depend on the organ system involved.

DIFFERENTIAL DIAGNOSIS

Differentials for leiomyosarcoma depend on the organ systems involved.

DIAGNOSIS

Definitive diagnosis is based on histologic examination of a biopsy specimen, with appropriate immunohistochemical staining.

MANAGEMENT

Surgical excision is considered the most appropriate primary treatment. Leiomyosarcomas are aggressive, with recurrence and metastasis to local lymph nodes and lungs commonly reported.

CONGENITAL ETHMOID CARCINOMA

KEY POINTS

- Aggressive tumor of the ethmoid region.
- Common clinical signs include nasal discharge and respiratory stridor.
- Endoscopy of the upper airway will identify the mass.
- Surgical removal is the best treatment.

DEFINITION/OVERVIEW

This tumor involves the ethmoid region of the nasal passages. Neoplasms of this region are often characterized by an insidious onset and are malignant. The one report in the literature is in a 4-day-old foal.

ETIOLOGY/PATHOPHYSIOLOGY

The etiology is unknown.

CLINICAL PRESENTATION

Clinical signs may include uni- or bilateral malodorous, hemorrhagic, or mucopurulent nasal discharge. Both inspiratory and expiratory stridor, with decreased airflow through the nostrils, and tachypnea may be evident. Occasionally, a cough will be present. If the lesion is extensive, facial asymmetry or deformity may be present. Due to the aggressive nature of these tumors and the local tissue destruction, secondary bacterial infections usually develop.

DIFFERENTIAL DIAGNOSIS

Differential diagnoses for an ethmoid carcinoma are progressive ethmoidal hematoma, nasal cyst, bacterial/viral rhinitis, sinusitis, and abscess.

DIAGNOSIS

Imaging of the ethmoid region is critical in differentiating ethmoid carcinoma from other conditions. Endoscopy of the upper airway will identify a mass in the ethmoid region and possibly define the extent of the mass. Radiography is very reliable in determining the size and potential additional structural involvement, such as the sinuses and septum. A definitive diagnosis is based on biopsy and histopathology of the mass.

MANAGEMENT

The best treatment is surgical removal of the mass. The prognosis is based on the size and involvement of local tissues. Overall the prognosis is guarded.

PHEOCHROMOCYTOMA

KEY POINTS

- Rare tumor involving the adrenal gland.
- Clinical signs due to overproduction of catecholamines.
- Diagnosis is difficult, therefore rule out other differentials.
- The prognosis is guarded due to rapid progression of clinical signs.

DEFINITION/OVERVIEW

Pheochromocytoma is a rare tumor involving the adrenal gland. Most reports are in adults, although a 6-month-old foal was diagnosed with a malignant tumor. These tumors may be benign or malignant and functional or nonfunctional.

ETIOLOGY/PATHOPHYSIOLOGY

The etiology is unknown. The tumor affects the adrenal medullary chromaffin cells that derive from the neuroectoderm. Functional tumors produce excessive amounts of catecholamines (norepinephrine and epinephrine). There is a report of a nonfunctional atypical tumor causing compression on the spinal cord and resulting in clinical signs.

CLINICAL PRESENTATION
Clinical signs of a functional tumor are tachycardia, colic, and apprehension. Dilated pupils, muscle tremors, and excessive sweating may also be noted. The clinical signs of a nonfunctional tumor are variable and may not be evident until the mass causes compression on the spinal cord, resulting in neurologic signs.

DIFFERENTIAL DIAGNOSIS
Differential diagnoses of a functional tumor are a mechanical or functional GI lesion and rabies. Differential diagnoses for the clinical signs noted with a nonfunctional tumor are viral/bacterial meningitis, osteomyelitis of vertebrae, a vertebral body abscess (VBA), and cervical compressive myelopathy.

DIAGNOSIS
Diagnosis can be difficult and other disorders should be ruled out. Changes in the hemogram are nonspecific and include a mature neutrophilia, a lymphopenia, and an elevated packed cell volume (PCV). Blood chemistry may show hyperglycemia, elevated creatine kinase (CK), and azotemia, all of which are nonspecific findings. Blood or urinary catecholamine levels may be diagnostic, although the results take several days to obtain. Normal catecholamine levels are known in the adult horse, but not in the pediatric patient.

MANAGEMENT
The best treatment is surgical resection and possibly use of alpha-receptor antagonists. Often, the individual has a rapid clinical course and euthanasia is the only course of action.

OSTEOSARCOMA

KEY POINTS
- Appears to be an aggressive tumor in foals.
- Lameness and facial deformity are common clinical signs.
- Definitive diagnosis is based on biopsy of the lesion.
- Surgical excision is feasible, but the tumor often returns.

DEFINITION/OVERVIEW
Osteosarcoma is a malignant tumor of bone. These tumors are predominantly found on the head, but have also been reported on the limbs and ribs. The metastatic rate is low. In two cases involving foals the condition progressed very rapidly.

ETIOLOGY/PATHOPHYSIOLOGY
The etiology is unknown, but predisposing factors may include trauma, viral agents, exposure to radiation, and genetic influences. These tumors produce unmineralized bone matrix, which may mineralize to produce new bone.

CLINICAL PRESENTATION
Clinical signs depend on the area affected, but include lameness and facial deformity.

DIFFERENTIAL DIAGNOSIS
Differential diagnoses for osteosarcoma include an abscess, osteomyelitis, septic joint, trauma, and other neoplasia.

DIAGNOSIS
Radiographs of the affected area reveal destruction of the cortex and formation of new bone in the periosteum. The margins of the lesion are not smooth and a "starburst" pattern may be noted. Biopsy is the only means of definitive diagnosis. If the mass is not easily accessible, the biopsy may need to be performed under general anesthesia.

MANAGEMENT
Treatment options are limited. The tumor usually recurs after surgical excision. Radiation therapy does not cure the condition, but it may relieve pain and retard the growth rate. Overall, the prognosis is poor.

HEPATOCELLULAR CARCINOMA

KEY POINTS
- Rare tumor of the liver.
- Clinical signs are weight loss and weakness.
- Biopsy is the only means of diagnosis.
- Prognosis is poor.

DEFINITION/OVERVIEW
Primary liver tumors are rare in horses. There are several reports of hepatocellular carcinoma in young horses (435) and even in a fetus.

ETIOLOGY/PATHOPHYSIOLOGY
The etiology is unknown, although there may be an association with exposure to environmental carcinogens such as aflatoxins.

CLINICAL PRESENTATION
Clinical signs may include weight loss, weakness, and inappetence. In one report, hemoperitoneum was noted.

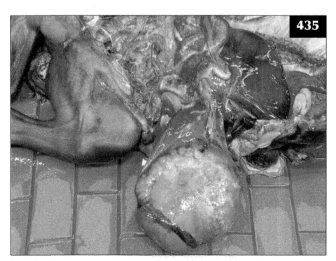

435 Hepatic tumor in a newborn foal. (Courtesy of L. Kennedy.)

DIFFERENTIAL DIAGNOSIS

Differential diagnoses for hepatocellular carcinoma include bacterial hepatitis, toxic insult to the liver, or other neoplasia (lymphoma).

DIAGNOSIS

Hematology and serum chemistry may indicate erythrocytosis, an increase in aspartate aminotransferase (AST), sorbitol dehydrogenase (SDH), and lactate dehydrogenase (LDH) levels; hyperbilirubinemia (predominantly unconjugated bilirubin); and extreme hypoglycemia. Abdominocentesis can be performed for cytologic analysis, although neoplastic cells are rarely noted. Ultrasound of the liver may be normal or reveal changes in the echogenicity of the liver or a solitary mass or multiple masses. Biopsy of the liver is the only means of an antemortem diagnosis (**178**).

MANAGEMENT

The prognosis is grave because most individuals are systemically compromised at the time of presentation. Supportive therapy may be given, including dietary management with low protein.

TERATOMA

KEY POINTS
- Tumor made up of different tissue types.
- Most commonly involve the testes.
- May be found intra-abdominal.
- Surgical removal is the treatment of choice.

DEFINITION/OVERVIEW

A teratoma is a germ cell tumor derived from pluripotential cells and made up of elements of different types of tissue from one or more of the three germ cell layers. These tumors are usually multicystic and contain bone, cartilage, glandular epithelium, nervous tissue, hair, and teeth. Teratomas are most commonly found in the testes (scrotal and cryptorchid) and are benign. There are reports of ovarian teratomas found in adults. Teratocarcinomas are very rare, but have a high rate of metastasis.

ETIOLOGY/PATHOPHYSIOLOGY

Teratomas contain only mature germ cell tissue; teratocarcinomas are composed of both mature and primitive germ cell tissue.

CLINICAL PRESENTATION

An enlarged testis may be noted on physical examination, although a teratoma may not be noted until the colt is due to be castrated. It is possible that the presence of the tumor may prevent normal descent of the testes. One case report describes signs of abdominal discomfort with an abdominal testicular teratoma due to obstruction of the small colon.

DIFFERENTIAL DIAGNOSIS

Differentials for a teratoma should include abscess and other tumors.

DIAGNOSIS

A teratoma can be definitively diagnosed on biopsy and histopathologic evaluation. The location of the tumor and the

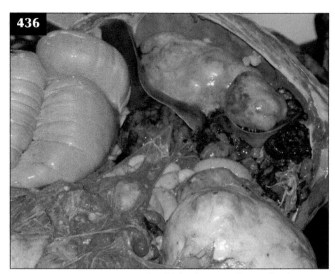

436 Teratoma in a 9-month-old foal. Note the multiple abdominal masses. (Courtesy of L. Kennedy).

presence of multiple tissue types may lead to a tentative diagnosis (**436**). A transabdominal ultrasound may reveal an intra-abdominal mass.

MANAGEMENT

The treatment of choice is complete surgical removal. Teratomas are normally well encapsulated and noninvasive to surrounding tissues. There have been reports of recurrence after removal, but this is rare.

HAMARTOMA

KEY POINTS
- A benign tumor, which can be found in different organs.
- Results from abnormal formation of normal tissue.
- Often asymptomatic.
- Diagnosis is based on biopsy.

DEFINITION/OVERVIEW

A hamartoma is a benign tumor of an organ composed of tissue elements normally found at that site, but that are growing in a disorganized mass. They occur in different parts of the body and are most often asymptomatic and undetected unless seen on an image taken for another reason. In the literature there are reports of an ovarian interstitial cell hamartoma, a pulmonary hamartoma, and a vascular hamartoma in a foal.

ETIOLOGY/PATHOPHYSIOLOGY

Hamartomas result from an abnormal formation of normal tissue, although the underlying reasons for the abnormality are not fully understood. They grow along with, and at the same rate as, the organ from whose tissue they are made and, unlike cancerous tumors, only rarely invade or compress surrounding structures significantly. Hamartomas are benign, but can cause problems due to their location; they may partially obstruct any organ in the body.

CLINICAL PRESENTATION

Hamartomas are often asymptomatic and can be incidental findings. However, if certain organ systems are involved (e.g., the lungs), clinical signs may be present.

DIFFERENTIAL DIAGNOSIS

Differential diagnosis for hamartoma includes an abscess and other tumors.

DIAGNOSIS

Definitive diagnosis is based on the results of a biopsy and histopathologic evaluation. Hamartomas may be noted on ultrasound performed for another reason, but the diagnosis can only be based on biopsy.

MANAGEMENT

Surgical resection is the treatment of choice, although it may not be a choice if the mass involves the lung.

HEMANGIOMA

KEY POINTS

- A benign skin tumor.
- Originates from endothelial cells.
- Diagnosis is based on histopathologic evaluation.
- Surgical resection is the best treatment.

DEFINITION/OVERVIEW

A hemangioma is a benign skin lesion. There have been several reports in the literature of the occurrence in young horses. Hemangioma is the most common benign tumor of human infants.

ETIOLOGY/PATHOPHYSIOLOGY

The tumor originates from endothelial cells and usually appears after birth.

CLINICAL PRESENTATION

Reports in the literature indicate a strong prevalence on the extremities.

DIFFERENTIAL DIAGNOSIS

Differentials include dermatologic disorders, septic arthritis, physitis, immune-mediated polysynovitis, or osteomyelitis.

DIAGNOSIS

Biopsy with histopathologic evaluation is the only means of obtaining a definitive diagnosis.

MANAGEMENT

Surgical resection is the best treatment; however, depending on the location, it may not be possible to resect the entire mass. These are benign tumors, but recurrence after removal is possible.

HEMANGIOSARCOMA

KEY POINTS

- A highly invasive malignant tumor.
- Originates from endothelial cells.
- Surgical resection is the best treatment.
- Evaluation of adjacent structures is warranted due to aggressive nature.

DEFINITION/OVERVIEW

Hemangiosarcoma is a highly invasive malignant neoplasm of endothelial cells. It is rare in the equine pediatric patient.

ETIOLOGY/PATHOPHYSIOLOGY

The tumor originates from endothelial cells and typically has a good vascular supply.

CLINICAL PRESENTATION

Hemangiosarcomas present as a swelling in the extremities in the area of the joint or tendon sheath or as lameness. In dogs there are reports of severe hemorrhage due to the tumor rupturing.

DIFFERENTIAL DIAGNOSIS

Differentials include trauma, other skin disorders, septic tenosynovitis, septic arthritis, immune-mediated polysynovitis, and osteomyelitis.

DIAGNOSIS

A definitive diagnosis is based on a biopsy and histopathologic analysis.

MANAGEMENT

Surgical resection of the entire mass, if possible, is the best treatment. This tumor is very aggressive, so radiographs of the adjacent bony structures and lymph node biopsy may be warranted.

CONGENITAL PAPILLOMA

KEY POINTS

- A benign epithelial tumor.
- May be single or multiple masses.
- Diagnosis is based on biopsy.
- Surgical excision is the best treatment.

DEFINITION/OVERVIEW

Papilloma refers to a benign epithelial tumor. There is one report in the literature documenting congenital papillomas in five foals.

ETIOLOGY/PATHOPHYSIOLOGY

A virus or an unexplained abnormal formation of normal tissue can cause papillomas.

CLINICAL PRESENTATION

The masses are pedunculated, with a roughened, wart-like or smooth cauliflower-like surface. There may be a single lesion or multiple lesions. Single lesions are most commonly noted on the forelimb, lip, and face, whereas multiple lesions are on the trunk.

DIFFERENTIAL DIAGNOSIS

Differential diagnosis includes other epithelial tumors.

Diagnosis

Biopsy with histopathologic evaluation is the only means of obtaining a definitive diagnosis.

Management

Surgical excision is the only treatment option.

FURTHER READING

Acland HM, Orsini JA, Elkins S et al. (1984) Congenital ethmoid carcinoma in a foal. *Journal of the American Veterinary Medical Association* 184: 979–980.

Allison N, Moeller RB (1999) Bilateral testicular leiomyosarcoma in a stallion. *Journal of Veterinary Diagnostics Investigation* 11: 179–182.

Cox JH, DeBowes RM, Leipold HW (1989) Congenital malignant melanomas in two foals. *Journal of the American Veterinary Medical Association* 194: 945–947.

Dunkle BM, DelPiero F, Kraus BM et al. (2004) Congenital cutaneous, oral and periarticular hemangiosarcoma in a 9-day-old Rocky Mountain horse. *Journal of Veterinary Internal Medicine* 18: 252–255.

Foley GL, Valentine BA, Kincaid AL (1991) Congenital and acquired melanocytomas (benign melanomas) in eighteen young horses. *Veterinary Pathology* 28: 363–369.

Froscher BG, Power HT (1982) Malignant pheochromocytoma in a foal. *Journal of the American Veterinary Medical Association* 181: 494–496.

Haley PJ, Spraker T (1983) Lymphosarcoma in an aborted fetus. *Veterinary Pathology* 20: 647–649.

Henry M, Prasse K, White S (1989) Hemorrhagic diathesis caused by multiple myeloma in a three-month-old foal. *Journal of the Veterinary Medical Association* 194: 392–394.

Hewes CA, Sullins KE (2006) Use of cisplatin-containing biodegradable beads for treatment of cutaneous neoplasia in equidae: 59 cases (2000–2004). *Journal of the Veterinary Medical Association* 229: 1617–1622.

Hong CB (1996) Congenital polyalveolar lobe in three foals. *Journal of Comparative Pathology* 115: 85–88.

Livesey MA, Wilkie IW (1986) Focal and multifocal osteosarcoma in two foals. *Equine Veterinary Journal* 18: 407–410.

Machida N, Tanaka Y, Taya K et al. (2001) An ovarian interstitial cell hamartoma in a newborn foal. *Journal of Comparative Pathology* 125: 322–325.

Morris DD, Bloom JC, Roby KA et al. (1984) Eosinophilic myeloproliferative disorder in a horse. *Journal of the American Veterinary Association* 185: 993–996.

Parks AH, Wyn-Jones G, Cox JE et al. (1986) Partial obstruction of the small colon associated with an abdominal testicular teratoma in a foal. *Equine Veterinary Journal* 18: 342–343.

Pollock PJ, Prendergast M, Callanan JJ et al. (2002) Testicular teratoma in a three-day-old thoroughbred foal. *Veterinary Record* 150: 348–350.

Roby KA, Beech J, Bloom JC et al. (1990) Hepatocellular carcinoma associated with erythrocytosis and hypoglycemia in a yearling filly. *Journal of the American Veterinary Association* 196: 465–467.

Savage CJ (Ed.) (1998) Neoplasia. *Veterinary Clinics of North America: Equine Practice* 14: 517–533.

Schmotzer WB, Hultgren BD, Watrous BJ et al. (1987) Nasomaxillary fibrosarcoma in three young horses. *Journal of the American Veterinary Association* 191: 437–439.

Seahorn TL, Carter GK, Morris EL et al. (1988) Lymphosarcoma in a foal: A case report. *Equine Veterinary Science* 8: 317–319.

Pharmacology

Bonnie S. Barr

OVERVIEW

Pharmacologic differences exist between a 1-day-old foal, a 7-day-old foal, and a 1-month-old foal. These differences are due to the rapid physiologic and metabolic adaptations that occur during the first few days of life. By 1 week of age, foals are usually relatively mature and by 1 month of age they have metabolic and excretory capabilities similar to an adult. However, because relative body fluid and fat reserves are still different at this age, drug disposition may be altered.

There are several physiologic considerations that must be kept in mind when attempting drug therapy in a neonate. Dosages must be frequently adjusted due to the rapidly changing body weight of the neonate. Foals less than 1 week of age have an altered absorption capacity, which is due to several factors including the absence of an established luminal microbial population, altered gastric and duodenal pH concentration, and a larger absorptive capacity. Bioavailability after intramuscular administration may also differ in foals due to variations in tissue water and lipid content, as well as local blood flow.

Neonates have an increased total body water and extracellular fluid volume. This difference means that for some drugs (beta-lactams, aminoglycosides, NSAIDS) serum concentrations are lower in neonates/foals because of a larger volume of distribution. In addition, the blood–brain barrier is incomplete during the first few days of life, thereby enhancing drug penetration into the central nervous system (CNS).

ALTERED METABOLISM

This feature primarily applies to lipid-soluble and nonpolar drugs, which undergo extensive hepatic metabolism to more polar compounds before excretion by the kidney or liver. Minor contributions to metabolism also exist from the gastrointestinal (GI) mucosa, kidney, endothelium, skin, and lung. Examples of compounds that undergo extensive hepatic metabolism include chloramphenicol, methylxanthines, trimethoprim, sulfonamides, erythromycin, rifampin, metronidazole, and barbiturates. Although not studied specially in foals, hepatic phase I (hydrolysis, oxidation, and reduction) and phase II (acetylation, glucuronide and sulfate conjugation) reactions have decreased activity in neonates. Indirect evidence for this exists in foals because the elimination half-life of many drugs decreases rapidly during the first week post partum.

ALTERED ELIMINATION

The kidneys, through glomerular filtration and tubular secretion, are the primary route of elimination for polar and ionized drugs such as beta-lactam and aminoglycoside antibiotics. The hepatic metabolites of nonpolar drugs are also eliminated through renal mechanisms. Biliary excretion is of secondary importance. Renal function is relatively mature in 2- to 4-day-old foals, as evidenced in studies of glomerular filtration rate and renal plasma flow. Thus, renal elimination is not significantly different in neonates. A small degree of maturation does occur during the first few days of life, as evidenced by a more rapid clearance of aminoglycosides in foals from 1 to 10 days of age. Because of the low urinary pH in foals, the reabsorption of weak base may be reduced, whereas that of acids may be increased.

ANTIMICROBIAL DRUGS

AMINOGLYCOSIDES

DEFINITION/OVERVIEW
Aminoglycosides are bactericidal antimicrobials used to treat Gram-negative infections. Current recommendations for use of aminoglycosides in horses include a high dose and once-daily administration. This protocol yields a higher peak plasma concentration of the drug and leads to more effective and rapid bactericidal potential compared with previous multiple-daily dosing administrations. Elimination of aminoglycosides is through glomerular filtration. The two most commonly used aminoglycosides are gentamicin and amikacin.

METHOD OF ACTION
Aminoglycosides bind irreversibly to 30S bacterial ribosome and interfere with translation of messenger RNA, distort codon–anticodon interaction, and impede translocation, thus inhibiting protein synthesis.

SPECTRUM OF ACTIVITY
Aminoglycosides are active against Gram-negative bacteria, but have limited activity against most Gram-positive bacteria. *Staphylococcus aureus* is sensitive to aminoglycosides, but it is seldom used to treat these infections. Aminoglycosides are not effective against anaerobes.

Uses/indications

Aminoglycosides, especially gentamicin, are commonly used as pre- and postoperative therapy. They are usually administered in combination with a beta-lactam as a first choice for broad-spectrum coverage to treat septicemia, pneumonia, peritonitis, soft tissue injuries, and bone injuries. Amikacin is reserved for Gram-negative infections that are not sensitive to cheaper aminoglycosides, although amikacin will often be used initially with penicillin to treat septic neonates. Because aminoglycosides may achieve high concentrations in the urine, they are a used to treat urinary tract infections.

Dosages

See *Table 76.*

Adverse effects

Aminoglycosides are well known for their nephrotoxic and ototoxic effects. The toxicity of these agents is dose related. The nephrotoxic effects are due to accumulation of the agent within the proximal tubules of the kidney. Because neonates are often severely compromised, it is advisable to perform therapeutic monitoring to ensure that peak therapeutic concentrations are achieved and to prevent

Table 76. Antimicrobial drugs

Drug	Dose	Route	Frequency
Amikacin	20–30 mg/kg	i/v or i/m	q24h (monitor renal function)
Amoxicillin	20–30 mg/kg	p/o	q8h (poorly absorbed after 3 weeks of age)
Ampicillin sodium	10–50 mg/kg	i/v	q6–8h
Azithromycin	10 mg/kg	p/o	q24h for first 5 days then q48h
Cefazolin	11–20 mg/kg	i/v or i/m	q6–12h
Cephalexin	10 mg/kg	p/o	q6h
Cefuroxime	10–15 mg/kg	p/o	q8–12h
Ceftriaxone	20–50 mg/kg	i/v or i/m	q12h
Ceftiofur sodium	2–10 mg/kg	i/v	q6–12h
	2–5 mg/kg	i/m	q12–24h
Ceftiofur crystalline free acid	6.6 mg/kg	i/m	every 4 days (for 2 doses)
	13.2 mg/kg	s/q	q48–72h (for neonatal foal; <4 weeks of age). Note: for severe infections administer 5 mg/kg ceftiofur sodium i/v or s/q along with first dose of ceftiofur crystalline free acid.
Cefotaxime	20–50 mg/kg	i/v	q6–8h
Ceftazidime	30–50 mg/kg	i/v	q6–12h
Cefpodoxime proxetil	10 mg/kg	p/o	q6–12h
Cefepime	11 mg/kg	i/v	q8h
Chloramphenicol sodium	25 mg/kg	i/v	q6h (q12h in foals <5 days succinate of age)
Chloramphenicol palmitate	40–50 mg/kg	p/o	q6h (q12h in foals <5 days of age)
Clarithromycin	7.5 mg/kg	p/o	q12h
Doxycycline	10 mg/kg	p/o	q12h
Enrofloxacin	5.5 mg/kg	i/v	q24h
	7.5 mg/kg	p/o	q24h
Erythromycin ethylsuccinate, stearate, or estolate	25 mg/kg	p/o	q6–8h
Erythromycin phosphate	37.5 mg/kg	p/o	q12h
Gamithromycin	6 mg/kg	i/m	Weekly
Gentamycin	6.6–8.8 mg/kg	i/v or i/m	q24h (monitor renal function)
Imipenem	10 mg/kg	i/v	q6h
Meropenem	5–10 mg/kg	i/v	q6–8h

(Continued)

Table 76. (*Continued*) Antimicrobial drugs

Drug	Dose	Route	Frequency
Metronidazole	15–25 mg/kg	p/o	q8–12h
	25–35 mg/kg	per rectum	q6–12h
	15 mg/kg	i/v	q8–12h
Minocycline	3–4 mg/kg	p/o	q12h
Oxytetracycline	6.6–10 mg/kg	i/v	q12–24h
Penicillin G procaine	20,000–40,000 IU/kg	i/m	q12h
Potassium penicillin	20,000–40,000 IU/kg	i/v	q6h
Rifampin	5 mg/kg	p/o	q12h
Sodium ampicillin	20 (10–50) mg/kg	i/v	q6–8h
Sodium penicillin	20,000–50,000 IU/kg	i/v	q6h
Ticarcillin	50 mg/kg	i/v	q6h
Timentin	50 mg/kg	i/v	q6h
Trimethoprim-sulfadiazine	24 mg/kg	p/o	q12h
Trimethoprim sulfamethoxazole	30 mg/kg	p/o	q12h (5 mg/kg of the trimethoprim portion)
Vancomycin	6 mg/kg	i/v	q8h (dilute and give over 1 h)

an accumulation of toxic concentrations. If the peak concentration of the drug is high, 36-hour dosing may be necessary if the patient is to remain on the aminoglycoside or until renal function is determined to be normal. Serum creatinine levels should be monitored frequently. Other risk factors for nephrotoxicity include age, fever, sepsis, and dehydration. Nephrotoxicity is manifested by azotemia, an increase in blood urea nitrogen (BUN), and a decrease in urine specific gravity (SG). Proteinuria and cells or casts may also be seen in the urine. Nephrotoxicity is usually reversible once the drug is discontinued. Ototoxic effects have not been reported in foals, but they have been reported in other species. Aminoglycosides should be used with caution in foals with neuromuscular disorders, especially botulism, due to their neuromuscular blocking activity (by inhibiting prejunctional acetylcholine release, thus decreasing motor end plate sensitivity to acetylcholine).

BETA-LACTAMS

Definition/overview
Beta-lactam antibiotics include the penicillins and cephalosporins. They are bactericidal and are all derivatives of 6-aminopenicillanic acid. The penicillins have a low systemic toxicity. They are commonly used to treat systemic disease in foals because of their low systemic toxicity and their effectiveness against a wide range of equine pathogens. Renal excretion is vital for the removal of beta-lactams from the body.

Method of action
Beta-lactams inhibit the cross-linking of peptidoglycan by binding to the enzyme responsible for cell wall synthesis.

Spectrum of activity
Penicillins
Benzyl penicillins include procaine penicillin, sodium penicillin, and potassium penicillin and are most effective against Gram-positive bacteria, particularly streptococci, and some anaerobes. Aminobenzyl penicillins have an increased activity against many Gram-negative aerobes and include ampicillin. Ticarcillin and timentin, which are carboxy penicillins, have greater activity against many Gram-negative organisms of the family Enterobacteriaecae (including *Pseudomonas aeruginosa*). These antimicrobials can be inactivated by enzymes produced by bacteria (beta-lactamase), although several antimicrobials have been manufactured with a beta-lactamase inhibitor.

Cephalosporins
The cephalosporins are classified as first, second, third, and fourth generation based on the chronology of their development and on general features of antimicrobial activity. Cephalosporins are effective against most anaerobes, though not against *Bacteroides fragilis*.

First-generation cephalosporins are effective against many Gram-positive organisms and are moderately effective against Gram-negative organisms and most anaerobes. First-generation cephalosporins include cefazolin and cephalexin.

Second-generation cephalosporins such as cefuroxime and cefaxitin have a more expanded activity against Gram-negative enteric bacteria and moderate activity against Gram-positive bacteria. These antibiotics are more effective against anaerobes and more resistant to beta-lactamases.

Third-generation cephalosporins have an even more extended Gram-negative coverage, with similar Gram-positive coverage to that of the second generation. Ceftiofur, cefotaxime, and ceftazidime are commonly used third-generation cephalosporins.

Fourth-generation cephalosporins have an extended spectrum of activity against both Gram-positive and Gram-negative bacteria and have a greater resistance to beta-lactamases than the third-generation cephalosporins. Cefepime is the only fourth-generation cephalosporin used in the equine patient.

USES/INDICATIONS

In the pediatric patient, beta-lactams are the first line of defense for the treatment of systemic disease. In neonatal foals, beta-lactams are often used in combination with an aminoglycoside to treat septicemia. Penicillins, due to their spectrum of activity against Gram-positive organisms, are used to treat respiratory infections. These antimicrobials are commonly used in pre- and postoperative cases. In addition, they are also the first line of treatment for peritonitis, soft tissue injury, and orthopedic injury.

Cephalosporins are also used in pre- and postsurgical cases. Many are commonly used for soft tissue and bone infections. Ceftiofur is used for the treatment of respiratory infections and detectable levels are reported in synovial fluid, peritoneal fluid, urine, and pleural fluid. Third-generation cephalosporins, except ceftiofur, obtain therapeutic levels in cerebrospinal fluid (CSF) and thus are used for treatment of meningitis. Third-generation cephalosporins are often used in the treatment of hospital-acquired infections. Fourth-generation cephalosporins can be used in the treatment of severe septicemia and many cross the blood–brain barrier and are therefore used to treat meningitis.

DOSAGES
See *Table 76*.

ADVERSE EFFECTS

Beta-lactams, especially the penicillins, have minimal toxic effects. Hypersensitivity reactions, which range from hives and skin eruptions to anaphylaxis, are the most common adverse reactions. Procaine penicillin given intravenously can result in a severe anaphylactic reaction or death. Penicillin-induced immune-mediated anemia, although uncommon, is reported in horses and results in extravascular and intravascular hemolysis and detection of anti-penicillin antibodies in the serum (Coombs hemolytic anemia). The most common complication associated with the use of cephalosporins is GI disturbances.

CARBAPENEM

DEFINITION/OVERVIEW

Carbapenem antibiotics (which are also beta-lactams) are structurally very similar to penicillins and cephalosporins, except that they have a broader antibacterial spectrum. Two commonly used are imipenem and meropenem. Both are bactericidal agents and are eliminated primarily by renal mechanisms.

METHOD OF ACTION

Imipenem and meropenem, like the other beta-lactams, have an affinity and bind to most penicillin-binding protein sites, thus inhibiting bacterial cell wall synthesis. These antibiotics are also beta-lactamase resistant.

SPECTRUM OF ACTIVITY

Carbapenem antibiotics are broad-spectrum and effective against a wide variety of bacteria including Gram-positive aerobic bacteria, Gram-negative aerobic bacteria, and anaerobic bacteria (including *Bacteroides fragilis* and *Clostridium difficile*). Imipenem is combined with cilastatin, a deactivating enzyme inhibitor, to protect it from degradation by the kidneys.

USES/INDICATIONS

Due to its expanded spectrum and the desire to avoid generation of resistance, carbapenem antibiotics are only used to treat serious infections when other antibiotics are ineffective. Carbapenems are distributed widely throughout the body, with the exception of the CSF. They are most commonly used to treat septicemia in neonates.

DOSAGES
See *Table 76*.

ADVERSE EFFECTS

There is little information available regarding adverse effects in the foal. In other species, possible adverse effects include GI disturbances, CNS toxicity, and hypersensitivity.

CHLORAMPHENICOL

DEFINITION/OVERVIEW

Chloramphenicol is a bacteriostatic antimicrobial that has a broad spectrum of coverage. Chloramphenicol is metabolized in the liver to an inactive form and excreted by the kidneys.

METHOD OF ACTION

Chloramphenicol inhibits bacterial protein synthesis by reversibly binding to the 50S subunit of the ribosome of the bacteria. Because of its high lipid solubility, this antibiotic readily penetrates bacterial cells and is effective against intracellular organisms.

SPECTRUM OF ACTIVITY

Chloramphenicol is effective against Gram-positive organisms, Gram-negative organisms, and anaerobes. Chloramphenicol is administered orally and intravenously, although the intravenous formulation is expensive.

USES/INDICATIONS

Chloramphenicol is used for a variety of infections in foals including pneumonia, septicemia, peritonitis, soft tissue injuries, abscesses, bone injuries, and meningitis.

DOSAGES
See *Table 76*.

ADVERSE EFFECTS

The use of chloramphenicol brings with it the potential human health risk of aplastic anemia. In patients with liver impairment, the dose may need to be reduced.

FLUOROQUINOLONES

DEFINITION/OVERVIEW

Fluoroquinolones are broad-spectrum bactericidal agents. The most commonly used fluoroquinolones in equine medicine are enrofloxacin and ciprofloxacin. Because of the potential athletic-restricting side effect, these agents should not be used in the pediatric patient unless there is no alternative, and then used only with the informed consent of the owner. Fluoroquinolones are eliminated by both renal and nonrenal mechanisms.

METHOD OF ACTION

Fluoroquinolones inhibit the bacterial DNA gyrase or the topoisomerase i/v enzyme, thereby inhibiting DNA replication and transcription.

SPECTRUM OF ACTIVITY

Fluoroquinolones have good activity against many Gram-negative bacilli and cocci and variable activity against streptococci. Other organisms susceptible to fluoroquinolones include *Brucella* spp., *Staphylococcus* spp., *Mycobacterium* spp., and *Mycoplasma* spp. These drugs have weak activity against most anaerobes.

USES/INDICATIONS

Fluoroquinolones are seldom used in equine pediatric patients because of the potential for arthropathy. Fluoroquinolones are widely distributed to most body systems and can enter cells easily; therefore, they are often used to treat intracellular pathogens.

DOSAGES

See *Table 76*.

ADVERSE EFFECTS

In the pediatric patient, fluoroquinolones can cause articular cartilage loss with joint distension. GI disturbances have been reported with oral administration of enrofloxacin.

MACROLIDES

DEFINITION/OVERVIEW

Macrolides are generally bacteriostatic, but may be bactericidal at higher doses. Erythromycin is an antibiotic and also a prokinetic agent. The poor absorption and adverse effects associated with erythromycin led to the development of the synthetic macrolides, azithromycin, and clarithromycin. These newer macrolides have better pharmacokinetic properties and an improved spectrum of activity and are better tolerated. Gamithromycin, a long-acting macrolide used to treat respiratory disease in cattle, has been used to treat *Rhodococcus equi*. In general, the main route of elimination for the macrolide agents is biliary excretion.

METHOD OF ACTION

Macrolides inhibit bacterial protein synthesis by binding to the 50S ribosomal subunit of the bacteria.

SPECTRUM OF ACTIVITY

Erythromycin is effective against Gram-positive cocci and bacilli. Some Gram-negative organisms are also susceptible to erythromycin. Erythromycin is distributed widely into the intracellular and extracellular spaces, but it does not cross the blood–brain barrier. Azithromycin and clarithromycin are effective against most Gram-positive aerobes, but are more active than erythromycin against Gram-negative bacteria. Clarithromycin is active against *Mycobacterium* species. Macrolides achieve high concentrations in phagocytes and are therefore actively transported to the site of infections.

USES/INDICATIONS

In foals, azithromycin and clarithromycin, usually along with rifampin, are used to treat *R. equi* infections (see *Table 76*). Gamithromycin maintains adequate levels in pulmonary epithelial lining fluid (PELF) and phagocytic cells but noninferior to azithromycin/rifampin. The macrolides may also be used to treat other infections such as *Lawsonia intracellularis*.

DOSAGES

See *Table 76*.

ADVERSE EFFECTS

Macrolides can cause GI disturbances (e.g., diarrhea), which may be due to an overgrowth of *Clostridium difficile*. Hyperthermia with associated respiratory distress and tachypnea has been reported to develop in foals. This adverse effect is believed to be due to suppression of the normal sweating mechanism. Gamithromycin administration resulted in lameness/discomfort due to irritation at the administration site. The macrolide agents should not be used in conjunction with chloramphenicol or any other antimicrobial that binds at bacterial ribosomes.

METRONIDAZOLE

DEFINITION/OVERVIEW

Metronidazole is a synthetic antibacterial and antiprotozoal agent. It is bactericidal against susceptible bacteria. The major route of elimination is by the kidneys.

METHOD OF ACTION

Metronidazole disrupts the DNA and nucleic acid synthesis of the bacteria.

SPECTRUM OF ACTIVITY

Metronidazole has activity against most obligate anaerobes including the following species: *Bacteroides* (including *B. fragilis*), *Fusobacterium*, *Veillonella*, *Clostridium*, *Peptococcus*, and *Peptostreptococcus*.

USES/INDICATIONS

Metronidazole is commonly used to treat anaerobic infections including pneumonia, abscesses, and soft tissue infections. In foals, metronidazole is the treatment of choice for clostridial diarrhea.

DOSAGES
See *Table 76*.

ADVERSE EFFECTS
Adverse effects include inappetence and CNS signs (ataxia). These are rarely reported in the foal.

RIFAMPIN

DEFINITION/OVERVIEW
Rifampin is most commonly used in conjunction with erythromycin, azithromycin, or clarithromycin to treat *R. equi* pneumonia in foals. It is bactericidal. In humans the drug is used to treat *Mycobacterium tuberculosis*. Rifampin is metabolized in the liver and eliminated by biliary excretion.

METHOD OF ACTION
Rifampin inhibits the formation of nucleic acids in the bacteria by inhibiting DNA-dependent RNA polymerase and suppressing initiation of chain formation for RNA synthesis. It does not inhibit the mammalian RNA polymerase enzyme.

SPECTRUM OF ACTIVITY
Rifampin is active against most Gram-positive organisms and some Gram-negative organisms. It has also been effective against some anaerobes. Rifampin also has some antifungal and antiviral activity.

USES/INDICATIONS
At the present time the most common use of rifampin is in the treatment of *R. equi* pneumonia along with erythromycin, azithromycin, or clarithromycin. Rifampin is lipid soluble and obtains high levels in phagocytic cells and abscesses, thus it can also be used to treat abscesses caused by other bacterium. Rifampin must be administered in combination with another antimicrobial to prevent development of resistance.

DOSAGES
See *Table 76*.

ADVERSE EFFECTS
Adverse effects are rare. Occasionally, discolored (red-orange colored) urine has been reported. It is possible that with long-term use an increase of liver enzymes may be noted due to rifampin inducing hepatic microsomal enzymes.

TETRACYCLINES

DEFINITION/OVERVIEW
Tetracyclines are bacteriostatic antibiotics; they include oxytetracycline, tetracycline, doxycycline and minocycline. Elimination of these drugs is by glomerular filtration.

METHOD OF ACTION
Tetracyclines inhibit protein synthesis of the bacteria by reversibly binding to the 30S ribosomal subunit of the bacteria.

SPECTRUM OF ACTIVITY
Tetracyclines have a broad spectrum of activity. They are effective against Gram-positive and Gram-negative bacteria. *Rickettsia* spp., *Mycoplasma* spp., and *Ehrlichia* spp. are also sensitive to tetracyclines.

USES/INDICATIONS
Tetracyclines are widely distributed in the body, except for the CSF. The most common use of oxytetracycline in the neonatal foal is treatment of flexural limb deformities. In older foals, tetracyclines may be used in the treatment of pneumonia, abscesses, or soft tissue injuries. Minocycline does get good concentrations in the CSF.

DOSAGES
See *Table 76*.

ADVERSE EFFECTS
Adverse effects include GI disturbances (diarrhea) and nephrotoxicity. In the compromised neonate, careful monitoring of renal parameters (serum creatinine and urine SG) should be performed. Intravenous administration has been associated with cardiovascular collapse, most likely related to chelation of calcium. It is advisable to dilute the antibiotic prior to giving it intravenously. Tetracyclines may cause tendon laxity; therefore, they must be used with caution.

TRIMETHOPRIM–SULFONAMIDE COMBINATIONS

DEFINITION/OVERVIEW
Trimethoprim–sulfonamide is a combination of trimethoprim (a pyrimidine) and sulfadiazine, sulfadoxine, or sulfamethoxazole. The use of the two drugs together developed as a result of the widespread resistance to sulfonamides. On their own, sulfonamides are bacteriostatic agents and trimethoprim is bactericidal, but in combination the two are bactericidal. The synergy of the two antimicrobials results in the minimum inhibitory concentration of each antimicrobial being lower. This broad-spectrum combination can be used orally or intravenously and is excreted by the kidneys.

METHOD OF ACTION
The sulfonamide blocks the conversion of para-aminobenzoic acid (PABA) to dihydrofolic acid (DFA), and trimethoprim blocks the conversion of DFA to tetrahydrofolic acid by inhibiting dihydrofolate reductase. The end result is the blockage of two essential pathways in the biosynthesis of nucleic acids and proteins in the bacteria.

SPECTRUM OF ACTIVITY
The combination of trimethoprim with sulfonamide results in a broader spectrum of activity including Gram-negative organisms, Gram-positive organisms, and protozoa. The combination is reported to have little activity against most anaerobes.

USES/INDICATIONS
This combination is sometimes used as a first-line antimicrobial for respiratory tract infections, urinary tract infections, and soft tissue injury. It is widely distributed throughout the body and readily penetrates CSF, ocular fluids, and synovial fluids. Its activity is

hindered in the presence of purulent material and therefore it may be of little value in the presence of abscessation. Unfortunately, some streptococci, especially *Streptococcus zooepidemicus*, have developed resistance to this combination.

DOSAGES
See *Table 76*.

ADVERSE EFFECTS
Adverse effects with usage of the trimethoprim–sulfonamide combination include GI disturbances, especially diarrhea. Long-term usage may result in hematologic effects such as anemia or leukopenia due to the inhibition of folic acid synthesis. Intravenous administration has been associated with excitation, muscle fasciculations, cardiovascular collapse, and death. Administration of alpha-2 agonist sedatives can result in severe reactions when the animal is being treated with the intravenous form of the agent.

VANCOMYCIN

DEFINITION/OVERVIEW
Vancomycin has been reserved as a drug of "last resort," used only after treatment with other agents has failed. The primary mechanism of excretion is through the kidneys.

METHOD OF ACTION
Vancomycin disrupts the synthesis of the bacterial cell wall in Gram-positive bacteria.

SPECTRUM OF ACTIVITY
Vancomycin is effective against Gram-positive organisms such as methicillin-resistant *Staphylococcus aureus* and *Clostridium* species.

USES/INDICATIONS
Vancomycin is reserved for the treatment of serious, life-threatening infections by Gram-positive bacteria that are unresponsive to other agents. It is very important for the bacteria to be sensitive to

vancomycin. Overuse or inappropriate use will result in the development of resistant bacteria.

DOSAGES
See *Table 76*.

ADVERSE EFFECTS
Potential adverse effects include nephrotoxicity and ototoxicity. Nephrotoxicity is more likely in foals that are compromised, especially neonates. Therefore, it is important to monitor renal function and avoid administration with other nephrotoxic drugs.

ANTIULCER MEDICATIONS

LIQUID ANTACID COMPOUNDS

DEFINITION/OVERVIEW
Liquid antacids include magnesium hydroxide, aluminum hydroxide, and calcium carbonate and are involved in neutralization of luminal acid. The efficacy in foals has been debated.

METHOD OF ACTION
Liquid antacids decrease gastric acid pH by neutralization of luminal acid. They exchange cations for anions, thus removing H+ activity from gastric milieu.

USES/INDICATIONS
Liquid antacids are used in the treatment of esophagitis, gastric ulcers, and gastritis. Studies have shown that to be effective, these drugs need to be administered every 2 hours.

DOSAGES
See *Table 77*.

ADVERSE EFFECTS
Constipation has been noted during the use of aluminum- and calcium-containing antacids. Diarrhea or frequent loose stools has been observed during the use of those containing magnesium. Prolonged use may result in interference with the absorption of electrolytes.

Table 77. Antiulcer medications

Drug	Dose	Route	Frequency
Cimetidine	10–20 mg/kg	p/o	q6–8h
	6.6 mg/kg	i/v	q4–6h
Liquid antacids	0.5–1.0 mL/kg	p/o	q2h
Omeprazole	1 mg/kg	p/o	q24h (prevention)
	4 mg/kg	p/o	q24h (treatment)
Ranitidine	5–10 mg/kg	p/o	q8–12h
	1.5 mg/kg	i/v	q8h
Sucralfate	20–40 mg/kg	p/o	q6–12h

OMEPRAZOLE

DEFINITION/OVERVIEW
Omeprazole is used in the treatment and prevention of GI ulceration. It is a proton pump inhibitor.

METHOD OF ACTION
Omeprazole is a proton pump inhibitor that exerts its action by selectively and irreversibly binding to parietal cell enzyme H+K$^+$ ATPase. This enzyme catalyzes the exchange of H+ for K$^+$ ions in the final step of HCl production by parietal cells. The binding of omeprazole to this enzyme effectively decreases acid secretion regardless of the stimulus to the cell. Omeprazole irreversibly binds to H+K$^+$ ATPase for the life of the parietal cell. Therefore, it is suitable for once-a-day administration.

USES/INDICATION
Omeprazole is used in foals for the treatment and prevention of gastric and duodenal ulcers or to treat gastric erosions caused by ulcerogenic drugs (i.e., aspirin).

DOSAGES
See *Table 77*.

ADVERSE EFFECTS
Adverse effects are unlikely with omeprazole. There is one report of a horse developing urticaria after receiving omeprazole.

RANITIDINE/CIMETIDINE

DEFINITION/OVERVIEW
Ranitidine and cimetidine are histamine type 2 receptor antagonists that are used in the treatment and prophylaxis of gastric ulcers. Ranitidine is more potent than cimetidine.

METHOD OF ACTION
Both act at the histamine type 2 receptors of the gastric parietal cells by competitively inhibiting histamine, thereby decreasing gastric acid output both during basal conditions and when stimulated by food, pentagastrin, histamine, or insulin. Ranitidine may increase gastric emptying by inhibiting acetylcholinesterase, which would result in an increased amount of acetylcholine available at muscarinic receptors.

USES/INDICATIONS
Ranitidine and cimetidine are used in foals for the treatment or prophylaxis of gastric and duodenal ulcers. The bioavailability of ranitidine is adequate when administered orally or intravenously. Antacids may decrease the absorption of ranitidine; therefore, these two medications should be given at different times, at least 2 hours apart. When administered orally the bioavailability of cimetidine is variable; intravenous administration results in better bioavailability. Ranitidine is used more often than cimetidine.

DOSAGES
See *Table 77*.

ADVERSE EFFECTS
Ranitidine has minimal adverse effects. Cimetidine may inhibit hepatic metabolism of certain drugs such as phenytoin, metronidazole, theophylline, and diazepam, thus caution is advised when administering these drugs in combination.

SUCRALFATE (MUCOSAL PROTECTANTS)

DEFINITION/OVERVIEW
Sucralfate is a mucosal protectant that acts locally in the treatment of gastric ulcers.

METHOD OF ACTION
Sucralfate is a complex polysaccharide that is composed of sucrose octasulfate and aluminum hydroxide. Sucralfate binds to negatively charged particles in the ulcerated mucosa, forming an acid-resistant layer that protects against acid and pepsin. It has been shown to enhance normal gastric defense mechanisms by stimulating mucus and bicarbonate production, deactivating pepsin, and promoting mucosal blood flow through stimulation of endogenous prostaglandins. Sucralfate is believed to enhance epithelial healing and stimulate cell proliferation.

USES/INDICATION
Sucralfate has been used in the treatment of oral, esophageal, gastric, and duodenal ulcers. It has also been employed to prevent drug-induced (i.e., aspirin) gastric erosions. Sucralfate may be an alternative for ulcer prophylaxis in severely compromised neonates in which there is an increased risk of pathogenic gastric colonization.

DOSAGES
See *Table 77*.

ADVERSE EFFECTS
Adverse effects are uncommon. Occasionally, constipation may be noted in foals.

OTHER GASTROINTESTINAL DRUGS

BISMUTH SUBSALICYLATE

DEFINITION/OVERVIEW
Bismuth subsalicylate is used as an antidiarrheal agent and GI protectant.

METHOD OF ACTION
Bismuth subsalicylate is cleaved in the small intestine into bismuth carbonate and salicylate. The bismuth portion coats the mucosa and has anti-endotoxic effects. The salicylate portion has antiprostaglandin activity, which may contribute to its effectiveness and reduce symptoms associated with secretory diarrheas.

USES/INDICATIONS
Bismuth subsalicylate is used in the equine pediatric patient to treat diarrhea. Care should be taken to stagger this drug with

other oral medications in order to avoid nonspecific binding and reduction in the bioavailability of the concurrently administered drugs.

DOSAGES
See *Table 77*.

ADVERSE EFFECTS
Bismuth subsalicylate may cause change in fecal color to a gray-black or greenish-black. Occasionally, bismuth subsalicylate has caused constipation to occur in the young pediatric patient. Bismuth subsalicylate may delay the absorption of other drugs; therefore, it should not be administered with other oral drugs.

DI-TRI-OCTAHEDRAL SMECTITE

DEFINITION/OVERVIEW
Di-tri-octahedral (DTO) smectite is an absorbent that can bind and reduce the absorption of endotoxin. It has also been shown to neutralize the toxins of *Clostridium difficile* and *Clostridium perfringens*.

METHOD OF ACTION
DTO smectite is a natural hydrated aluminomagnesium silicate. Positively charged organic cations, such as endotoxins or exotoxins, bind to the negatively charged surface of DTO smectite, thus neutralizing the toxic effects of the endotoxin or exotoxin.

USES/INDICATIONS
DTO smectite is used in the treatment and prevention of enterocolitis, especially in cases caused by *C. perfringens* or *C. difficile*.

DOSAGES
See *Table 78*.

ADVERSE EFFECTS
DTO smectite may delay the absorption of some drugs, but experimentally there is no delay in the absorption of metronidazole.

ANTICONVULSANT MEDICATIONS

DIAZEPAM

DEFINITION/OVERVIEW
Diazepam is a benzodiazepine derivative that possesses anxiolytic, anticonvulsant, sedative, skeletal muscle relaxant, and amnestic properties. It is the most commonly used drug in neonates for short-term control of generalized seizure activity and sedation. It has a rapid onset of action and relatively few adverse effects.

METHOD OF ACTION
The mechanism of action of diazepam is due to increased release of and/or facilitation of gamma-aminobutyric acid (GABA) activity, which is an inhibitory neurotransmitter in the CNS. It provides excellent sedation and muscle relaxation, with minimal cardiovascular effects. The subcortical levels of the CNS (primarily limbic, thalamic, and hypothalamic) are depressed by diazepam.

USES/INDICATIONS
Diazepam is used in the neonate for short-term control of generalized seizure activity. If the seizures persist after 2–3 doses, another anticonvulsant medication should be administered. It can also be used as a sedative in the compromised neonate for short procedures such as catheter placement.

DOSAGES
See *Table 79*.

Table 78. Other gastrointestinal drugs

Drug	Dose	Route	Frequency
Bismuth subsalicylate	0.5–1 mL/kg	p/o	q4–6h
DTO smectite	45 mL of powder mixed with water	p/o	q6–12h

Table 79. Anticonvulsant medications

Drug	Dose	Route	Frequency
Diazepam	0.05–0.4 mg/kg	i/v	May repeat in 20–30 min
Midazolam	0.1–0.2 mg/kg 0.02–0.1 mg/kg/hr	i/v bolus CRI	
Phenobarbital	5–25 mg/kg	i/v	Administer over 20 min
	2–10 mg/kg	p/o	q12h (maintenance)
Phenytoin	1–5 mg/kg	i/v or p/o	q4h
	1–5 mg/kg	p/o	q12h (maintenance)
Potassium bromide	25 mg/kg	p/o	q24h; 20% increase/ decrease every 2 weeks as needed
Primidone	1–2 g	p/o	Initial dose
	1 g	p/o	q12–24h (maintenance)

ADVERSE EFFECTS

There are no serious adverse effects and few drug interactions.

MIDAZOLAM

DEFINITION/OVERVIEW

Midazolam is a short-acting benzodiazepine CNS depressant. It is shorter acting than diazepam and used in patients that have intractable seizures.

METHOD OF ACTION

The mechanism of action of midazolam is an increased release of the neurotransmitter GABA, which is the major inhibitory neurotransmitter in the CNS.

USES/INDICATIONS

Midazolam is used to treat seizure activity in pediatric patients that are refractory to diazepam and phenobarbital.

DOSAGES

See *Table 79*.

ADVERSE EFFECTS

In humans, midazolam has been associated with respiratory depression and hypotension, therefore midazolam should only be used in a controlled hospital setting under close monitoring.

PHENOBARBITAL

DEFINITION/OVERVIEW

Phenobarbital is a barbiturate with anticonvulsant, sedative, and hypnotic properties. It is used to treat seizures in foals, especially those that are refractory to diazepam or when benzodiazepine treatment is contraindicated.

METHOD OF ACTION

The actions of phenobarbital are attributed to its specific ability to depress the motor centers of the cerebral cortex, limit the spread of seizure activity, and elevate seizure threshold.

USES/INDICATIONS

Phenobarbital is used in the neonatal foal and older foal for the treatment of recurrent or persistent seizure disorders.

DOSAGES

See *Table 79*.

ADVERSE EFFECTS

Administration of phenobarbital may result in respiratory depression, hypothermia, and hypotension, so careful monitoring of these parameters must be performed, especially in the compromised neonate. Oral absorption of phenobarbital in the newborn foal is expected to be more rapid than in the adult due to enhanced absorption by the neonatal gut. This drug has a long half-life in neonates; therefore, it may be useful to monitor peak and trough drug concentrations.

If the foal has been on the drug long term, slow weaning may be necessary because abrupt withdrawal can precipitate seizures. There

is potential for interaction with other drugs because phenobarbital results in induction of the hepatic microsomal enzyme system. In the neonatal foal the following adverse effects can occur: respiratory depression, hypothermia, and hypotension. Phenobarbital may also cause upper airway obstruction.

PHENYTOIN

DEFINITION/OVERVIEW

Phenytoin is an anticonvulsant that is also occasionally used to control recurrent seizures associated with hypoxic ischemic encephalopathy (HIE) in the neonatal foal. No studies of the bioavailability in foals have been performed. The pharmacokinetics of phenytoin in the pediatric patient has not been determined.

METHOD OF ACTION

The primary site of action appears to be the motor cortex, where the spread of seizure activity is inhibited. Excessive stimulation or environmental changes can alter the sodium gradient, which may lower the threshold for seizure spread. Phenytoin stabilizes the threshold against hyperexcitability by possibly promoting sodium efflux from neurons. There is also a reduction of post-tetanic potentiation at synapses, thus preventing cortical seizure activity and reducing activity of the brainstem centers.

USES/INDICATIONS

Phenytoin is used to treat seizure activity that is refractory to benzodiazepines or phenobarbital.

DOSAGES

See *Table 79*.

ADVERSE EFFECTS

Marked depression is the primary adverse effect of phenytoin administration; therefore, drug levels may need to be monitored. The liver is the chief site of biotransformation, therefore patients with impaired liver function should be monitored closely and have their liver values evaluated.

POTASSIUM BROMIDE

DEFINITION/OVERVIEW

Potassium bromide is a very old anticonvulsant and sedative. It is rarely used in equine pediatric patients, but may be used if seizures are multiple, frequent, or difficult to control with other anticonvulsants.

METHOD OF ACTION

The action of potassium bromide is due to the bromide ion. Its mechanism of action is not fully understood, but presumably it competes for and replaces chloride in the cell (and the neuron), thus increasing the electronegativity of the cell and hyperpolarizing it.

USES/INDICATIONS

Potassium bromide is used as therapy in pediatric patients in which the seizures are refractory to other anticonvulsant drugs. The liver does not metabolize potassium bromide, therefore it may be safer for foals with severe liver disease.

DOSAGES

See *Table 79.*

ADVERSE EFFECTS

Adverse effects in the horse are not reported, but in the dog they include sedation, ataxia, increased urination, and rare skin disorders. Overdose can be treated with administration of sodium chloride, which will increase elimination from the kidneys.

PRIMIDONE

DEFINITION/OVERVIEW

Primidone is an anticonvulsant that may be used in cases that are refractory to other anticonvulsant medications.

METHOD OF ACTION

Primidone stimulates the action of GABA in the CNS. It is metabolized to phenylethylmalonamide and phenobarbital. These agents are known to raise the seizure threshold and alter seizure patterns.

USES/INDICATIONS

Primidone can be used to treat seizure activity in equine pediatric patients when other anticonvulsant medications are not effective.

DOSAGES

See *Table 79.*

ADVERSE EFFECTS

The efficacy of primidone in pediatric patients has not been determined. Possible adverse effects include respiratory depression, hypothermia, and hypotension, and primidone may cause upper airway obstruction.

ANTI-INFLAMMATORY MEDICATION

CORTICOSTEROIDS

DEFINITION/OVERVIEW

Corticosteroids are a group of drugs that are produced naturally and synthetically. They are classified as glucocorticoids, mineralocorticoids, and adrenal sex hormones. Glucocorticoids have a variety of pharmacologic effects including anti-inflammatory, immunosuppressive, metabolic, and endocrine properties. The most commonly used synthetic glucocorticoids are prednisolone, methylprednisolone sodium succinate, prednisolone sodium succinate, and dexamethasone.

METHOD OF ACTION

The anti-inflammatory activity of glucocorticoids is mediated by the inhibition of the cyclooxygenase and lipoxygenase pathways. Blockage of these pathways results in a variety of anti-inflammatory effects including stabilization of cellular membranes, decreased vascular permeability, inhibition of leukocyte migration, and adherence and inhibition of platelet aggregation. Glucocorticoids suppress the immune system by effecting leukocytes, macrophages, and cell-mediated immunity, and they also affect protein, fat, and carbohydrate metabolism. Cortisol, produced by the anterior pituitary, is a very potent, naturally occurring glucocorticoid that is carefully regulated in the body and can be affected by endogenously administered glucocorticoids.

USES/INDICATIONS

Glucocorticoids are used to treat immune reactions such as anaphylaxis and hypersensitivity, spinal cord injury, and, occasionally, other types of trauma.

DOSAGES

See *Table 80.*

Table 80. Anti-inflammatory medications

Drug	Dose	Route	Frequency
Aspirin	10–100 mg/kg	p/o	q24h
Dexamethasone	0.05–0.2 mg/kg	i/v, i/m, or p/o	q12–24h
DMSO	0.1–1 g/kg	i/v	q12–24h (as a 10% solution)
Firocoxib	0.1 mg/kg	p/o	q24h
Flunixin meglumine	1 mg/kg	i/v	q12–24h
	0.25 mg/kg	i/v	q8h (anti-endotoxic dose)
Ketoprofen	2.2 mg/kg	i/v	q12–24h
Methylprednisolone sodium succinate	5–30 mg/kg	i/v	As required
Phenylbutazone	2.2–4.4 mg/kg	i/v or p/o	q12–24h
Prednisolone	0.25–1.0 mg/kg	p/o	q12–24h
Prednisolone sodium succinate	0.25–2.5 mg/kg	i/v	q6h or as required

ADVERSE EFFECTS

Glucocorticoids suppress the immune system, resulting in the potential for the development of opportunistic fungal or bacterial infections. In the adult, glucocorticoids can cause laminitis. Sudden withdrawal of exogenous glucocorticoids has resulted in adrenal insufficiency.

DIMETHYL SULFOXIDE

DEFINITION/OVERVIEW

Dimethyl sulfoxide (DMSO) is an organic solvent commonly used to treat inflammation resulting from CNS trauma or soft tissue injuries. The pharmacologic effects of DMSO are diverse and include anti-inflammatory, anti-ischemic, antimicrobial, and analgesic properties.

METHOD OF ACTION

The anti-inflammatory effects of DMSO are a result of the trapping of free radicals, including free radical hydroxide, its metabolite dimethyl sulfide (DMS), and free radical oxygen. Free radicals are released from neutrophils and macrophages as a response to inflammation, or they are released from cells injured by ischemia or ionizing radiation. DMSO also serves as a carrier agent in promoting percutaneous absorption of other compounds that normally would not penetrate the skin. It has weak antibacterial activity and, possibly, topical antifungal activity. DMSO appears to be more effective as an anti-inflammatory agent when used for acute inflammation rather than chronic conditions. The membrane stabilizing property of DMSO reduces release of inflammatory mediators. DMSO may slow conductance in nerve fibers, thus providing analgesia for certain kinds of pain. Finally, DMSO has diuretic properties.

USES/INDICATIONS

DMSO has been used systemically to treat transient ischemic conditions, CNS trauma, and cerebral edema. In addition, it has been used topically to reduce acute soft tissue swelling.

DOSAGES

See *Table 80*.

ADVERSE EFFECTS

Minimal adverse effects have been reported. DMSO can cause hemolysis and pigmenturia when given intravenously; therefore, to minimize this adverse effect a <20% solution should be given. If the foal is dehydrated or severely compromised, close monitoring of serum creatinine should be carried out.

NONSTEROIDAL ANTI-INFLAMMATORY DRUGS

DEFINITION/OVERVIEW

NSAIDs are the most commonly used drugs for the control of pain and inflammation in horses. The most frequently used ones are flunixin meglumine, phenylbutazone, ketoprofen, aspirin, and firocoxib.

METHOD OF ACTION

NSAIDs irreversibly inhibit the enzyme cyclooxygenase, which converts arachidonic acid to eicosanoids (prostaglandins, thromboxanes, and protacycline). Blocking these eicosanoids results in analgesic, anti-inflammatory, antipyretic, antithrombotic, and anti-endotoxic effects. Three forms of cyclooxygenase have been documented: COX-1, COX-2, and COX-3. COX-1 is required for normal tissue homeostasis, COX-2 is responsible for the inflammatory response, and COX-3 may have a role in inflammation-induced fever. Ideally, anti-inflammatory agents to target COX-2 (and possible COX-3) would have less adverse effects.

USES/INDICATIONS

Flunixin meglumine is most commonly used in the alleviation of inflammation and pain associated with visceral pain in horses with colic. It is also used in the treatment of other conditions including colitis, respiratory disease, ophthalmic inflammatory conditions, laminitis, endotoxic shock, general surgery, and soft tissue injuries. Low-dose therapy with flunixin meglumine is very effective at preventing the clinical signs of endotoxemia. Phenylbutazone is used extensively to treat a wide variety of musculoskeletal disorders. It is less effective as a treatment for endotoxemia than flunixin meglumine. Ketoprofen is used to treat various causes of pain and inflammation. Aspirin is the most effective NSAID for antiplatelet therapy and may be beneficial in the treatment of thrombophlebitis, laminitis, and verminous arteritis. Firocoxib is a newer NSAID that primarily inhibits COX-2, making it safer with fewer side effects.

DOSAGES

See *Table 80*. Flunixin meglumine and phenylbutazone are rapidly absorbed following oral administration and both are available in an intravenous form. The duration of action is up to 36 hours with flunixin meglumine and 24 hours with phenylbutazone. Phenylbutazone has a longer half-life in neonates; therefore, it may only need to be administered once daily. Ketoprofen is only administered intravenously because of its poor bioavailability if given orally. Aspirin is only available in the oral form. Firocoxib is rapidly absorbed following oral administration.

ADVERSE EFFECTS

The adverse effects of NSAIDs are due to the cyclooxygenase inhibition in tissues where prostaglandins are beneficial and protective. Those tissues most affected are the GI tract and the kidneys. In the GI tract, NSAIDs lead to ulcer formation due to increased acidity, decreased mucosal blood flow, and decreased mucus production. The effects on the kidneys include decreased blood flow and glomerular filtration rate, resulting in acute renal failure. Bleeding tendencies may result due to decreased platelet function, specifically with aspirin therapy. Neonates are more prone to toxic effects of nonsteroidal drugs in general. Foals with pre-existing GI ulcers and renal, hepatic, or hematologic disease should be closely monitored if these drugs have to be administered. Ketoprofen is considered to be safer than flunixin meglumine and phenylbutazone. Because firocoxib is COX-2 selective, it is safer than other NSAIDS. Adverse reactions may occur with intramuscular injections and include localized swelling, stiffness, or sweating. This method of injection is not recommended in foals, especially neonates.

RESPIRATORY DRUGS

CAFFEINE

DEFINITION/OVERVIEW
Caffeine can be used as a respiratory stimulant in cases of hypoventilation in the foal.

METHOD OF ACTION
Caffeine stimulates the central respiratory center.

USES/INDICATIONS
Caffeine can be used in equine neonates that suffer from neonatal hypercapnia secondary to HIE, resulting in depression of central respiratory receptors. Caffeine should not be used if the hypercapnia is compensation for metabolic alkalosis and the pH is not low (this should be treated by correcting the electrolyte imbalances).

DOSAGES
See *Table 81*.

ADVERSE EFFECTS
Adverse effects may include restlessness, hyperactivity, and tachycardia.

CLENBUTEROL

DEFINITION/OVERVIEW
Clenbuterol is a bronchodilator that may also act as an expectorant by reducing the viscosity of mucus, increasing airway ciliary wave motion for clearance, and reducing inflammation.

METHOD OF ACTION
Clenbuterol is a beta-2 adrenergic agonist that binds to the beta-2 adrenoceptors in airway smooth muscle to induce increased intracellular concentrations of cyclic adenosine monophosphate, resulting in smooth muscle relaxation and bronchodilation.

USES/INDICATIONS
Clenbuterol, administered orally, is often used as an adjunct in the treatment of pneumonia.

DOSAGES
See *Table 81*.

ADVERSE EFFECTS
Clenbuterol overdose can cause anxiety, tachycardia, sweating, and muscle trembling.

DOXAPRAM

DEFINITION/OVERVIEW
Doxapram is a respiratory stimulant.

METHOD OF ACTION
Doxapram is a general CNS stimulant in which the medullary respiratory centers are directly stimulated. The result is a transient increase in respiratory rate and volume without increases in arterial oxygenation. Doxapram increases the work associated with respiration, resulting in increased oxygen consumption and carbon dioxide production.

USES/INDICATIONS
Doxapram is used to stimulate respiration during and after general anesthesia and for respiratory stimulation associated with CNS disease.

DOSAGES
See *Table 81*.

ADVERSE EFFECTS
Possible adverse effects include hypertension, arrhythmias, hyperventilation, and seizures. Doxapram should not be used as a substitute for aggressive mechanical respiratory support and oxygen therapy, especially in cases of cardiopulmonary resuscitation. Doxapram should be used in the neonate with caution because of increased oxygen consumption and carbon dioxide production, which may worsen hypoxemia and acid–base abnormalities.

Table 81. Respiratory drugs

Drug	Dose	Route	Frequency
Caffeine	10 mg/kg loading dose, then 2.5–10 mg/kg	p/o or per rectum	q12–24h
Clenbuterol	0.8–3.2 µg/kg	p/o	q12h
Doxapram	0.5 mg/kg. For hypoventilating foals short term: 0.02–0.05 mg/kg/min diluted infusion for a few hours (total amount 400 mg)	i/v as needed	
Glycopyrrolate	0.0022 mg/kg (for bronchodilation)	i/v	q8h

CARDIAC DRUGS

ATROPINE

DEFINITION/OVERVIEW
Atropine is an anticholinergic agent used to treat sinus bradycardia and vagally induced arrhythmias.

METHOD OF ACTION
Atropine acts by increasing sinus node activity and atrioventricular (AV) node conduction.

USES/INDICATIONS
Atropine is used to treat vagally induced bradyarrhythmias, sinus bradycardia, sinus arrest, and AV block.

DOSAGES
See *Table 82*.

ADVERSE EFFECTS
Due to its vagolytic effects, atropine can cause a decrease in GI tract motility, resulting in signs of abdominal discomfort. Atropine can also cause CNS adverse effects such as stimulation, drowsiness, ataxia, seizures, and respiratory depression. Atropine has also been reported to cause abnormal cardiac rhythms.

DIGOXIN

DEFINITION/OVERVIEW
Digoxin is a cardiac glycoside extracted from the foxglove plant. It is widely used in the treatment of various cardiac conditions. It is both a positive inotrope and a negative chronotrope.

METHOD OF ACTION
Digoxin increases myocardial contractility (inotropism) by inhibiting the Na+/K+ ATPase pump in the sarcoplasmic reticulum of myocardial cells. Inhibition of this pump results in the intracellular accumulation of calcium and dose-dependent increases in cardiac contractility. Digoxin is also a negative chronotrope, slowing the heart rate by increasing parasympathetic tone and slowing AV conduction. This results in improved cardiac filling and increased cardiac output.

USES/INDICATIONS
Digoxin is used prior to administration of quinidine in patients with atrial fibrillation and a high resting heart rate. Digoxin is also used to treat other supraventricular tachycardias and congestive heart failure.

DOSAGES
See *Table 82*.

Table 82. Cardiac drugs

Drug	Dose/route/frequency
Atropine	0.005–0.01 mg/kg i/v
Digoxin	0.0022 mg/kg i/v q12h
	0.011 mg/kg p/o q12h
Dobutamine	3–40 µg/kg/minute i/v CRI
Dopamine	3–20 µg/kg/minute i/v CRI
Epinephrine	0.01–0.02 mg/kg i/v single doses repeatedly for CPR
	0.2–2 µg/kg/minute i/v CRI for hypotension
Glycopyrrolate	0.005–0.01 mg/kg i/v
Lidocaine	0.1–0.25 mg/kg as a bolus, repeat up to total of 0.5 mg/kg in 10–15 min; or 1.3 mg/kg i/v loading dose, then 0.05 mg/kg/min i/v CRI
Magnesium sulfate	4 mg/kg i/v bolus every 2 min to a maximum of 50 mg/kg
	2 mg/kg/min i/v CRI to a maximum of 50 mg/kg
Norepinephrine	0.2–3 µg/kg/min i/v CRI
Procainamide	1 mg/kg/min i/v to a maximum of 20 mg/kg
	25–35 mg/kg p/o q8h
Propanolol	0.03 mg/kg i/v 0.38–0.78 mg/kg p/o q8h
Quinidine	1.1–2.2 mg/kg i/v every 10 min until either conversion to normal sinus rhythm gluconate occurs or until a total dose of 12 mg/kg has been administered
Quinidine sulfate	22 mg/kg via nasogastric tube every 2 h until either conversion to normal sinus rhythm occurs, a total of 5 doses have been administered, significant QRS complex prolongation occurs to >25% of the pretreatment duration, or other life-threatening complications occur. If failure to convert and no adverse effects, continue at 22 mg/kg p/o q6h. Some cases take over 350 g to convert.

ADVERSE EFFECTS

Digoxin has a low margin of safety and variations can exist between individuals in oral bioavailability, distribution, or elimination of the drug. Peak (1–2 hour) and trough (12 hour) plasma concentrations should be maintained at a steady state within the therapeutic range of 0.5–2 ng/mL. Digoxin toxicity causes depression, anorexia, colic, diarrhea, or cardiac arrhythmias, therefore plasma concentrations should be closely monitored. The kidneys eliminate digoxin, so close monitoring should occur in foals with renal impairment.

DOBUTAMINE

DEFINITION/OVERVIEW

Dobutamine is a beta-1 adrenergic agonist and positive inotropic agent used in the treatment of hypotension.

METHOD OF ACTION

Dobutamine acts on cardiac beta-1 adrenergic receptors to increase myocardial contractility, stroke volume, and cardiac output.

USES/INDICATIONS

Dobutamine is used to treat hypotension secondary to decreased myocardial contractility and severe bradycardia. Marked increases in heart rate and blood pressure may occur, therefore the administration of dobutamine should be carefully controlled via an infusion pump and the dose titrated to effect. Heart rate and rhythm and blood pressure should also be closely monitored. Dobutamine is useful in shock patients when fluid therapy alone has not restored acceptable arterial BP, cardiac output, or tissue perfusion. It is also used for short-term treatment of heart failure.

DOSAGES

See *Table 82* and Chapter 2 (Shock, Resuscitation, Fluid and Electrolyte Therapy, pp. 26–27).

ADVERSE EFFECTS

Dobutamine administration should be discontinued if severe tachycardia (>50% increase), arrhythmias, or hypertension develops. Because of the drug's short duration of action, temporarily halting therapy is usually all that is required to reverse these effects.

DOPAMINE

DEFINITION/OVERVIEW

Dopamine is a catecholamine with alpha adrenergic, beta adrenergic, and dopaminergic effects. It is a precursor to norepinephrine and is produced naturally by the body. Dopamine produces positive chronotropic and inotropic effects on the myocardium, resulting in increased heart rate and cardiac contractility. This is accomplished directly by exerting an agonist action on beta adrenergic receptors and indirectly by causing release of norepinephrine from storage sites in sympathetic nerve endings.

METHOD OF ACTION

At very low intravenous doses (0.5–2.0 µg/kg/min), dopamine acts predominantly on dopaminergic receptors and dilates the renal, mesenteric, coronary, and intracerebral vascular beds. At doses from 2–10 µg/kg/min, dopamine also stimulates beta-1 adrenergic receptors. The net effect at this dose range is to exert positive cardiac inotropic activity and increase organ perfusion, renal blood flow, and urine production (heart rate, myocardial contractility, and cardiac output increase). At these lower doses, systemic vascular resistance (SVR) remains largely unchanged. At higher doses (>10–12 µg/kg/min), the dopaminergic effects are overridden by alpha effects. Systemic peripheral resistance is increased and hypotension may be corrected in cases where SVR is diminished (peripheral vasoconstriction, increase in SVR and BP). Renal and peripheral blood flow is thus decreased. The onset of action is within 5 minutes and persists for less than 10 minutes after the infusion has stopped.

USES/INDICATIONS

Dopamine is used to correct the hemodynamic imbalances present in shock after adequate fluid volume replacement, to treat oliguric renal failure, and as adjunctive therapy for the treatment of acute heart failure. The dose of dopamine should be titrated to effect. It should be administered via an infusion pump, with continuous monitoring of heart rate, heart rhythm, BP, and urine output.

DOSAGES

See *Table 82* and Chapter 2 (Shock, Resuscitation, Fluid and Electrolyte Therapy, p. 28).

ADVERSE EFFECTS

The most frequent adverse effects are tachycardia and arrhythmias.

EPINEPHRINE

DEFINITION/OVERVIEW

Epinephrine is a catecholamine used systemically for treating anaphylaxis and cardiac resuscitation. It is a "fight or flight" hormone, which is naturally released from the adrenal gland. The hormone boosts the supply of oxygen and energy-giving glucose to the brain and muscles.

METHOD OF ACTION

Epinephrine is an alpha and beta adrenergic agent. Stimulation of the beta adrenergic receptors results in cardiac effects including direct stimulation of the heart (increases heart rate and contractility) and increases in systolic BP. Total peripheral resistance is decreased due to the beta effects. In addition, epinephrine relaxes smooth muscle in the bronchi and the iris, antagonizes the effects of histamine, increases glycogenolysis, and raises blood sugar levels.

USES/INDICATIONS

Epinephrine is used in the treatment for anaphylaxis and in cardiac resuscitation. It can be administered intravenously, intratracheally, or via an endotracheal tube. It is available in different concentrations, so it is important to know what concentration of the drug is being administered. Heart rate, heart rhythm, BP, and urine output should be monitored continuously.

DOSAGES

See *Table 82* and Chapter 2 (Shock, Resuscitation, Fluid and Electrolyte Therapy, p. 27).

ADVERSE EFFECTS

Possible adverse effects include hypertension and arrhythmias.

GLYCOPYRROLATE

DEFINITION/OVERVIEW

Glycopyrrolate is used to treat bradyarrhythmias and as a broncho-dilator. It is an anticholinergic agent similar to atropine, although with less adverse effects.

METHOD OF ACTION

Glycopyrrolate inhibits the action of acetylcholine on structures innervated by postganglionic cholinergic nerves and on smooth muscles that respond to acetylcholine but lack cholinergic innervation.

USES/INDICATIONS

Glycopyrrolate is used to treat bradyarrhythmias, sinus bradycardia, sinus arrest, and AV block. It is also used as a bronchodilator and to control excessive pharyngeal, tracheal, and bronchial secretions.

DOSAGES

See *Tables 81* and *82*.

ADVERSE EFFECTS

Adverse effects include signs of abdominal discomfort secondary to a decrease in GI motility. Glycopyrrolate is less arrhythmogenic than atropine and rarely causes adverse CNS effects.

LIDOCAINE

DEFINITION/OVERVIEW

Lidocaine has many uses including as an antiarrhythmic agent, a local and topical anesthetic agent, and a prokinetic agent.

METHOD OF ACTION

Lidocaine is considered to be a membrane-stabilizing agent by blocking fast sodium channels. Most of lidocaine's antidysrhythmic effect is on the Purkinje fibers and ventricular myocardium.

USES/INDICATIONS

Lidocaine is used to treat ventricular arrhythmias, in particular ventricular tachycardia and ventricular premature complexes. It is not effective orally and when given intravenously a loading dose must be give prior to a CRI.

DOSAGES

See *Table 82*.

ADVERSE EFFECTS

The most commonly reported adverse effects are CNS signs, including drowsiness, depression, ataxia, and muscle tremors.

MAGNESIUM SULFATE

DEFINITION/OVERVIEW

Magnesium sulfate is used to treat ventricular and supraventricular arrhythmias. In some experimental studies, when given prior to the asphyxia injury, magnesium sulfate has been shown to prevent or reduce hypoxic brain injury.

METHOD OF ACTION

Magnesium sulfate is a physiologic calcium channel blocker and is a cofactor in a variety of enzyme systems. By blocking calcium influx or by maintaining cellular enzymatic reactions magnesium sulfate may protect neuronal structure and function.

USES/INDICATIONS

Magnesium sulfate is used to treat ventricular tachycardia. It is slower acting than lidocaine. Also used as a possible prevention or therapy for HIE.

DOSAGES

See *Table 82*. For therapy for HIE: 50 mg/kg/h for 1 hour, then 25 mg/kg/h constant rate infusion (CRI) for up to 3 days.

ADVERSE EFFECTS

With excessive use or overdose, clinical signs of hypermagnesemia may be noted (e.g., muscle weakness, cardiovascular effects, and neurologic effects). When administered after asphyxia injury, there is no effect or evidence of harm.

NOREPINEPHRINE

DEFINITION/OVERVIEW

Norepinephrine is an alpha and beta-1 agonist used to treat hypotension.

METHOD OF ACTION

Norepinephrine increases heart rate and cardiac output due to its beta-1 adrenergic effects. The alpha adrenergic effects cause an increase in vascular tone and, therefore, SVR.

USES/INDICATIONS

Norepinephrine is used to treat hypotension. Heart rate, heart rhythm, BP, and urine output should be carefully monitored during norepinephrine infusion. The dose should be titrated to effect.

DOSAGES

See *Table 82* and Chapter 2 (Shock Resuscitation, Fluid and Electrolyte Therapy, p. 27).

ADVERSE EFFECTS

Possible adverse effects are arrhythmias, decreased urine production, and hypertension.

PROCAINAMIDE

DEFINITION/OVERVIEW

Procainamide is a class 1A antidysrhythmic agent.

METHOD OF ACTION

Procainamide blocks potassium channels in myocardial cells, prolonging the duration of action potentials and slowing conduction through the myocardium.

USES/INDICATIONS

Intravenous procainamide is used to treat refractory cases of ventricular tachycardia.

DOSAGES

See *Table 82*.

ADVERSE EFFECTS

Possible adverse effects include hypersensitivity reaction or an abnormal rhythm.

PROPANOLOL

DEFINITION/OVERVIEW

Propanolol is a class II antidysrhythmic agent.

METHOD OF ACTION

Propanolol inhibits both cardiac beta-1 and vascular beta-1 receptors. It also inhibits bronchial beta-2 receptors.

USES/INDICATIONS

Propanolol is used to treat unresponsive tachyarrhythmias including rapid supraventricular tachycardia and atrial flutter/fibrillation.

DOSAGES

See *Table 82*.

ADVERSE EFFECTS

Possible adverse effects include depression, lethargy, weakness, bradycardia, AV block, hypotension, and bronchoconstriction.

QUINIDINE

DEFINITION/OVERVIEW

Quinidine is an anti-arrhythmic agent that depresses myocardial excitability, conduction velocity, and contractility.

METHOD OF ACTION

Quinidine is classified as a class 1 anti-arrhythmic agent. Quinidine affects various ion channels in the myocardium. The overall result is to slow conduction and prolong the effective refractory period, resulting in interruption or prevention of re-entrant arrhythmias and arrhythmias due to increased automaticity. Its indirect actions include a vagolytic (positive chronotropic) effect and peripheral vasodilation secondary to alpha adrenoceptor antagonism.

USES/INDICATIONS

Quinidine is indicated for the treatment of atrial fibrillation in horses with no clinical or echocardiographic signs of heart failure. Quinidine is available in an oral (sulfate) or intravenous form (gluconate). The prognosis for successful conversion is excellent in patients with a duration of atrial fibrillation of <3–4 months, a resting heart rate <60 beats per minute (bpm), and no signs of heart failure. The prognosis for successful conversion decreases and the likelihood of recurrence increases with longer duration of the disease.

DOSAGES

See *Table 82*. Intravenous quinidine gluconate is used to treat horses with recent onset (less than 7 days) of atrial fibrillation. Patients with atrial fibrillation of longer than 7 days or who have not responded to initial intravenous treatment are treated with oral quinidine sulfate. Several different treatment regimes exist for the use of quinidine sulfate, but the protocol shown in *Table 82* is the one commonly used.

ADVERSE EFFECTS

After quinidine therapy, horses may show signs of depression or inappetence, which does not indicate toxicity. Signs of toxicity include swelling of the nasal mucosa, paraphimosis, ataxia, diarrhea, and colic. Cardiovascular adverse effects include cardiac dysrhythmias that can be life threatening, therefore it is important to perform a continuous electrocardiogram (ECG) during treatment.

PROKINETICS DRUGS

OVERVIEW

Prokinetic drugs are agents that facilitate or enhance the net movement of feed material down the length of the intestinal tract. The control of intestinal motility is complex and involves a combination of central innervation, autonomic innervation, and the enteric nervous system. Effective coordination and modulation of motility requires both sympathetic and parasympathetic input, along with several hormones. Prokinetic drugs promote motility by either augmenting the pathway that stimulates motility or attenuating the inhibitory neurons that predominantly suppress activity. These agents generally act by increasing the release or availability of ACh from cholinergic pathways, increasing activity at dopamine-1 and 5-hydroxytryptamine-4 (5-HT-4) receptors, and antagonizing inhibitory neurotransmitters or stimulating noncholinergic and nonadrenergic molecules that promote contractile activity. The efficacy of many of these agents has not been reported in the equine pediatric patient and most information has been extrapolated from studies done in adults.

BETHANECOL CHLORIDE

DEFINITION/OVERVIEW

Bethanecol chloride is a muscarinic cholinergic agonist used to treat postoperative ileus.

METHOD OF ACTION

Bethanecol chloride causes contraction of GI smooth muscle through stimulation of muscarinic receptors. It stimulates gastric emptying and gastric motility, therefore it is used more often in proximal GI disorders.

USES/INDICATIONS

Bethanecol chloride is used to treat gastric atony and ileus associated with gastroesophageal ulceration.

17

Table 83. Prokinetic drugs

Drug	Dose/route/frequency
Bethanecol chloride	0.3–0.4 mg/kg p/o q6–8h
	0.025–0.1 mg/kg s/c q6–8h
Cisapride	0.5–0.8 mg/kg p/o q6–8h
Erythromycin lactobionate	2.2 mg/kg i/v q6h (give each dose over 60 min in 1 L of saline)
Lidocaine	1.3 mg/kg i/v loading dose, then 0.05 mg/kg/min i/v CRI
Metoclopramide	0.1–0.25 mg/kg/h i/v CRI; 0.02–0.1 mg/kg i/v q6h (give each dose over 60 min in 1 L of saline);
	0.1–0.2 mg/kg s/q q6–8h

DOSAGES

See *Table 83*.

ADVERSE EFFECTS

The reported possible adverse effects are diarrhea, inappetence, salivation, and colic.

CISAPRIDE

DEFINITION/OVERVIEW

Cisapride is a second-generation benzamide that is used as a prokinetic agent. It lacks the extrapyramidal adverse effects of metoclopramide, although there are conflicting reports on its efficacy.

METHOD OF ACTION

Cisapride enhances the release of ACh from postganglionic neurons in the myenteric plexus through stimulation of 5HT-4 receptors. It has been reported to affect motility from the gastroesophageal sphincter to the descending colon.

USES/INDICATIONS

Cisapride could be used to treat motility disorder from the proximal GI tract to large colon stasis. Unfortunately, it is only available in the oral form, which is not useful in the treatment of postoperative ileus, especially if the foal is refluxing.

DOSAGES

See *Table 83*.

ADVERSE EFFECTS

In humans, cisapride has caused fatal cardiac dysrhythmias, although this adverse effect has not been reported in horses.

ERYTHROMYCIN

DEFINITION/OVERVIEW

Erythromycin is a macrolide antibiotic that at a lower dose has prokinetic properties.

METHOD OF ACTION

Erythromycin promotes intestinal motility by initiating the migrating motor complexes through motilin receptors. Motilin is an intestinal hormone whose release is naturally stimulated through vagal influences and the passage of feed through the duodenum. Erythromycin acts on motilin receptors on smooth muscle and on enteric cholinergic neurons to stimulate release of ACh, and it is through its neuronal receptors that it induces the migrating motor complexes. This drug has been reported to stimulate small intestinal, cecal, and colonic progressive motility.

USES/INDICATIONS

A low dose of erythromycin is used to treat postoperative small intestinal ileus and large intestinal stasis. Prolonged use may induce receptor downregulation, resulting in the tissues becoming refractory to treatment.

DOSAGES

See *Table 83*.

ADVERSE EFFECTS

Even at a low dose, diarrhea is a reported adverse effect.

LIDOCAINE

DEFINITION/OVERVIEW

Lidocaine is used to treat postoperative ileus because of its prokinetic properties, but also because of its anti-inflammatory and analgesic properties. In addition, it is used as an antiarrhythmic agent and local anesthetic.

METHOD OF ACTION

The stimulatory effect of lidocaine on intestinal function is believed to be the result of blockade of inhibitory sympathetic and parasympathetic reflexes, anti-inflammatory properties, inhibition of free radical formation, reduction in circulating catecholamines, and direct stimulation of the smooth muscles. Lidocaine exhibits anti-inflammatory properties by inhibiting granulocyte migration and release of lysosomal enzymes. The systemic administration of lidocaine is also thought to attenuate the perception of pain significantly by depressing the spiking activity, amplitude, and conduction time of myelinated A fibers and unmyelinated C fibers.

USES/INDICATIONS
Lidocaine is used to treat postoperative small intestinal ileus and large intestinal stasis. Following an intravenous bolus, the onset of action is generally within 2 minutes and has a duration of action of 10–20 minutes. A loading dose is given prior to beginning a CRI. If the CRI is stopped for >20 minutes, the loading dose must be administered again to allow for the proper therapeutic effects. For postoperative ileus, lidocaine is usually administered for 24 hours or longer.

DOSAGES
See *Table 83*.

ADVERSE EFFECTS
The most commonly reported adverse effects are CNS signs including drowsiness, depression, and mild to moderate ataxia and muscle tremors. Once the drug is discontinued these signs resolve quickly.

METOCLOPRAMIDE

DEFINITION/OVERVIEW
Metoclopramide is a first-generation benzamide that is used to treat postoperative ileus.

METHOD OF ACTION
Metoclopramide's main mechanism of action is release of ACh from postsynaptic cholinergic nerves in the GI tract by activation of 5-HT-4 receptors, which results in activation of GI smooth muscle. In addition, metoclopramide antagonizes the inhibitory effects of dopamine on GI smooth muscle. It is also an alpha-2 receptor antagonist.

USES/INDICATIONS
Metoclopramide is used to treat postoperative small intestinal ileus. A few reports indicate more contractility in the proximal part of the intestinal tract.

DOSAGES
See *Table 83*.

ADVERSE EFFECTS
Intravenous metoclopramide administration has been associated with extrapyramidal adverse effects such as sedation, excitement, involuntary muscle spasms, and behavioral changes. The adverse effects are due to metoclopramide's ability to cross the blood–brain barrier and antagonize dopaminergic receptors.

RENAL DRUGS

FUROSEMIDE

DEFINITION/OVERVIEW
Furosemide is a loop diuretic used in many species for the treatment of congestive cardiomyopathy, pulmonary edema, udder edema, hypercalcemic nephropathy, and uremia, as adjunctive therapy in hyperkalemia, and, occasionally, as an antihypertensive agent. It is also used in racehorses to prevent/reduce exercise-induced pulmonary hemorrhage.

METHOD OF ACTION
The mechanism of action of furosemide is blockage of the Na+/K+/2Cl- cotransporter in the ascending loop of Henle, resulting in reduced absorption of electrolytes. Furosemide also reduces the absorption of sodium and chloride in the proximal and distal tubules, resulting in increased excretion of water, sodium, chloride, potassium, calcium, magnesium, hydrogen, bicarbonate, and phosphate.

USES/INDICATIONS
Furosemide is used as a diuretic in cases of acute renal failure to induce or increase urine output. It is also used to reduce edema associated with congestive heart failure and to treat acute pulmonary edema.

DOSAGES
See *Table 84*. The intravenous dose used to treat oliguric acute renal failure is 1–2 mg/kg q6h. If an increase in urine production is not observed, a larger dose (4–6 mg/kg) can be administered. In the treatment of pulmonary or cardiac edema, 0.5–3 mg/kg can be administered q6–12h intravenously, intramuscularly, or orally.

ADVERSE EFFECTS
Excessive diuresis may cause dehydration and blood volume reduction. Careful monitoring of the electrolyte status should be carried out if furosemide is administered more than once or if the pediatric patient is severely compromised.

Table 84. Renal drugs

Drug	Dose/route/frequency
Furosemide	1–2 mg/kg i/v q6h
Mannitol	0.25–2.0 mg/kg as a 20% solution i/v over 30–60 min q6h
Phenazopyridine	4 mg/kg p/o q8–12h

MANNITOL

DEFINITION/OVERVIEW

Mannitol is an osmotic diuretic used to treat oliguric renal failure, to reduce intraocular and intracerebral pressures, to enhance urinary excretion of some toxins, and, with other diuretics, to rapidly reduce edema or ascites.

METHOD OF ACTION

Mannitol is filtered at the glomerulus and poorly reabsorbed in the tubule. The increased osmolarity of the glomerular filtrate hinders tubular reabsorption of water. Excretion of sodium and chloride is also enhanced. Mannitol does not enter the eye or CNS, but it can decrease intraocular and CSF pressure through its osmotic effects.

DOSAGES

See *Table 84*.

ADVERSE EFFECTS

Fluid and electrolyte imbalances are the most severe adverse effects generally encountered during mannitol therapy. Mannitol is contraindicated in pediatric patients with anuric renal failure, severe dehydration, intracranial bleeding, severe pulmonary congestion, or pulmonary edema.

PHENAZOPYRIDINE

DEFINITION/OVERVIEW

Phenazopyridine is an agent that has a specific local analgesic effect in the urinary tract, promptly relieving burning and pain. It is available in tablet form.

METHOD OF ACTION

The exact mechanism of action is unknown, but phenazopyridine is excreted in the urine and has a direct topical analgesic effect on the mucosal lining of the urinary tract.

USES/INDICATIONS

Phenazopyridine helps relieve pain, burning, urgency, and frequency caused by irritation of the lower urinary tract mucosa due to infection, trauma, surgery, or passage of catheters.

DOSAGES

See *Table 84*.

ADVERSE EFFECTS

Phenazopyridine causes a distinct color change in the urine to a dark orange to reddish color.

ANTIFUNGAL DRUGS

DEFINITION/OVERVIEW

There are various antifungal agents used in the treatment and prevention of fungal infections. Pharmacokinetics and therapeutic data for antifungal agents in adult horses and foals are limited. Despite this lack of information, antifungals have been used topically and systemically. There are two types of antifungal agents used in equine medicine: the azoles (fluconazole, miconazole, itraconazole, ketoconazole) and the polyenes (amphotericin B).

METHOD OF ACTION

The azole antifungal agents are synthetic compounds that are classified as imidazoles (miconazole and ketoconazole) and triazoles (itraconazole and fluconazole). They inhibit the fungal ergosterol synthesis in the cell membranes by interfering with the cytochrome P-450 enzyme system. The polyene antifungal agents bind to sterols in the fungal cell membrane, resulting in change in membrane permeability, which leads to cell death.

USES/INDICATIONS

Miconazole is only used topically to treat ophthalmologic or dermatologic problems caused by the common dermatophytes *Candida albicans* and *Malassezia furfur*. If administered systemically, it is toxic. Ketoconazole is poorly absorbed; therefore, it is not used for systemic infections. Instead, ketoconazole is used for topical infections such as those caused by dermatophytes and *Candida albicans*. Fluconazole is absorbed well after oral administration and reaches adequate concentrations in plasma, CSF, synovial fluid, aqueous humor, and urine. It is effective against histoplasmosis, coccidioidomycosis, cryptococcosis, blastomycosis, *Microsporum* spp., *Trichophyton* spp., and several *Candida* spp. Itraconazole is effective against the same fungal organisms as fluconazole with the addition of *Asperillus* spp. Administration of itraconazole solution is superior to the capsules. Amphotericin B is administered intravenously and is active against many species of fungi.

DOSAGES

See *Table 85*.

Table 85. Antifungal drugs

Drug	Dose	Route/frequency
Amphotericin B	0.3–1.0 mg/kg	i/v in 1 L of 5% dextrose over 30 min every other day
Fluconazole	5 mg/kg	Loading dose of 14 mg/kg p/o followed by maintenance dose of 5 mg/kg p/o q24h
Itraconazole	3–5 mg/kg	p/o q12–24h

ADVERSE EFFECTS

Amphotericin B can cause renal failure; therefore, kidney function should be closely monitored while it is being administered. Little is known about the adverse effects of the other antifungal agents.

ANTIVIRAL DRUGS

VALACYCLOVIR

DEFINITION/OVERVIEW

Valacyclovir is an antiviral drug. It is a prodrug that is completely converted to acyclovir and L-valine. It is better absorbed than acyclovir.

METHOD OF ACTION

Valacyclovir inhibits viral DNA replication.

USES/INDICATIONS

Valacyclovir is used in the treatment of EHV infections.

DOSAGES

Loading dose of 27 mg/kg/p/o q8h for 2 days, then maintenance dose of 18 mg/kg/p/o q12h.

ADVERSE EFFECTS

No adverse effects have been reported in horses.

SEDATIVES

BUTORPHANOL

DEFINITION/OVERVIEW

Butorphanol is used to produce analgesia and augment the sedation produced by other agents.

METHOD OF ACTION

Butorphanol, like other opioid analgesics, combines with opioid receptors in the CNS and in other organs.

USES/INDICATIONS

Butorphanol is most often used in combination with other sedatives or tranquilizers. In the younger foal, a small amount of butorphanol can be administered in cases of abdominal discomfort.

DOSAGES

See *Tables 86* and *87*.

ADVERSE EFFECTS

Butorphanol can cause increased locomotor activity and ataxia. If given at an extremely high dose, CNS excitement may occur.

Table 86. Sedatives

Drug	Dose/route
Butorphanol	0.01–0.04 mg/kg i/v
	0.02–0.08 mg/kg i/m
Diazepam	0.05–0.4 mg/kg i/v (only on foals <4 weeks old)
Xylazine	0.2–0.5 mg/kg i/v or i/m

Table 87. Sedation and anesthesia

Special considerations with foals:

- Young foals (<1 month of age) have rapidly changing cardiovascular and pulmonary physiology which must be taken into consideration.
- Cardiac output in foals is highly dependent on heart rate. Avoid bradycardia.
- Mean arterial pressure (MAP) in neonatal foal under general anesthesia is usually lower than an older foal.
- Foals are insensitive to hypercarbia and hypoxia and thus are prone to hypoventilation.
- Hepatic and renal function is immature in the foal until approximately 3 months of age.

Sedation:

- Foals < 2 weeks of age: Diazepam or midazolam (0.1–0.2 mg/kg i/v) generally provides excellent sedation and muscle relaxation.
- Older healthy foals (>2 weeks of age): Xylazine (0.2–0.5 mg/kg i/v) provides more reliable sedation
- Older critically ill foal: Diazepam or midazolam (0.1–0.2 mg/kg i/v) may be a more suitable option for sedation. This dose can be repeated as necessary.
- To provide analgesia and improve the quality of sedation butorphanol (0.02–0.1 mg/kg) can be administered i/v or i/m.
- For short procedures (i.e., joint tap or flush), ketamine (1.8–2.2 mg/kg i/v) will maintain anesthesia for approximately 15–20 min.
- For longer procedures, triple drip (guaifenesin+ketamine+xylazine) can be used as a maintenance anesthetic. Deliver a slow drip rate to effect.

(Continued)

Table 87. (*Continued*) Sedation and anesthesia

General anesthesia (GA) with inhalant agents:

- Induction with benzodiazepines (neonate) or xylazine (older foal) and ketamine
- Maintenance with isoflurane or sevoflurane

Monitoring:

- Palpation of peripheral pulse and auscultation of heart
- EKG/ECG—continuous or intermittent
- Indirect (tail cuff or cuff placed on forearm or dorsal metatarsal artery) or direct BP measurement
- Temperature (foals are prone to hypothermia)
- Oxygenation—arterial blood gas or pulse oximetry
- Neonatal foals undergoing long procedure—evaluate blood glucose

---

XYLAZINE/DETOMIDINE

DEFINITION/OVERVIEW

Xylazine and detomidine are sedatives and analgesics with muscle relaxant properties. Detomidine is more potent than xylazine.

METHOD OF ACTION

Xylazine and detomidine are alpha-2 adrenergic agonists that mediate sedation and analgesia through the brain and spinal alpha-2 receptors. Stimulation of the alpha-2 receptors results in a reduction of excitatory neurotransmitters by inhibiting the release of norepinephrine.

USES/INDICATIONS

Xylazine and detomidine are used to provide standing chemical restraint and to provide analgesia, as well as sedatives prior to general anesthesia. They are used most widely to treat colic.

DOSAGES

See *Tables 86 and 87.*

ADVERSE EFFECTS

Xylazine and detomidine cause respiratory depression and bradycardia, therefore they should not be used, or used with caution, in foals that are compromised or have respiratory disease. Xylazine and detomidine also depress thermoregulatory mechanisms, usually resulting in hypothermia. When large doses are given intravenously, muscle relaxation and ataxia may be severe. Despite appearing heavily sedated, foals can be aroused and may be aggressive. Often the foal will sweat. Intracarotid injection will result in seizure and collapse.

ANTI-ENDOTOXIC DRUGS

PENTOXIFYLLINE

DEFINITION/OVERVIEW

Pentoxifylline is a methyl xanthine derivative that is used in humans as a hemorrheologic agent (an agent that affects blood viscosity). It has also been shown to have beneficial effects in the treatment of endotoxemia.

METHOD OF ACTION

Pentoxifylline improves capillary blood flow by reducing blood viscosity and increasing red blood cell (RBC) deformability. In the treatment of endotoxemia, pentoxifylline inhibits the production of tumor necrosis factor, decreases thromboxane B2 concentration and tissue thromboplastin activity, and increases concentration of 6-keto-protaglandin-F1.

USES/INDICATIONS

In patients with GI disorders that are or may become endotoxic, pentoxifylline may be used in conjunction with other anti-endotoxic medications. Due to its hemorrheologic effects, pentoxifylline has also been used in cases of laminitis.

DOSAGES

See *Tables 88 and 89.*

ADVERSE EFFECTS

No adverse effects have been reported in horses, although minimal research on pentoxifylline use has been done in the pediatric patient.

Table 88. Anti-endotoxic drugs

Drug	Dose/route/frequency
Pentoxifylline	7.5–8.5 mg/kg p/o q8–12h
Polymixin B	3,000–6,000 U/kg in 1 L of fluids q6–8h

Table 89. Other drugs

Drug	Indications	Dose/route/frequency
Yunnan Baiyao	Control hemorrhage	8 mg/kg p/o q6–24h
ε-Aminocaproic acid	Control hemorrhage (inhibitor of fibrinolysis)	Bolus: 20–40 mg/kg i/v q6h (diluted) CRI 3.5 mg/kg/min for 20 min then 0.25 mg/kg/min
N-butylscopolammonium bromide	Spasmolytic analgesic	0.3 mg/kg (once) Side effects: Can cause ileus/colic and tachycardia

POLYMIXIN B

DEFINITION/OVERVIEW
Polymixin B is a broad-spectrum antibiotic that is used for its anti-endotoxic properties. It is rarely used as an antibiotic because of severe adverse effects.

METHOD OF ACTION
Polymixin B binds to and neutralizes endotoxins.

USES/INDICATIONS
Polymixin B is used in patients with severe endotoxemia, most often associated with GI disorders.

DOSAGES
See *Tables 88 and 89.*

ADVERSE EFFECTS
The low dose used for the treatment of endotoxemia has minimal adverse effects. In patients with severe dehydration or renal compromise, polymixin B should be used with caution. At high doses, polymixin B can cause respiratory paralysis and nephrotoxicity.

FURTHER READING

Baggot JD (1994) Drug therapy in the neonatal foal. *Vet Clin North Am Equine Pract* 10: 87–107.

Barton MH (2000) Use of polymixin B for treatment of endotoxemia in horses. *Comp Cont Educ Pract* 22: 1056–1059.

Baskett A, Barton MH, Norton N, Anders B, Moore JN (1997) Effect of pentoxifylline, flunixin meglumine, and their combination on a model of endotoxemia in horses. *Am J Vet Res* 58: 1291–1299.

Fischer B, Clark-Price S (2015) Anesthesia of the equine neonate in health and disease. *Vet Clin North Am Equine Pract* 31: 567–586.

Giguere S, Prescot JF, Dowling PM (Eds.) (2013) *Antimicrobial Therapy in Veterinary Medicine,* 5th ed. Wiley, Oxford, UK.

Hildebrand F, Venner M, Giguere S (2015) Efficacy of gamithromycin for treatment of foals with mild to moderate bronchopneumonia. *J Vet Intern Med* 59: 333–338.

Hovanessian N, Davis JL, McKenzie III HC, Hodgson JL, Crisman MV (2014) Pharmacokinetics and safety of firocoxib after oral administration of repeated consecutive doses to neonatal foal. *J Vet Pharm Ther* 37: 243–251.

Magdesian KG (2017) Antimicrobial pharmacology for the neonatal foal. *Vet Clin North Am Equine Pract* 33: 47–65.

Norman WM, Court MH, Greenblatt DJ (1997) Age-related changes in pharmacokinetic disposition of diazepam in foals. *Am J Vet Res* 53: 878–880.

Plumb DC (2015) *Veterinary Drug Handbook,* 8th ed. Wiley-Blackwell, Hoboken, NJ.

Robertson SA (2005) Sedation and general anaesthesia of the foal. *Equine Vet Educ* 7: 94–101.

Soma LR, Uboh CE, Guan F, Birks EK, Teleis DC, Rudy JA, Tsang DS, Watson AO (2001) Disposition, elimination and bioavailability of phenytoin and its major metabolite in horses. *Am J Vet Res* 62: 483–489.

Whittem T (1999) Clinical pharmacology and therapeutics. *Vet Clin North Am: Equine Pract* 15: 1–782.

Pediatric Nutrition

18

Bonnie S. Barr

KEY POINTS

- Young foals nurse 7–10 times per hour. The frequency gradually decreases as the foal grows older. They begin to eat solid food within a few days of age and will consume significant amounts by 2 months of age.
- Weight gain for a healthy foal is 1.2–1.6 kg/day in the first month and gradually declines to about 1.0 kg/day at 4 months of age.
- An ill neonatal foal (<1 month of age) may require nutritional intervention sooner than a suckling foal (>1 month of age) due to limited body reserves.
- The best route to provide supplemental nutrition is by the enteral route, although certain circumstances warrant the parenteral route.

A healthy full-term neonate should stand and suckle strongly from the mare within 2–3 hours of birth. The foal then develops a regular feeding pattern involving periods of nursing/eating and periods of resting and exercise. Young foals nurse 7–10 times per hour. The frequency gradually decreases as the foal grows older. Milk provides all the necessary nutrients, cells, enzymes, hormones, and multiple minerals and vitamins that the very young foal requires. The foal is born immunologically naive because the epitheliochorial placentation does not allow transfer of maternal immunoglobulins to the fetus. Colostrum contains many soluble and cellular components that likely play a role in neonatal immunity and intestinal maturation (*Table 90*). Foals, especially those confined in a stall, will begin to eat solid food within a few days, but milk is the primary source of nutrition. A normal, healthy neonatal foal consumes roughly 15% of body weight as milk in the first 24 hours, increasing to 20%–23% by day 2 and up to 25% by day 7. By 5 weeks of age foals spend more than 20% of their time grazing or eating non-milk foods. As the foal matures the capacity for fiber digestion increases and by 6 months of age the foal is receiving less than 30% of the total nutritional requirement in the form of milk.

The neonatal foal is born with minimal energy stores. Glycogen, stored in the liver and muscle, is one source of energy for the neonate. Energy is also derived from endogenous fat. Both glycogen and fat are limited in the newborn foal, thus these energy stores can be exhausted within a day. It has been estimated that a healthy neonatal foal's energy requirement is about 120–150 kcal/bwt/day (bwt = body weight). The energy requirements of a healthy suckling foal are estimated to be 120 kcal/kg bwt/day at 3 weeks of age, then 80–100 kcal/kg bwt/day at 1 month to weaning (*Table 91*). Weight gain during the first month is roughly 1.2–1.6 kg/day then gradually declines to about 1.0 kg/day at 4 months of age. The aim is for a steady growth rate and a lean foal rather than a foal that is obese.

In the earliest stages of life a foal's nutritional requirements are met with mare's milk. Mare's milk is higher in carbohydrates (lactose) and lower in fat content than that of most species. Milk production peaks around 2 months of lactation and then declines. Most foals will eat solid food within a few days and will consume significant amounts of hay, pasture, and grain by 2–3 months of age. There is limited research to assess the optimal nutrient intake for a 2–3 month old foal but reports indicate that a ration of 14%–15% crude protein, 0.7% calcium, and 0.4% phosphate is adequate. Specific nutrient requirements for feeding foals older than 3 months of age have been documented in the National Research Council's Nutrient Requirements for the Horse.

Foals are born without bacteria in the gastrointestinal (GI) tract, but colonization begins rapidly with a mature microbial

Table 90. Colostrum's soluble and cellular components

Soluble components	Cellular components
Immunoglobulins	Lymphocytes
Hormones	Macrophages
Growth factors	Neutrophils
Cytokines	Epithelial cells
Lactoferrin	
CD-14	
Lysozymes	
Other enzymes	

Table 91. Energy requirements of the foal

Neonatal healthy foal: 120–150 kcal/kg bwt/day
A 3-week old healthy foal: 120 kcal/kg bwt/day
A 1 month to weanling healthy foal: 80–100 kcal/kg bwt/day
Critically ill neonatal foal: 50 kcal/kg bwt/day

community present by the sixth week of life. The process of foaling exposes the newborn to environmental bacterial from the mare's vagina, feces, and saliva. Young foals frequently consume the mare's fresh feces. This behavior serves as a direct inoculation of viable GI microbes. *Lactobacilli*, Enterobacteriaceae, *Streptococci*, *Staphylococci*, and Clostridia have been isolated from feces of foals as young as 3 days of age. Cellulolytic bacteria have been detected in low levels from the feces of 3–5 day old neonates. By 12 weeks of age cellulolytic and lactic acid bacteria are present in feces at levels similar to mature horses. Overall, the timeline of the microbial establishment of the GI tract is consistent with the time at which plant-based feeds become important in the diet of the foal. As hindgut function increases, a shift in the primary energy substrate also occurs from ingested carbohydrates absorbed in the small intestine to volatile fatty acids produced by fermentation that are absorbed from the large intestines.

NUTRITIONAL SUPPORT OF THE SICK FOAL

Nutritional needs of the sick foal depend on several factors including the age of the foal, severity of the illness, and reason for illness, as well as the involvement of other systemic factors. Foals with mild transient illness will continue to nurse and be able to maintain proper caloric intake. A neonatal foal that stops nursing or is unable to nurse may require nutritional intervention sooner than a suckling foal due to the limitation of body reserves. The presence of GI abnormalities such as ileus or abdominal distention may warrant extra nutrition because the foal is unable to nurse. Foals with profuse watery diarrhea due to osmotic diarrhea often suffer from gas accumulation and abdominal distension. In the neonatal foal limited nutrient intake can be secondary to asphyxia gut injuries resulting in mucosal injury and milk intolerance. Failure to provide adequate nutritional support may also have a substantial negative influence on the immune response. Nutritional management of the foal also depends on the resources available, such as whether the foal will be hospitalized or managed on the farm.

Prior to developing a nutritional plan the foal must be triaged and stabilized (see Chapter 2). Every effort must be made to correct electrolyte, acid–base, and hydration status of the patient. Once the foal has been stabilized attention can be given to determining if there is a need for nutritional support and the best way to go about providing it. Neonatal foals that stop nursing or have secondary GI problems should be supplemented because of limited energy reserves in the form of glycogen and fat. Profound hypoglycemia can occur in the neonatal foal if deprived of energy intake even for a few hours. Suckling foals that stop nursing and are in good body condition may not require supplementation as soon as the neonate. But even after 24–36 hours of inappetence a suckling foal will benefit from extra calories. In a recent report the resting energy requirements in critically ill neonatal foals was documented to be approximately 50 kcal/kg bwt/day, which is about one-third the energy requirements for the growing, active, normal neonatal foal. Interestingly, this study also noted that the surviving critically ill neonatal foal's resting energy requirements normalized to healthy neonatal foal values prior to discharge from the hospital. Nutritional supplementation can be provided either enterally or parenterally. The best route and most natural is the enteral route, although certain circumstances warrant the parenteral route.

ENTERAL NUTRITION

Benefits of enteral nutrition

Results from numerous animal and human studies support enteral nutrition as superior to parenteral nutrition. Food in the GI tract has an important role in preserving normal physiology, especially related to immune function and systemic inflammation. Animal models have demonstrated that enteral nutrition lowers the risk of infection by preserving GI tract integrity and enhancing its ability to provide an immunocompetent barrier to prevent invasion by pathogenic microorganisms. The intestinal barrier is maintained by the enterocytes that play a major role in digestion and immunologic protection. Enterocytes are responsible for brush border digestion and absorption of nutrients. Amino acids, specifically glutamine, are the enterocytes' main source of fuel. But glucose and fatty acids can also be utilized by enterocytes. Enterocytes also provide a barrier against microbial translocation across the bowel wall into the systemic circulation and behave as true immunocompetent cells by reacting to antigens.

Studies have shown that after just a few days of complete bowel rest, progressive atrophy of the intestinal tract occurs. The lack of food produces a state of "luminal starvation" that adversely affects the enterocytes. The consequences of enterocyte starvation are characterized by intestinal mucosal atrophy, decreased absorption of nutrients, loss of tight junctions between enterocytes, impaired immune functions, and an increased risk for translocation of bacteria. Enteral nutrition helps to maintain the functional integrity of the bowel, prevent translocation of bacteria, and subsequent sepsis. Therefore, even if the GI tract cannot be used to meet complete needs, small amounts of enteral feeding may be helpful. Numerous studies with pre-term human infants have documented the beneficial outcomes of minimal enteral feedings (trophic feedings) including decreased hospitalization, faster transition to complete oral feedings, fewer infants with feeding intolerance, and a reduction in sepsis. An experimental study in mice noted that small amounts of enteral nutrition paired with parenteral nutrition prevented and reversed some of the changes in the GI mucosa that are typically noted with lack of enteral nutrition.

Sources of enteral nutrition

It has been well documented that fresh mare's milk is the preferred source of enteral nutrition in the neonatal foal. Advantages of this source of enteral feeding include physiologic stimulation leading to normal metabolic regulation, preservation of GI mucosa integrity, and important trophic substances (including epidermal growth factor and insulin-like growth factors) that stimulate normal growth and development. If fresh mare's milk is not available, frozen mare's milk is the next best alternative followed by milk replacer. Several commercial milk replacers that mimic mare's milk are available (*Table 92*). Side effects of milk replacer are diarrhea, colic, and soft feces. If not diluted adequately, constipation, dehydration, and hypernatremia can occur. To avoid these side effects it is best to read directions carefully, slowly switch to milk replacer, and not change brands once a foal is started on a particular brand. Milk from another species can be used if there are no other options. Mare's milk is noted to be higher in carbohydrates or lactose and lower in fat content than cow's or goat's milk (*Table 93*). The composition of mare's milk changes throughout lactation with the fat, protein, calcium, and phosphorous levels decreasing. Goat's milk is higher in fat, total

Table 92. Nutrient content of various brands of milk replacer

Nutrient	Foal Lac (Pet-Ag)	Mare's Milk Plus (Buckeye)	Foals First Milk Replacer Powder (Progressive Nutrition)	Mare's Match Foal Milk Replacer (Land O'Lakes)	Mare Replacer Powder (Kalmbach Feeds)	Mare's Milk Replacer (Baileys Horse Feeds)
Crude protein (%)	19.5	21	21	24	21	21
Crude fat (%)	14	14	14	16	14	14
Crude fiber (%)	0.1	0.15	0.4	0.15	0.15	0.05
Calcium (max %)	1.20	1.20	1.20	1.15	1.1	1
Phosphorous (%)	0.75	0.65	0.7	0.6	0.65	0.65

Table 93. Composition of mare's, cow's, and goat's milk (during first 4 weeks of lactation)

Nutrient	Mare	Cow	Goat
Crude protein (%)	25	27	25
Crude fat (%)	17	38	31
Crude fiber (%)	0	0	0
Total solids (dry matter [DM] %)	10.7	12.5	13.5
Calcium (%)	1.1	1.1	1.0

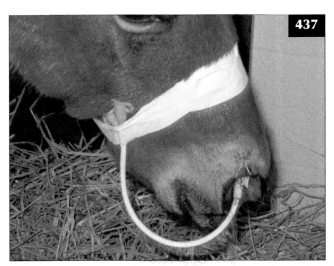

437 Small-diameter feeding tube (Kangaroo™ Feeding Tube, Covidien, Mansfield, MA).

solids, and gross energy than mare's milk and is easier to digest than cow's milk. Most foals will accept a goat milk diet and exhibit satisfactory growth. Cow's milk can be fed to foals but it is lower in carbohydrates than mare's milk and has twice the fat content, which can lead to diarrhea due to poor digestibility. If cow's milk is used, it is best to feed 2% milk and add dextrose, which will increase the carbohydrate content. The addition of 40 mL of 50% dextrose solution to each quart of milk or a 2 ounce package of jam/jelly pectin per 3 quarts of milk will satisfactorily increase the carbohydrate content. Those products that contain sucrose, such as honey, corn syrup, or table sugar, should not be used because will cause diarrhea and colic.

Routes to provide enteral nutrition

Physiologically the best route for providing milk is by normal suckling. Other methods utilized to provide milk include bottle or bowl feeding or feeding through a nasogastric tube. Placement of a small-diameter indwelling nasogastric tube is well tolerated by foals (437). In the neonatal foal small volumes of milk should be started and if tolerated, the volume gradually increased over several days. Ideally the foal should be fed at least every 2 hours (438). A good starting point is 5% of body weight for the first 24 hours. If this volume is well tolerated (i.e., the foal remains comfortable and exhibits no abdominal distension), then the volume can be increased until the

foal is able or willing to nurse (*Tables 94, 95*). In any case, the goal is to provide appropriate calories and protein.

Parenteral supplementation may be needed to completely satisfy caloric requirements. Suckling foals might prefer to eat hay instead of nurse. The addition of forage to the diet provides energy in the form of volatile fatty acids, maintains colonocyte health by the generation of butyric acid, and may decrease fecal water volume. In a majority of cases, preference for hay over milk is only temporary and the foal will resume nursing within 24 hours. If a foal completely refuses to nurse or eat and has no additional GI problems that would prevent it from nursing or eating, an indwelling nasogastric tube can be placed for supplementation. Milk can be administered to the neonatal foal (less than 1 month of age) and a slurry of pelleted balanced creep/foal feed to the older suckling foal. This pelleted feed would need to be ground with the addition of water, a balanced electrolyte solution, or milk to form a slurry in a consistency that will go down a tube. The amount of foal feed to supplement per day is generally 1 lb (0.45 kg) per month of age or as per listed on the feed bag. This should be divided into several feedings and the foal should be closely monitored for complications. A commercially

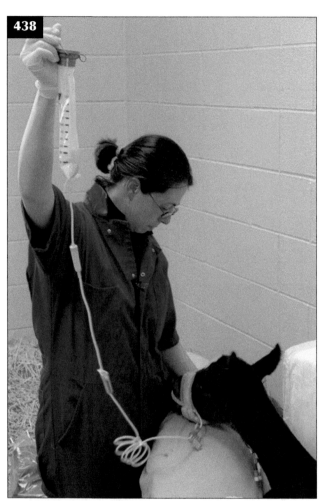

438

438 Feeding foal with gravity feeding bag (Kangaroo™ Gravity Feeding Bag, Covidien, Mansfield, MA).

Table 95. Example calculation of enteral feeding requirement

Example: 20% bwt/day for a 50 kg foal

50 kg × 20% = 10 kg = 10 L

Goal: Feed every 2 hours

10 L ÷ 12 = 0.833 L or 833 mL/feeding

833 mL/feeding = 27 oz/feeding

Volume will need to be reevaluated daily as the foal gains weight.

Table 94. Enteral nutrition numbers to know

Normal foal consumes 20%–25% body weight in milk per day.

Stall-confined sick foal consumes about 12%–15% body weight in milk per day.

1 oz = 30 mL

16 oz = 1 lb

1 kg = 1 L

Mare's milk = 0.57 kcal/mL

---

formulated enteral nutrition made by Platinum Performance has been used by this author for older foals.

Possible complications of enteral feeding include overfeeding resulting in gastric distension and colic, diarrhea, esophageal irritation, or aspiration pneumonia. Additional fluids intravenously or orally may need to be administered based on the foal's hydration status and if ongoing losses are present. It is unlikely that supplementation by nasogastric tube will be needed because most foals will continue to consume some type of enteral nutrition on their own.

Based on the above information the best route to provide the foal with nutrition is to allow the foal to nurse or eat. Foals with severe abdominal distention, ileus, septic shock, or colic will benefit from a brief period of feed restriction. The addition of parenteral nutrition will depend on the age of the foal and length of time the foal will be restricted from enteral nutrition. As soon as the foal's condition stabilizes and the GI tract is ready, enteral feeding should be reintroduced. This introduction can be an intermittent allowance to nurse or, in the case of an older foal, the addition of handfuls of hay. The introduction period should be short, for instance, every 2–4 hours provide an enteral form of nutrition with the final goal of return to full feed/milk in 24–36 hours. If the foal is receiving parenteral nutrition, the rate can be decreased by one-half, then discontinued once the foal is back to full enteral nutrition.

PARENTERAL NUTRITION

Parenteral nutrition is indicated for foals with poor GI function and intolerance to enteral feeding. The goal of parenteral nutrition is to provide enough nutritional support to avoid energy depletion during a phase of disease in which enteral nutrition is not an option or to provide supplemental nutrition when full enteral nutrition cannot be tolerated. Carbohydrates and lipids are the primary sources of energy used in parenteral nutrition solutions, whereas amino acids are added to meet protein requirements.

Dextrose supplementation

Carbohydrate-containing fluid solutions represent the simplest means of providing intravenous nutrition to foals and all compromised foals will benefit from endogenous glucose support. Before birth the normal fetus receives all of its glucose needs from the placenta. The blood glucose value of a newborn foal may be low (30–40 mg/dL) with the lowest value occurring about 2–4 hours after birth, but once glucogenesis begins the value will normalize. With fetal distress resulting from placentitis or poor nutrient intake by the mare, glucogenesis may begin while *in utero* and the foal might be born with a high blood glucose value. Newborn foals suffering from perinatal disease can have a hard time making a normal transition from relying on the placenta for glucose to providing their own glucose and will benefit from endogenous supplementation. Supplying energy in the form of dextrose decreases the need for catabolism, which allows the foal's metabolic energy to be focused on recovery rather than support.

The caloric content of a 50% dextrose solution is 1.7 kcal/g. Carbohydrate-containing solutions can be administered for a short period of time in the younger foal (24–48 hours) and longer in the older foal (2–3 days) because dextrose-containing fluids are an incomplete nutritional source. There are several commercially available products with dextrose or one can compound a dextrose solution by adding 50% dextrose (500 mg of dextrose/mL) to an isotonic polyionic fluid used for routine fluids support. Dextrose in 5% water is not a good choice as a maintenance solution because of the absence of electrolytes, and is primarily useful in providing free water to patients suffering from hyperosmolar conditions. A 50% dextrose solution can be administered without dilution using an infusion pump, as long as additional isotonic fluids are being administered concurrently to meet the patient's hydration needs and to avoid endothelial injury caused by the hypertonic nature of this solution. The primary fluid needs of the patient can be met with isotonic fluids and it will be easier to adjust fluid rate in response to the patient's hydration needs without affecting the nutritional needs of the patient. The transfer rate of glucose from the placenta to the fetus has been estimated in several species to be between 4 and 8 mg/kg/min of glucose, thus this is the appropriate rate of the dextrose-containing fluids for the neonate. The severely septic neonate may require more. The rate similar to an adult, 0.5–2 mg/kg/min, is appropriate for the suckling foal (*Tables 96, 97*).

Dextrose and amino acid supplementation

After 24–48 hours of dextrose-containing fluids, the nutritional plan should be revisited to determine if the foal can tolerate enteral nutrition. In addition to vital parameters and hydration status, the presence or absence of GI motility, frequency of fecal output, and consistency of feces should be considered in the assessment. If continued parenteral nutrition is required, a more complete solution that contains amino acids and possibly lipids should be administered. Since the metabolic response to injury and sepsis is to increase protein degradation in muscle tissue, the addition of a protein source reduces this catabolic response. Protein supplementation provides essential and nonessential amino acids.

The most commonly used protein solutions provide approximately 4.0 kcal/gm of protein. A commercially premixed standardized combination of a 50% dextrose solution and 8.5% amino acid

---

Table 96. Sample calculation of dextrose supplementation for a neonatal foal

50 kg newborn foal

Goal: 4 mg/kg bwt/min (range 4–8 mg/kg bwt/min)

50 kg × 4 mg/kg bwt/min = 200 mg/min

200 mg/min × 60 min/h = 12,000 mg/h

Using a 5% dextrose solution = 50 mg/mL of dextrose

12,000 mg/h ÷ 50 mg/mL = 240 mL/h

Constant rate infusion (CRI) = 240 mL/h of 5% dextrose

Table 97. Sample calculation of dextrose supplementation for a 5-week-old foal

Constant rate infusion (CRI):

115 kg 5-week-old foal

Goal: 0.5 mg/kg bwt/min (range 0.5–2 mg/kg bwt/min)

115 kg × 0.5 mg/kg bwt/min = 57.5 mg/min

57.5 mg/min × 60 min/h = 3450 mg/h

Bolus:

From the above calculation, the hourly amount of dextrose is 3,450 mg/h.

3,450 mg/h × 24 h = 82,800 mg/day

If administering fluids every 4 hours then would need to administer 13,800 mg every 4 hour.

This would be 28 mL of 50% dextrose at each treatment time (or every 4 hours) added to fluids.

50% dextrose = 500 mg/mL of dextrose

Remember: This is an incomplete nutritional source, so only utilize for a short period of time.

---

solution is available and has been utilized in the author's practice. Another option is to purchase the solutions separately and aseptically mix them in a sterile parenteral nutrition bag. The following formula is well tolerated by the foal: 1,500 mL 50% dextrose and 1,500 mL 8.5% amino acids. The caloric density of this solution is 1.02 kcal/mL (*Table 98*). This solution should be diluted in an isotonic solution or sterile water for administration because the combination of dextrose and amino acids is hypertonic and potentially harsh on the vein.

Total parenteral nutrition supplementation

The greatest benefit to the addition of lipids is providing more calories than dextrose alone or dextrose and amino acids. Foals, especially neonatal foals, utilize lipids readily as an energy source when it is provided. Lipid emulsions contain primarily long-chain triglycerides and provide a concentrated source of calories at 9–11 kcal per gram. Another benefit is that lipid emulsions are isotonic and help reduce total osmolarity when added to glucose and amino acid mixtures. Critical illness may result in protein catabolism and muscle wasting as a result of the release of cytokines and catabolic hormones. Thus it is important to minimize protein breakdown by providing enough carbohydrates and lipids. A rule of thumb is to provide at least 100–200 nonprotein calories (carbohydrate and lipids) per gram of nitrogen in the parenteral nutrition formula.

Solutions composed of 10 g/kg/day of dextrose, 2 g/kg/day of amino acids, and 1 g/kg/day of lipids are well tolerated by the foal. The volume of each nutrient is calculated based on the proportion of energy derived from dextrose and lipids, as well as the grams of protein that the foal requires. Once the final volume is determined, an hourly infusion rate is calculated by dividing the total volume in milliliters by 24 hours. This approach will calculate the anticipated

Table 98. Sample calculation with dextrose and amino acid mixture

115 kg 6-week-old foal

Goal: 80 kcal/kg bwt/day

Mixture of 1,500 mL of 50% dextrose and 1,500 mL of 8.5% amino acids

Caloric density of the above mixture = 1.02 kcal/mL

80 kcal/kg bwt/day × 115 kg = 9200 kcal/day

9,200 kcal/day ÷ 1.02 kcal/mL = 9020 mL/day

9020 mL/day ÷ 24 h = 376 mL/h as target rate

Start around one-quarter to one-third of this rate, then increase every 4–6 hours until target rate is achieved.

Table 99. Parenteral nutrition numbers to know

Glucose: 3.4 kcal/g

Amino acids: 4.0 kcal/g

Lipids: 9–11 kcal/g

6.25 g amino acids = 1 g nitrogen

Nonprotein nitrogen calories/g
nitrogen = dextrose calories + lipid calories/(grams amino acids/6.35)

non protein calories per gram of nitrogen 100:1 to 200:1

Table 100. Example calculation of TPN based on 10-2-1 formula for neonatal foal

Formula:

Dextrose—10 g/kg/day using a 50% dextrose solution (0.5 g/mL)

Amino Acids—2 g/kg/day using a 10% amino acid solution (0.1 g/mL)

Lipids—1 g/kg/day using a 20% lipid solution (0.2 g/mL)

For a 50 kg foal:

Dextrose—10 g/kg/day × 50 kg = 500 g/day ÷ 0.5 g/mL = 1,000 mL/day

Amino acids—2 g/kg/day × 50 kg = 100 g/day ÷ 0.1 g/mL = 1,000 mL/day

Lipids—1 g/kg/day × 50 kg = 50 g/day ÷ 0.2 g/mL = 250 mL/day

TOTAL: 2,250 mL/day ÷ 24 h = target rate 94 mL/h

Table 101. TPN formulations for the foal

Composition, caloric density

Formula 1:

900 mL 50% dextrose solution, 1.19 kcal/mL

1,400 mL 8.5% amino acids solution

900 mL 20% lipid solution

Formula 2:

1,500 mL 50% dextrose solution, 1.08 kcal/mL

2,000 mL 8.5% amino acids solution

500 mL 20% lipid solution

Formula 3:

1,000 mL 50% dextrose solution, 1.13 kcal/mL

1,000 mL 10% amino acids solution

250 mL 20% lipid solution

metabolic needs of the individual patient but is complex and involves various calculations (*Tables 99, 100*). Another approach is to utilize one of the several basic formulas that have been described for use in the foal. These formulas can easily be prepared aseptically (*Tables 101, 102*). Premade mixtures of intravenous multivitamins can be added to parenteral nutrition. These products contain the fat-soluble vitamins A, D, and E, which are solubilized in an aqueous medium, permitting intravenous administration. The B-complex vitamins, including thiamine, folic acid, pantothenic acid, and niacin, are also found in these commercial vitamin products. Thiamine (vitamin B1) is a component of thiamine pyrophosphate and is an essential cofactor in carbohydrate metabolism. Vitamin B complex can be added directly to the parenteral nutrition solution. Supplemental electrolytes can be added to the maintenance crystalloid fluids.

Administration of parenteral nutrition

Parenteral nutrition can safely be administered by an intravenous catheter placed aseptically in the jugular vein. Proper catheter management is extremely important. The solutions used for parenteral nutrition are hypertonic and can cause injury to the vascular endothelium resulting in phlebitis or thrombosis. Multi-lumen catheters allow for 1 lumen to be dedicated to infusion of the solution, thus minimizing the risks of contamination (**439, 440**). Parenteral nutrition should be delivered at a constant rate using an infusion pump to avoid fluctuations in glucose delivery and metabolic complications, and the actual volume of parenteral nutrition delivered to the patient should be carefully monitored and recorded (**441**). To allow for insulin and other physiological parameters to adapt to the solution, parenteral nutrition administration should be started at one-quarter of the target rate. The rate should then be gradually

Table 102. Sample calculation of total parenteral nutrition for neonatal foal

50 kg newborn foal

Goal: 50 kcal/kg bwt/day

Using formula 3 from Table 101 with caloric density of 1.13 kcal/mL:

50 kcal/kg bwt/day × 50 kg = 2,500 kcal/day

2,500 kcal/day ÷ 1.13 kcal/mL = 2,212 mL/day

2,212 mL/day ÷ 24 h = 92 mL/h as target rate

Start around one-quarter of this rate, then increase every 4–6 hours until target rate is reached.

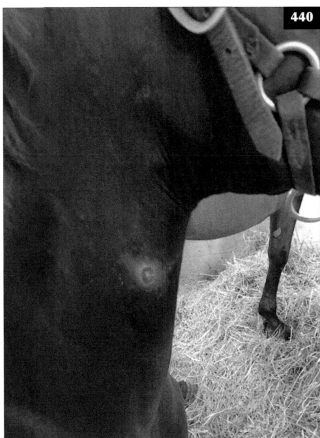

440 Infected jugular vein.

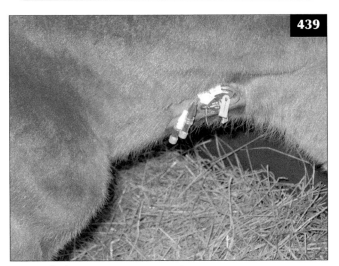

439 Multi-lumen intravenous catheter.

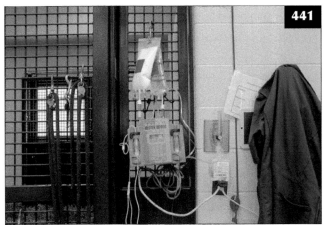

441 Total parenteral nutrition (TPN) on fluid pump.

increased every 4–6 hours, depending on the blood glucose values, until the target rate is reached.

In the early stage of parenteral nutritional therapy the foal must be frequently monitored. In addition to the physical examination and vital signs, blood glucose concentrations should be monitored. A dextrometer purchased from a human pharmacy provides a cheap and accurate assessment of blood glucose values. Initially, the blood glucose concentration should be monitored every 2–4 hours until the patient is at the target rate of parenteral nutrition then the frequency can be decreased. Blood glucose should be maintained between 90 and 180 mg/dL (**442**). The frequency of monitoring blood glucose concentration depends on the age and stability of the patient, with the very critically ill neonatal foal often requiring more frequent monitoring. Urine output should be monitored constantly with intermittent monitoring of urine glucose. In some cases glucosuria and diuresis are observed when blood glucose levels exceed 180 mg/dL, indicating that the administration rate should be adjusted. Some critically ill foals, usually neonatal foals, are intolerant of even a conservative rate of dextrose because of insulin resistance. Foals with persistently increased values, above 180–200 mg/dL for more than 4–6 hours, may benefit from exogenous insulin therapy.

Clearance of lipids can be impaired in the severely compromised foal and triglyceride concentrations of >200 mg/dL have been associated with non-survival. Monitoring the blood sample for lipemia or elevated triglyceride value is important in certain cases. Lipid administration should be discontinued (or decreased) if lipemia is noted or the triglyceride value is persistently elevated. Since electrolyte abnormalities are a common occurrence in critically ill foals, frequent monitoring of electrolytes should be performed. Hypokalemia is common in foals receiving intravenous nutrition because glucose and insulin administration reduce extracellular potassium concentrations.

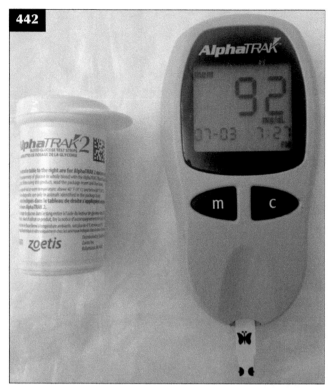

442 Dextrometer (AlphaTrak blood glucose monitoring system by Zoetis, Parsippany, NJ).

Table 103. Complications with parenteral nutrition

Jugular vein phlebitis or thrombophlebitis

Hyperglycemia

Glucosuria/osmotic diuresis

Hyperlipidemia

Electrolyte imbalances

Metabolic acidosis or sodium abnormalities can occur in critically ill foals secondary to GI losses (diarrhea or gastric reflux) (*Table 103*).

Intermittent (bolus) fluids with dextrose supplementation

In certain instances a constant rate of infusion of fluids and parenteral nutrition is not feasible and fluids will need to be bolused. Depending on the age of the foal and severity of the illness, fluids can be administered every 2–6 hours over a period of 30 minutes. To provide supplemental calories, dextrose can be added to the maintenance fluids. In order to prevent significant hyperglycemia, a 1%–2.5% dextrose solution in isotonic polyionic fluids can be administered slowly over a period of 20–30 minutes. Based on this author's experience, this amount of dextrose will not result in significant hyperglycemia. Because dextrose is an incomplete nutritional source, this type of supplementation should be provided for a short period of time or with enteral nutrition. Once the foal has been stabilized, the amount of maintenance fluids to administer at each bolus can be calculated by estimating the total volume the foal would receive in a 24-hour period and dividing by the frequency of administration. If there are additional fluid losses from diarrhea or gastric reflux, a daily estimate of the ongoing losses will need to be added to the maintenance amount. The volume will need to be changed daily as the foal's condition improves or worsens (*Table 97*).

Assessment of adequate nutrition being provided

It is important to assess the response to the nutritional support. The ideal way would be daily weight on a walk-on scale, but this is impractical because of the expense of a walk-on scale and the risk of contamination of the scale with an infectious agent. A weight tape can be used but it is not as accurate in a young foal. Similar to adults the body scoring system established by Henneke et al. (1983) can be used to provide a general idea of whether body condition is being lost or maintained. This system is based on visual appraisal and body palpation of six areas including along the neck, along the withers, topline, tailhead, ribs, and behind the shoulder. The foal's ideal body condition score is between 5 and 7, with the goal of seeing the foal's ribs as it moves. Daily monitoring of these parameters will serve as a guide to determine if the nutritional plan is appropriate. Trends in either direction but, most importantly, evidence of body condition loss can help one determine if a modification of the nutritional plan is required (*Tables 104, 105*).

Table 104. Example calculation of nutritional requirement for a weak newborn foal

50 kg newborn foal

Day 1:

Parenteral nutrition with dextrose solution

Goal: 4 mg/kg bwt/min (range 4–8 mg/kg bwt/min)

50 kg × 4 mg/kg bwt/min = 200 mg/min

200 mg/min × 60 min/h = 12,000 mg/h

10% dextrose solution = 100 mg/mL of dextrose

12,000 mg/h ÷ 100 mg/mL = 120 mL/h

Infusion rate = 120 mL/h of 10% dextrose

Enteral nutrition:

Example: 5% bwt/day for a 50 kg foal

50 kg × 5% = 2.5 kg = 2.5 L or 2,500 mL

Goal is to feed every 2 hours

2,500 mL ÷ 12 = 208 mL/feeding

208 mL/feeding = 7 oz/feeding

Day 2:

If the foal is tolerating oral feeding increase to 10% bwt/day and decrease the parenteral nutrition by one-half. The ultimate goal is to discontinue the parenteral nutrition on day 3 and increase the oral feedings (or hopefully the foal is nursing) to 15%–20% bwt/day.

Table 105. One method of feeding a healthy orphaned foal

Days 1–3	Feed 32 ounces of milk every 3 hours.
Days 4–7	Feed 42 ounces of milk every 3 hours.
Week 2	Feed 48 ounces of milk every 3 hours.
Week 3	Feed 58 ounces of milk every 4 hours with free choice of hay and milk pellets.
Week 4	Feed 64 ounces of milk every 4 hours with free choice of hay and milk pellets.
Week 5	Feed 64–72 ounces of milk every 6 hours and free choice of hay and milk pellets.
Week 6	Continue with milk, hay, and milk pellets as in week 5 but introduce grain mixture. Begin with 0.5 pounds of creep grain mixture per 100 pounds (45 kg) of body weight daily.
Weeks 8–10	Continue milk, milk pellets, and hay as in week 5 but gradually increase the amount of grain mixture to 1–1.5 lb of creep grain mixture per 100 lb (45 kg) of body weight.
Weeks 11–14	Reduce milk by 16 ounces per day. The goal is to have the foal completely weaned from milk by the end of week 12 or 13. Continue with milk pellets, grain mixture, and hay. Wean from milk pellets by 4 months of age.

A normal, healthy neonatal foal consumes roughly 15% of body weight as milk in the first 24 hours, increasing to 20%–23% by day 2 and up to 25% by day 7. Multiple small feedings are indicated and more closely mimic natural feedings. Thus the total quantity of milk should be divided into eight feedings daily the first 1–2 weeks of life. From the second week to the fourth, the milk can be divided into six feedings daily. The transition should be made slowly. If the foal displays signs of abdominal discomfort or diarrhea the amount may need to be decreased or initially fed more frequently.

Monitor the foal's attitude, appetite, hydration, and urine output. If diarrhea or constipation occurs, the frequency of feeding, quality of feeding, procedures used for mixing replacers, and cleanliness of feeding equipment should be monitored. Often, reducing the quantity of milk fed, with a concurrent increase in feeding frequency, alleviates many problems.

REFERENCES

Earing JE, Durig AC, Gellin, GL, Lawrence LM, Flythe MD (2012) Bacterial colonization of the equine gut; Comparison of mare and foal pairs by PCR-DGGE. *Adv in Microbiol* 2: 79–86.

Hansen TO (1990) Nutritional support: Parenteral feeding. In: *Equine Clinical Neonatology* (Koterba AM, Drummond WH, Kosch PC, Eds.). Lea & Febiger, Philadelphia, PA, pp. 747–762.

Henneke DR, Potter GD, Kreider JL, Yeates, BF (1983) Relationship between condition score, physical measurements, and body fat percentages in mares. *Equine Vet J* 15: 371–372.

Hollis AR, Furr MO, Magdesian KG, Axon, JE, Ludlow V, Boston RC, Corley KT (2008) Blood glucose concentration in critically ill neonatal foals. *J Vet Intern Med* 5: 1223–1227.

Jose-Cunilleras E, Viu J, Corradini I, Armengou L, Cesarini C, Monreal L (2012) Energy expenditure of critically ill neonatal foals. *Equine Vet J* 44: 48–51.

Krause JB, McKenzie HC (2007) Parenteral nutrition in foals: A retrospective study of 45 cases (2000–2004). *Equine Vet J* 39: 74–78.

Lawrence LA, Lawrence TJ (2009) Development of the equine gastrointestinal tract. In: *Advances in Equine Nutrition IV* (Pagan JD, Ed.). Nottingham University Press, Nottingham, UK, pp. 173–183.

Martin RG, McMeniman NP, Dowsett, KF (1992) Milk and water intakes of foals sucking grazing mares. *Equine Vet J* 24: 295–299.

McKenzie 3rd HC, Geor RJ (2009) Feeding management of sick neonatal foals. *Vet Clin North Am Equine Pract* 25: 109–119.

Miron N, Cristea V (2012) Enterocytes: Active cells in tolerance to food and microbial antigens in the gut. *Clin Exp Immunol* 167: 405–412.

National Research Council (2007) *Nutrient Requirements of Horses*, 6th rev. ed. National Academies Press, Washington, DC.

Ousey JC, Holdstock N, Rossdale PD, McArthur AJ (1996) How much energy do sick neonatal foals require compared with healthy foals? *Pferdeheilkunde* 12: 231–237.

Ousey JC, Prandi S, Zimmer J, Holdstock N, Rossdale PD (1997) Effects of various feeding regimens on the energy balance of equine neonates. *Am J Vet Res* 58: 1243–1253.

Stoneham SJ, Morresey PR, Ousey J (2016) Nutritional management and practical feeding of the orphan foal. *Equine Vet Ed*. First published January 16. doi:10.1111/eve.12546.

Case Studies

19

Laurie Metcalfe and Bonnie S. Barr

PREMATURE NEONATAL FOAL WITH SEPSIS

HISTORY

A 6-hour-old American Saddlebred filly weighing approximately 26 kg presented to the clinic. The filly was 310 days gestation and the mare had been treated for placentitis for 1 month.

PHYSICAL EXAMINATION

The filly was recumbent but alert and would occasionally struggle in an attempt to stand. Vital parameters were as follows: temperature 97°F (36°C), heart rate 56 beats per minute (bpm), and respiratory rate 28 breaths per minute. Mucous membranes were bright pink and injected. The respiratory pattern was normal with no abnormal lung sounds. A normal cardiac rhythm was present but a faint physiologic flow murmur was auscultated. There was blepharospasm of the left eye and the conjunctiva was hyperemic in both eyes. The extremities were cool and peripheral pulses weak. Gastrointestinal (GI) motility was quiet. The hair coat was short and silky and the forehead domed. The suckle reflex was weak. When assisted to stand there was flexor laxity of all fetlocks (**443**).

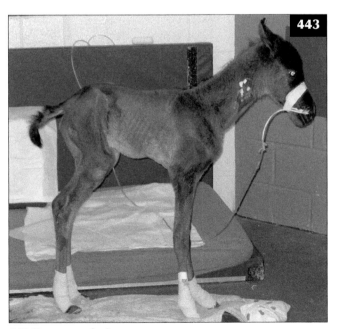

443 Premature foal.

DIAGNOSTICS AND INITIAL TRIAGE

Indirect blood pressures were performed and the mean arterial pressure (MAP) was 48. Five milligrams of diazepam was administered and an intravenous catheter was placed aseptically in the jugular vein. Blood was collected for blood culture, complete blood count (CBC), fibrinogen, chemistry panel, and blood glucose with the following results: white blood cell (WBC) 3,600 cells/µL, creatinine (Cr) 1.4 mg/dL, packed cell volume (PCV) 45%, total protein 4.1 g/dl, and blood glucose 31 mg/dL. An indwelling nasal oxygen cannula was sutured in the right nostril along with a nasogastric feeding tube. Intranasal oxygen was started at 5 L/min. A bolus of polyionic fluids with 20 mL of 50% dextrose, dimethyl sulfoxide (DMSO) (1 g/kg as a 10% solution), and thiamine (10 mg/kg) was administered over 20 minutes. The cardiovascular status and indirect blood pressures were reevaluated and indicated improvement in perfusion. Antimicrobials, potassium penicillin (30,000 IU/kg i/v q6h), and amikacin (30 mg/kg i/v q24h), were administered. Fluorescein stain of both eyes identified a large corneal ulcer in the center of the left eye. A sepsis score was performed using information from the initial physical examination and the value was 13, suggesting that the filly was septic.

TREATMENT PLAN

With the initial assessment the diagnosis was premature foal (*Table 106*) with septicemia. Treatment included proper nursing care, continuation of antimicrobial agents, and intranasal oxygen administration. A pint of colostrum was administered (30 mL every hour until the pint was gone) by indwelling nasogastric tube. Nutritional needs were met by enteral and parenteral routes. Enteral trophic feedings consisted of 1/2 oz (15 mL) of milk every 2 hours for 12 hours by nasogastric tube, which was started after all of the colostrum was administered. Parenteral nutrition included administration of 10% intravenous dextrose solution at rate 6 mg/kg/min. Vital parameters were closely monitored and the final part of the plan was proper nursing care (*Table 107*).

CASE PROGRESSION

Because the filly was not strong enough to nurse after 24 hours, parenteral nutrition was changed to total parenteral nutrition (TPN). Radiographs of carpi and tarsi were obtained and indicated incomplete ossification of the cuboidal bones (**444**).

Results of blood culture were positive revealing *Enterobacter cloacae* (antibiotic sensitivity—amikacin, ceftiofur, chloramphenicol,

Table 106. Prematurity

• Prematurity is the result of a pre-term birth.

• Most veterinary texts define prematurity by a gestational length less than 320 days but due to the variability in each mare's gestational length it is best to base diagnosis on clinical characteristics.

• Clinical characteristics of prematurity include:

  ○ Low birth weight

  ○ Small frame and may appear thin with poor muscle development

  ○ General muscle weakness; delayed time to stand

  ○ Short, silky hair coat

  ○ Domed forehead

  ○ Floppy ears—poor ear cartilage development

  ○ Weak suckle

  ○ Poor thermoregulation

  ○ Periarticular laxity

  ○ Flexor laxity occasionally contracture

  ○ Usually hypotonia; occasionally hypertonia

  ○ Soft rib cage and high compliance to chest wall

  ○ Low compliance of lungs; stiff lungs; respiratory distress secondary to fatigue

  ○ GI dysfunction

  ○ Delayed maturation of renal function and low urine output

  ○ Entropion with secondary corneal ulcers

  ○ Poor glucose regulation

• Causes of pre-term birth:

  ○ Placental problems—infectious or noninfectious problems; twins

  ○ Maternal problems—systemic illness, chronic problems, malnutrition

  ○ Early induction or C-section based on inaccurate breeding dates, catastrophic medical problem with mare

  ○ Idiopathic

• Treatment:

  ○ Treatment may include antibiotics, fluids, proper nutritional management, plasma, respiratory and cardiovascular support.

  ○ Each body system must be critically examined for signs of dysfunction.

  ○ Successful outcomes are dependent not only on careful management of identified problems but on predicting problems that may arise later.

  ○ Prognosis depends on how early the foal was born and the number of problems encountered.

ceftriaxone, timentin, ceftazidime). The antimicrobial agent was changed to ceftiofur only. Daily serial WBC counts were monitored and the value decreased then improved to a normal range with the change in antimicrobials. The filly slowly became stronger and was able to stand without assistance. Enteral feedings were increased and parenteral nutrition was decreased. The filly was encouraged to nurse and the enteral feedings were decreased. Once the filly was strong enough to get up/down and nurse, all supplemental nutrition was decreased. The filly was discharged after 14 days of hospitalization. Recommended treatment at the farm included restricted/limited exercise and topical treatment of the corneal ulcers. A follow-up evaluation a month later revealed the corneal ulcer had healed and there was complete ossification of the cuboidal bones.

Table 107. Nursing care

Environmental factors that should be considered with respect to neonatal care include:

• Well-padded area and mattress to minimize decubitus ulceration and self-injury

• Large enough stall to safely work around the mare

• Ability to separate the mare and foal to prevent nursing as needed

• Equipment that is easy to clean and disinfect to prevent transmission of disease

Nursing factors related to the neonatal foal include:

• Frequent, thorough, physical examinations and vital checks including the following:

  ○ Positive or negative changes in mentation, strength, ability to stand, and suckle

  ○ Presence of cutaneous sores, ulcers, or injuries

  ○ Evidence of fecal and urinary output

  ○ Umbilical and ocular health

• Assistance with thermoregulation as needed; small increments of change work best

• Warmed, loosely layered blankets

• Warmed or cooled intravenous fluids

• Tall tube socks on extremities

• Bair Hugger™

• Gently warmed, well-mixed rice or fluid bags

• Changes to recumbency to minimize the occurrence of decubitus ulcers and pneumonia; fractured ribs or musculoskeletal disorders may limit, or prevent, recumbency changes

• Skin care; frequent removal fecal and urine stains to prevent scalding

• Assistance to sit in sternal recumbency and stand if nonambulatory

• Assistance to move around the stall to develop strength and muscle tone if ambulatory

• Careful attention to nutritional intake, ability to handle feedings and guidance to nurse

• Management of indwelling or accessory items including:

  ○ Intravenous catheters and fluid lines

  ○ Urinary catheters, nasogastric tubes, and oxygen cannulas

  ○ Bandages, splints, casts, incisions, or drains

  ○ Muzzles—rotate dry muzzles if bruxism and sialorrhea is exhibited

Nursing factors related to the mare include:

• Maintaining a continuous but safe bond with the foal, even if access is limited

• Adequate nutrition for lactation ± maintenance of a pregnancy

• Continued attention to postpartum health of the mare, including mammary health

Source: Courtesy of Andrea Whittle.

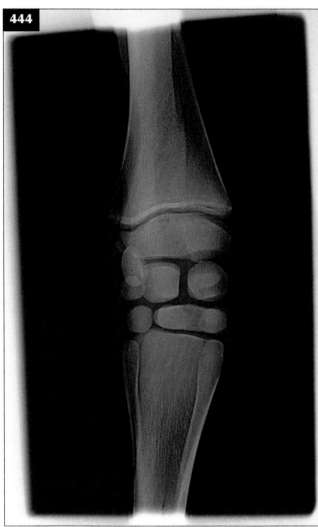

444 Dorsopalmar radiograph of carpus from premature foal demonstrating incomplete ossification of cuboidal bones.

WEAK FOAL

HISTORY

A 5-hour-old, 45 kg Thoroughbred colt of 330 days gestation presented at a large, well-managed breeding farm for failure to stand and nurse. Dam was a maiden mare that sustained a displaced pelvic fracture diagnosed by ultrasound and rectal palpation 2 days prior. Mare was significantly distressed and very painful with heart rate consistently >60 bpm. Mare was unable to ambulate effectively around stall and went into labor without demonstrating any typical signs of impending parturition. Mare foaled standing up and developed little to no udder prior to delivery.

PHYSICAL EXAMINATION

On examination, foal was weak, unable to stand without assistance and had a poor suckle reflex. Rectal temperature was 99°F (37.2°C), heart rate was 88 bpm, respiratory rate was 40 breaths per minute with clear lungs and mucous membranes light pink

but tacky, and foal had sunken eyes consistent with dehydration. Hind pasterns demonstrated significant laxity but no contractures or rib fractures. Colt had normal GI motility and had passed appropriate meconium. Foal was mentally inappropriate at that time, with periods of intermittent depression and lack of affinity for the mare. Primary differential was hypoxic ischemic encephalopathy (HIE)/neonatal maladjustment syndrome (NMS).

DIAGNOSTICS AND INITIAL TRIAGE

Blood work was submitted with the following results: WBC was 7,200 cells/µL with a 31.4% PCV and a 0.0 serum amyloid A (SAA). Creatine kinase (CK) was 1,800 units per liter (U/L), consistent with recumbency and Cr was 8.1 mg/dL, consistent with placental insufficiency. Ultrasound examination revealed no significant abnormalities in thorax or abdomen.

TREATMENT PLAN

An indwelling enteral feeding tube was placed to facilitate enteral feedings, starting with 4 oz (120 mL) of colostrum q1h (derived from farm stock obtained from other foaling mares with excess colostrum) for a total of 24 oz (720 mL). When colostrum administration was complete, the foal was gradually worked up to 9 oz (270 mL) of goat's milk diluted with water at a 1:1 ratio q2h, with instructions to discontinue enteral feedings if it became uncomfortable or distended (**445**). On day 1, an intravenous catheter was placed in the right jugular vein. Foal was administered 1L i/v hyperimmunized plasma (*Rhodococcus equi*, rotavirus) given as routine protocol to all foals housed on farm. This was immediately followed by a 1L i/v bolus of lactated Ringer's solution (LRS) with 50 mL of 90% DMSO, vitamin C (100 mg/kg), and thiamine (20 mg/kg) added as an anti-inflammatory/antioxidant treatment. In addition, one dose of ketoprofen (2.2 mg/kg) was administered intravenously following fluid administration. Colt continued 1L i/v boluses of LRS q4h until Cr was rechecked on day 2. Antimicrobial treatment was started using ceftiofur (10 mg/kg i/v q12h). Farm personnel were instructed to assist foal up q1h and allow the foal to attempt to nurse, although supply was

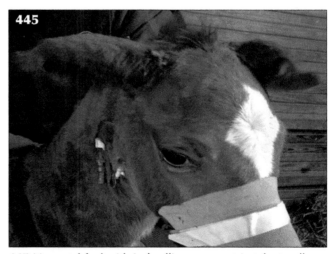

445 Neonatal foal with indwelling nasogastric tube to allow for supplemental oral feedings.

questionable. Arrangements were made to acquire a nursemare for the foal as the mare's prognosis was guarded.

CASE PROGRESSION

At recheck on day 2, foal was stronger, brighter, and had gained the ability to stand and ambulate unassisted. Colt had a strong suckle and was latching onto nursemare despite the mare's unwillingness to accept the foal. Antioxidant/anti-inflammatory 1 L i/v bolus was repeated and fluids reduced to 1 L q6h as Cr had fallen to 3.7 mg/dL. Foal had also become leukopenic (WBC 3,700 cells/μL) and anemic (PCV 22.2%) with a 636.7 mg/dL immunoglobulin G (IgG), despite receiving a large amount of good-quality colostrum and 1 L plasma. Antimicrobials were continued and enteral feedings reduced to 10 oz (300 mL) q4h to encourage nursing from mare until gradually discontinued overnight. On day 3, foal was strong but was reported to have slowly lost interest in nursing, becoming slightly dull and lethargic. Foal was mentally not as appropriate as the previous day. Ultrasound of the thorax revealed no significant abnormalities, although ultrasound of the abdomen identified slight liquid ingesta in the large colon. Ceftiofur was discontinued and to provide more broad-spectrum coverage potassium penicillin (40,000 IU/kg i/v q6h) and amikacin (25 mg/kg i/v q24h) were administered. In addition, metronidazole (15 mg/kg p/o q8h) and sucralfate (20 mg/kg p/o q6h) were added and small enteral feedings (4 oz q1h) were reinstituted until foal returned to proper nursing. Foal never displayed any signs of abdominal discomfort or distention. On day 4, colt was bright, alert, responsive, and aggressively nursing from nursemare that had since accepted the foal. Feeding tube was removed and IV fluids discontinued. Clinically, foal was improving daily, despite remaining leukopenic and anemic (*Table 108*). Intravenous antibiotics and metronidazole were continued for 7 days, then discontinued. Catheter was removed and foal switched to oral doxycycline (10 mg/kg p/o q12h) and rifampin (5 mg/kg p/o q12h) as well as adding omeprazole (1 mg/kg p/o q24h). Sucralfate was continued. Foal remained on this treatment protocol for 2 weeks until WBC was >5,000. Foal recovered uneventfully and had no further issues. Incidentally, foal's dam recovered uneventfully as well.

NEONATAL FOAL—HYPOXIC ISCHEMIC ENCEPHALOPATHY SUSPECT

HISTORY

An 8-hour-old, 60 kg Thoroughbred filly of 340 days gestation was evaluated. Foaling was not normal, with premature placental separation noted. The filly initially was able to sit sternal soon after birth and was able to stand within 1 hour. But the filly was not able to nurse. The referring veterinarian had given colostrum via a nasogastric tube and supplemental feedings were continued. The filly also was reported to not have a suckle reflex and appeared to walk in circles.

PHYSICAL EXAMINATION

The filly was standing. Vital parameters were within normal limits. Auscultation of the heart and lungs was normal. The suckle reflex was weak and the filly was hyperresponsive to the touch and walking large circles in the stall. There was no joint effusion and the umbilical stump was dry. GI motility was quiet and the filly was observed to have passed meconium at the farm.

DIAGNOSTICS AND INITIAL TRIAGE

Five milligrams of diazepam was administered and an intravenous catheter was placed aseptically in the jugular vein. Blood was collected for blood culture, a CBC, chemistry panel, blood glucose, and blood lactate value. WBC was 10,200 cells/μL, lactate 4.4 mmol/L, Cr 2.3 mg/dL, IgG 2702 mg/dL, and blood glucose 196 mg/dL. A bolus (1 L over 20 min) of polyionic fluids was administered with 10% solution of DMSO and thiamine (20 mg/kg). An indwelling nasogastric tube was placed to allow for feedings. Intravenous antimicrobials including potassium penicillin (22,000 IU/kg q6h) and amikacin (30 mg/kg q24h) were administered.

TREATMENT PLAN

Based on history (premature placental separation) and clinical signs, the diagnosis was HIE. The goal of the treatment plan was

Table 108. Serial blood work results – Weak foal case

	Day 1	Day 2	Day 3	Day 7	Day 14	Day 21
PCV (%)	31.4	22.2	26.3	24.3	23.1	30.4
WBC	7,200	3,700	4,600	4,900	4,000	5,600
TP (g/dL)	5.2	5.3	5.5	5.5	5.0	4.8
Fibrinogen (mg/dL)	200	300	300	400	300	300
Cr (mg/dL)	8.1	3.7	1.6	0.8	0.9	1.2
Other	CK1800 U/L SAA 0.0 μg/mL	IgG 636.7 mg/dL	SAA 69 μg/mL	SAA 0.0 μg/mL	SAA 0.0 μg/mL	SAA 0.0 μg/mL

supportive care with frequent monitoring for secondary problems. Treatment included continuing the current antimicrobial agents and oral feedings (starting at 5% body weight [bwt], then increasing to 10% over 12 hours). For the first 24 hours the filly was also supplemented with an intravenous fluid bolus of polyionic fluids (0.5 L every 4 h). Vital parameters, urine production, and worsening of the neurologic signs were closely monitored. Blood glucose was monitored 3–4 times a day, Cr value daily, and CBC every 3 days.

CASE PROGRESSION

On day 1 the filly was noticeable less hyperresponsive and continued to intermittently walk in circles. A strong suckle was noted but the filly showed no interest in nursing from the mare. The blood lactate (1.8 mmol/L) and Cr (1.4 mg/dl) had decreased to normal values. Treatment remained the same, except the fluid boluses were discontinued. By day 2 the filly was noted to be nursing. Checking the udder after the filly nursed confirmed that the filly was nursing the mare out. The filly was no longer circling and was noted to be playing in the stall. The oral feeding and blood glucose monitoring were discontinued but prophylactic antibiotic treatment continued. The filly was discharged on day 4 to continue 2 more days of antibiotics. Follow-up reports at 2 weeks and 1 month after discharge revealed the filly to be doing well.

NEONATAL FOAL—HYPOXIC ISCHEMIC ENCEPHALOPATHY (SEIZURES)

HISTORY

A 6-hour-old, 41 kg Thoroughbred filly of 320 days gestation was evaluated for weakness. The foaling was reported to have been normal. The only other significant historical information was

that at around 280 days of gestation the mare had been treated for severe enterocolitis, which required hospitalization. The filly initially was able to sit sternal soon after birth but needed assistance to stand. Bank colostrum was syringed to the foal by the farm manager because the mare had minimal udder development.

PHYSICAL EXAMINATION

The filly was bright and alert. Vital parameters were temperature 99°F (37.2°C), heart rate 120 bpm, and respiratory rate 24 breaths per minute. Auscultation of the heart revealed a physiologic flow murmur with a normal rhythm. Peripheral pulses were strong. Respiratory rate and effort were normal for a foal of this age. Palpation of the rib cage did not identify rib fractures. Extremities were warm to the touch. Meconium was noted to have been passed. The filly was attempting to stand but could only do so with assistance. The suckle reflex was poor.

DIAGNOSTICS AND INITIAL TRIAGE

Five milligrams of diazepam was administered intravenously and a double-lumen wire-guided intravenous catheter was placed aseptically in the jugular vein. Blood was collected for blood culture, CBC, fibrinogen, chemistry panel, glucose, and lactate values (*Table 109*). A 1 L bolus (over 20 min) of polyionic fluids was administered with DMSO (0.5 g/kg as 10% solution) and thiamine (20 mg/kg). An indwelling nasogastric tube was placed to allow for feedings. Intravenous antimicrobials including potassium penicillin (30,000 IU/kg q6h) and amikacin (30 mg/kg q24h) were administered.

TREATMENT PLAN

The initial assessment of the foal indicated that it was weak and compromised, most likely secondary to *in-utero* compromise/insufficiency

Table 109. Serial blood values – Neonatal Foal – HIE (Seizure) case

	Admit	Day 1	Day 2	Day 3	Day 4	Day 6	Day 9
WBC (cells/μL)	8,000		12,400	16,000		8,200	9,900
Fibrinogen (mg/dL)	500					500	500
PCV (%)	39					31	34
Total protein (g/dL)	5.5					6	5.8
Cr (mg/dL)	2.2		1.1			0.8	0.5
Lactate (mmol/L)							
Other	IgG 270 mg/dL; SAA 0	IgG 540 mg/dL		SAA 99 μg/mL		SAA 0	SAA 0
Sodium (mmol/L)	137		151	158	149	139	
Potassium (mmol/L)	4.5		3.7	3.8	3.5	4.5	
Ionized calcium (mmol/L)	6.3		7	7.1	6.5	6.9	
Chloride (mmol/L)	92		105	115	103	95	
Bicarbonate (mmol/L)	23		23	30	24	30	

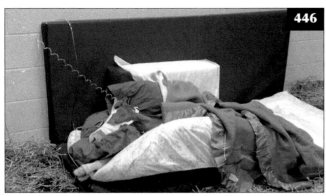

446 Compromised neonatal foal sleeping on foal bed maintained in sternal recumbency.

due to the mare's systemic illness a few weeks prior to parturition. The goal of the treatment plan was supportive care with frequent monitoring for secondary problems. Treatment included continuing the current antimicrobial agents and beginning oral feedings (starting at 5% bwt). Supplemental nutrition of 10% dextrose solution was administered intravenously at a rate of 5 mg/kg/h. Vital parameters, urine production, and any sign of worsening of the clinical symptoms were noted. Blood glucose values were monitored every 4 hours, along with providing proper nursing and supportive care (**446**). The dynamic nature of these cases may result in the need to modify the treatment plan based on the clinical picture, thus it is important to monitor the patient closely.

Case progression

Day 1: Initially vital parameters were normal and the filly still required assistance to stand. The suckle reflex was improving. Early in the evening the filly's attitude was reported to be quieter, with occasional stretching. About an hour after the noted attitude change, a grand mal seizure occurred characterized by paddling and opisthotonos (**447**).

Modification of treatment: Antiseizure medications were administered, including an initial 5 mg of diazepam intravenously. Even with the administration of a second dose of diazepam the seizure activity continued, thus a

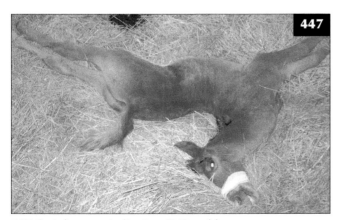

447 Opisthotonos indicating CNS problems.

constant rate infusion (CRI) of midazolam (0.04 mg/kg/h) was started. An indwelling nasal oxygen cannula was placed for supplemental oxygen administration. Oral feedings were decreased to trophic feedings (0.5 oz/15 mL every 2 h). In order to provide additional calories, parenteral nutrition was changed from 10% dextrose solution to TPN. LRS with the addition of 20 mEq/L potassium chloride was administered (rate 2 mL/kg/h). The filly was maintained in sternal position on a "foal bed" (**446**) with minimal stimulation to allow it to quietly rest.

Day 2: The filly remained quiet and sedated on the foal bed. Blood electrolyte panel indicated an increase in the serum sodium value. Because foals are designed to live on a low-sodium milk diet, neonatal kidneys can have a hard time with the larger sodium load found in some replacement fluids. To decrease the sodium load, the intravenous fluids were changed to a lower sodium maintenance fluid (Normosol™-M and 5% dextrose). The filly was febrile (103°F/39.4°C) in the evening, thus one dose of firocoxib (0.1 mg/kg) was administered.

Day 3: In an effort to determine the source of the fever, an ultrasound of the thorax and abdomen was performed. The thorax indicated pneumonia characterized by bilateral diffuse comet tails and an area of consolidation on the right side. Pneumonia as a secondary complication in compromised neonates is not uncommon. Nebulization three times a day with ceftiofur (1.1 mg/kg), albuterol (0.01 mg/kg), and sterile water was added to the treatment. The midazolam was discontinued and with gentle stimulation the filly was encouraged to begin to "wake-up." Oral feedings were increased (3% bwt/day).

Day 4–9: Filly progressively became stronger with no signs of recurrence of seizure activity. The oral feedings were gradually increased and the intravenous TPN and fluids were decreased and finally discontinued. Within 36 hours the filly was strong enough to get up without assistance and nurse. Once the filly was nursing well the oral feedings were discontinued. Follow-up blood work indicated a return to normal values of WBC, SAA, and electrolytes (*Table 109*).

Day 10: Follow-up ultrasound of the thorax revealed improvement, fewer comet tails, and a decrease in the size of the area of consolidation. Thus the nebulization was discontinued. The filly was discharged to return to the farm to continue intravenous antibiotics. On follow-up examination about 5 days after discharge, the filly was reported to be doing well, physical examination and ultrasound of the lungs were normal. All treatments were discontinued.

PNEUMONIA: *RHODOCOCCUS EQUI*

History
A 30-day-old, 100 kg Paint Horse colt was evaluated due to fevers and an increased respiratory rate and effort. The colt had been healthy since birth. Another foal had recently died suddenly. The farm has a history of suspected *Rhodococcus equi* pneumonia cases.

PHYSICAL EXAMINATION

The colt was quiet and alert. Vital parameters were as follows: temperature 104°F (40°C), heart rate 80 bpm, and respiratory rate 60 breaths per minute. Auscultation of the lungs identified abnormal lung sounds on the left characterized by wheezes and on the right side the lung sounds were decreased. There was a slight increased respiratory effort. No nasal discharge was present. The mucous membranes were bright pink with a capillary refill time (CRT) of about 2 seconds. The rest of the physical examination was unremarkable.

DIAGNOSTICS AND INITIAL TRIAGE

Blood work was submitted with the following results: WBC 21,000 cells/μL; fibrinogen 600 mg/dL; and no significant abnormalities on the chemistry panel. Ultrasound of the thorax identified an area of consolidated lung on the right (**448**) and several smaller abscesses on the left (**449**). A transtracheal aspirate (TTA) was performed through an endoscope using a triple-guarded catheter. The sample was submitted for cytology and bacterial culture.

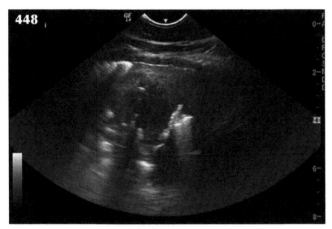

448 Ultrasonogram of consolidated lung.

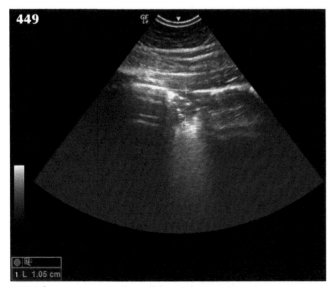

449 Ultrasonogram of small lung abscess (1 cm).

The cytology identified numerous neutrophils and intra- and extracellular coccobacilli-shaped bacteria.

TREATMENT PLAN

With the history of prior *R. equi* cases on the farm and TTA cytology (coccobacilli-shaped bacteria), the antibiotic selection was as follows: azithromycin (10 mg/kg daily p/o for 5 days, then every other day) and rifampin (5 mg/kg p/o q12h). Flunixin meglumine (1.1 mg/kg) was administered for the fever. Omeprazole (1 mg/kg p/o q24h) was also administered because the foal was stressed and receiving a nonsteroidal anti-inflammatory agent.

CASE PROGRESSION

The results of the bacterial culture were reported in 48 hours and identified *R. equi*, which was sensitive to macrolide and rifampin antibiotics. Follow-up evaluations were done daily for the first 6 days, then every 2 weeks afterward. After 6 weeks of treatment the antibiotics were discontinued. Follow-up evaluations and blood work were performed every 2 weeks when the antibiotics were discontinued (*Table 110*). The thoracic lesions identified on ultrasound gradually resolved and after 6 weeks of treatment only a few comet tails were noted.

PNEUMONIA WITH INTERSTITIAL COMPONENT

HISTORY

A 3-month-old, 200 kg Thoroughbred colt presented on a large, well-managed Thoroughbred breeding farm with a 2-day history of low-grade fevers and coughing. Foal was reported to have a mildly increased respiratory rate and effort.

PHYSICAL EXAMINATION

Foal had a 102.4°F (39.1°C) temperature at examination with mild/moderately increased respiratory rate and effort, including an abdominal component. A moderate amount of mucopurulent nasal discharge was present. Lungs were harsh with increased bronchovesicular sounds bilaterally, and foal coughed when held off. Respiratory rate was 44, but foal was otherwise bright and nursing well.

DIAGNOSTICS AND INITIAL TRIAGE

Blood work was submitted with the following results: moderately elevated WBC at 16,100 cells/μL; all else within normal limits. Ultrasound exam of the thorax revealed several small 0.5 cm abscesses with pleural irregularities (comet tails) diffusely within all lung fields, confirming a definite inflammatory component. No pleural effusion was present.

TREATMENT PLAN

Initially intravenous flunixin meglumine (1.1 mg/kg) was administered. Antibiotic selection was doxycycline (10 mg/kg p/o q12h) and rifampin (5 mg/kg p/o q12h), which was administered for 10 days. Adjunctive treatment included clenbuterol (0.8 mcg/kg p/o q12h) for 6 days, flunixin meglumine (1.1 mg/kg p/o q24h) for 5 days, and omeprazole (1 mg/kg p/o q24h) for 10 days.

Table 110. Serial results: Pneumonia R. equi case

Day	Temperature (°F/°C)	Respiratory rate (breaths per min)	WBC (cells/µL)	Fibrinogen (g/dL)	Comments
1	104.5/40.2	60–70			
2	104/40	60–70			
3	102.7/39.3	30–40	23,800	600	
4	101.7/38.7	30–50			
5	102.3/39	20–40			
6	101.1/38.4	20–30	19,000	600	
7	101.5/38.6	20–30			
14	101.3/38.5	20–30	17,800	500	
30	100.8/38.2	20–30			
45	99.6/37.5	20	12,700	500	Discontinued antibiotics
60	100.3/37.9	20–30	11,200	400	
75	99.5/37.5	20	9,800	200	

CASE PROGRESSION

Foal was reexamined on day 10, and was afebrile and no longer coughing. No nasal discharge was present, there were no abnormal lungs sounds on auscultation, and respiratory rate and effort were normal. WBC had decreased (13,700 cells/µL) and the fibrinogen value was normal. Medications were discontinued and recheck ultrasound of the lungs demonstrated resolution of the abnormalities. On day 25, colt presented with a 1-day history of fever. Foal had a 104°F (40°C) temperature and a significantly increased respiratory rate (64 breaths per minute) and effort with a distinct abdominal component. On auscultation, there were wheezes bilaterally that were audible without holding off. Ultrasound of the thorax revealed diffuse coalescing comet tails throughout, with a single 1 cm abscess (**450**). Based on the ultrasound and auscultation

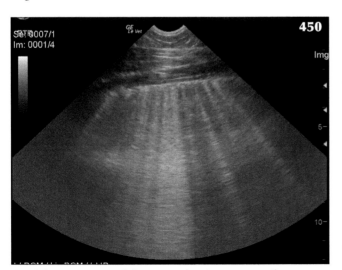

450 Ultrasonogram of thorax coalescing comet tails.

finding, a suspected diagnosis of interstitial pneumonia was made. A TTA was obtained via endoscope, and nasal swabs submitted for respiratory viral polymerase chain reaction (PCR) testing (equine influenza virus, equine herpesvirus 1 and 4, and equine rhinitis A and B virus). An intravenous catheter was placed and the foal started on potassium penicillin (22,000 IU/kg i/v q6h), gentamicin (6.6 mg/kg i/v q24h), clenbuterol (0.8 mcg p/o q12h), flunixin meglumine (1.1 mg/kg p/o q12h), omeprazole (1 mg/kg p/o q24h), and a decreasing dose of oral dexamethasone, following a single injectable dose on day 25 (0.05 mg/kg i/v). The foal was nebulized using a farm-owned Flexineb™ nebulizer three times a day with ceftiofur (1 mg/kg) and albuterol (0.01 mg/kg) (**451**). On day 28, TTA bacterial culture results yielded *Streptococcus equi* ssp. *zooepidemicus*, which was sensitive to penicillin, ceftiofur, doxycycline, and chloramphenicol. All viral testing was negative. The colt was rechecked at day 32, following one week of intravenous antibiotics and found to be responding well to treatment (*Table 111*). Intravenous antibiotics were discontinued and changed to oral doxycycline (10 mg/kg q12h), while the foal continued to be weaned off of dexamethasone (down to 0.02 mg/kg p/o q24h) and flunixin meglumine (0.05 mg/kg q24h). Nebulization was decreased to twice a day (*Table 112*). By day 40, antibiotics were discontinued and anti-inflammatory agents gradually stopped. Nebulization was continued once daily for 7 more days and the foal recovered uneventfully.

DIARRHEA: ROTAVIRUS

HISTORY

A 4-month-old, 220 kg Thoroughbred filly presented on a large, well-managed Thoroughbred breeding farm with a 2-day history of fever, lethargy, and diarrhea. Several other foals in the group had

451

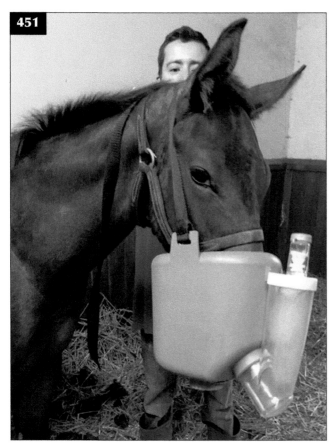

451 Foal being nebulized (Flexineb™, Galway, Ireland).

Table 112. Medications for nebulization

Drug	Dose	Frequency
Antibiotics		
Ceftiofur sodium	1 mg/kg (OR)	q6–12h
	2.2 mg/kg	q24h
Gentamycin	2 mg/kg	q24h
Bronchodilators		
Albuterol Sulfate	0.001– 0.01 mg/kg	q6–24h
Anti-inflammatory agents		
Dexamethasone	0.01– 0.02 mg/kg	q12–24h
Fluticasone	2–4 mcg/kg	q12h–24h
Mucolytic agents		
Sterile water or saline	2–5 mL/ 50 kg	q6–24h
N-acetylcysteine	4–8 mg/kg	q12–24h

presented with similar clinical signs that week. Farm had history of widespread rotavirus infection affecting foals 30–120 days of age.

PHYSICAL EXAMINATION
Normally difficult to handle, the filly was quiet and depressed on examination. Vital parameters were as follows: temperature 103°F (39.4°C), heart rate 84 bpm, and respiratory rate 36 breaths per minute. The mare's udder was engorged and dripping milk. Filly's hindquarters were covered in profuse gray/green foul-smelling liquid diarrhea. Lungs were harsh bilaterally on auscultation with

occasional cough when held off, and mild mucopurulent nasal discharge. Mucous membranes were pink but tacky with a CRT of 2.5 seconds, and foal was clinically dehydrated. On auscultation GI motility was markedly decreased, nearly silent.

DIAGNOSTICS AND INITIAL TRIAGE
Initial blood work performed prior to replacement fluids involved CBC, fibrinogen, electrolytes, and creatinine. PCV was elevated at 45% and Cr high at 2.8 mg/dL, confirming dehydration. Electrolytes were generally low with sodium 124 mmol/L, potassium 3.1 mmol/L, chloride 89 mmol/L, and bicarbonate

Table 111. Serial results – Pneumonia (Interstitial Component Case)

Day	Temperature (°F/°C)	Respiratory rate (breaths per min)	WBC (cells/µL)	Fibrinogen (g/dL)
Day 1	102.4/39.1	44	16,100	300
Day 10	100.9/38.3	28	13,700	300
Day 25	104.0/40	64	14,900	200
Day 32	100.2/37.9	36	12,300	400
Day 40	100.0/37.8	20	11,600	400

Table 113. Serial results – Diarrhea: Rotavirus

Day	WBC (cells/μL)	Fib (mg/dL)	Cr (mg/dL)
1	8800	500	2.8
2	5200	500	1.6
8	17000	400	1.0

20 mmol/L. Ultrasound of the thorax revealed moderate changes on the pleural surface bilaterally within cranioventral lung lobes, while an abdominal ultrasound easily imaged an edematous colon full of liquid ingesta. The diagnosis was enterocolitis. A fecal sample was collected and submitted for real-time PCR testing for the common GI pathogens.

TREATMENT PLAN

An intravenous catheter was placed and an initial 6 L bolus of LRS administered, followed by 2 L every 4 hours administered by farm personnel. Additional treatments included metronidazole (15 mg/kg p/o q12h), lactase enzyme supplement (18,000 IU p/o q6h), sucralfate (20 mg/kg p/o q6h), omeprazole (3 mg/kg p/o q24h), and a probiotic. Due to the pulmonary changes, ceftiofur (2.2 mg/kg i/v q12h) was also administered. One dose of flunixin meglumine (1.1 mg/kg) was given following fluids. All treatments were administered by farm personnel.

CASE PROGRESSION

At recheck the following day, filly was afebrile, brighter, and nursing more consistently. Mucous membranes were no longer tacky and foal was clinically well hydrated. Heart rate was 60 bpm and GI motility was increased from day 1, however, still hypomotile. Diarrhea had decreased in frequency and amount, but consistency remained liquid. Blood Cr value was normal. Fluids were slowly reduced over the next 2 days while diarrhea continued to resolve. Treatments were continued for 7 days, and filly returned to being bright, feisty, and difficult to handle. Real-time PCR results from the fecal sample were positive for rotavirus, with all other pathogens negative. Even though the WBC was still increased on day 8, the filly was clinically normal so the treatments were discontinued and the filly made an uneventful recovery (*Table 113*).

LAWSONIA INTRACELLULARIS

HISTORY

A 9-month-old, 300 kg, weanling Thoroughbred colt presented at a Thoroughbred breeding farm for 2-day history of fever (102.6°F/39°C), diarrhea, mild throatlatch edema, and inappetence. The colt was housed in an area believed to be endemic for *Lawsonia intracellularis* (LI), where 4 of 13 weanlings exhibited clinical signs over a period of 3 weeks, with this colt showing the most severe signs. Owners noted that colt's clinical condition had recently deteriorated.

PHYSICAL EXAMINATION

On examination, the colt was depressed and febrile, with profuse watery diarrhea. The colt was tachycardic at 64 bpm. No abnormal lungs sounds were noted on auscultation but borborygmi were extremely hypermotile, with colt exhibiting periods of mild discomfort. The colt was moderately clinically dehydrated with tacky mucous membranes and a CRT of 2.5–3 seconds. The colt was very thin over topline and ribs, and hips were quite prominent. There was mild but not marked throatlatch edema. The colt was eating hay and drinking water, but uninterested in grain. The primary differential was LI.

DIAGNOSTICS AND INITIAL TRIAGE

Blood work was submitted with the following results: WBC 8,600 cells/μL, total protein (TP) 5.0 g/dL, fibrinogen 800 mg/dL, albumin 1.5 g/dL, and Cr 1.2 mg/dL (*Table 114*). Ultrasound of the abdomen revealed mild amount of anechoic free fluid, thick-walled (>0.5 cm) small intestine (**452**) and a colon full of liquid ingesta. A fecal sample was collected and submitted for real-time PCR testing for the common GI pathogens.

TREATMENT PLAN

Due the colt's initial degree of dehydration, an intravenous catheter was placed and a 7 L bolus of LRS administered. Since LI

Table 114. Serial blood values – LI case

Day	WBC (cells/μL)	TP (g/dL)	Fibrinogen (mg/dL)	Albumin (g/dL)
1	8,600	5.0	800	1.5
3	13,600	5.4	600	1.7
20	6,300	4.9	400	1.6
38	11,000	6.5	400	2.3

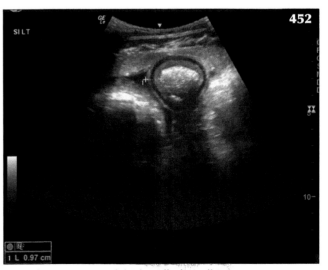

452 Ultrasonogram of thick-walled small intestine.

was the suspected diagnosis, oxytetracycline (10 mg/kg diluted in fluids) was administered. Flunixin meglumine was administered (1.1 mg/kg i/v) for the fever and additional treatments included metronidazole (20 mg/kg p/o q12h), sucralfate (20 mg/kg p/o q6h), omeprazole (3 mg/kg p/o q24h), di-tri-octahedral (DTYO) smectite supplement, and a probiotic. The following day, 1,000 mL 6% hydroxyethyl starch 130/0.4 in 0.9% sodium chloride injection and 2 L of plasma were administered. The treatment plan consisted of intravenous oxytetracycline for 5 days, followed by a change to doxycycline (10 mg/kg p/o q12h) if diarrhea subsided.

CASE PROGRESSION

Over the next few days, fevers subsided and the colt slowly improved in attitude and appetite. Blood work stabilized following colloid administration. Diarrhea ceased by day 5. The intravenous catheter was removed and a course of doxycycline initiated. Bio-Sponge® was discontinued, but all other oral medication continued. On day 9, the results of the real-time PCR confirmed the diagnosis of LI. Doxycycline was given for a 10-day course, then discontinued as the colt remained afebrile with an improving appetite.

On day 20, the colt presented again with a 1-day history of significant throatlatch edema and marked weight loss over topline and hips. The colt was quiet with a good appetite and normal, formed feces, however, lying down frequently. Blood work indicated TP and albumin had again decreased (*Table 114*). An additional 3-day course of tetracycline (10 mg/kg i/v q24h) was administered, along with 1,000 mL hetastarch and 2 L plasma. A 14-day course of doxycycline (10 mg/kg p/o q12h) was administered. Adjunctive supplements included fish oil (omega-3) and a hindgut buffer. The colt eventually gained weight and improved satisfactorily in condition.

UMBILICAL REMNANT INFECTION

HISTORY

A 4-day-old, 60 kg Thoroughbred colt presented on a large, well-managed Thoroughbred farm with a 1-day history of fever, depression, and anorexia. The colt had a history of initial failure of passive transfer (IgG 313 mg/dL at 12 hours). On subsequent blood draw 24 hours following 1 L hyperimmune plasma administration, IgG was 680 mg/dL. New foal exam 4 days prior was unremarkable with the exception of a thickened but dry external umbilical remnant with a very large body wall defect.

PHYSICAL EXAMINATION

On examination, the colt was dull and the dam's udder was swollen and dripping milk. Temperature was 103.5°F (40°C), with a heart rate of 96 bpm. Mucous membranes were pink, however, slightly tacky with a CRT <2.0. Foal was mildly tachypneic (48 breaths per minute) but no abnormal lungs sounds were evident on auscultation. External umbilical remnant remained thick and swollen, though markedly reduced from initial new foal exam. No drainage was observed or available for culture. The rest of the physical examination was unremarkable.

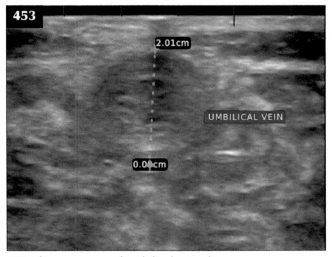

453 Ultrasonogram of umbilical vein abscess.

DIAGNOSTICS AND INITIAL TRIAGE

Initial blood work revealed a marked leukocytosis (WBC 20,300 cells/μL); increased from WBC (10,600 cells/μL) at 12 hours of age. Fibrinogen was normal (200 mg/dL), however, SAA was increased (>3,000 μg/mL). Ultrasound of the thorax demonstrated mild pleural roughening cranioventrally on the right side, with the left side unremarkable. Ultrasound of the abdomen revealed normal small intestine and colon with no evidence of impending diarrhea. A very large umbilical vein was imaged (**453**) approximately 2 cm cranial to the external umbilical remnant. Umbilical arteries and urachus measured within normal limits. A presumptive diagnosis of an infected umbilical vein remnant was made and a treatment plan initiated.

TREATMENT PLAN

Foal was initially given firocoxib (0.27 mg/kg i/v) as an antipyretic. An intravenous catheter was placed, and the foal started on potassium penicillin (40,000 IU/kg i/v q6h), amikacin (25 mg/kg i/v q24h), omeprazole (3 mg/kg p/oq24h), and a daily oral probiotic. All medications were administered by farm personnel.

CASE PROGRESSION

Colt was reexamined 5 days after initial examination. The colt had been afebrile since initiating intravenous antibiotics, and external umbilical remnant appeared less swollen. The colt was bright, alert, and nursing well. Blood work revealed a now normal WBC and improved SAA, but increased fibrinogen (*Table 115*). Umbilical ultrasound demonstrated a large umbilical vein still measuring nearly 2 × 2 cm in diameter. Since the intravenous catheter had been removed that morning, the decision was made to switch to broad-spectrum oral antibiotics. Chloramphenicol (50 mg/kg p/o q6h) and metronidazole (20 mg/kg p/o q12h) were started and the penicillin and amikacin were discontinued. The foal did well on the oral antibiotics, remained afebrile, and was rechecked 1 week later. The external umbilical remnant appeared almost normal, and the foal still bright, alert, and nursing well. All joints still palpated within normal limits and the foal was sound. Blood work

Table 115. Serial blood values – Umbilical Remnant infection case

Day	PCV (%)	WBC (cells/μL)	Fibrinogen (mg/dL)	SAA (μg/dL)
1	39.4	20,300	200	>3,000
6	30.2	6,000	600	1,020
12	28.6	7,000	600	44
18	28.5	5,400	500	0

Table 116. Umbilical vein measurements

Day	Umbilical vein measurements (normal <1 cm)
1	1.7 × 2.0 cm
6	2.0 × 2.0 cm
12	1.0 × 1.3 cm
18	0.88 × 0.85 cm

Table 117. Synovial fluid results

Day	WBC (cells/μL)	TP (g/dL)	Comments
Admit	163,600	4.8	
1	101,000		
2	60,700		
3	20,300		Last day of lavage
5	15,200	2.5	Only synovial fluid sample collected for analysis
6	12,200		Only synovial fluid sample collected for analysis

indicated an improved SAA but fibrinogen remained increased. Recheck ultrasound demonstrated that the umbilical vein size had reduced (1 × 1.3 cm). Treatment was continued for an additional week. At that time blood work had improved and ultrasound revealed that the umbilical vein size had decreased (*Table 116*). Antibiotics were discontinued at that time, and the foal recovered without any further complications.

SEPTIC ARTHRITIS

History
A 6-week-old, 80 kg Thoroughbred colt was evaluated for lameness and fever.

Physical examination
The colt's attitude was bright and alert. Vital parameters were as follows: temperature 102.5°F (39.2°C), heart rate 88 bpm, and respiratory rate 28 breaths per minute. Grade 4 lameness in the right front was noted along with a moderate amount of effusion in the fetlock. The colt was nursing well. No additional abnormalities were noted on the physical examination.

Diagnostics and initial triage
Blood work revealed the following abnormalities: WBC 19,600 cells/μL and fibrinogen 600 mg/dL. Radiographs of the right front fetlock were performed and no bony lesions were identified. Arthrocentesis of the right front fetlock was performed to collect synovial fluid for analysis and bacterial culture. Results of the synovial fluid sample are as follows: WBC 163,600 cells/μL and TP 4.8 mg/dL.

Treatment plan
The diagnosis was septic arthritis in the right front fetlock. The foal was placed under general anesthesia and the joint was lavaged with 1–2 L physiologic saline and 500 mg amikacin was instilled into the joint. A bandage was placed on the limb afterward. The following systemic antibiotics were administered: potassium penicillin (22,000 IU/kg i/v q6h) and gentamicin (6.6 mg/kg i/v q24h). Flunixin meglumine (1.1 mg/kg IV q24h) was administered for its anti-inflammatory and analgesic properties, and omeprazole (1 mg/kg p/o q24h) was also administered.

Case progression
The foal was evaluated daily for lameness and joint effusion. Temperature was monitored three times a day, synovial fluid samples were obtained daily. The joint was lavaged daily for 3 days, with antibiotics instilled into the joint after each lavage (*Table 117*). The bacterial culture yielded no growth. Systemic antibiotics were continued for 5 days past the last joint lavage.

Index

Note: Page numbers in *italics* refer to figures or tables.